2018
HCPCS Level II

Carol J. Buck
MS, CPC, CCS-P

Former Program Director
Medical Secretary Programs
Northwest Technical College
East Grand Forks, Minnesota

ELSEVIER

ELSEVIER

3251 Riverport Lane
St. Louis, Missouri 63043

2018 HCPCS LEVEL II, STANDARD EDITION   ISBN: 978-0-323-43073-9

Notices

Knowledge and best practice in this field are constantly changing. As new research and experience broaden our understanding, changes in research methods, professional practices, or medical treatment may become necessary.

Practitioners and researchers must always rely on their own experience and knowledge in evaluating and using any information, methods, compounds, or experiments described herein. In using such information or methods they should be mindful of their own safety and the safety of others, including parties for whom they have a professional responsibility.

With respect to any drug or pharmaceutical products identified, readers are advised to check the most current information provided (i) on procedures featured or (ii) by the manufacturer of each product to be administered, to verify the recommended dose or formula, the method and duration of administration, and contraindications. It is the responsibility of practitioners, relying on their own experience and knowledge of their patients, to make diagnoses, to determine dosages and the best treatment for each individual patient, and to take all appropriate safety precautions.

To the fullest extent of the law, neither the Publisher nor the authors, contributors, or editors, assume any liability for any injury and/or damage to persons or property as a matter of products liability, negligence or otherwise, or from any use or operation of any methods, products, instructions, or ideas contained in the material herein.

International Standard Book Number: 978-0-323-43073-9

Content Strategist: Brandi Graham
Content Development Manager: Luke Held
Associate Content Development Specialist: Anna Miller
Publishing Services Manager: Jeffrey Patterson
Project Manager: Lisa A. P. Bushey
Designer: Maggie Reid

Printed in the United States of America

Last digit is the print number: 9   8   7   6   5   4   3   2   1

Working together
to grow libraries in
developing countries

www.elsevier.com • www.bookaid.org

DEVELOPMENT OF THIS EDITION

Lead Technical Editor

Jenna Price, BA, CPC
President
Price Editorial Services, LLC
St. Louis, Missouri

Technical Collaborators

Jackie Grass Koesterman, CPC
Coding and Reimbursement Specialist
Grand Forks, North Dakota

Patricia Cordy Henricksen, MS, CHCA, CPC-I, CPC, CCP-P, ACS-PM
AAPC/AHIMA Approved ICD-10-CM Trainer
Auditing, Coding, and Education Specialist
Soterion Medical Services/Merrick Management
Lexington, Kentucky

Nancy Maguire, ACS, CRT, PCS, FCS, HCS-D, APC, AFC
Physician Consultant for Auditing and Education
Palm Bay, Florida

DEDICATION

To all who require of themselves the highest level of accuracy, integrity, and professionalism. You enhance our profession and are a tremendous asset to health care. May this manual be of assistance to you.
With Greatest Admiration.

Carol J. Buck, MS, CPC, CCS-P

LOVE YOUR HEART

Classification of Blood Pressure	Systolic Blood Pressure (mmHg)	Diastolic Blood Pressure (mmHg)		Symptoms of Organ Damage	Follow-Up Recommendation	Recommended Nurse Action
Normal	<120	And	<80		Re-check yearly or as recommended by doctor	Give BP Guide and Love Your Heart Handout
Elevated	120-129	And	<80		Follow up with your doctor within 3 months	Give BP Guide and Love Your Heart Handout
Hypertension, Stage 1	130-139	Or	80-89		Follow up with doctor within 1 month; call 2-1-1 if you do not have insurance to find a community health center near you	Give BP Guide and Love Your Heart Handout; if uninsured, refer to on-site County eligibility worker/recommend they call 2-1-1
Hypertension, Stage 2	≥140	Or	≥90		Follow up with doctor immediately; call 2-1-1 if you do not have insurance to find a community health center near you	Give BP Guide and Love Your Heart Handout; if uninsured, refer to on-site County eligibility worker/recommend they call 2-1-1
Hypertensive Urgency	≥180	And/Or	≥120	No		
Hypertensive Emergency	≥180	And/Or	≥120	Yes	Call 9-1-1 or go to the Emergency Department	Call 9-1-1

And remember to be active, eat healthy and don't smoke!
Visit LOVEYOURHEARTSD.org to learn more.

DATE	BLOOD PRESSURE	PULSE

CONTENTS

Updates will be posted on
codingupdates.com when available.

Check the Centers for Medicare and Medicaid Services
(www.cms.gov/Manuals/IOM/list.asp) website and
codingupdates.com for full and select IOMs.

INTRODUCTION

2018 HCPCS quarterly updates available on the companion website at: www.codingupdates.com

The Centers for Medicare and Medicaid Services (CMS) (formerly Health Care Financing Administration [HCFA]) Healthcare Common Procedure Coding System (HCPCS) is a collection of codes and descriptors that represent procedures, supplies, products, and services that may be provided to Medicare beneficiaries and to individuals enrolled in private health insurance programs. The codes are divided as follows:

Level I: Codes and descriptors copyrighted by the American Medical Association's (AMA's) Current Procedural Terminology, ed. 4 (CPT-4). These are five-position numeric codes representing physician and nonphysician services.

Level II: Includes codes and descriptors copyrighted by the American Dental Association's current dental terminology, seventh edition (CDT-7/8). These are five-position alpha-numeric codes comprising the D series. All other Level II codes and descriptors are approved and maintained jointly by the alpha-numeric editorial panel (consisting of CMS, the Health Insurance Association of America, and the Blue Cross and Blue Shield Association). These are five-position alpha-numeric codes representing primarily items and nonphysician services that are not represented in the Level I codes.

Level III: The CMS eliminated Level III local codes. See Program Memorandum AB-02-113.

Headings are provided as a means of grouping similar or closely related items. The placement of a code under a heading does not indicate additional means of classification, nor does it relate to any health insurance coverage categories.

HCPCS also contains modifiers, which are two-position codes and descriptors used to indicate that a service or procedure that has been performed has been altered by some specific circumstance but not changed in its definition or code. Modifiers are grouped by the levels. Level I modifiers and descriptors are copyrighted by the AMA. Level II modifiers are HCPCS modifiers. Modifiers in the D series are copyrighted by the ADA.

HCPCS is designed to promote uniform reporting and statistical data collection of medical procedures, supplies, products, and services.

HCPCS Disclaimer

Inclusion or exclusion of a procedure, supply, product, or service does not imply any health insurance coverage or reimbursement policy.

HCPCS makes as much use as possible of generic descriptions, but the inclusion of brand names to describe devices or drugs is intended only for indexing purposes; it is not meant to convey endorsement of any particular product or drug.

Updating HCPCS

The primary updates are made annually. Quarterly updates are also issued by CMS.

GUIDE TO USING THE 2018 HCPCS LEVEL II CODES

Medical coding has long been a part of the health care profession. Through the years medical coding systems have become more complex and extensive. Today, medical coding is an intricate and immense process that is present in every health care setting. The increased use of electronic submissions for health care services only increases the need for coders who understand the coding process.

2018 HCPCS Level II was developed to help meet the needs of today's coder.

All material adheres to the latest government versions available at the time of printing.

Annotated

Throughout this text, revisions and additions are indicated by the following symbols:

◄ **New:** Additions to the previous edition are indicated by the color triangle.

⊃ **Revised:** Revisions within the line or code from the previous edition are indicated by the color arrow.

✔ **Reinstated** indicates a code that was previously deleted and has now been reactivated.

✖ ~~deleted~~ words have been removed from this year's edition.

HCPCS Symbols

⊕ **Special coverage instructions** apply to these codes. Usually these special coverage instructions are included in the Internet Only Manuals (IOM). References to the IOM locations are given in the form of Medicare Pub. 100 reference numbers listed below the code. IOM select references are located at codingupdates.com.

⊘ **Not covered or valid by Medicare** is indicated by the "No" symbol. Usually the reason for the exclusion is included in the Internet Only Manuals (IOM) select references at codingupdates.com.

✳ **Carrier discretion** is an indication that you must contact the individual third-party payers to find out the coverage available for codes identified by this symbol.

Ⓑ Bill Part B MAC.

Ⓓ Bill DME MAC.

Color typeface terms within the Table of Drugs and tabular section are terms added by the publisher and do not appear in the official code set. Information supplementing the official HCPCS Index produced by CMS is *italicized*.

SYMBOLS AND CONVENTIONS

HCPCS Symbols

Special coverage instructions apply to these codes. Usually these instructions are included in the Internet Only Manuals (IOM). References to the IOM locations are given in the form of Medicare Pub. 100 reference numbers listed below the code. IOM select references are located at codingupdates.com.

⊕ **L3540**   Miscellaneous shoe additions, sole, full

IOM: 100-2, 15, 290

The Internet Only Manuals (IOM) give instructions regarding use of the code. IOM select references are located at codingupdates.com.

Not covered or valid by Medicare is indicated by the "No" symbol. Usually the reason for the exclusion is included in the IOM references located at codingupdates.com.

⊘ **A65331**   Gradient compression stocking, thigh length, 18–30 mm Hg, each

IOM: 100-02, 15, 130; 100-03, 4, 280.1

Carrier discretion is an indication that you must contact the individual third-party payers for the coverage for these codes.

✳ **A6154**   Wound pouch, each

A4650   Implantable radiation dosimeter; each Ⓑ

Bill Part B MAC.

A4606   Oxygen probe for use with oximeter device; replacement Ⓑ

Bill DME MAC.

Codes shown are for illustration purposes only and may not be current codes.

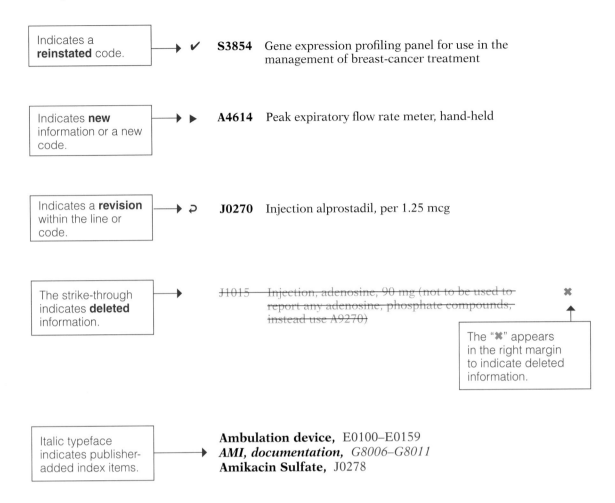

Indicates a **reinstated** code.	✔ **S3854**	Gene expression profiling panel for use in the management of breast-cancer treatment
Indicates **new** information or a new code.	▶ **A4614**	Peak expiratory flow rate meter, hand-held
Indicates a **revision** within the line or code.	↻ **J0270**	Injection alprostadil, per 1.25 mcg

The strike-through indicates **deleted** information.

~~J1015   Injection, adenosine, 90 mg (not to be used to report any adenosine, phosphate compounds, instead use A9270)~~   ✖

The "✖" appears in the right margin to indicate deleted information.

Italic typeface indicates publisher-added index items.

Ambulation device, E0100–E0159
AMI, documentation, G8006–G8011
Amikacin Sulfate, J0278

Codes shown are for illustration purposes only and may not be current codes.

2018 HCPCS UPDATES

2018 HCPCS New/Revised/Deleted Codes and Modifiers

HCPCS quarterly updates are posted on the companion website (www.codingupdates.com) when available.

NEW CODES/MODIFIERS

FY	E0954	G9907	G9933	G9963	J7345
JG	G0511	G9908	G9934	G9964	J9022
QQ	G0512	G9909	G9935	G9965	J9023
TB	G0513	G9910	G9936	G9966	J9203
VM	G0514	G9911	G9937	G9967	J9285
X1	G0515	G9912	G9938	G9968	K0553
X2	G0516	G9913	G9939	G9969	K0554
X3	G0517	G9914	G9940	G9970	L3761
X4	G0518	G9915	G9941	G9974	L7700
X5	G9890	G9916	G9942	G9975	L8625
ZC	G9891	G9917	G9943	G9976	L8694
C9014	G9892	G9918	G9944	G9977	P9073
C9015	G9893	G9919	G9945	J0565	P9100
C9016	G9894	G9920	G9946	J0604	Q0477
C9024	G9895	G9921	G9947	J0606	Q2040
C9028	G9896	G9922	G9948	J1428	Q4176
C9029	G9897	G9923	G9949	J1555	Q4177
C9488	G9898	G9924	G9954	J1627	Q4178
C9492	G9899	G9925	G9955	J1726	Q4179
C9493	G9900	G9926	G9956	J1729	Q4180
C9738	G9901	G9927	G9957	J2326	Q4181
C9745	G9902	G9928	G9958	J2350	Q4182
C9746	G9903	G9929	G9959	J3358	
C9747	G9904	G9930	G9960	J7210	
C9748	G9905	G9931	G9961	J7211	
E0953	G9906	G9932	G9962	J7296	

REVISED CODES/MODIFIERS

Change in Long Description	G9758	Q4162	J0132	J3489	**Change in Short Description**
Q5	G9762	Q4163	J0215	J7191	E1639
Q6	G9763		J0365	J7196	G8430
G8442	G9764	**Change in Administrative Data Field**	J0400	J7309	G8433
G8535	G9765	A4575	J0470	J7310	G8938
G8540	G9785	E0446	J0583	J7320	G9256
G8808	G9786		J0720	J7328	G9257
G8869	G9794	**Change in Payment**	J0725	J7508	G9258
G8880	G9814	A4421	J0833	J7513	G9259
G8939	G9815	A9586	J0884	J8510	G9260
G8941	G9816	A9606	J0888	J8650	G9261
G8967	G9817	C1822	J1110	J8700	G9262
G8968	G9840	C2613	J1130	J9151	G9384
G8969	G9841	C2623	J1205	J9185	G9541
G9227	G9843	C2624	J1324	J9200	G9716
G9263	J7321	C9248	J1730	J9208	G9717
G9313	L3760	C9447	J1945	J9213	G9744
G9348	L8618	E0575	J2020	J9219	G9745
G9504	L8624	E0950	J2260	J9263	G9784
G9607	L8691	G0458	J2358	J9351	J2274
G9624	Q4132	J0120	J2510	Q2009	
G9637	Q4133	J0130	J2670	Q4121	
G9638	Q4148		J2730	Q4172	
G9656	Q4156		J3355	Q5102	
	Q4158		J3365	Q9950	

DELETED CODES/MODIFIERS

CP	G0202	G0503	G8696	G8947	G9496
SZ	G0204	G0504	G8697	G8971	J1725
A9599	G0206	G0505	G8698	G8972	J9300
C9140	G0364	G0507	G8879	G9381	P9072
C9483	G0502				

ADDED AND DELETED DURING 2017

C9484	C9487	C9491	Q9984	Q9986	Q9988
C9485	C9489	C9494	Q9985	Q9987	Q9989
C9486	C9490				

HCPCS 2018
INDEX

A

Abatacept, J0129
Abciximab, J0130
Abdomen
    dressing holder/binder, A4462
    pad, low profile, L1270
Abduction control, each, L2624
Abduction restrainer, *A4566*
Abduction rotation bar, foot, L3140–L3170
    adjustable shoe style positioning device, L3160
    including shoes, L3140
    plastic, heel-stabilizer, off-shelf, L3170
    without shoes, L3150
AbobotulinumtypeA, J0586
Absorption dressing, A6251–A6256
Access, site, occlusive, device, *G0269*
Access system, A4301
Accessories
    ambulation devices, E0153–E0159
      crutch attachment, walker, E0157
      forearm crutch, platform attachment, E0153
      leg extension, walker, E0158
      replacement, brake attachment, walker, E0159
      seat attachment, walker, E0156
      walker, platform attachment, E0154
      wheel attachment, walker, per pair, E0155
    artificial kidney and machine; (see also ESRD),
      E1510–E1699
      adjustable chair, ESRD patients, E1570
      automatic peritoneal dialysis system,
      intermittent, E1592
      bath conductivity meter, hemodialysis, E1550
      blood leak detector, hemodialysis,
      replacement, E1560
      blood pump, hemodialysis, replacement, E1620
      cycler dialysis machine, peritoneal, E1594
      deionizer water system, hemodialysis, E1615
      delivery/instillation charges, hemodialysis
      equipment, E1600
      hemodialysis machine, E1590
      hemostats, E1637
      heparin infusion pump, hemodialysis, E1520
      kidney machine, dialysate delivery system, E1510
      peritoneal dialysis clamps, E1634
      portable travel hemodialyzer, E1635
      reciprocating peritoneal dialysis system, E1630
      replacement, air bubble detector,
      hemodialysis, E1530
      replacement, pressure alarm, hemodialysis, E1540
      reverse osmosis water system, hemodialysis, E1610
      scale, E1639
      sorbent cartridges, hemodialysis, E1636
      transducer protectors, E1575
      unipuncture control system, E1580
      water softening system, hemodialysis, E1625
      wearable artificial kidney, E1632

Accessories *(Continued)*
    beds, E0271–E0280, E0300–E0326
      bed board, E0273
      bed, board/table, E0315
      bed cradle, E0280
      bed pan, standard, E0275
      bed side rails, E0305–E0310
      bed-pan fracture, E0276
      hospital bed, extra heavy duty, E0302, E0304
      hospital bed, heavy duty, E0301–E0303
      hospital bed, pediatric, electric, E0329
      hospital bed, safety enclosure frame, E0316
      mattress, foam rubber, E0272
      mattress, innerspring, E0271
      over-bed table, E0274
      pediatric crib, E0300
      powered pressure-reducing air mattress, E0277
    wheelchairs, E0950–E1030, E1050–E1298,
      E2300–E2399, K0001–K0109
      accessory tray, E0950
      arm rest, E0994
      back upholstery replacement, E0982
      calf rest/pad, E0995
      commode seat, E0968
      detachable armrest, E0973
      elevating leg rest, E0990
      headrest cushion, E0955
      lateral trunk/hip support, E0956
      loop-holder, E0951–E0952
      manual swingaway, E1028
      manual wheelchair, adapter, amputee, E0959
      manual wheelchair, anti-rollback device, E0974
      manual wheelchair, anti-tipping device, E0971
      manual wheelchair, hand rim with
      projections, E0967
      manual wheelchair, headrest extension, E0966
      manual wheelchair, lever-activated, wheel
      drive, E0988
      manual wheelchair, one-arm drive
      attachment, E0958
      manual wheelchair, power add-on, E0983–E0984
      manual wheelchair, push activated power
      assist, E0986
      manual wheelchair, solid seat insert, E0992
      medial thigh support, E0957
      modification, pediatric size, E1011
      narrowing device, E0969
      No. 2 footplates, E0970
      oxygen related accessories, E1352–E1406
      positioning belt/safety belt/pelvic strap, E0978
      power-seating system, E1002–E1010
      reclining back addition, pediatric size
      wheelchair, E1014
      residual limb support system, E1020
      safety vest, E0980
      seat lift mechanism, E0985
      seat upholstery replacement, E0981
      shock absorber, E1015–E1018

◀ **New** ⟳ **Revised** ✔ **Reinstated** ~~deleted~~ **Deleted**

Accessories *(Continued)*
  wheelchairs *(Continued)*
    shoulder harness strap, E0960
    ventilator tray, E1029–E1030
    wheel lock brake extension, manual, E0961
    wheelchair, amputee, accessories, E1170–E1200
    wheelchair, fully inclining, accessories,
    E1050–E1093
    wheelchair, heavy duty, accessories, E1280–E1298
    wheelchair, lightweight, accessories, E1240–E1270
    wheelchair, semi-reclining, accessories,
    E1100–E1110
    wheelchair, special size, E1220–E1239
    wheelchair, standard, accessories, E1130–E1161
   whirlpool equipment, E1300–E1310
Ace type, elastic bandage, *A6448–A6450*
Acetaminophen, J0131
Acetazolamide sodium, J1120
Acetylcysteine
  inhalation solution, J7604, J7608
  injection, J0132
Activity, therapy, *G0176*
Acyclovir, J0133
Adalimumab, J0135
Additions to
  fracture orthosis, L2180–L2192
    abduction bar, L2300–L2310
    adjustable motion knee joint, L2186
    anterior swing band, L2335
    BK socket, PTB and AFO, L2350
    disk or dial lock, knee flexion, L2425
    dorsiflexion and plantar flexion, L2220
    dorsiflexion assist, L2210
    drop lock, L2405
    drop lock knee joint, L2182
    extended steel shank, L2360
    foot plate, stirrup attachment, L2250
    hip joint, pelvic band, thigh flange, pelvic belt, L2192
    integrated release mechanism, L2515
    lacer custom-fabricated, L2320–L2330
    lift loop, drop lock ring, L2492
    limited ankle motion, L2200
    limited motion knee joint, L2184
    long tongue stirrup, L2265
    lower extremity orthrosis, L2200–L2397
    molded inner boot, L2280
    offset knee joint, L2390
    offset knee joint, heavy duty, L2395
    Patten bottom, L2370
    pelvic and thoracic control, L2570–L2680
    plastic shoe insert with ankle joints, L2180
    polycentric knee joint, L2387
    pre-tibial shell, L2340
    quadrilateral, L2188
    ratchet lock knee extension, L2430
    reinforced solid stirrup, L2260
    rocker bottom, custom fabricated, L2232
    round caliper/plate attachment, L2240

Additions to *(Continued)*
  fracture orthosis (Continued)
    split flat caliper stirrups, L2230
    straight knee joint, heavy duty, L2385
    straight knee, or offset knee joints, L2405–L2492
    suspension sleeve, L2397
    thigh/weight bearing, L2500–L2550
    torsion control, ankle joint, L2375
    torsion control, straight knee joint, L2380
    varus/valgus correction, L2270–L2275
    waist belt, L2190
  general additions, orthosis, L2750–L2999
    lower extremity, above knee section, soft
    interface, L2830
    lower extremity, concentric adjustable torsion style
    mechanism, L2861
    lower extremity, drop lock retainer, L2785
    lower extremity, extension, per extension, per
    bar, L2760
    lower extremity, femoral length sock, L2850
    lower extremity, full kneecap, L2795
    lower extremity, high strength, lightweight material,
    hybrid lamination, L2755
    lower extremity, knee control, condylar pad, L2810
    lower extremity, knee control, knee cap, medial or
    lateral, L2800
    lower extremity orthrosis, non-corrosive finish, per
    bar, L2780
    lower extremity orthrosis, NOS, L2999
    lower extremity, plating chrome or nickel, per
    bar, L2750
    lower extremity, soft interface, below knee, L2820
    lower extremity, tibial length sock, L2840
    orthotic side bar, disconnect device, L2768
Adenosine, J0151, J0153
Adhesive, A4364
  bandage, A6413
  disc or foam pad, A5126
  remover, A4455, A4456
  support, breast prosthesis, A4280
  wound, closure, G0168
Administration, chemotherapy, *Q0083–Q0085*
  both infusion and other technique, Q0085
  infusion technique only, Q0084
  other than infusion technique, Q0083
Administration, Part D
  vaccine, hepatitis B, G0010
  vaccine, influenza, G0008
  vaccine, pneumococcal, G0009
Administrative, Miscellaneous and Investigational,
  A9000–A9999
  alert or alarm device, A9280
  artificial saliva, A9155
  DME delivery set-up, A9901
  exercise equipment, A9300
  external ambulatory insulin delivery system, A9274
  foot pressure off loading/supportive device, A9283
  helmets, A8000–A8004

◀ **New**   ⇄ **Revised**   ✔ **Reinstated**   ~~deleted~~ **Deleted**

Administrative, Miscellaneous and Investigational
(Continued)
home glucose disposable monitor, A9275
hot-water bottle, ice cap, heat wrap, A9273
miscellaneous DME, NOS, A9999
miscellaneous DME supply, A9900
monitoring feature/device, stand-alone or integrated, A9279
multiple vitamins, oral, per dose, A9153
non-covered item, A9270
non-prescription drugs, A9150
pediculosis treatment, topical, A9180
radiopharmaceuticals, A9500–A9700
reaching grabbing device, A9281
receiver, external, interstitial glucose monitoring system, A9278
sensor, invasive, interstitial continuous glucose monitoring, A9276
single vitamin/mineral trace element, A9152
spirometer, non-electronic, A9284
transmitter, interstitial continuous glucose monitoring system, A9277
wig, any type, A9282
wound suction, disposable, A9272
Admission, observation, *G0379*
Ado-trastuzumab, J9354
Adrenalin, J0171
Advanced life support, *A0390, A0426, A0427, A0433*
ALS2, A0433
ALS emergency transport, A0427
ALS mileage, A0390
ALS, non-emergency transport, A0426
Aerosol
compressor, E0571–E0572
compressor filter, A7013–A7014, K0178–K0179
mask, A7015, K0180
Aflibercept, J0178
AFO, E1815, E1830, L1900–L1990, L4392, L4396
Afstyla, J7210 ◀
Agalsidase beta, J0180
Aggrastat, J3245
A-hydroCort, J1710
Aid, hearing, *V5030–V5263*
Aide, home, health, *G0156, S9122, T1021*
home health aide/certified nurse assistant, in home, S9122
home health aide/certified nurse assistant, per visit, T1021
home health or hospital setting, G0156
Air bubble detector, dialysis, E1530
Air fluidized bed, E0194
Air pressure pad/mattress, E0186, E0197
Air travel and nonemergency transportation, A0140
Alarm
not otherwise classified, A9280
pressure, dialysis, E1540
Alatrofloxacin mesylate, J0200
Albumin, human, P9041, P9042

Albuterol
all formulations, inhalation solution, J7620
all formulations, inhalation solution, concentrated, J7610, J7611
all formulations, inhalation solution, unit dose, J7609, J7613
Alcohol, A4244
Alcohol wipes, A4245
Alcohol/substance, assessment, *G0396, G0397, H0001, H0003, H0049*
alcohol abuse structured assessment, greater than 30 min., G0397
alcohol abuse structured assessment, 15–30 min., G0396
alcohol and/or drug assessment, Medicaid, H0001
alcohol and/or drug screening; laboratory analysis, Medicaid, H0003
alcohol and/or drug screening, Medicaid, H0049
Aldesleukin (IL2), J9015
Alefacept, J0215
Alemtuzumab, J0202
Alert device, A9280
Alginate dressing, A6196–A6199
alginate, pad more than 48 sq. cm, A6198
alginate, pad size 16 sq. cm, A6196
alginate, pad size more than 16 sq. cm, A6197
alginate, wound filler, sterile, A6199
Alglucerase, J0205
Alglucosidase, J0220
Alglucosidase alfa, J0221
Alphanate, J7186
Alpha-1–proteinase inhibitor, human, J0256, J0257
Alprostadil
injection, J0270
urethral supposity, J0275
ALS mileage, *A0390*
Alteplase recombinant, J2997
Alternating pressure mattress/pad, A4640, E0180, E0181, E0277
overlay/pad, alternating, pump, heavy duty, E0181
powered pressure-reducing air mattress, E0277
replacement pad, owned by patient, A4640
Ambulance, A0021–A0999
air, A0430, A0431, A0435, A0436
conventional, transport, one way, fixed wing, A0430
conventional, transport, one way, rotary wing, A0431
fixed wing air mileage, A0435
rotary wing air mileage, A0436
disposable supplies, A0382–A0398
ALS routine disposable supplies, A0398
ALS specialized service disposable supplies, A0394
ALS specialized service, esophageal intubation, A0396
BLS routine disposable, A0832
BLS specialized service disposable supplies, defibrillation, A0384, A0392
non-emergency transport, fixed wing, S9960
non-emergency transport, rotary wing, S9961
oxygen, A0422

◀ **New**   ↻ **Revised**   ✔ **Reinstated**   ~~deleted~~ **Deleted**

Ambulation device, E0100–E0159

brake attachment, wheeled walker replacement, E0159

cane, adjustable or fixed, with tip, E0100

cane, quad or three prong, adjustable or fixed, with tip, E0105

crutch attachment, walker, E0157

crutch forearm, each, with tips and handgrips, E0111

crutch substitute, lower leg platform, with or without wheels, each, E0118

crutch, underarm, articulating, spring assisted, each, E0117

crutches forearm, pair, tips and handgrips, E0110

crutches, underarm, other than wood, pair, with pads, tips and handgrips, E0114

crutches, underarm, other than wood, with pad, tip, handgrip, with or without shock absorber, each, E0116

crutches, underarm, wood, each, with pad, tip and handgrip, E0113

leg extensions, walker, set (4), E0158

platform attachment, forearm crutch, each, E0153

platform attachment, walker, E0154

seat attachment, walker, E0156

walker, enclosed, four-sided frame, wheeled, posterior seat, E0144

walker, folding, adjustable or fixed height, E0135

walker, folding, wheeled, adjustable or fixed height, E0143

walker, heavy duty, multiple braking system, variable wheel resistance, E0147

walker, heavy duty, wheeled, rigid or folding, E0149

walker, heavy duty, without wheels, rigid or folding, E0148

walker, rigid, adjustable or fixed height, E0130

walker, rigid, wheeled, adjustable or fixed height, E0141

walker, with trunk support, adjystable or fixed height, any, E0140

wheel attachment, rigid, pick up walker, per pair, E0155

Amikacin Sulfate, J0278

Aminolevulinate, J7309

Aminolevulinic, J7345 ◄

Aminolevulinic acid HCl, J7308

Aminophylline, J0280

Amiodarone HCl, J0282

Amitriptyline HCl, J1320

Ammonia N-13, A9526

Ammonia test paper, A4774

Amniotic membrane, V2790

Amobarbital, J0300

Amphotericin B, J0285

Lipid Complex, J0287–J0289

Ampicillin

sodium, J0290

sodium/sulbactam sodium, J0295

Amputee

adapter, wheelchair, E0959

prosthesis, L5000–L7510, L7520, L7900, L8400–L8465

above knee, L5200–L5230

Amputee (Continued)

prosthesis (Continued)

additions to exoskeletal knee-shin systems, L5710–L5782

additions to lower extremity, L5610–L5617

additions to socket insert and suspension, L5654–L5699

additions to socket variations, L5630–L5653

additions to test sockets, L5618–L5629

additions/replacements feet-ankle units, L5700–L5707

ankle, L5050–L5060

below knee, L5100–L5105

component modification, L5785–L5795

endoskeletal, L5810–L5999

endoskeleton, below knee, L5301–L5312

endoskeleton, hip disarticulation, L5331–L5341

fitting endoskeleton, above knee, L5321

fitting procedures, L5400–L5460

hemipelvectomy, L5280

hip disarticulation, L5250–L5270

initial prosthesis, L5500–L5505

knee disarticulation, L5150–L5160

male vacuum erection system, L7900

partial foot, L5000–L5020

preparatory prosthesis, L5510–L5600

prosthetic socks, L8400–L8485

repair, prosthetic device, L7520

tension ring, vacuum erection device, L7902

upper extremity, battery components, L7360–L7368

upper extremity, other/repair, L7400–L7510

upper extremity, preparatory, elbow, L6584–L6586

upper limb, above elbow, L6250

upper limb, additions, L6600–L6698

upper limb, below elbow, L6100–L6130

upper limb, elbow disarticulation, L6200–L6205

upper limb, endoskeletal, above elbow, L6500

upper limb, endoskeletal, below elbow, L6400

upper limb, endoskeletal, elbow disarticulation, L6450

upper limb, endoskeletal, interscapular thoracic, L6570

upper limb, endoskeletal, shoulder disarticulation, L6550

upper limb, external power, device, L6920–L6975

upper limb, interscapular thoracic, L6350–L6370

upper limb, partial hand, L6000–L6025

upper limb, postsurgical procedures, L6380–L6388

upper limb, preparatory, shoulder, interscapular, L6588–L6590

upper limb, preparatory, wrist, L6580–L6582

upper limb, shoulder disarticulation, L6300–L6320

upper limb, terminal devices, L6703–L6915, L7007–L7261

upper limb, wrist disarticulation, L6050–L6055

◄ **New**   ↻ **Revised**   ✔ **Reinstated**   ~~deleted~~ **Deleted**

Amputee (*Continued***)**

stump sock, L8470–L8485

  single ply, fitting above knee, L8480

  single ply, fitting, below knee, L8470

  single ply, fitting, upper limb, L8485

wheelchair, E1170–E1190, E1200, K0100

  detachable arms, swing away detachable elevating footrests, E1190

  detachable arms, swing away detachable footrests, E1180

  detachable arms, without footrests or legrest, E1172

  detachable elevating legrest, fixed full length arms, E1170

  fixed full length arms, swing away detachable footrest, E1200

  heavy duty wheelchair, swing away detachable elevating legrests, E1195

  without footrests or legrest, fixed full length arms, E1171

Amygdalin, J3570

Anadulafungin, J0348

Analysis

  semen, G0027

Angiography, iliac, artery, *G0278*

Angiography, renal, non-selective, *G0275*

  non-ophthalmic fluorescent vascular, C9733

  reconstruction, G0288

Anistreplase, J0350

Ankle splint, recumbent, K0126–K0130

Ankle-foot orthosis (AFO), L1900–L1990, L2106–L2116, L4361, L4392, L4396

  ankle gauntlet, custom fabricated, L1904

  ankle gauntlet, prefabricated, off-shelf, L1902

  double upright free plantar dorsiflexion, olid stirrup, calf-band/cuff, custom, L1990

  fracture orthosis, tibial fracture, thermoplastic cast material, custom, L2106

  multiligamentus ankle support, prefabricated, off-shelf, L1906

  plastic or other material, custom fabricated, L1940

  plastic or other material, prefabricated, fitting and adjustment, L1932, L1951

  plastic or other material, with ankle joint, prefabricated, fitting and adjustment, L1971

  plastic, rigid anterior tibial section, custom fabricated, L1945

  plastic, with ankle joint, custom, L1970

  posterior, single bar, clasp attachment to shoe, L1910

  posterior, solid ankle, plastic, custom, L1960

  replacement, soft interface material, static AFO, L4392

  single upright free plantar dorsiflection, solid stirrup, calf-band/cuff, custom, L1980

  single upright with static or adjustable stop, custom, L1920

  spiral, plastic, custom fabricated, L1950

  spring wire, dorsiflexion assist calf band, L1900

  static or dynamic AFO, adjustable for fit, minimal ambulation, L4396

Ankle-foot orthosis (*Continued*)

  supramalleolar with straps, custom fabricated, L1907

  tibial fracture cast orthrosis, custom, L2108

  tibial fracture orthrosis, rigid, prefabricated, fitting and adjustment, L2116

  tibial fracture orthrosis, semi-rigid, prefabricated, fitting and adjustment, L2114

  tibial fracture orthrosis, soft prefabricated, fitting and adjustment, L2112

  walking boot, prefabricated, off-the-shelf, L4361

Anterior-posterior-lateral orthosis, L0700, L0710

Antibiotic, *G8708–G8712*

  antibiotic not prescribed or dispensed, G8712

  patient not prescribed or dispensed antibiotic, G8708

  patient prescribed antibiotic, documented condition, G8709

  patient prescribed or dispensed antibiotic, G8710

  prescribed or dispensed antibiotic, G8711

Antidepressant, documentation, G8126–G8128

Anti-emetic, oral, J8498, J8597, Q0163–Q0181

  antiemetic drug, oral NOS, J8597

  antiemetic drug, rectal suppository, NOS, J8498

  diphenhydramine hydrochloride, 50 mg, oral, Q0163

  dolasetron mesylate, 100 mg, oral, Q0180

  dronabinol, 2.5 mg, Q0167

  granisetron hydrochloride, 1 mg, oral, Q0166

  hydroxyzine pomoate, 25 mg, oral, Q0177

  perphenazine, 4 mg, oral, Q0175

  prochlorperazine maleate, 5 mg, oral, Q0164

  promethazine hydrochloride, 12.5 mg, oral, Q0169

  thiethylperazine maleate, 10 mg, oral, Q0174

  trimethobenzamide hydrochloride, 250 mg, oral, Q0173

  unspecified oral dose, Q0181

Anti-hemophilic factor (Factor VIII), J7190–J7192

Anti-inhibitors, per I.U., J7198

Antimicrobial, prophylaxis, documentation, *G8201*

Anti-neoplastic drug, NOC, J9999

Antithrombin III, J7197

Antithrombin recombinant, J7196

Apomorphine, J0364

Appliance

  cleaner, A5131

  pneumatic, E0655–E0673

    non-segmental pneumatic appliance, E0655, E0660, E0665, E0666

    segmental gradient pressure, pneumatic appliance, E0671–E0673

    segmental pneumatic appliance, E0656–E0657, E0667–E0670

Application, heat, cold, *E0200–E0239*

  electric heat pad, moist, E0215

  electric heat pad, standard, E0210

  heat lamp with stand, E0205

  heat lamp without stand, E0200

  hydrocollator unit, pads, E0225

  hydrocollator unit, portable, E0239

  infrared heating pad system, E0221

  non-contact wound warming device, E0231

◀ **New**   ⟳ **Revised**   ✔ **Reinstated**   ~~deleted~~ **Deleted**

Application, heat, cold *(Continued)*
  paraffin bath unit, E0235
  phototherapy (bilirubin), E0202
  pump for water circulating pad, E0236
  therapeutic lightbox, E0203
  warming card, E0232
  water circulating cold pad with pump, E0218
  water circulating heat pad with pump, E0217
Aprotinin, J0365
Aqueous
  shunt, L8612
  sterile, J7051
ARB/ACE therapy, G8473–G8475
Arbutamine HCl, J0395
Arch support, L3040–L3100
  hallus-valgus night dynamic splint, off-shelf, L3100
  intralesional, J3302
  non-removable, attached to shoe, longitudinal, L3070
  non-removable, attached to shoe, longitudinal/
    metatarsal, each, L3090
  non-removable, attached to shoe, metatarsal, L3080
  removable, premolded, longitudinal, L3040
  removable, premolded, longitudinal/metatarsal,
    each, L3060
  removable, premolded, metatarsal, L3050
Arformoterol, J7605
Argatroban, J0883–J0884
Aripiprazole, J0400, J0401, J1942
Arm, wheelchair, E0973
Arsenic trioxide, J9017
Arthrography, injection, sacroiliac, joint,
    G0259, G0260
Arthroscopy, knee, surgical, G0289, S2112
  chondroplasty, different compartment, knee, G0289
  harvesting of cartilage, knee, S2112
Artificial
  Cornea, L8609
  kidney machines and accessories; (see also
    Dialysis), E1510–E1699
  larynx, L8500
  saliva, A9155
Asparaginase, J9019–J9020
Aspirator, VABRA, A4480
Assessment
  alcohol/substance; (see also Alcohol/substance,
    assessment), G0396, G0397, H0001,
    H0003, H0049
  assessment for hearing aid, V5010
  audiologic, V5008–V5020
  cardiac output, M0302
  conformity evaluation, V5020
  fitting/orientation, hearing aid, V5014
  hearing screening, V5008
  repair/modification hearing aid, V5014
  speech, V5362–V5364
Assistive listening devices and accessories,
    V5281–V5290
  FMlDM system, monaural, V5281

Astramorph, J2275
Atezolizumab, J9022 ◀
Atherectomy, PTCA, C9602, C9603
Atropine
  inhalation solution, concentrated, J7635
  inhalation solution, unit dose, J7636
Atropine sulfate, J0461
Attachment, walker, E0154–E0159
  brake attachment, wheeled walker,
    replacement, E0159
  crutch attachment, walker, E0157
  leg extension, walker, E0158
  platform attachment, walker, E0154
  seat attachment, walker, E0156
  wheel attachment, rigid pick up walker, E0155
Audiologic assessment, V5008–V5020
Auditory osseointegrated device, L8690–L8694 ↻
Aurothioglucose, J2910
Avelumab, J9023 ◀
Azacitidine, J9025
Azathioprine, J7500, J7501
Azithromycin injection, J0456

B

Back supports, L0621–L0861, L0960
  lumbar orthrosis, L0625–L0627
  lumbar orthrosis, sagittal control, L0641–L0648
  lumbar-sacral orthrosis, L0628–L0640
  lumbar-sacral orthrosis, sagittal-coronal control,
    L0640, L0649–L0651
  sacroiliac orthrosis, L0621–L0624
Baclofen, J0475, J0476
Bacterial sensitivity study, P7001
Bag
  drainage, A4357
  enema, A4458
  irrigation supply, A4398
  urinary, A4358, A5112
Bandage, conforming
  elastic, >5", A6450
  elastic, >3", <5", A6449
  elastic, load resistance 1.25 to 1.34 foot pounds, >3",
    <5", A6451
  elastic, load resistance <1.35 foot pounds, >3",
    <5", A6452
  elastic, <3", A6448
  non-elastic, non-sterile, >5", A6444
  non-elastic, non-sterile, width greater than or equal
    to 3", <5", A6443
  non-elastic, non-sterile, width <3", A6442
  non-elastic, sterile, >5", A6447
  non-elastic, sterile, >3" and <5", A6446
Basiliximab, J0480
Bath, aid, E0160–E0162, E0235, E0240–E0249
  bath tub rail, floor base, E0242
  bath tub wall rail, E0241

◀ **New**   ↻ **Revised**   ✔ **Reinstated**   ~~deleted~~ **Deleted**

Bath, aid *(Continued)*
  bath/shower chair, with/without wheels, E0240
  pad for water circulating heat unit,
    replacement, E0249
  paraffin bath unit, portable, E0235
  raised toilet seat, E0244
  sitz bath chair, E0162
  sitz type bath, portable, with faucet
    attachment, E0161
  sitz type bath, portable, with/without
    commode, E0160
  toilet rail, E0243
  transfer bench, tub or toilet, E0248
  transfer tub rail attachment, E0246
  tub stool or bench, E0245
Bathtub
  chair, E0240
  stool or bench, E0245, E0247–E0248
  transfer rail, E0246
  wall rail, E0241–E0242
Battery, L7360, L7364–L7368
  charger, E1066, L7362, L7366
  replacement for blood glucose monitor,
    A4233–A4236
  replacement for cochlear implant device, L8618,
    L8623–L8625 ↻
  replacement for TENS, A4630
  ventilator, A4611–A4613
BCG live, intravesical, J9031
Beclomethasone inhalation solution, J7622
Bed
  accessories, E0271–E0280, E0300–E0326
    bed board, E0273
    bed cradle, E0280
    bed pan, fracture, metal, E0276
    bed pan, standard, metal, E0275
    mattress, foam rubber, E0272
    mattress innerspring, E0271
    over-bed table, E0274
    power pressure-reducing air mattress, E0277
  air fluidized, E0194
  cradle, any type, E0280
  drainage bag, bottle, A4357, A5102
  hospital, E0250–E0270, E0300–E0329
  pan, E0275, E0276
  rail, E0305, E0310
  safety enclosure frame/canopy, E0316
Behavioral, health, treatment services (Medicaid),
    H0002–H2037
  activity therapy, H2032
  alcohol/drug services, H0001, H0003, H0005–H0016,
    H0020–H0022, H0026–H0029, H0049–H0050,
    H2034–H2036
  assertive community treatment, H0040
  community based wrap-around services,
    H2021–H2022
  comprehensive community support, H2015–H2016
  comprehensive medication services, H2010

Behavioral, health, treatment services (Medicaid)
    (Continued)
  comprehensive multidisciplinary evaluation, H2000
  crisis intervention, H2011
  day treatment, per diem, H2013
  day treatment, per hour, H2012
  developmental delay prevention activities, dependent
    child of client, H2037
  family assessment, H1011
  foster care, child, H0041–H0042
  health screening, H0002
  hotline service, H0030
  medication training, H0034
  mental health clubhouse services, H2030–H2031
  multisystemic therapy, juveniles, H2033
  non-medical family planning, H1010
  outreach service, H0023
  partial hospitalization, H0035
  plan development, non-physician, H0033
  prenatal care, at risk, H1000–H1005
  prevention, H0024–H0025
  psychiatric supportive treatment, community,
    H0036–H0037
  psychoeducational service, H2027
  psychoscial rehabilitation, H2017–H2018
  rehabilitation program, H2010
  residential treatment program, H0017–H0019
  respite care, not home, H0045
  self-help/peer services, H0039
  sexual offender treatment, H2028–H2029
  skill training, H2014
  supported employment, H2024–H2026
  supported housing, H0043–H0044
  therapeutic behavioral services, H2019–H2020
Behavioral therapy, cardiovascular disease, *G0446*
Belatacept, J0485
Belimumab, J0490
Belt
  belt, strap, sleeve, garment, or covering, any
    type, A4467
  extremity, E0945
  ostomy, A4367
  pelvic, E0944
  safety, K0031
  wheelchair, E0978, E0979
Bench, bathtub; (see also Bathtub), E0245
Bendamustine HCl ↻
  Bendeka, 1 mg, J9034 ◄
  Treanda, 1 mg, J9033 ◄
Benesch boot, L3212–L3214
Benztropine, J0515
Beta-blocker therapy, *G9188–G9192*
Betadine, A4246, A4247
Betameth, J0704
Betamethasone
  acetate and betamethasone sodium
    phosphate, J0702
  inhalation solution, J7624

Bethanechol chloride, J0520

Bevacizumab, J9035, Q2024

Bezlotoxumab, J0565 ◀

Bifocal, glass or plastic, V2200–V2299

aniseikonic, bifocal, V2218

bifocal add-over 3.25 d, V2220

bifocal seg width over 28 mm, V2219

lenticular, bifocal, myodisc, V2215

lenticular lens, V2221

specialty bifocal, by report, V2200

sphere, bifocal, V2200–V2202

spherocylinder, bifocal, V2203–V2214

Bilirubin (phototherapy) light, E0202

Binder, A4465

Biofeedback device, E0746

Bioimpedance, electrical, cardiac output, M0302

Biosimilar (infliximab), Q5102

Biperiden lactate, J0190

Bitolterol mesylate, inhalation solution

concentrated, J7628

unit dose, J7629

Bivalirudin, J0583

***Bivigam, 500 mg,* J1556**

Bladder calculi irrigation solution, Q2004

Bleomycin sulfate, J9040

Blood

count, G0306, G0307, S3630

complete CBC, automated, without platelet count, G0307

complete CBC, automated without platelet count, automated WBC differential, G0306

eosinophil count, blood, direct, S3630

fresh frozen plasma, P9017

glucose monitor, E0607, E2100, E2101, *S1030, S1031, S1034*

blood glucose monitor, integrated voice synthesizer, E2100

blood glucose monitor with integrated lancing/blood sample, E2101

continuous noninvasive device, purchase, S1030

continuous noninvasive device, rental, S1031

home blood glucose monitor, E0607

glucose test, A4253

glucose, test strips, dialysis, A4772

granulocytes, pheresis, P9050

ketone test, A4252

leak detector, dialysis, E1560

leukocyte poor, P9016

mucoprotein, P2038

platelets, P9019

platelets, irradiated, P9032

platelets, leukocytes reduced, P9031

platelets, leukocytes reduced, irradiated, P9033

platelets, pheresis, P9034, P9073, P9100 ↻

platelets, pheresis, irradiated, P9036

platelets, pheresis, leukocytes reduced, P9035

platelets, pheresis, leukocytes reduced, irradiated, P9037

Blood *(Continued)*

pressure monitor, A4660, A4663, A4670

pump, dialysis, E1620

red blood cells, deglycerolized, P9039

red blood cells, irradiated, P9038

red blood cells, leukocytes reduced, P9016

red blood cells, leukocytes reduced, irradiated, P9040

red blood cells, washed, P9022

strips, A4253

supply, P9010–P9022

testing supplies, A4770

tubing, A4750, A4755

Blood collection devices accessory, A4257, E0620

***BMI,* G8417–G8422**

Body jacket

scoliosis, L1300, L1310

***Body mass index,* G8417–G8422**

Body sock, L0984

Bond or cement, ostomy skin, A4364

Bone

density, study, G0130

Boot

pelvic, E0944

surgical, ambulatory, L3260

Bortezomib, J9041

Brachytherapy radioelements, Q3001

brachytherapy, LDR, prostate, G0458

brachytherapy planar source, C2645

brachytherapy, source, hospital outpatient, C1716–C1717, C1719

Breast prosthesis, L8000–L8035**,** L8600

adhesive skin support, A4280

custom breast prosthesis, post mastectomy, L8035

garment with mastectomy form, post mastectomy, L8015

implantable, silicone or equal, L8600

mastectomy bra, with integrated breast prosthesis form, unilateral, L8001

mastectomy bra, with prosthesis form, bilateral, L8002

mastectomy bra, without integrated breast prosthesis form, L8000

mastectomy form, L8020

mastectomy sleeve, L8010

nipple prosthesis, L8032

silicone or equal, with integral adhesive, L8031

silicone or equal, without integral adhesive, L8030

Breast pump

accessories, A4281–A4286

adapter, replacement, A4282

cap, breast pump bottle, replacement, A4283

locking ring, replacement, A4286

polycarbonate bottle, replacement, A4285

shield and splash protector, replacement, A4284

tubing, replacement, A4281

electric, any type, E0603

heavy duty, hospital grade, E0604

manual, any type, E0602

◀ **New** ↻ **Revised** ✔ **Reinstated** ~~deleted~~ **Deleted**

Breathing circuit, A4618
Brentuximab Vedotin, J9042
Brompheniramine maleate, J0945
Budesonide inhalation solution, J7626, J7627, J7633, J7634
Bulking agent, L8604, L8607
Buprenorphine hydrochlorides, J0592
Buprenorphine/Naloxone, J0571–J0575
Burn, compression garment, A6501–A6513
  bodysuit, head-foot, A6501
  burn mask, face and/or neck, A6513
  chin strap, A6502
  facial hood, A6503
  foot to knee length, A6507
  foot to thigh length, A6508
  glove to axilla, A6506
  glove to elbow, A6505
  glove to wrist, A6504
  lower trunk, including leg openings, A6511
  trunk, including arms, down to leg openings, A6510
  upper trunk to waist, including arm openings, A6509
Bus, nonemergency transportation, A0110
Busulfan, J0594, J8510
Butorphanol tartrate, J0595
Bypass, graft, coronary, artery
  surgery, S2205–S2209

C

C-1 Esterase Inhibitor, J0596–J0598
Cabazitaxel, J9043
Cabergoline, oral, J8515
Cabinet/System, ultraviolet, E0691–E0694
  multidirectional light system, 6 ft. cabinet, E0694
  timer and eye protection, 4 foot, E0692
  timer and eye protection, 6 foot, E0693
  ultraviolet light therapy system, treatment area 2 sq ft., E0691
Caffeine citrate, J0706
Calcitonin-salmon, J0630
Calcitriol, J0636, *S0169*
Calcium
  disodium edetate, J0600
  gluconate, J0610
  glycerophosphate and calcium lactate, J0620
  lactate and calcium glycerophosphate, J0620
  leucovorin, J0640
Calibrator solution, A4256
Canakinumab, J0638
Cancer, screening
  cervical or vaginal, G0101
  colorectal, G0104–G0106, G0120–G0122, G0328
    alternative to screening colonoscopy, barium enema, G0120
    alternative to screening sigmoidoscopy, barium enema, G0106
    barium enema, G0122

Cancer, screening (Continued)
  colorectal (Continued)
    colonoscopy, high risk, G0105
    colonoscopy, not at high-risk, G0121
    fecal occult blood test-1–3 simultaneous, G0328
    flexible sigmoidoscopy, G0104
  prostate, G0102, G0103
Cane, E0100, E0105
  accessory, A4636, A4637
Canister
  disposable, used with suction pump, A7000
  non-disposable, used with suction pump, A7001
Cannula, nasal, A4615
Capecitabine, oral, J8520, J8521
Capsaicin patch, J7336
Carbidopa 5 mg/levodopa 20 mg enteral suspension, J7340
Carbon filter, A4680
Carboplatin, J9045
Cardia Event, recorder, implantable, E0616
Cardiokymography, Q0035
Cardiovascular services, M0300–M0301
  Fabric wrapping abdominal aneurysm, M0301
  IV chelation therapy, M0300
Cardioverter-defibrillator, G0448
Care, coordinated, G9001–G9011, H1002
  coordinated care fee, home monitoring, G9006
  coordinated care fee, initial rate, G9001
  coordinated care fee, maintenance rate, G9002
  coordinated care fee, physician coordinated care oversight, G9008
  coordinated care fee, risk adjusted high, initial, G9003
  coordinated care fee, risk adjusted low, initial, G9004
  coordinated care fee, risk adjusted maintenance, G9005
  coordinated care fee, risk adjusted maintenance, level 3, G9009
  coordinated care fee, risk adjusted maintenance, level 4, G9010
  coordinated care fee, risk adjusted maintenance, level 5, G9011
  coordinated care fee, scheduled team conference, G9007
  prenatal care, at-risk, enhanced service, care coordination, H1002
Care plan, G0162
Carfilzomib, J9047
Carmustine, J9050
Case management, T1016, T1017
Caspofungin acetate, J0637
Cast
  hand restoration, L6900–L6915
  materials, special, A4590
  supplies, A4580, A4590, Q4001–Q4051
    body cast, adult, Q4001–Q4002
    cast supplies, (e.g. plaster), A4580
    cast supplies, unlisted types, Q4050

◄ **New** ⟳ **Revised** ✔ **Reinstated** ~~deleted~~ **Deleted**

Cast (Continued)
    supplies (Continued)
        finger splint, static, Q4049
        gauntlet cast, adult, Q4013–Q4014
        gauntlet cast, pediatric, Q4015–Q4016
        hip spica, adult, Q4025–Q4026
        hip spica, pediatric, Q4027–Q4028
        long arm cast, adult, Q4005–Q4006
        long arm cast, pediatric, Q4007–Q4008
        long arm splint, adult, Q4017–Q4018
        long arm splint, pediatric, Q4019–Q4020
        long leg cast, adult, Q4029–Q4030
        long leg cast, pediatric, Q4031–Q4032
        long leg cylinder cast, adult, Q4033–Q4034
        long leg cylinder cast, pediatric, Q4035–Q4036
        long leg splint, adult, Q4041–Q4042
        long leg splint, pediatric, Q4043–Q4044
        short arm cast, adult, Q4009–Q4010
        short arm cast, pediatric, Q4011–Q4012
        short arm splint, adult, Q4021–Q4022
        short arm splint, pediatric, Q4023–Q4024
        short leg cast, adult, Q4037–Q4038
        short leg cast, pediatric, Q4039–Q4040
        short leg splint, adult, Q4045–Q4046
        short leg splint, pediatric, Q4047–Q4048
        shoulder cast, adult, Q4003–Q4004
        special casting material (fiberglass), A4590
        splint supplies, miscellaneous, Q4051
    thermoplastic, L2106, L2126
Caster
    front, for power wheelchair, K0099
    wheelchair, E0997, E0998
Catheter, A4300–A4355
    anchoring device, A4333, A4334, A5200
    cap, disposable (dialysis), A4860
    external collection device, A4327–A4330,
        A4347–A7048
    female external, A4327–A4328
    indwelling, A4338–A4346
    insertion tray, A4354
    insulin infusion catheter, A4224
    intermittent with insertion supplies, A4353
    irrigation supplies, A4355
    male external, A4324, A4325, *A4326*, A4348
    oropharyngeal suction, A4628
    starter set, A4329
    trachea (suction), A4609, A4610, A4624
    transluminal angioplasty, C2623
    transtracheal oxygen, A4608
    vascular, A4300–A4301
Catheterization, specimen collection, P9612, P9615
CBC, G0306, G0307
Cefazolin sodium, J0690
Cefepime HCl, J0692
Cefotaxime sodium, J0698
Ceftaroline fosamil, J0712
Ceftazidime, J0713, J0714
Ceftizoxime sodium, J0715

Ceftolozane 50 mg and tazobactam 25 mg, J0695
Ceftriaxone sodium, J0696
Cefuroxime sodium, J0697
CellCept, K0412
Cellular therapy, M0075
Cement, ostomy, A4364
Centrifuge, A4650
Centruroides Immune F(ab), J0716
Cephalin Floculation, blood, P2028
Cephalothin sodium, J1890
Cephapirin sodium, J0710
Certification, physician, home, health (per calendar
        month), G0179–G0182
    Physician certification, home health, G0180
    Physician recertification, home health, G0179
    Physician supervision, home health, complex care,
        30 min or more, G0181
    Physician supervision, hospice 30 min or
        more, G0182
Certolizumab pegol, J0717
Cerumen, removal, G0268
Cervical
    cancer, screening, G0101
    cytopathology, G0123, G0124, G0141–G0148
        screening, automated thin layer, manual
        rescreening, physician supervision, G0145
        screening, automated thin layer preparation,
        cytotechnologist, physician interpretation, G0143
        screening, automated thin layer preparation,
        physician supervision, G0144
        screening, by cytotechnologist, physician
        supervision, G0123
        screening, cytopathology smears, automated
        system, physician interpretation, G0141
        screening, interpretation by physician, G0124
        screening smears, automated system, manual
        rescreening, G0148
        screening smears, automated system, physician
        supervision, G0147
    halo, L0810–L0830
    head harness/halter, E0942
    orthosis, L0100–L0200
        cervical collar molded to patient, L0170
        cervical, flexible collar, L0120–L0130
        cervical, multiple post collar, supports,
        L0180–L0200
        cervical, semi-rigid collar, L0150–L0160, L0172, L0174
        cranial cervical, L0112–L0113
    traction, E0855, E0856
Cervical cap contraceptive, A4261
Cervical-thoracic-lumbar-sacral orthosis (CTLSO),
    L0700, L0710
Cetuximab, J9055
Chair
    adjustable, dialysis, E1570
    lift, E0627
    rollabout, E1031
    sitz bath, E0160–E0162

◀ New   ⟳ Revised   ✔ Reinstated   deleted Deleted

Chair *(Continued)*
  transport, E1035–E1039
    chair, adult size, heavy duty, greater than 300 pounds, E1039
    chair, adult size, up to 300 pounds, E1038
    chair, pediatric, E1037
    multi-positional patient transfer system, extra-wide, greater than 300 pounds, E1036
    multi-positional patient transfer system, up to 300 pounds, E1035
Chelation therapy, M0300
Chemical endarterectomy, M0300
Chemistry and toxicology tests, P2028–P3001
Chemotherapy
  administration (hospital reporting only), Q0083–Q0085
  drug, oral, not otherwise classified, J8999
  drugs; (see also drug by name), J9000–J9999
Chest shell (cuirass), E0457
Chest Wall Oscillation System, E0483
  hose, replacement, A7026
  vest, replacement, A7025
Chest wrap, E0459
Chin cup, cervical, L0150
Chloramphenicol sodium succinate, J0720
Chlordiazepoxide HCl, J1990
Chloromycetin sodium succinate, J0720
Chloroprocaine HCl, J2400
Chloroquine HCl, J0390
Chlorothiazide sodium, J1205
Chlorpromazine HCl, J3230
  Chlorpromazine HCL, 5 mg, oral, Q0161
Chorionic gonadotropin, J0725
Choroid, lesion, destruction, *G0186*
Chromic phosphate P32 suspension, A9564
Chromium CR-51 sodium chromate, A9553
Cidofovir, J0740
Cilastatin sodium, imipenem, J0743
Cinacalcet, J0604 ◄
Ciprofloxacin
  for intravenous infusion, J0744
  octic suspension, J7342
Cisplatin, J9060
Cladribine, J9065
Clamp
  dialysis, A4918
  external urethral, A4356
Cleanser, wound, A6260
Cleansing agent, dialysis equipment, A4790
Clofarabine, J9027
Clonidine, J0735
Closure, wound, adhesive, tissue, *G0168*
Clotting time tube, A4771
Clubfoot wedge, L3380
Cochlear prosthetic implant, L8614
  accessories, L8615–L8617, *L8618*
  batteries, L8621–L8624

Cochlear prosthetic implant *(Continued)*
  replacement, L8619, L8627–L8629
    external controller component, L8628
    external speech processor and controller, integrated system, L8619
    external speech processor, component, L8627
    transmitting coil and cable, integrated, L8629
Codeine phosphate, J0745
Cold/Heat, application, E0200–E0239
  bilirubin light, E0202
  electric heat pad, moist, E0215
  electric heat pad, standard, E0210
  heat lamp with stand, E0205
  heat lamp, without stand, E0200
  hydrocollator unit, E0225
  hydrocollator unit, portable, E0239
  infrared heating pad system, E0221
  non-contact wound warming device, E0231
  paraffin bath unit, E0235
  pump for water circulating pad, E0236
  therapeutic lightbox, E0203
  warming card, non-contact wound warming device, E0232
  water circulating cold pad, with pump, E0218
  water circulating heat pad, with pump, E0217
Colistimethate sodium, J0770
Collagen
  meniscus implant procedure, G0428
  skin test, G0025
  urinary tract implant, L8603
  wound dressing, A6020–A6024
Collagenase, Clostridium histolyticum, J0775
Collar, cervical
  multiple post, L0180–L0200
  nonadjust (foam), L0120
Colorectal, screening, cancer, *G0104–G0106, G0120–G0122, G0328*
Coly-Mycin M, J0770
Comfort items, A9190
Commode, E0160–E0175
  chair, E0170–E0171
  lift, E0172, E0625
  pail, E0167
  seat, wheelchair, E0968
Complete, blood, count, *G0306, G0307*
Composite dressing, A6200–A6205
Compressed gas system, E0424–E0446
  oximeter device, E0445
  portable gaseous oxygen system, purchase, E0430
  portable gaseous oxygen system, rental, E0431
  portable liquid oxygen, rental, container/ supplies, E0434
  portable liquid oxygen, rental, home liquefier, E0433
  portable liquid oxygen system, purchase, container/ refill adapter, E0435
  portable oxygen contents, gaseous, 1 month, E0443
  portable oxygen contents, liquid, 1 month, E0444

Compressed gas system *(Continued)*
  stationary liquid oxygen system, purchase, use of reservoir, E0440
  stationary liquid oxygen system, rental, container/ supplies, E0439
  stationary oxygen contents, gaseous, 1 month, E0441
  stationary oxygen contents, liquid, 1 month, E0442
  stationary purchase, compressed gas system, E0425
  stationary rental, compressed gaseous oxygen system, E0424
  topical oxygen delivery system, NOS, E0446
Compression
  bandage, A4460
  burn garment, A6501–A6512
  stockings, A6530–A6549
Compressor, E0565, E0650–E0652, E0670–E0672
  aerosol, E0572, E0575
  air, E0565
  nebulizer, E0570–E0585
  pneumatic, E0650–E0676
Conductive gel/paste, *A4558*
Conductivity meter, bath, dialysis, E1550
Conference, team, *G0175, G9007, S0220, S0221*
  coordinate care fee, scheduled team conference, G9007
  medical conference /physician/interdisciplinary team, patient present, 30 min, S0220
  medical conference physician/interdisciplinary team, patient present, 60 min, S0221
  scheduled interdisciplinary team conference, patient present, G0175
Congo red, blood, P2029
Consultation, S0285, S0311, T1040, T1041
  Telehealth, G0425–G0427
Contact layer, A6206–A6208
Contact lens, V2500–V2599
Continent device, A5081, A5082, A5083
Continuous glucose monitoring system
  receiver, A9278, *S1037*
  sensor, A9276, *S1035*
  transmitter, A9277, *S1036*
Continuous passive motion exercise device, E0936
Continuous positive airway pressure device(CPAP), E0601
  compressor, K0269
Contraceptive
  cervical cap, A4261
  condoms, A4267, A4268
  diaphragm, A4266
  intratubal occlusion device, A4264
  intrauterine, copper, J7300
  intrauterine, levonorgestrel releasing, J7296–J7298, J7301 ⮌
  patch, J7304
  spermicide, A4269
  supply, A4267–A4269
  vaginal ring, J7303
Contracts, maintenance, ESRD, A4890

Contrast, *Q9951–Q9969*
  HOCM, Q9958–Q9964
  injection, iron based magnetic resonance, per ml, Q9953
  Injection, non-radioactive, non-contrast, visualization adjunct, Q9968
  injection, octafluoropropane microspheres, per ml, Q9956
  injection, perflexane lipid microspheres, per ml, Q9955
  injection, perflutren lipid microspheres, per ml, Q9957
  LOCM, Q9965–Q9967
  LOCM, 400 or greater mg/ml iodine, per ml, Q9951
  oral magnetic resonance contrast, Q9954
  Tc-99m per study dose, Q9969
Contrast material
  injection during MRI, A4643
  low osmolar, A4644–A4646
Coordinated, care, *G9001–G9011*
  CORF, registered nurse- face-face, G0128
Corneal tissue processing, V2785
Corset, spinal orthosis, L0970–L0976
  LSO, corset front, L0972
  LSO, full corset, L0976
  TLSO, corset front, L0970
  TLSO, full corset, L0974
Corticorelin ovine triflutate, J0795
Corticotropin, J0800
Corvert, (see Ibutilide fumarate)
Cosyntropin, J0833, J0834
Cough stimulating device, A7020, E0482
Counseling
  alcohol misuse, G0443
  cardiovascular disease, G0448
  obesity, G0447
  sexually transmitted infection, G0445
Count, blood, *G0306, G0307*
Counterpulsation, external, *G0166*
Cover, wound
  alginate dressing, A6196–A6198
  foam dressing, A6209–A6214
  hydrogel dressing, A6242–A6248
  non-contact wound warming cover, and accessory, A6000, E0231, E0232
  specialty absorptive dressing, A6251–A6256
CPAP (continuous positive airway pressure) device, E0601
  headgear, K0185
  humidifier, A7046
  intermittent assist, E0452
Cradle, bed, E0280
Crib, E0300
Cromolyn sodium, inhalation solution, unit dose, J7631, J7632
Crotalidae polyvalent immune fab, J0840
Crutches, E0110–E0118
  accessories, A4635–A4637, K0102
  crutch substitute, lower leg, E0118

◀ New   ⮌ Revised   ✔ Reinstated   ~~deleted~~ Deleted

Crutches *(Continued)*
   forearm, E0110–E0111
   underarm, E0112–E0117
Cryoprecipitate, each unit, P9012
CTLSO, L0700, L0710, L1000–L1120
   addition, axilla sling, L1010
   addition, cover for upright, each, L1120
   addition, kyphosis pad, L1020
   addition, kyphosis pad, floating, L1025
   addition, lumbar bolster pad, L1030
   addition, lumbar rib pad, L1040
   addition, lumbar sling, L1090
   addition, outrigger, L1080
   addition, outrigger bilateral, vertical
      extensions, L1085
   addition, ring flange, L1100
   addition, ring flange, molded to patient model, L1110
   addition, sternal pad, L1050
   addition, thoracic pad, L1060
   addition, trapezius sling, L1070
   anterior-posterior-lateral control, molded to patient
      model (CTLSO), L0710
   cervical, thoracic, lumbar, sacral orthrosis
      (CTLSO), L0700
   furnishing initial orthrosis, L1000
   immobilizer, infant size, L1001
   tension based scoliosis orthosis, fitting, L1005
Cuirass, E0457
Culture sensitivity study, P7001
Cushion, wheelchair, E0977
Cyanocobalamin Cobalt C057, A9559
Cycler dialysis machine, E1594
Cyclophosphamide, J9070
   oral, J8530
Cyclosporine, J7502, J7515, J7516
Cytarabine, J9100
   liposome, J9098
Cytomegalovirus immune globulin
   (human), J0850
***Cytopathology, cervical or vaginal,** G0123, G0124,*
   G0141–G0148

D

Dacarbazine, J9130
Daclizumab, J7513
Dactinomycin, J9120
Dalalone, J1100
Dalbavancin, 5mg, J0875
Dalteparin sodium, J1645
Daptomycin, J0878
Daratumumab, J9145
Darbepoetin Alfa, J0881–J0882
Daunorubicin
   Citrate, J9151
   HCl, J9150
DaunoXome, (see Daunorubicin citrate)

Decitabine, J0894
Decubitus care equipment, E0180–E0199
   air fluidized bed, E0194
   air pressure mattress, E0186
   air pressure pad, standard mattress, E0197
   dry pressure mattress, E0184
   dry pressure pad, standard mattress, E0199
   gel or gel-like pressure pad mattress,
      standard, E0185
   gel pressure mattress, E0196
   heel or elbow protector, E0191
   positioning cushion, E0190
   power pressure reducing mattress overlay, with
      pump, E0181
   powered air flotation bed, E0193
   pump, alternating pressure pad,
      replacement, E0182
   synthetic sheepskin pad, E0189
   water pressure mattress, E0187
   water pressure pad, standard mattress, E0198
Deferoxamine mesylate, J0895
Defibrillator, external, E0617, K0606
   battery, K0607
   electrode, K0609
   garment, K0608
Degarelix, J9155
Deionizer, water purification system, E1615
Delivery/set-up/dispensing, A9901
Denileukin diftitox, J9160
Denosumab, J0897
***Density, bone, study,** G0130*
Depo-estradiol cypionate, J1000
***Dermal filler injection,** G0429*
Desmopressin acetate, J2597
***Destruction, lesion, choroid,** G0186*
Detector, blood leak, dialysis, E1560
***Developmental testing,** G0451*
***Devices, other orthopedic,** E1800–E1841*
   assistive listening device, V5267–V5290
Dexamethasone
   acetate, J1094
   inhalation solution, concentrated, J7637
   inhalation solution, unit dose, J7638
   intravitreal implant, J7312
   oral, J8540
   sodium phosphate, J1100
Dextran, J7100
Dextrose
   saline (normal), J7042
   water, J7060, J7070
Dextrose, 5% in lactated ringers infusion, J7121
Dextrostick, A4772
Diabetes
   evaluation, G0245, G0246
   shoes (fitting/modifications), A5500–A5508
      deluxe feature, depth-inlay shoe, A5508
      depth inlay shoe, A5500
      molded from cast patient's foot, A5501

◀ **New**   ⭯ **Revised**   ✔ **Reinstated**   ~~deleted~~ **Deleted**

Diabetes *(Continued)*
  shoes (fitting/modifications) (Continued)
    shoe with metatarsal bar, A5505
    shoe with off-set heel(s), A5506
    shoe with rocker or rigid-bottom rocker, A5503
    shoe with wedge(s), A5504
    specified modification NOS, depth-inlay shoe, A5507
  training, outpatient, G0108, G0109

Diagnostic
  florbetaben, Q9983
  flutemetamol F18, Q9982
  mammography, digital image, G9899, G9900
  radiology services, R0070–R0076

Dialysate
  concentrate additives, A4765
  solution, *A4720–A4728*
  testing solution, A4760

Dialysis
  air bubble detector, E1530
  bath conductivity, meter, E1550
  chemicals/antiseptics solution, A4674
  disposable cycler set, A4671
  emergency, G0257
  equipment, E1510–E1702
  extension line, A4672–A4673
  filter, A4680
  fluid barrier, E1575
  home, S9335, S9339
  kit, A4820
  pressure alarm, E1540
  shunt, A4740
  supplies, A4650–A4927
  tourniquet, A4929
  unipuncture control system, E1580
  unscheduled, G0257
  venous pressure clamp, A4918

Dialyzer, A4690

Diaper, T1500, T4521–T4540, T4543, T4544
  adult incontinence garment, A4520, A4553
  incontinence supply, rectal insert, any type,
    each, A4337

Diazepam, J3360
Diazoxide, J1730
Diclofenac, J1130
Dicyclomine HCl, J0500
Diethylstilbestrol diphosphate, J9165
Digoxin, J1160
Digoxin immune fab (ovine), J1162
Dihydroergotamine mesylate, J1110
Dimenhydrinate, J1240
Dimercaprol, J0470
Dimethyl sulfoxide (DMSO), J1212
Diphenhydramine HCl, J1200
Dipyridamole, J1245

Disarticulation
  lower extremities, prosthesis, L5000–L5999
    above knee, L5200–L5230
    additions exoskeletal-knee-shin system, L5710–L5782

Disarticulation *(Continued)*
  lower extremities, prosthesis *(Continued)*
    additions to lower extremities, L5610–L5617
    additions to socket insert, L5654–L5699
    additions to socket variations, L5630–L5653
    additions to test sockets, L5618–L5629
    additions/replacements, feet-ankle units,
    L5700–L5707
    ankle, L5050–L5060
    below knee, L5100–L5105
    component modification, L5785–L5795
    endoskeletal, L5810–L5999
    endoskeletal, above knee, L5321
    endoskeletal, hip disarticulation, L5331–L5341
    endoskeleton, below knee, L5301–L5312
    hemipelvectomy, L5280
    hip disarticulation, L5250–L5270
    immediate postsurgical fitting, L5400–L5460
    initial prosthesis, L5500–L5505
    knee disarticulation, L5150–L5160
    partial foot, L5000–L5020
    preparatory prosthesis, L5510–L5600
  upper extremities, prosthesis, L6000–L6692
    above elbow, L6250
    additions to upper limb, L6600–L6698
    below elbow, L6100–L6130
    elbow disarticulation, L6200–L6205
    endoskeletal, below elbow, L6400
    endoskeletal, interscapular thoracic, L6570–L6590
    endoskeletal, shoulder disarticulation, L6550
    immediate postsurgical procedures, L6380–L6388
    interscapular/thoracic, L6350–L6370
    partial hand, L6000–L6026
    shoulder disarticulation, L6300–L6320
    wrist disarticulation, L6050–L6055

Disease
  status, oncology, G9063–G9139

Dispensing, fee, pharmacy, G0333,
  Q0510–Q0514, S9430
  dispensing fee inhalation drug(s), 30 days, Q0513
  dispensing fee inhalation drug(s), 90 days, Q0514
  inhalation drugs, 30 days, as a beneficiary, G0333
  initial immunosuppressive drug(s), post
    transplanr, G0510
  oral anti-cancer, oral anti-emetic,
    immunosuppressive, first prescription, Q0511
  oral anti-cancer, oral anti-emetic,
    immunosuppressive, subsequent
    preparation, Q0512

Disposable supplies, ambulance, A0382, A0384,
  A0392–A0398

DME
  miscellaneous, A9900–A9999
    DME delivery, set up, A9901
    DME supple, NOS, A9999
    DME supplies, A9900

DMSO, J1212
Dobutamine HCl, J1250

◀ **New**   ⟳ **Revised**   ✔ **Reinstated**   ~~deleted~~ **Deleted**

Docetaxel, J9171

Documentation

   antidepressant, G8126–G8128

   blood pressure, G8476–G8478

   bypass, graft, coronary, artery, documentation,
     G8160–G8163

   CABG, G8160–G8163

   dysphagia, G8232

   dysphagia, screening, G8232, V5364

   ECG, 12–lead, G8705, G8706

   eye, functions, G8315–G8333

   influenza, immunization, G8482–G8484

   pharmacologic therapy for osteoporosis, G8635

   physician for DME, G0454

   prophylactic antibiotic, G8702, G8703

   prophylactic parenteral antibiotic, G8629–G8632

   prophylaxis, DVT, G8218

   prophylaxis, thrombosis, deep, vein, G8218

   urinary, incontinence, G8063, G8267

Dolasetron mesylate, J1260

Dome and mouthpiece (for nebulizer), A7016

Dopamine HCl, J1265

Doripenem, J1267

**Dornase alpha, inhalation solution, unit dose
form,** J7639

Doxercalciferol, J1270

Doxil, J9001

Doxorubicin HCl, J9000, J9002

Drainage

   bag, A4357, A4358

   board, postural, E0606

   bottle, A5102

Dressing; (see also Bandage), A6020–A6406

   alginate, A6196–A6199

   collagen, A6020–A6024

   composite, A6200–A6205

   contact layer, A6206–A6208

   foam, A6209–A6215

   gauze, A6216–A6230, A6402–A6406

   holder/binder, A4462

   hydrocolloid, A6234–A6241

   hydrogel, A6242–A6248

   specialty absorptive, A6251–A6256

   transparent film, A6257–A6259

   tubular, A6457

   wound, K0744–K0746

Droperidol, J1790

   and fentanyl citrate, J1810

Dropper, A4649

Drugs; (see also Table of Drugs)

   administered through a metered dose inhaler, J3535

   antiemetic, J8498, J8597, Q0163–Q0181

   chemotherapy, J8500–J9999

   disposable delivery system, 50 ml or greater per
     hour, A4305

   disposable delivery system, 5 ml or less per
     hour, A4306

   immunosuppressive, J7500–J7599

Drugs *(Continued)*

   infusion supplies, A4221, A4222, A4230–A4232

   inhalation solutions, J7608–J7699

   non-prescription, A9150

   not otherwise classified, J3490, J7599, J7699, J7799,
     J7999, J8499, J8999, J9999

   oral, NOS, J8499

   prescription, oral, J8499, J8999

Dry pressure pad/mattress, E0179, **E0184,** E0199

Durable medical equipment (DME), E0100–E1830,
   K Codes

   additional oxygen related equipment, E1352–E1406

   arm support, wheelchair, E2626–E2633

   artificial kidney machines/accessories, E1500–E1699

   attachments, E0156–E0159

   bath and toilet aides, E0240–E0249

   canes, E0100–E0105

   commodes, E0160–E0175

   crutches, E0110–E0118

   decubitus care equipment, E0181–E0199

   DME, respiratory, inexpensive, purchased,
     A7000–A7509

   gait trainer, E8000–E8002

   heat/cold application, E0200–E0239

   hospital beds and accessories, E0250–E0373

   humidifiers/nebulizers/compressors, oxygen IPPB,
     E0550–E0585

   infusion supplies, E0776–E0791

   IPPB machines, E0500

   jaw motion rehabilitation system, E1700–E1702

   miscellaneous, E1902–E2120

   monitoring equipment, home glucose, E0607

   negative pressure, E2402

   other orthopedic devices, E1800–E1841

   oxygen/respiratory equipment, E0424–E0487

   pacemaker monitor, E0610–E0620

   patient lifts, E0621–E0642

   pneumatic compressor, E0650–E0676

   rollout chair/transfer system, E1031–E1039

   safety equipment, E0700–E0705

   speech device, E2500–E2599

   suction pump/room vaporizers, E0600–E0606

   temporary DME codes, regional carriers,
     K0000–K9999

   TENS/stimulation device(s), E0720–E0770

   traction equipment, E0830–E0900

   trapeze equipment, fracture frame, E0910–E0948

   walkers, E0130–E0155

   wheelchair accessories, E2201–E2397

   wheelchair, accessories, E0950–E1030

   wheelchair, amputee, E1170–E1200

   wheelchair cusion/protection, E2601–E2621

   wheelchair, fully reclining, E1050–E1093

   wheelchair, heavy duty, E1280–E1298

   wheelchair, lightweight, E1240–E1270

   wheelchair, semi-reclining, E1100–E1110

   wheelchair, skin protection, E2622–E2625

   wheelchair, special size, E1220–E1239

◄ New   ⊃ Revised   ✔ Reinstated   ~~deleted~~ Deleted

Durable medical equipment *(Continued)*
wheelchair, standard, E1130–E1161
whirlpool equipment, E1300–E1310
Duraclon, (see Clonidine)
Dyphylline, J1180
Dysphagia, screening, documentation, G8232, V5364
Dystrophic, nails, trimming, G0127

E

Ear mold, V5264, *V5265*
Ecallantide, J1290
Echocardiography injectable contrast material, A9700
ECG, 12–lead, G8704
Eculizumab, J1300
ED, visit, G0380–G0384
Edetate
calcium disodium, J0600
disodium, J3520
Educational Services
chronic kidney disease, G0420, G0421
Eggcrate dry pressure pad/mattress, E0184, E0199
EKG, G0403–G0405
Elbow
disarticulation, endoskeletal, L6450
orthosis (EO), E1800, L3700–L3740, L3760, L3761 ↻
dynamic adjustable elbow flexion device, E1800
elbow arthrosis, L3702–L3766
protector, E0191
Electric hand, L7007–L7008
Electric, nerve, stimulator, transcutaneous, A4595, E0720–E0749
conductive garment, E0731
electric joint stimulation device, E0762
electrical stimulator supplies, A4595
electromagnetic wound treatment device, E0769
electronic salivary reflex stimulator, E0755
EMG, biofeedback device, E0746
functional electrical stimulator, nerve and/or muscle groups, E0770
functional stimulator sequential muscle groups, E0764
incontinence treatment system, E0740
nerve stimulator (FDA), treatment nausea and vomiting, E0765
osteogenesis stimulator, electrical, surgically implanted, E0749
osteogenesis stimulator, low-intensity ultrasound, E0760
osteogenesis stimulator, non-invasive, not spinal, E0747
osteogenesis stimulator, non-invasive, spinal, E0748
radiowaves, non-thermal, high frequency, E0761
stimulator, electrical shock unit, E0745
stimulator for scoliosis, E0744
TENS, four or more leads, E0730
TENS, two lead, E0720

Electrical stimulation device used for cancer treatment, E0766
Electrical work, dialysis equipment, A4870
Electrodes, per pair, A4555, A4556
Electromagnetic, therapy, G0295, G0329
Electronic medication compliance, T1505
Elevating leg rest, K0195
Elliotts b solution, J9175
Elotuzumab, J9176
Emergency department, visit, G0380–G0384
EMG, E0746
Eminase, J0350
Endarterectomy, chemical, M0300
Endoscope sheath, A4270
Endoskeletal system, addition, L5848, L5856–L5857, L5925, *L5961*, L5969
Enema, bag, A4458
Enfuvirtide, J1324
Enoxaparin sodium, J1650
Enteral
feeding supply kit (syringe) (pump) (gravity), B4034–B4036
formulae, B4149–B4156, *B4157–B4162*
nutrition infusion pump (with alarm) (without), B9000, **B9002**
therapy, supplies, B4000–B9999
enteral and parenteral pumps, B9002–B9999
enteral formula/medical supplies, B0434–B4162
parenteral solutions/supplies, B4164–B5200
Epinephrine, J0171
Epirubicin HCl, J9178
Epoetin alpha, J0885, Q4081
Epoetin beta, J0887–J0888
Epoprostenol, J1325
Equipment
decubitus, E0181–E0199
exercise, A9300, E0935, E0936
orthopedic, E0910–E0948, E1800–E8002
oxygen, E0424–E0486, E1353–E1406
pump, E0781, E0784, E0791
respiratory, E0424–E0601
safety, E0700, E0705
traction, E0830–E0900
transfer, E0705
trapeze, E0910–E0912, E0940
whirlpool, E1300, E1310
Erection device, tension ring, L7902
Ergonovine maleate, J1330
Eribulin mesylate, J9179
Ertapenem sodium, J1335
Erythromycin lactobionate, J1364
ESRD (End-Stage Renal Disease); (see also Dialysis)
machines and accessories, E1500–E1699
adjustable chair, ESRD, E1570
centrifuge, dialysis, E1500
dialysis equipment, NOS, E1699
hemodialysis, air bubble detector, replacement, E1530
hemodialysis, bath conductivity meter, E1550

◀ **New**   ↻ **Revised**   ✔ **Reinstated**   ~~deleted~~ **Deleted**

ESRD *Continued*

  hemodialysis, blood leak detector, replacement, E1560
  hemodialysis, blood pump, replacement, E1620
  hemodialysis equipment, delivery/instillation charges, E1600
  hemodialysis, heparin infusion pump, E1520
  hemodialysis machine, E1590
  hemodialysis, portable travel hemodialyzer system, E1635
  hemodialysis, pressure alarm, E1540
  hemodialysis, reverse osmosis water system, E1615
  hemodialysis, sorbent cartridges, E1636
  hemodialysis, transducer protectors, E1575
  hemodialysis, unipuncture control system, E1580
  hemodialysis, water softening system, E1625
  hemostats, E1637
  peritoneal dialysis, automatic intermittent system, E1592
  peritoneal dialysis clamps, E1634
  peritoneal dialysis, cycler dialysis machine, E1594
  peritoneal dialysis, reciprocating system, E1630
  scale, E1639
  wearable artificial kidney, E1632
 plumbing, A4870
 supplies, A4651–A4929
  acetate concentrate solution, hemodialysis, A4708
  acid concentrate solution, hemodialysis, A4709
  activated carbon filters, hemodialysis, A4680
  ammonia test strip, dialysis, A4774
  automatic blood pressure monitor, A4670
  bicarbonate concentrate, powder, hemodialysis, A4707
  bicarbonate concentrate, solution, A4706
  blood collection tube, vaccum, dialysis, A4770
  blood glucose test strip, dialysis, A4772
  blood pressure cuff only, A4663
  blood tubing, arterial and venous, hemodialysis, A4755
  blood tubing, arterial or venous, hemodialysis, A4750
  chemicals/antiseptics solution, clean dialysis equipment, A4674
  dialysate solution, non-dextrose, A4728
  dialysate solution, peritoneal dialysis, A4720–A4726, A4760–A4766
  dialyzers, hemodialysis, A4690
  disposable catheter tips, peritoneal dialysis, A4860
  disposable cycler set, dialysis machine, A4671
  drainage extension line, dialysis, sterile, A4672
  extension line easy lock connectors, dialysis, A4673
  fistula cannulation set, hemodialysis, A4730
  injectable anesthetic, dialysis, A4737
  occult blood test strips, dialysis, A4773
  peritoneal dialysis, catheter anchoring device, A4653

ESRD *(Continued)*

 supplies *(Continued)*
  protamine sulfate, hemodialysis, A4802
  serum clotting timetube, dialysis, A4771
  shunt accessory, hemodialysis, A4740
  sphygmomanometer, cuff and stethoscope, A4660
  syringes, A4657
  topical anesthetic, dialysis, A4736
  treated water, peritoneal dialysis, A4714
  "Y set" tubing, peritoneal dialysis, A4719

Estrogen conjugated, J1410

Estrone (5, Aqueous), J1435

Etelcalcetide, J0606 ◀

Eteplirsen, J1428 ◀

Ethanolamine oleate, J1430

Etidronate disodium, J1436

Etonogestrel implant system, J7307

Etoposide, J9181
 oral, J8560

Euflexxa, J7323

Evaluation
 conformity, V5020
 contact lens, S0592
 diabetic, G0245, G0246
 footwear, G8410–G8416
 hearing, S0618, V5008, V5010
 hospice, G0337
 multidisciplinary, H2000
 nursing, T1001
 ocularist, S9150
 performance measurement, S3005
 resident, T2011
 speech, S9152
 team, T1024

Everolimus, J7527

Examination
 gynecological, S0610–S0613
 ophthalmological, S0620, S0621
 pinworm, Q0113

Exercise
 class, S9451
 equipment, A9300

External
 ambulatory infusion pump, E0781, E0784
 ambulatory insulin delivery system, A9274
 power, battery components, L7360–L7368
 power, elbow, L7160–L7191
 urinary supplies, A4356–A4359

Extremity
 belt/harness, E0945
 traction, E0870–E0880

Eye
 case, V2756
 functions, documentation, G8315–G8333
 lens (contact) (spectacle), V2100–V2615
 pad, patch, A6410–A6412
 prosthetic, V2623, V2629
 service (miscellaneous), V2700–V2799

◀ New   ⊃ Revised   ✔ Reinstated   ~~deleted~~ Deleted

F

Face tent, oxygen, A4619
Faceplate, ostomy, A4361
Factor IX, J7193, J7194, J7195, J7200–J7202
Factor VIIA coagulation factor, recombinant, J7189, J7205
Factor VIII, anti-hemophilic factor, J7182, J7185, J7190–J7192, J7207, J7209
Factor X, J7175 ↻
Factor XIII, anti-hemophilic factor, J7180, J7188
Factor XIII, A-subunit, J7181
Family Planning Education, H1010
Fee
  coordinated care, G9001–G9011
  dispensing, pharmacy, G0333, Q0510–Q0514, S9430
Fentanyl citrate, J3010
  and droperidol, J1810
Fern test, Q0114
Ferumoxytol, Q0138, Q0139
Filgrastim (G-CSF & TBO), J1442, J1447, Q5101
Filler, wound
  alginate dressing, A6199
  foam dressing, A6215
  hydrocolloid dressing, A6240, A6241
  hydrogel dressing, A6248
  not elsewhere classified, A6261, A6262
Film, transparent (for dressing), A6257–A6259
Filter
  aerosol compressor, A7014
  dialysis carbon, A4680
  ostomy, A4368
  tracheostoma, A4481
  ultrasonic generator, A7014
Fistula cannulation set, A4730
Flebogamma, J1572
Florbetapir F18, A9586
Flowmeter, E0440, E0555, E0580
Floxuridine, J9200
Fluconazole, injection, J1450
Fludarabine phosphate, J8562, J9185
Fluid barrier, dialysis, E1575
Flunisolide inhalation solution, J7641
Fluocinolone, J7311, J7313
Fluorodeoxyglucose F-18 FDG, A9552
Fluorouracil, J9190
Fluphenazine decanoate, J2680
Foam
  dressing, A6209–A6215
  pad adhesive, A5126
Folding walker, E0135, E0143
Foley catheter, A4312–A4316, A4338–A4346
  indwelling catheter, specialty type, A4340
  indwelling catheter, three-way, continuous irrigation, A4346
  indwelling catheter, two-way, all silicone, A4344

Foley catheter *(Continued)*
  indwelling catheter, two-way latex, A4338
  insertion tray with drainage bag, A4312
  insertion tray with drainage bag, three-way, continuous irrigation, A4316
  insertion tray with drainage bag, two-way latex, A4314
  insertion tray with drainage bag, two-way, silicone, A4315
  insertion tray without drainage bag, A4313
Fomepizole, J1451
Fomivirsen sodium intraocular, J1452
Fondaparinux sodium, J1652
Foot care, G0247
Footdrop splint, L4398
Footplate, E0175, E0970, L3031
Footwear, orthopedic, L3201–L3265
  additional charge for split size, L3257
  Benesch boot, pair, child, L3213
  Benesch boot, pair, infant, L3212
  Benesch boot, pair, junior, L3214
  custom molded shoe, prosthetic shoe, L3250
  custom shoe, depth inlay, L3230
  ladies shoe, hightop, L3217
  ladies shoe, oxford, L3216
  ladies shoe, oxford/brace, L3224
  mens shoe, depth inlay, L3221
  mens shoe, hightop, L3222
  mens shoe, oxford, L3219
  mens shoe, oxford/brace, L3225
  molded shoe, custom fitted, Plastazote, L3253
  non-standard size or length, L3255
  non-standard size or width, L3254
  Plastazote sandal, L3265
  shoe, hightop, child, L3206
  shoe, hightop, infant, L3204
  shoe, hightop, junior, L3207
  shoe molded/patient model, Plastazote, L3252
  shoe, molded/patient model, silicone, L3251
  shoe, oxford, child, L3202
  shoe, oxford, infant, L3201
  shoe, oxford, junior, L3203
  surgical boot, child, L3209
  surgical boot, infant, L3208
  surgical boot, junior, L3211
  surgical boot/shoe, L3260
Forearm crutches, E0110, E0111
Formoterol, J7640
  fumarate, J7606
Fosaprepitant, J1453
Foscarnet sodium, J1455
Fosphenytoin, Q2009
Fracture
  bedpan, E0276
  frame, E0920, E0930, E0946–E0948
    attached to bed/weights, E0920
    attachments for complex cervical traction, E0948
    attachments for complex pelvic traction, E0947

◄ New   ↻ Revised   ✔ Reinstated   ~~deleted~~ Deleted

Fracture (*Continued*)
  frame (*Continued*)
    dual, cross bars, attached to bed, E0946
    free standing/weights, E0930
  orthosis, L2106–L2136, L3980–L3984
    ankle/foot orthosis, fracture, L2106–L2128
    KAFO, fracture orthosis, L2132–L2136
    upper extremity, fracture orthosis, L3980–L3984
  orthotic additions, L2180–L2192, L3995
    addition to upper extremity orthosis, sock,
    fracture, L3995
    additions lower extremity fracture, L2180–L2192
Fragmin, (see Dalteparin sodium), *J1645*
Frames (spectacles), V2020, V2025
  Deluxe frame, V2025
  Purchases, V2020
Fulvestrant, J9395
Furosemide, J1940

G

Gadobutrol, A9585
Gadofosveset trisodium, A9583
Gadoxetate disodium, A9581
Gait trainer, E8000–E8002
Gallium Ga67, A9556
Gallium nitrate, J1457
Galsulfase, J1458
Gamma globulin, J1460, J1560
  injection, gamma globulin (IM), 1cc, J1460
  injection, gamma globulin, (IM), over 10cc, J1560
Gammagard liquid, J1569
Gammaplex, J1557
Gamunex, J1561
Ganciclovir
  implant, J7310
  sodium, J1570
Garamycin, J1580
Gas system
  compressed, E0424, E0425
  gaseous, E0430, E0431, E0441, E0443
  liquid, E0434–E0440, E0442, E0444
Gastric freezing, hypothermia, *M0100*
Gatifloxacin, J1590
Gauze; (see also Bandage)
  impregnated, A6222–A6233, A6266
  non-impregnated, A6402–A6404
Gefitinib, J8565
Gel
  conductive, A4558
  pressure pad, E0185, E0196
Gemcitabine HCl, J9201
Gemtuzumab ozogamicin, J9203 ↻
Generator
  neurostimulator (implantable), high frequency, C1822
  ultrasonic with nebulizer, E0574–E0575 ↻

Gentamicin (Sulfate), J1580
Glasses
  air conduction, V5070
  binaural, V5120–V5150
    behind the ear, V5140
    body, V5120
    glasses, V5150
    in the ear, V5130
  bone conduction, V5080
  frames, V2020, V2025
  hearing aid, V5230
Glaucoma
  screening, G0117, G0118
Gloves, A4927
Glucagon HCl, J1610
Glucose
  monitor includes all supplies, K0553 ◀
  monitor with integrated lancing/blood sample
    collection, E2101
  monitor with integrated voice
    synthesizer, E2100
  receiver (monitor) dedicated, K0554 ◀
  test strips, A4253, A4772
Gluteal pad, L2650
Glycopyrrolate, inhalation solution,
  concentrated, J7642
Glycopyrrolate, inhalation solution, unit
  dose, J7643
Gold
  sodium thiomalate, J1600
Golimumab, J1602
Gomco drain bottle, A4912
Gonadorelin HCl, J1620
Goserelin acetate implant; (see also
  Implant), J9202
Grab bar, trapeze, E0910, E0940
Grade-aid, wheelchair, E0974
Gradient, compression stockings, *A6530–A6549*
  below knee, 18–30 mmHg, A6530
  below knee, 30–40 mmHg, A6531
  below knee, thigh length, 18–30 mmHg, A6533
  full length/chap style, 18–30 mmHg, A6536
  full length/chap style, 30–40 mmHg, A6537
  full length/chap style, 40–50 mmHg, A6538
  garter belt, A6544
  non-elastic below knee, 30–50 mmhg, A6545
  sleeve, NOS, A6549
  thigh length, 30–40 mmHg, A6534
  thigh length, 40–50 mmHg, A6535
  waist length, 18–30 mmHg, A6539
  waist length, 30–40 mmHg, A6540
  waist length, 40–50 mmHg, A6541
Granisetron HCl, J1626
  XR, J1627 ◀
Gravity traction device, E0941
Gravlee jet washer, A4470
Guidelines, practice, oncology, *G9056–G9062*

◀ New   ↻ Revised   ✔ Reinstated   ~~deleted~~ Deleted

H

Hair analysis (excluding arsenic), P2031
Halaven, Injection, eribulin mesylate, 0.1 mg, J9179
Hallus-Valgus dynamic splint, L3100
Hallux prosthetic implant, L8642
Halo procedures, L0810–L0860
  addition HALO procedure, MRI compatible
    systems, L0859
  addition HALO procedure, replacement liner, L0861
  cervical halo/jacket vest, L0810
  cervical halo/Milwaukee type orthosis, L0830
  cervical halo/plaster body jacket, L0820
Haloperidol, J1630
  decanoate, J1631
Halter, cervical head, E0942
Hand finger orthosis, prefabricated, L3923
Hand restoration, L6900–L6915
  orthosis (WHFO), E1805, E1825, L3800–L3805,
    L3900–L3954
  partial prosthesis, L6000–L6020
  partial hand, little and/or ring finger
    remaining, L6010
  partial hand, no finger, L6020
  partial hand, thumb remaining, L6000
  transcarpal/metacarpal or partial hand
    disarticulation prosthesis, L6025
  rims, wheelchair, E0967
Handgrip (cane, crutch, walker), A4636
Harness, E0942, E0944, E0945
Headgear (for positive airway pressure device), K0185
Hearing
  aid, V5030–V5267, V5298
    aid-body worn, V5100
    assistive listening device, V5268–V5274,
    V5281–V5290
    battery, use in hearing device, V5266
    dispensing fee, binaural, V5160
    dispensing fee, monaural hearing aid, any
    type, V5241
    dispensing fee, unspecified hearing aid, V5090
    ear impression, each, V5275
    ear mold/insert, disposable, any type, V5265
    ear mold/insert, not disposable, V5264
    glasses, air conduction, V5070
    glasses, bone conduction, V5080
    hearing aid, analog, binaural, CIC, V5248
    hearing aid, analog, binaural, ITC, V5249
    hearing aid, analog, monaural, CIC, V5242
    hearing aid, analog, monaural, ITC, V5243
    hearing aid, BICROS, V5210–V5240
    hearing aid, binaural, V5120–V5150
    hearing aid, CROS, V5170–V5200
    hearing aid, digital, V5254–V5261
    hearing aid, digitally programmable, V5244–V5247,
    V5250–V5253

Hearing *(Continued)*
  aid (Continued)
    hearing aid, disposable, any type, binaural, V5263
    hearing aid, disposable, any type, monaural, V5262
    hearing aid, monaural, V5030–V5060
    hearing aid, NOC, V5298
    hearing aid or assistive listening device/supplies/
    accessories, NOS, V5267
    hearing service, miscellaneous, V5299
    semi-implantable, middle ear, V5095
  assessment, S0618, V5008, V5010
  devices, L8614, V5000–V5299
  services, V5000–V5999
Heat
  application, E0200–E0239
  infrared heating pad system, A4639, E0221
  lamp, E0200, E0205
  pad, A9273, E0210, E0215, E0237, E0249
Heater (nebulizer), E1372
Heavy duty, wheelchair, E1280–E1298, K0006,
  K0007, K0801–K0886
  detachable arms, elevating legrests, E1280
  detachable arms, swing away detachable
    footrest, E1290
  extra heavy duty wheelchair, K0007
  fixed full length arms, elevating legrest, E1295
  fixed full length arms, swing away detachable
    footrest, E1285
  heavy duty wheelchair, K0006
  power mobility device, not coded by DME PDAC or
    no criteria, K0900
  power operated vehicle, group 2, K0806–K0808
  power operated vehicle, NOC, K0812
  power wheelchair, group 1, K0813–K0816
  power wheelchair, group 2, K0820–K0843
  power wheelchair, group 3, K0848–K0864
  power wheelchair, group 4, K0868–K0886
  power wheelchair, group 5, pediatric, K0890–K0891
  power wheelchair, NOC, K0898
  power-operated vehicle, group 1, K0800–K0802
  special wheelchair seat depth and/or width, by
    construction, E1298
  special wheelchair seat depth, by upholstery, E1297
  special wheelchair seat height from floor, E1296
Heel
  elevator, air, E0370
  protector, E0191
  shoe, L3430–L3485
  stabilizer, L3170
Helicopter, ambulance; (see also Ambulance)
Helmet
  cervical, L0100, L0110
  head, A8000–A8004
Hemin, J1640
Hemipelvectomy prosthesis, L5280
Hemi-wheelchair, E1083–E1086
Hemodialysis machine, E1590

◀ **New**   ⊃ **Revised**   ✔ **Reinstated**   ~~deleted~~ **Deleted**

Hemodialysis, vessel mapping, *G0365*
Hemodialyzer, portable, E1635
Hemofil M, J7190
Hemophilia clotting factor, J7190–J7198
 anti-inhibitor, per IU, J7198
 anti-thrombin III, human, per IU, J7197
 Factor IX, complex, per IU, J7194
 Factor IX, purified, non-recombinant, per IU, J7193
 Factor IX, recombinant, J7195
 Factor VIII, human, per IU, J7190
 Factor VIII, porcine, per IU, J7191
 Factor VIII, recombinant, per IU, NOS, J7192
 injection, antithrombin recombinant, 50 i.u., J7196
 NOC, J7199
Hemostats, A4850, *E1637*
Hemostix, A4773
Hepagam B
 IM, J1571
 IV, J1573
Heparin
 infusion pump, dialysis, E1520
 lock flush, J1642
 sodium, J1644
Hepatitis B, vaccine, administration, *G0010*
Hep-Lock (U/P), J1642
Hexalite, A4590
High osmolar contrast material, Q9958–Q9964
 HOCM, 400 or greater mg/ml iodine, Q9964
 HOCM, 150–199 mg/ml iodine, Q9959
 HOCM, 200–249 mg/ml iodine, Q9960
 HOCM, 250–299 mg/ml iodine, Q9961
 HOCM, 300–349 mg/ml iodine, Q9962
 HOCM, 350–399 mg/ml iodine, Q9963
 HOCM, up to 149 mg/ml iodine, Q9958
Hip
 disarticulation prosthesis, L5250, L5270
 orthosis (HO), L1600–L1690
Hip-knee-ankle-foot orthosis (HKAFO),
 L2040–L2090
Histrelin
 acetate, J1675
 implant, J9225
HKAFO, L2040–L2090
Home
 certification, home health, G0180
 glucose, monitor, E0607, E2100, E2101,
  S1030, S1031
 health, aide, G0156, S9122, T1021
 health, aide, in home, per hour, S9122
 health, aide, per visit, T1021
 health, clinical, social worker, G0155
 health, hospice, each 15 min, G0156
 health, occupational, therapist, G0152
 health, physical therapist, G0151
 health, physician, certification, G0179–G0182
 health, respiratory therapy, S5180, S5181
 recerticication, home health, G0179
 supervision, home health, G0181

Home *(Continued)*
 supervision, hospice, G0182
 therapist, speech, S9128
Home Health Agency Services, T0221, *T1022*
 care improvement home visit assessment, G9187
Home sleep study test, *G0398–G0400*
HOPPS, *C1000–C9999*
Hospice care
 assisted living facility, Q5002
 hospice facility, Q5010
 inpatient hospice facility, Q5006
 inpatient hospital, Q5005
 inpatient psychiatric facility, Q5008
 long term care facility, Q5007
 nursing long-term facility, Q5003
 patient's home, Q5001
 skilled nursing facility, Q5004
Hospice, evaluation, pre-election, *G0337*
Hospice physician supervision, *G0182*
Hospital
 bed, E0250–E0304, E0328, E0329
 observation, G0378, G0379
 outpatient clinic visit, assessment , G0463
Hospital Outpatient Payment System, *C1000–C9999*
Hot water bottle, A9273
Human fibrinogen concentrate, J7178
Humidifier, A7046, E0550–E0563
 durable, diring IPPB treatment, E0560
 durable, extensive, IPPB, E0550
 durable glass bottle type, for regulator, E0555
 heated, used with positive airway pressure
  device, E0562
 non-heated, used with positive airway
  pressure, E0561
 water chamber, humidifier, replacement, positive
  airway device, A7046
Hyalgan, J7321
Hyalomatrix, *Q4117*
Hyaluronan, J7326, J7327
 gel-Syn, J7328
 genvisc, J7320
 hymovis, *J7322*
Hyaluronate, sodium, J7317
Hyaluronidase, J3470
 ovine, J3471–J3473
Hydralazine HCl, J0360
Hydraulic patient lift, E0630
Hydrocollator, E0225, E0239
Hydrocolloid dressing, A6234–A6241
Hydrocortisone
 acetate, J1700
 sodium phosphate, J1710
 sodium succinate, J1720
Hydrogel dressing, A6231–A6233, A6242–A6248
Hydromorphone, J1170
Hydroxyprogesterone caproate, J1725–J1726,
 J1729 ⊋
Hydroxyzine HCl, J3410

◄ New   ⊋ Revised   ✔ Reinstated   ~~deleted~~ Deleted

Hygienic item or device, disposable or non-disposable, any type, each, A9286
Hylan G-F 20, J7322
Hyoscyamine Sulfate, J1980
Hyperbaric oxygen chamber, topical, A4575
Hypertonic saline solution, J7130, *J7131*

I

Ibandronate sodium, J1740
Ibuprofen, J1741
Ibutilide Fumarate, J1742
Icatibant, J1744
Ice
  cap, E0230
  collar, E0230
Idarubicin HCl, J9211
Idursulfase, J1743
Ifosfamide, J9208
Iliac, artery, angiography, G0278
Iloprost, Q4074
Imaging, PET, G0219, G0235
  any site, NOS, G0235
  whole body, melanoma, non-covered indications, G0219
Imiglucerase, J1786
Immune globulin, J1575
  Bivigam, 500 mg, J1556
  Cuvitru, J1555 ◀
  Flebogamma, J1572
  Gammagard liquid, J1569
  Gammaplex, J1557
  Gamunex, J1561
  HepaGam B, J1571
  Hizentra, J1559
  Intravenous services, supplies and accessories, Q2052
  NOS, J1566
  Octagam, J1568
  Privigen, J1459
  Rho(D), J2788, J2790, *J2791*
  Rhophylac, J2791
  Subcutaneous, J1562
Immunosuppressive drug, not otherwise classified, J7599
Implant
  access system, A4301
  aqueous shunt, L8612
  breast, L8600
  buprenorphine implant, J0570
  cochlear, L8614, L8619
  collagen, urinary tract, L8603
  dextranomer/hyaluronic acid copolymer, L8604
  ganciclovir, J7310
  hallux, L8642
  infusion pump, programmable, E0783, E0786
    implantable, programmable, E0783
    implantable, programmable, replacement, E0786
  joint, L8630, L8641, L8658

Implant *(Continued)*
  joint *(Continued)*
    interphalangeal joint spacer, silicone or equal, L8658
    metacarpophalangeal joint implant, L8630
    metatarsal joint implant, L8641
  lacrimal duct, A4262, A4263
  metacarpophalangeal joint, L8630
  metatarsal joint, L8641
  neurostimulator pulse generator, L8679, L8681–L8688
  not otherwise specified, L8699
  ocular, L8610
  ossicular, L8613
  osteogenesis stimulator, E0749
  percutaneous access system, A4301
  replacement implantable intraspinal catheter, E0785
  synthetic, urinary, L8606
  urinary tract, L8603, L8606
  vascular graft, L8670
Implantable radiation dosimeter, A4650
Impregnated gauze dressing, A6222–A6230, *A6231–A6233*
Incobotulinumtoxin a, J0588
Incontinence
  appliances and supplies, A4310, A4331, A4332, A4360, A5071–A5075, *A5081–A5093,* A5102–A5114
  garment, A4520, T4521–T4543
    adult sized disposable incontinence product, T4522–T4528
    any type, e.g. brief, diaper, A4520
    pediatric sized disposable incontinence product, T4529–T4532
    youth sized disposable incontinence product, T4533–T4534
  supply, A4335, A4356–A4360
    bedside drainage bag, A4357
    disposable external urethral clamp/compression device, A4360
    external urethral clamp or compression device, A4356
    incontinence supply, miscellaneous, A4335
    urinary drainage bag, leg or abdomen, A4358
  treatment system, E0740
Indium IN-111
  carpromab pendetide, A9507
  ibritumomab tiuxetan, A9542
  labeled autologous platelets, A9571
  labeled autologous white blood cells, A9570
  oxyquinoline, A9547
  pentetate, A9548
  pentetreotide, A9572
  satumomab, A4642
Infliximab injection, J1745
Influenza
  afluria, Q2035
  agriflu, Q2034
  flulaval, Q2036
  fluvirin, Q2037
  fluzone, Q2038
  immunization, documentation, G8482–G8484

◀ **New** ↻ **Revised** ✔ **Reinstated** ~~deleted~~ **Deleted**

Influenza (*Continued*)
  not otherwise specified, Q2039
  vaccine, administration, G0008
  virus vaccine, Q2034–Q2039
Infusion
  pump, ambulatory, with administrative
    equipment, E0781
  pump, heparin, dialysis, E1520
  pump, implantable, E0782, E0783
  pump, implantable, refill kit, A4220
  pump, insulin, E0784
  pump, mechanical, reusable, E0779, E0780
  pump, uninterrupted infusion of
    Epiprostenol, K0455
  replacement battery, A4602
  saline, J7030–J7060
  supplies, A4219, A4221, A4222, A4225,
    A4230–A4232, E0776–E0791
  therapy, other than chemotherapeutic drugs, Q0081
Inhalation solution; (see also drug name),
    J7608–J7699, Q4074
Injection device, needle-free, A4210
Injections; (see also drug name), J0120–J7320,
    J7321–J7330, J9032, J9039, J9271, J9299,
    J9308, Q9950
  ado-trastuzumab emtansine, 1 mg, J9354
  aripiprazole, extended release, J0401
  arthrography, sacroiliac, joint, G0259, G0260
  carfilzomib, 1 mg, J9047
  certolizumab pegol, J0717
  dermal filler (LDS), G0429
  filgrastim, J1442
  interferon beta-1a, IM, Q3027
  interferon beta-1a, SC, Q3028
  omacetaxtine mepesuccinate, 0.01 mg, J9262
  pertuzumb, 1 mg, J9306
  sculptra, 0.5 mg, Q2028
  supplies for self-administered, A4211
  vincristine, 1 mg, J9371
  ziv-aflibercept, 1 mg, J9400
INR, monitoring, G0248–G0250
  demonstration prior to initiation, home INR, G0248
  physician review and interpretation, home INR, G0250
  provision of test materials, home INR, G0249
Insertion tray, A4310–A4316
Insulin, J1815, J1817, *S5550–S5571*
  ambulatory, external, system, A9274
  treatment, outpatient, G9147
Integra flowable wound matrix, Q4114
Interferon
  Alpha, J9212–J9215
  Beta-1a, J1826, Q3027, Q3028
  Beta-1b, J1830
  Gamma, J9216
Intermittent
  assist device with continuous positive airway
    pressure device, E0470–E0472
  limb compression device, E0676

Intermittent (*Continued*)
  peritoneal dialysis system, E1592
  positive pressure breathing machine
    (IPPB), E0500
Interphalangeal joint, prosthetic implant,
    L8658, L8659
Interscapular thoracic prosthesis
  endoskeletal, L6570
  upper limb, L6350–L6370
Intervention, alcohol/substance (not tobacco),
    G0396–G0397
Intervention, tobacco, G9016
Intraconazole, J1835
Intraocular
  lenses, V2630–V2632
Intrapulmonary percussive ventilation
    system, E0481
Intrauterine copper contraceptive, J7300
Inversion/eversion correction device, A9285
Iodine I-123
  iobenguane, A9582
  ioflupane, A9584
  sodium iodide, A9509, A9516
Iodine I-125
  serum albumin, A9532
  sodium iodide, A9527
  sodium iothalamate, A9554
Iodine I-131
  iodinated serum albumin, A9524
  sodium iodide capsule, A9517, A9528
  sodium iodide solution, A9529–A9531
Iodine Iobenguane sulfate I-131, A9508
Iodine swabs/wipes, A4247
IPD
  system, E1592
Ipilimumab, J9228
IPPB machine, E0500
Ipratropium bromide, inhalation solution, unit
    dose, J7644, J7645
Irinotecan, J9205, J9206
Iron
  Dextran, J1750
  sucrose, J1756
Irrigation solution for bladder calculi, Q2004
Irrigation supplies, A4320–A4322, A4355,
    A4397–A4400
  irrigation supply, sleeve, each, A4397
  irrigation syringe, bulb, or piston, each, A4320
  irrigation tubing set, bladder irrigation, A4355
  ostomy irrigation set, A4400
  ostomy irrigation supply, bag, A4398
  ostomy irrigation supply, cone/catheter, A4399
Irrigation/evacuation system, bowel
  control unit, E0350
  disposable supplies for, E0352
  manual pump enema, A4459
Isavuconazonium, J1833
Islet, transplant, G0341–G0343, S2102

◀ **New**   ↻ **Revised**   ✔ **Reinstated**   ~~deleted~~ **Deleted**

Isoetharine HCl, inhalation solution
concentrated, J7647, J7648
unit dose, J7649, J7650
Isolates, B4150, B4152
Isoproterenol HCl, inhalation solution
concentrated, J7657, J7658
unit dose, J7659, J7660
Isosulfan blue, Q9968
Item, non-covered, A9270
IUD, *J7300, S4989*
IV pole, each, E0776, K0105
Ixabepilone, J9207

J

Jacket
scoliosis, L1300, L1310
Jaw, motion, rehabilitation system, E1700–E1702
Jenamicin, J1580
Jetria, (ocriplasmin), J7316

K

Kadcyla, ado-trastuzumab emtansine, 1 mg, J9354
Kanamycin sulfate, J1840, J1850
Kartop patient lift, toilet or bathroom; (see also Lift), E0625
Ketorolac thomethamine, J1885
Kidney
ESRD supply, A4650–A4927
machine, E1500–E1699
machine, accessories, E1500–E1699
system, E1510
wearable artificial, E1632
Kits
enteral feeding supply (syringe) (pump) (gravity), B4034–B4036
fistula cannulation (set), A4730
parenteral nutrition, B4220–B4224
administration kit, per day, B4224
supply kit, home mix, per day, B4222
supply kit, premix, per day, B4220
surgical dressing (tray), A4550
tracheostomy, A4625
Knee
arthroscopy, surgical, G0289, S2112, S2300
knee, surgical, harvesting cartilage, S2112
knee, surgical, removal loose body, chondroplasty, different compartment, G0289
shoulder, surgical, thermally-induced, capsulorraphy, S2300
disarticulation, prosthesis, L5150, L5160
joint, miniature, L5826
orthosis (KO), E1810, L1800–L1885
dynamic adjustable elbow entension/flexion device, E1800

Knee *(Continued)*
orthosis *(Continued)*
dynamic adjustable knee extension/flexion device, E1810
static-progressive devices, E1801, E1806, E1811, E1816–E1818, E1831, E1841
Knee-ankle-foot orthosis (KAFO), L2000–L2039, L2126–L2136
addition, high strength, lightweight material, L2755
base procedure, used with any knee joint, double upright, double bar, L2020
base procedure, used with any knee joint, full plastic double upright, L2036
base procedure, used with any knee joint, single upright, single bar, L2000
foot orthrosis, double upright, double bar, without knee joint, L2030
foot orthrosis, single upright, single bar, without knee joint, L2010
Kovaltry, J7211 ◄
Kyphosis pad, L1020, L1025

L

Laboratory tests
chemistry, P2028–P2038
cephalin flocculation, blood, P2028
congo red, blood, P2029
hair analysis, excluding arsenic, P2031
mucoprotein, blood, P2038
thymol turbidity, blood, P2033
microbiology, P7001
miscellaneous, P9010–P9615, Q0111–Q0115
blood, split unit, P9011
blood, whole, transfusion, unit, P9010
catheterization, collection specimen, multiple patients, P9615
catheterization, collection specimen, single patient, P9612
cryoprecipitate, each unit, P9012
fern test, Q0114
fresh frozen plasma, donor retested, each unit, P9060
fresh frozen plasma (single donor), frozen within 8 hours, P9017
fresh frozen plasma, within 8–24 hours of collection, each unit, P9059
granulocytes, pheresis, each unit, P9050
infusion, albumin (human), 25%, 20 ml, P9046
infusion, albumin (human), 25%, 50 ml, P9047
infusion, albumin (human), 5%, 250 ml, P9045
infusion, albumin (human), 5%, 50 ml, P9041
infusion, plasma protein fraction, human, 5%, 250 ml, P9048
infusion, plasma protein fraction, human, 5%, 50 ml, P9043

◄ New ↻ Revised ✔ Reinstated ~~deleted~~ Deleted

Laboratory tests *(Continued)*

miscellaneous *(Continued)*

KOH preparation, Q0112

pinworm examinations, Q0113

plasma, cryoprecipitate reduced, each unit, P9044

plasma, pooled, multiple donor, frozen, P9023

platelet rich plasma, each unit, P9020

platelets, each unit, P9019

platelets, HLA-matched leukocytes reduced, apheresis/pheresis, each unit, P9052

platelets, irradiated, each unit, P9032

platelets, leukocytes reduced, CMV-neg, aphresis/pheresis, each unit, P9055

platelets, leukocytes reduced, each unit, P9031

platelets, leukocytes reduced, irradiated, each unit, P9033

platelets, pheresis, each unit, P9034

platelets, pheresis, irradiated, each unit, P9036

platelets, pheresis, leukocytes reduced, CMV-neg, irradiated, each unit, P9053

platelets, pheresis, leukocytes reduced, each unit, P9035

platelets, pheresis, leukocytes reduced, irradiated, each unit, P9037

post-coital, direct qualitative, vaginal or cervical mucous, Q0115

red blood cells, deglycerolized, each unit, P9039

red blood cells, each unit, P9021

red blood cells, frozen/deglycerolized/washed, leukocytes reduced, irradiated, each unit, P9057

red blood cells, irradiated, each unit, P9038

red blood cells, leukocytes reduced, CMV-neg, irradiated, each unit, P9058

red blood cells, leukocytes reduced, each unit, P9016

red blood cells, leukocytes reduced, irradiated, each unit, P9040

red blood cells, washed, each unit, P9022

travel allowance, one way, specimen collection, home/nursing home, P9603, P9604

wet mounts, vaginal, cervical, or skin, Q0111

whole blood, leukocytes reduced, irradiated, each unit, P9056

whole blood or red blood cells, leukocytes reduced, CMV-neg, each unit, P9051

whole blood or red blood cells, leukocytes reduced, frozen, deglycerol, washed, each unit, P9054

toxicology, P3000–P3001, Q0091

Lacrimal duct, implant

permanent, A4263

temporary, A4262

Lactated Ringer's infusion, J7120

Laetrile, J3570

Lancet, A4258, A4259

Language, screening, *V5363*

Lanreotide, J1930

Laronidase, J1931

Larynx, artificial, L8500

Laser blood collection device and accessory, A4257, E0620

LASIK, *S0800*

Lead investigation, T1029

Lead wires, per pair, A4557

Leg

bag, A4358, A5105, A5112

leg or abdomen, vinyl, with/without tubes, straps, each, A4358

urinary drainage bag, leg bag, leg/abdomen, latex, with/without tube, straps, A5112

urinary suspensory, leg bag, with/without tube, each, A5105

extensions for walker, E0158

rest, elevating, K0195

rest, wheelchair, E0990

strap, replacement, A5113–A5114

Legg Perthes orthosis, L1700–L1755

Newington type, L1710

Patten bottom type, L1755

Scottish Rite type, L1730

Tachdjian type, L1720

Toronto type, L1700

Lens

aniseikonic, V2118, V2318

contact, V2500–V2599

gas permeable, V2510–V2513

hydrophilic, V2520–V2523

other type, V2599

PMMA, V2500–V2503

scleral, gas, V2530–V2531

eye, V2100–V2615, V2700–V2799

bifocal, glass or plastic, V2200–V2299

contact lenses, V2500–V2599

low vision aids, V2600–V2615

miscellaneous, V2700–V2799

single vision, glass or plastic, V2100–V2199

trifocal, glass or plastic, V2300–V2399

variable asphericity, V2410–V2499

intraocular, V2630–V2632

anterior chamber, V2630

iris supported, V2631

new technology, category 4, IOL, Q1004

new technology, category 5, IOL, Q1005

posterior chamber, V2632

telescopic lens, C1840

low vision, V2600–V2615

hand held vision aids, V2600

single lens spectacle mounted, V2610

telescopic and other compound lens system, V2615

progressive, V2781

Lepirudin, J1945

Lesion, destruction, choroid, *G0186*

Leucovorin calcium, J0640

Leukocyte poor blood, each unit, P9016

Leuprolide acetate, J1950, J9217, J9218, J9219

for depot suspension, 7.5 mg, J9217

implant, 65 mg, J9219

◀ **New**   ⭑ **Revised**   ✔ **Reinstated**   ~~deleted~~ **Deleted**

Leuprolide acetate *(Continued)*
  injection, for depot suspension, per 3.75 mg, J1950
  per 1 mg, J9218
Levalbuterol, all formulations, inhalation solution
  concentrated, J7607, J7612
  unit dose, J7614, J7615
Levetiracetam, J1953
Levocarnitine, J1955
Levofloxacin, J1956
Levoleucovorin, J0641
Levonorgestrel, (contraceptive), implants and supplies, J7306
Levorphanol tartrate, J1960
Lexidronam, A9604
Lidocaine HCl, J2001
Lift
  patient (includes seat lift), E0621–E0635
    bathroom or toilet, E0625
    mechanism incorporated into a combination lift-chair, E0627
    patient lift, electric, E0635
    patient lift, hydraulic or mechanical, E0630
    separate seat lift mechanism, patient owned furniture, non-electric, E0629
    sling or seat, canvas or nylon, E0621
  shoe, L3300–L3334
    lift, elevation, heel, L3334
    lift, elevation, heel and sole, cork, L3320
    lift, elevation, heel and sole, Neoprene, L3310
    lift, elevation, heel, tapered to metatarsals, L3300
    lift, elevation, inside shoe, L3332
    lift, elevation, metal extension, L3330
Lightweight, wheelchair, E1087–E1090, E1240–E1270
  detachable arms, swing away detachable, elevating leg rests, E1240
  detachable arms, swing away detachable footrest, E1260
  fixed full length arms, swing away detachable elevating legrests, E1270
  fixed full length arms, swing away detachable footrest, E1250
  high strength, detachable arms desk, E1088
  high strength, detachable arms desk or full length, E1090
  high strength, fixed full length arms, E1087
  high strength, fixed length arms swing away footrest, E1089
Lincomycin HCl, J2010
Linezolid, J2020
Liquid barrier, ostomy, A4363
Listening devices, assistive, V5281–V5290
  personal blue tooth FM/DM, V5286
  personal FM/DM adapter/boot coupling device for receiver, V5289
  personal FM/DM binaural, 2 receivers, V5282
  personal FM/DM, direct audio input, V5285
  personal FM/DM, ear level receiver, V5284
  personal FM/DM monaural, 1 receiver, V5281

Listening devices, assistive (Continued)
  personal FM/DM neck, loop induction receiver, V5283
  personal FM/DM transmitter assistive listening device, V5288
  transmitter microphone, V5290
Lodging, recipient, escort nonemergency transport, A0180, A0200
LOPS, G0245–G0247
  follow-up evaluation and management, G0246
  initial evaluation and management, G0245
  routine foot care, G0247
Lorazepam, J2060
Loss of protective sensation, G0245–G0247
Low osmolar contrast material, Q9965–Q9967
LSO, L0621–L0640
Lubricant, A4332, A4402
Lumbar flexion, L0540
Lumbar-sacral orthosis (LSO), L0621–L0640
LVRS, services, G0302–G0305
Lymphocyte immune globulin, J7504, J7511

M

Machine
  IPPB, E0500
  kidney, E1500–E1699
Magnesium sulphate, J3475
Maintenance contract, ESRD, A4890
Mammography, screening, G9899, G9900
Mannitol, J2150, J7665
Mapping, vessel, for hemodialysis access, G0365
Marker, tissue, A4648
Mask
  aerosol, K0180
  oxygen, A4620
Mastectomy
  bra, L8000
  form, L8020
  prosthesis, L8030, L8600
  sleeve, L8010
Matristem, Q4118
  micromatrix, 1 mg, Q4118
Mattress
  air pressure, E0186
  alternating pressure, E0277
  dry pressure, E0184
  gel pressure, E0196
  hospital bed, E0271, E0272
  non-powered, pressure reducing, E0373
  overlay, E0371–E0372
  powered, pressure reducing, E0277
  water pressure, E0187
Measurement period
  left ventricular function testing, G8682
Mecasermin, J2170
Mechlorethamine HCl, J9230

◄ **New**   ⊃ **Revised**   ✔ **Reinstated**   ~~deleted~~ **Deleted**

Medicaid, codes, *T1000–T9999*
Medical and surgical supplies, A4206–A8999
Medical nutritional therapy, G0270, G0271
Medical services, other, M0000–M9999
Medroxyprogesterone acetate, J1050
Melphalan
    HCl, J9245
    oral, J8600
Mental, health, training services, G0177
Meperidine, J2175
    and promethazine, J2180
Mepivacaine HCl, J0670
Mepolizumab, J2182
Meropenem, J2185
Mesna, J9209
Metacarpophalangeal joint, prosthetic implant, L8630, L8631
Metaproterenol sulfate, inhalation solution
    concentrated, J7667, J7668
    unit dose, J7669, J7670
Metaraminol bitartrate, J0380
Metatarsal joint, prosthetic implant, L8641
Meter, bath conductivity, dialysis, E1550
Methacholine chloride, J7674
Methadone HCl, J1230
Methergine, J2210
Methocarbamol, J2800
Methotrexate
    oral, J8610
    sodium, J9250, J9260
Methyldopate HCl, J0210
Methylene blue, Q9968
Methylnaltrexone, J2212
Methylprednisolone
    acetate, J1020–J1040
      injection, 20 mg, J1020
      injection, 40 mg, J1030
      injection, 80 mg, J1040
    oral, J7509
    sodium succinate, J2920, J2930
Metoclopramide HCl, J2765
Micafungin sodium, J2248
Microbiology test, P7001
Midazolam HCl, J2250
Mileage
    ALS, A0390
    ambulance, A0380, A0390
Milrinone lactate, J2260
Mini-bus, nonemergency transportation, A0120
Minocycline hydrochloride, J2265
Miscellaneous and investigational, A9000–A9999
Mitomycin, J7315, J9280
Mitoxantrone HCl, J9293
MNT, G0270, G0271
Mobility device, physician, service, G0372
Modalities, with office visit, M0005–M0008
Moisture exchanger for use with invasive mechanical ventilation, A4483

Moisturizer, skin, A6250
Molecular pathology procedure, G0452
Monitor
    blood glucose, home, E0607
    blood pressure, A4670
    pacemaker, E0610, E0615
Monitoring feature/device, A9279
Monitoring, INR, G0248–G0250
    demonstration prior to initiation, G0248
    physician review and interpretation, G0250
    provision of test materials, G0249
Monoclonal antibodies, J7505
Morphine sulfate, J2270
    epidural or intrathecal use, J2274
Motion, jaw, rehabilitation system, E1700–E1702
    motion rehabilitation system, E1700
    replacement cushions, E1701
    replacement measuring scales, E1702
Mouthpiece (for respiratory equipment), A4617
Moxifloxacin, J2280
Mucoprotein, blood, P2038
Multiaxial ankle, L5986
Multidisciplinary services, H2000–H2001, T1023–T1028
Multiple post collar, cervical, L0180–L0200
    occipital/mandibular supports, adjustable, L0180
    occipital/mandibular supports, adjustable cervical bars, L0200
    SQMI, Guilford, Taylor types, L0190
Multi-Podus type AFO, L4396
Muromonab-CD3, J7505
Mycophenolate mofetil, J7517
Mycophenolic acid, J7518

N

Nabilone, J8650
Nails, trimming, dystrophic, G0127
Nalbuphine HCl, J2300
Naloxone HCl, J2310
Naltrexone, J2315
Nandrolone
    decanoate, J2320
Narrowing device, wheelchair, E0969
Nasal
    application device, K0183
    pillows/seals (for nasal application device), K0184
    vaccine inhalation, J3530
Nasogastric tubing, B4081, B4082
Natalizumab, J2323
Nebulizer, E0570–E0585
    aerosol compressor, E0571, *E0572*
    aerosol mask, A7015
    corrugated tubing, disposable, A7010
    filter, disposable, A7013
    filter, non-disposable, A7014
    heater, E1372

◄ **New** ⟳ **Revised** ✔ **Reinstated** ~~deleted~~ **Deleted**

Nebulizer *(Continued)*
  large volume, disposable, prefilled, A7008
  large volume, disposable, unfilled, A7007
  not used with oxygen, durable, glass, A7017
  pneumatic, administration set, A7003,
    A7005, A7006
  pneumatic, nonfiltered, A7004
  portable, E0570
  small volume, A7003–A7005
  ultrasonic, E0575
  ultrasonic, dome and mouthpiece, A7016
  ultrasonic, reservoir bottle, non-disposable, A7009
  water collection device, large volume
    nebulizer, A7012
Necitumumab, J9295
Needle, A4215
  bone marrow biopsy, C1830
  non-coring, A4212
  with syringe, A4206–A4209
Negative pressure wound therapy pump, E2402
  accessories, A6550
Nelarabine, J9261
Neonatal transport, ambulance, base rate, A0225
Neostigmine methylsulfate, J2710
Nerve, conduction, sensory, test, G0255
Nerve stimulator with batteries, E0765
Nesiritide injection, J2324, *J2325*
Neupogen, injection, filgrastim, 1 mcg, J1442
Neuromuscular stimulator, E0745
Neurophysiology, intraoperative, monitoring, G0453
Neurostimulator
  battery recharging system, L8695
  external antenna, L8696
  implantable pulse generator, L8679
  pulse generator, L8681–L8688
    dual array, non-rechargeable, with
    extension, L8688
    dual array, rechargeable, with extension, L8687
    patient programmer (external), replacement
    only, L8681
    radiofrequency receiver, L8682
    radiofrequency transmitter (external), sacral root
    receiver, bowel and bladder management, L8684
    radiofrequency transmitter (external), with
    implantable receiver, L8683
    single array, rechargeable, with extension, L8686
Nitrogen N-13 ammonia, A9526
NMES, E0720–E0749
Nonchemotherapy drug, oral, NOS, J8499
Noncovered services, A9270
Nonemergency transportation, A0080–A0210
Nonimpregnated gauze dressing, A6216–A6221,
  A6402–A6404
Nonprescription drug, A9150
Not otherwise classified drug, J3490, J7599, J7699,
  J7799, J8499, J8999, J9999, Q0181
NPH, J1820
NPWT, pump, E2402

NTIOL category 3, Q1003
NTIOL category 4, Q1004
NTIOL category 5, Q1005
Nursing care, T1030–T1031
Nursing service, direct, skilled, outpatient, G0128
Nusinersen, J2326 ◀
Nutrition
  enteral infusion pump, B9002
  parenteral infusion pump, B9004, B9006
  parenteral solution, B4164–B5200
  therapy, medical, G0270, G0271

O

O & P supply/accessory/service, L9900
Observation
  admission, G0379
  hospital, G0378
Occipital/mandibular support, cervical, L0160
Occlusive device, placement, G0269
Occupational, therapy, G0129, S9129
Ocrelizumab, J2350 ◀
Ocriplasmin, J7316
Octafluoropropane, Q9956
Octagam, J1568
Octreotide acetate, J2353, J2354
Ocular prosthetic implant, L8610
Ofatumumab, J9302
Olanzapine, J2358
Olaratumab, J9285 ◀
Omacetaxine Mepesuccinate, J9262
Omalizumab, J2357
OnabotulinumtoxinA, J0585
Oncology
  disease status, G9063–G9139
  practice guidelines, G9056–G9062
  visit, G9050–G9055
Ondansetron HCl, J2405
Ondansetron oral, Q0162
One arm, drive attachment, K0101
Ophthalmological examination, refraction, S0621
Oprelvekin, J2355
Oral device/appliance, E0485–E0486
Oral interface, A7047
Oral, NOS, drug, J8499
Oral/nasal mask, A7027
  nasal pillows, A7029
  oral cushion, A7028
Oritavancin, J2407
Oropharyngeal suction catheter, A4628
Orphenadrine, J2360
Orthopedic shoes
  arch support, L3040–L3100
  footwear, L3000–L3649, L3201–L3265
  insert, L3000–L3030
  lift, L3300–L3334
  miscellaneous additions, L3500–L3595

◀ **New** ⟳ **Revised** ✔ **Reinstated** ~~deleted~~ **Deleted**

Orthopedic shoes *(Continued)*
  positioning device, L3140–L3170
  transfer, L3600–L3649
  wedge, L3340–L3420
Orthotic additions
  carbon graphite lamination, L2755
  fracture, L2180–L2192, L3995
  halo, L0860
  lower extremity, L2200–L2999, L4320
  ratchet lock, L2430
  scoliosis, L1010–L1120, L1210–L1290
  shoe, L3300–L3595, L3649
  spinal, L0970–L0984
  upper limb, L3810–L3890, *L3900, L3901,*
    L3970–L3974, L3975–L3978, L3995
Orthotic devices
  ankle-foot (AFO); (see also Orthopedic shoes),
    E1815, E1816, E1830, L1900–L1990,
    L2102–L2116, L3160, L4361, *L4397*
  anterior-posterior-lateral, L0700, L0710
  cervical, L0100–L0200
  cervical-thoracic-lumbar-sacral (CTLSO),
    L0700, L0710
  elbow (EO), E1800, E1801, L3700–L3740,
    L3760–L3761, *L3762* ↻
  fracture, L2102–L2136, L3980–L3986
  halo, L0810–L0830
  hand, (WHFO), E1805, E1825, L3807,
    L3900–L3954, *L3956*
  hand, finger, prefabricated, L3923
  hip (HO), L1600–L1690
  hip-knee-ankle-foot (HKAFO), L2040–L2090
  interface material, E1820
  knee (KO), E1810, E1811, L1800–L1885
  knee-ankle-foot (KAFO); (see also Orthopedic
    shoes), L2000–L2038, L2126–L2136
  Legg Perthes, L1700–L1755
  lumbar, L0625–L0651
  multiple post collar, L0180–L0200
  not otherwise specified, L0999, L1499, L2999,
    L3999, L5999, L7499, L8039, L8239
  pneumatic splint, L4350–L4380
  pronation/supination, E1818
  repair or replacement, L4000–L4210
  replace soft interface material, L4390–L4394
  sacroiliac, L0600–L0620, *L0621–L0624*
  scoliosis, L1000–L1499
  shoe, (see Orthopedic shoes)
  shoulder (SO), L1840, L3650, L3674, *L3678*
  shoulder-elbow-wrist-hand (SEWHO), L3960–L3978
  side bar disconnect, L2768
  spinal, cervical, L0100–L0200
  spinal, DME, K0112–K0116
  thoracic, L0210, *L0220*
  thoracic-hip-knee-ankle (THKO), L1500–L1520
  toe, E1830
  wrist-hand-finger (WHFO), E1805, E1806, E1825,
    L3806–L3809, L3900–L3954, *L3956*

Orthovisc, J7324
Ossicula prosthetic implant, L8613
Osteogenesis stimulator, E0747–E0749, E0760
Ostomy
  accessories, A5093
  belt, A4396
  pouches, A4416–A4435, *A5056, A5057*
  skin barrier, A4401–A4449, *A4462*
  supplies, A4361–A4421, A5051–A5149, *A5200*
Otto Bock, prosthesis, *L7007*
Outpatient payment system, hospital, *C1000–C9999*
Overdoor, traction, *E0860*
Oxacillin sodium, *J2700*
Oxaliplatin, J9263
Oxygen
  ambulance, A0422
  battery charger, E1357
  battery pack/cartridge, E1356
  catheter, transtracheal, A7018
  chamber, hyperbaric, topical, A4575
  concentrator, E1390–E1391
  DC power adapter, E1358
  delivery system (topical), E0446 ◄
  equipment, E0424–E0486, E1353–E1406
  Liquid oxygen system, E0433
  mask, A4620
  medication supplies, A4611–A4627
  rack/stand, E1355
  regulator, E1352, E1353
  respiratory equipment/supplies, E0424–E0480,
    A4611–A4627, *E0481*
  supplies and equipment, E0425–E0444, E0455
  tent, E0455
  tubing, A4616
  water vapor enriching system, E1405, E1406
  wheeled cart, E1354
Oxymorphone HCl, J2410
Oxytetracycline HCl, J2460
Oxytocin, J2590

P

Pacemaker monitor, E0610, E0615
Paclitaxel, J9267
Paclitaxel protein-bound particles, J9264
Pad
  correction, CTLSO, L1020–L1060
  gel pressure, E0185, E0196
  heat, A9273, E0210, E0215, E0217, E0238, E0249
    electric heat pad, moist, E0215
    electric heat pad, standard, E0210
    hot water bottle, ice cap or collar, heat and/or cold
    wrap, A9273
    pad for water circulating heat unit, replacement
    only, E0249
    water circulating heat pad with pump, E0217
  orthotic device interface, E1820

◄ **New**   ↻ **Revised**   ✔ **Reinstated**   ~~deleted~~ **Deleted**

Pad *(Continued)*
sheepskin, E0188, E0189
water circulating cold with pump, E0218
water circulating heat unit, E0249
water circulating heat with pump, E0217
Pail, for use with commode chair, E0167
Pain assessment, G8730–G8732
Palate, prosthetic implant, L8618
Palifermin, J2425
Paliperidone palmitate, J2426
Palonosetron, J2469, J8655
Pamidronate disodium, J2430
Pan, for use with commode chair, E0167
Panitumumab, J9303
Papanicolaou screening smear(Pap), P3000,
P3001, Q0091
cervical or vaginal, up to 3 smears, by
technician, P3000
cervical or vaginal, up to 3 smears, physician
interpretation, P3001
obtaining, preparing and conveyance, Q0091
Papaverine HCl, J2440
Paraffin, A4265
bath unit, E0235
Parenteral nutrition
administration kit, B4224
pump, B9004, B9006
solution, B4164–B5200
compounded amino acid and carbohydrates, with
electrolytes, B4189–B4199, B5000–B5200
nutrition additives, homemix, B4216
nutrition administration kit, B4224
nutrition solution, amino acid, B4168–B4178
nutrition solution, carbohydrates, B4164, B4180
nutrition solution, per 10 grams, liquid, B4185
nutrition supply kit, homemix, B4222
supply kit, B4220, B4222
Paricalcitol, J2501
Parking fee, nonemergency transport, A0170
Partial Hospitalization, OT, G0129
Pasireotide long acting, J2502
Paste, conductive, A4558
Pathology and laboratory tests, miscellaneous,
P9010–P9615
Pathology, surgical, G0416
Patient support system, E0636
Patient transfer system, E1035–E1036
Pediculosis (lice) treatment, A9180
PEFR, peak expiratory flow rate meter, A4614
Pegademase bovine, J2504
Pegaptanib, J2503
Pegaspargase, J9266
Pegfilgrastim, J2505
Peginesatide, J0890
Pegloticase, J2507
Pelvic
belt/harness/boot, E0944
traction, E0890, E0900, E0947

Pemetrexed, J9305
Penicillin
G benzathine/G benzathine and penicillin G
procaine, J0558, J0561
G potassium, J2540
G procaine, aqueous, J2510
Pentamidine isethionate, J2545, J7676
Pentastarch, 10% solution, J2513
Pentazocine HCl, J3070
Pentobarbital sodium, J2515
Pentostatin, J9268
Peramivir, J2547
Percussor, E0480
Percutaneous access system, A4301
Perflexane lipid microspheres, Q9955
Perflutren lipid microspheres, Q9957
Peroneal strap, L0980
Peroxide, A4244
Perphenazine, J3310
Personal care services, T1019–T1021
home health aide or CAN, per visit, T1021
per diem, T1020
provided by home health aide or CAN, per
15 minutes, T1019
Pertuzumab, J9306
Pessary, A4561, A4562
PET, G0219, G0235, G0252
Pharmacologic therapy, G8633
Pharmacy, fee, G0333
Phenobarbital sodium, J2560
Phentolamine mesylate, J2760
Phenylephrine HCl, J2370
Phenytoin sodium, J1165
Phisohex solution, A4246
Photofrin, (see Porfimer sodium)
Photorefraction keratectomy, (PRK), S0810
Phototherapeutic keratectomy, (PTK), S0812
Phototherapy light, E0202
Phytonadione, J3430
Pillow, cervical, E0943
Pinworm examination, Q0113
Plasma
multiple donor, pooled, frozen, P9023, P9070
single donor, fresh frozen, P9017, P9071
Plastazote, L3002, L3252, L3253, L3265,
L5654–L5658
addition to lower extremity socket insert, L5654
addition to lower extremity socket insert, above
knee, L5658
addition to lower extremity socket insert, below
knee, L5655
addition to lower extremity socket insert, knee
disarticulation, L5656
foot insert, removable, plastazote, L3002
foot, molded shoe, custom fitted, plastazote, L3253
foot, shoe molded to patient model,
plastazote, L3252
plastazote sandal, L3265

◄ **New** ↻ **Revised** ✔ **Reinstated** ~~deleted~~ **Deleted**

Platelet, P9073, P9100 ↻
   concentrate, each unit, P9019
   rich plasma, each unit, P9020
Platelets, P9031–P9037, P9052–P9053, P9055
Platform attachment
   forearm crutch, E0153
   walker, E0154
Plerixafor, J2562
Plicamycin, J9270
Plumbing, for home ESRD equipment, A4870
Pneumatic
   appliance, E0655–E0673, L4350–L4380
   compressor, E0650–E0652
   splint, L4350–L4380
   ventricular assist device, Q0477, Q0480–Q0505 ↻
Pneumatic nebulizer
   administration set, small volume, filtered, A7006
   administration set, small volume,
      nonfiltered, A7003
   administration set, small volume, nonfiltered,
      nondisposable, A7005
   small volume, disposable, A7004
Pneumococcal
   vaccine, administration, G0009
Porfimer, J9600
Portable
   equipment transfer, R0070–R0076
   gaseous oxygen, K0741, K0742
   hemodialyzer system, E1635
   liquid oxygen system, E0433
   x-ray equipment, Q0092
Positioning seat, T5001
Positive airway pressure device, accessories,
   A7030–A7039, E0561–E0562
Positive expiratory pressure device, E0484
Post-coital examination, Q0115
Postural drainage board, E0606
Potassium
   chloride, J3480
   hydroxide preparation(KOH), Q0112
Pouch
   fecal collection, A4330
   ostomy, A4375–A4378, A5051–A5054, A5061–A5065
   urinary, A4379–A4383, A5071–A5075
Practice, guidelines, oncology, G9056–G9062
Pralatrexate, J9307
Pralidoxime chloride, J2730
Prednisolone
   acetate, J2650
   oral, J7510
Prednisone, J7512
Preparation kits, dialysis, A4914
Preparatory prosthesis, L5510–L5595
   chemotherapy, J8999
   nonchemotherapy, J8499
Pressure
   alarm, dialysis, E1540
   pad, A4640, E0180–E0199

Privigen, J1459
Procainamide HCl, J2690
Procedure
   HALO, L0810–L0861
   noncovered, G0293, G0294
   scoliosis, L1000–L1499
Prochlorperazine, J0780
Prolotherapy, M0076
Promazine HCl, J2950
Promethazine
   and meperdine, J2180
   HCl, J2550
Propranolol HCl, J1800
Prostate, cancer, screening, G0102, G0103
Prosthesis
   artificial larynx battery/accessory, L8505
   breast, L8000–L8035, L8600
   eye, L8610, L8611, V2623–V2629
   fitting, L5400–L5460, L6380–L6388
   foot/ankle one piece system, L5979
   hand, L6000–L6020, L6026
   implants, L8600–L8690
   larynx, L8500
   lower extremity, L5700–L5999, L8640–L8642
   mandible, L8617
   maxilla, L8616
   maxillofacial, provided by a non-physician,
      L8040–L8048
   miscellaneous service, L8499
   ocular, V2623–V2629
   repair of, L7520, L8049
   socks (shrinker, sheath, stump sock), L8400–L8485
   taxes, orthotic/prosthetic/other, L9999
   tracheo-esophageal, L8507–L8509
   upper extremity, L6000–L6999
   vacuum erection system, L7900
Prosthetic additions
   lower extremity, L5610–L5999
   upper extremity, L6600–L7405
Prosthetic, eye, V2623
Protamine sulfate, J2720
Protectant, skin, A6250
Protector, heel or elbow, E0191
Protein C Concentrate, J2724
Protirelin, J2725
Psychotherapy, group, partial hospitalization,
   G0410–G0411
Pulse generator, E2120
Pump
   alternating pressure pad, E0182
   ambulatory infusion, E0781
   ambulatory insulin, E0784
   blood, dialysis, E1620
   breast, E0602–E0604
   enteral infusion, B9000, B9002
   external infusion, E0779
   heparin infusion, E1520
   implantable infusion, E0782, E0783

◀ **New**   ↻ **Revised**   ✔ **Reinstated**   ~~deleted~~ **Deleted**

Pump (*Continued*)
  implantable infusion, refill kit, A4220
  infusion, supplies, A4230, A4232
  negative pressure wound therapy, E2402
  parenteral infusion, B9004, B9006
  suction, portable, E0600
  water circulating pad, E0236
  wound, negative, pressure, E2402
Purification system, E1610, E1615
Pyridoxine HCl, J3415

Q

Quad cane, E0105
Quinupristin/dalfopristin, J2770

R

Rack/stand, oxygen, E1355
Radiesse, Q2026
Radioelements for brachytherapy, Q3001
Radiological, supplies, *A4641, A4642*
Radiology service, R0070–R0076
Radiopharmaceutical diagnostic and therapeutic imaging agent, A4641, A4642, A9500–A9699
Radiosurgery, robotic, *G0339–G0340*
Radiosurgery, stereotactic, *G0339, G0340*
Rail
  bathtub, E0241, E0242, E0246
  bed, E0305, E0310
  toilet, E0243
Ranibizumab, J2778
Rasburicase, J2783
Reaching/grabbing device, A9281
Reagent strip, A4252
Reciprocating peritoneal dialysis system, E1630
Reclast, J3488, *J3489*
Reclining, wheelchair, *E1014, E1050–E1070, E1100–E1110*
Reconstruction, angiography, *G0288*
Red blood cells, P9021, P9022
Regadenoson, J2785
Regular insulin, *J1815,* J1820
Regulator, oxygen, E1353
Rehabilitation
  cardiac, S9472
  program, H2001
  psychosocial, H2017, H2018
  pulmonary, S9473
  system, jaw, motion, E1700–E1702
  vestibular, S9476
Removal, cerumen, *G0268*
Repair
  contract, ESRD, A4890
  durable medical equipment, E1340

Repair (*Continued*)
  maxillofacial prosthesis, L8049
  orthosis, L4000–L4130
  prosthetic, L7500, L7510
Replacement
  battery, A4630
  pad (alternating pressure), A4640
  tanks, dialysis, A4880
  tip for cane, crutches, walker, A4637
  underarm pad for crutches, A4635
Reslizumab, J2786
RespiGam, (see Respiratory syncytial virus immune globulin)
Respiratory
  DME, A7000–A7527
  equipment, E0424–E0601
  function, therapeutic, procedure, G0237–G0239, S5180–S5181
  supplies, A4604–A4629
Restraint, any type, E0710
Reteplase, J2993
Revascularization, *C9603–C9608*
Rho(D) immune globulin, human, J2788, J2790, J2791, J2792
Rib belt, thoracic, A4572, L0220
Rilanocept, J2793
RimabotulinumtoxinB, J0587
Ring, ostomy, A4404
Ringers lactate infusion, J7120
Risk-adjusted functional status
  elbow, wrist or hand, G8667–G8670
  hip, G8651–G8654
  lower leg, foot or ankle, G8655–G8658
  lumbar spine, G8659–G8662
  neck, cranium, mandible, thoracic spine, ribs, or other, G8671–G8674
  shoulder, G8663–G8666
Risperidone, J2794
Rituximab, J9310
Robin-Aids, L6000, L6010, L6020, L6855, L6860
Rocking bed, E0462
Rolapitant, J8670
Rollabout chair, E1031
Romidepsin, J9315
Romiplostim, J2796
Ropivacaine HCl, J2795
Rubidium Rb-82, A9555

S

Sacral nerve stimulation test lead, A4290
Safety equipment, E0700
  vest, wheelchair, E0980
Saline
  hypertonic, J7130, *J7131*
  infusion, J7030–J7060
  solution, A4216–A4218, J7030–J7050

◄ New   ⟳ Revised   ✔ Reinstated   ~~deleted~~ Deleted

Saliva
artificial, A9155
Samarium SM 153 Lexidronamm, A9605
Sargramostim (GM-CSF), J2820
Scale, E1639 ◄
Scoliosis, L1000–L1499
additions, L1010–L1120, L1210–L1290
Screening
alcohol misuse, G0442
cancer, cervical or vaginal, G0101
colorectal, cancer, G0104–G0106,
G0120–G0122, G0328
cytopathology cervical or vaginal, G0123, G0124,
G0141–G0148
depression, G0444
dysphagia, documentation, V5364
enzyme immunoassay, G0432
glaucoma, G0117, G0118
infectious agent antibody detection, G0433, G0435
language, V5363
mammography, digital image, G9899, G9900
prostate, cancer, G0102, G0103
speech, V5362
Sculptra, Q2028
Sealant
skin, A6250
Seat
attachment, walker, E0156
insert, wheelchair, E0992
lift (patient), E0621, E0627–E0629
upholstery, wheelchair, E0975, E0981
Sebelipase alfa , J2840
Secretin, J2850
Semen analysis, G0027
Semi-reclining, wheelchair, E1100, E1110
Sensitivity study, P7001
Sensory nerve conduction test, G0255
Sermorelin acetate, Q0515
Serum clotting time tube, A4771
Service
Allied Health, home health, hospice, G0151–G0161
behavioral health and/or substance abuse, H0001–H9999
hearing, V5000–V5999
laboratory, P0000–P9999
mental, health, training, G0177
non-covered, A9270
physician, for mobility device, G0372
pulmonary, for LVRS, G0302–G0305
skilled, RN/LPN, home health, hospice, G0162
social, psychological, G0409–G0411
speech-language, V5336–V5364
vision, V2020–V2799
SEWHO, L3960–L3974, L3975–L3978
SEXA, G0130
Sheepskin pad, E0188, E0189
Shoes
arch support, L3040–L3100
for diabetics, A5500–A5508

Shoes (Continued)
insert, L3000–L3030, L3031
lift, L3300–L3334
miscellaneous additions, L3500–L3595
orthopedic, L3201–L3265
positioning device, L3140–L3170
transfer, L3600–L3649
wedge, L3340–L3485
Shoulder
disarticulation, prosthetic, L6300–L6320, L6550
orthosis (SO), L3650–L3674
spinal, cervical, L0100–L0200
Shoulder sling, A4566
Shoulder-elbow-wrist-hand orthosis (SEWHO),
L3960–L3969, L3971–L3978
Shunt accessory for dialysis, A4740
aqueous, L8612
Sigmoidoscopy, cancer screening, G0104, G0106
Siltuximab, J2860
Sincalide, J2805
Sipuleucel-T, Q2043
Sirolimus, J7520
Sitz bath, E0160–E0162
Skin
barrier, ostomy, A4362, A4363, A4369–A4373,
A4385, A5120
bond or cement, ostomy, A4364
sealant, protectant, moisturizer, A6250
substitute, Q4100–Q4182 ⟳
Skyla, 13.5 mg, J7301
Sling, A4565
patient lift, E0621, E0630, E0635
Smear, Papanicolaou, screening, P3000,
P3001, Q0091
SNCT, G0255
Social worker, clinical, home, health, G0155
Social worker, nonemergency transport, A0160
Social work/psychological services, CORF, G0409
Sock
body sock, L0984
prosthetic sock, L8417, L8420–L8435, L8470,
L8480, L8485
stump sock, L8470–L8485
Sodium
chloride injection, J2912
ferric gluconate complex in sucrose, J2916
fluoride F-18, A9580
hyaluronate
Euflexxa, J7323
GELSYN-3, J7328 ◄
Hyalgan, J7321
Orthovisc, J7324
Supartz, J7321
Synvisc and Synvisc-One, J7325
Visco-3, J7321 ◄
phosphate P32, A9563
pyrophosphate, J1443
succinate, J1720

◄ **New**   ⟳ **Revised**   ✔ **Reinstated**   ~~deleted~~ **Deleted**

Solution
    calibrator, A4256
    dialysate, A4760
    elliotts b, J9175
    enteral formulae, B4149–B4156, *B4157–B4162*
    parenteral nutrition, B4164–B5200
Solvent, adhesive remover, A4455
Somatrem, J2940
Somatropin, J2941
Sorbent cartridge, ESRD, E1636
Special size, wheelchair, E1220–E1239
Specialty absorptive dressing, A6251–A6256
Spectacle lenses, V2100–V2199
Spectinomycin HCl, J3320
Speech assessment, V5362–V5364
Speech generating device, E2500–E2599
Speech, pathologist, G0153
Speech-Language pathology, services,
    V5336–V5364
Spherocylinder, single vision, V2100–V2114
    bifocal, V2203–V2214
    trifocal, V2303–V2314
Spinal orthosis
    cervical, L0100–L0200
    cervical-thoracic-lumbar-sacral (CTLSO), L0700, L0710
    DME, K0112–K0116
    halo, L0810–L0830
    multiple post collar, L0180–L0200
    scoliosis, L1000–L1499
    torso supports, L0960
Splint, A4570, L3100, L4350–L4380
    ankle, L4390–L4398
    dynamic, E1800, E1805, E1810, E1815, E1825,
      E1830, E1840
    footdrop, L4398
    supplies, miscellaneous, Q4051
Standard, wheelchair, E1130, K0001
Static progressive stretch, E1801, E1806, E1811,
    E1816, E1818, E1821
Status
    disease, oncology, G9063–G9139
STELARA, ustekinumab, 1 mg, J3357
Stent, transcatheter, placement, C9600, C9601
Stereotactic, radiosurgery, G0339, G0340
Sterile cefuroxime sodium, J0697
Sterile water, A4216–A4217
Stimulation, electrical, non-attended, G0281–G0283
Stimulators
    neuromuscular, E0744, E0745
    osteogenesis, electrical, E0747–E0749
    salivary reflex, E0755
    stoma absorptive cover, A5083
    transcutaneous, electric, nerve, A4595, E0720–E0749
    ultrasound, E0760
Stockings
    gradient, compression, A6530–A6549
    surgical, A4490–A4510
Stoma, plug or seal, A5081

Stomach tube, B4083
Streptokinase, J2995
Streptomycin, J3000
Streptozocin, J9320
Strip, blood glucose test, A4253–A4772
    urine reagent, A4250
Strontium-89 chloride, supply of, A9600
Study, bone density, G0130
Stump sock, L8470–L8485
Stylet, A4212
Substance/Alcohol, assessment, G0396, G0397,
    H0001, H0003, H0049
Succinylcholine chloride, J0330
Suction pump
    gastric, home model, E2000
    portable, E0600
    respiratory, home model, E0600
Sumatriptan succinate, J3030
Supartz, J7321
Supplies
    battery, A4233–A4236, A4601, A4611–A4613, A4638
    cast, A4580, A4590, Q4001–Q4051
    catheters, A4300–A4306
    contraceptive, A4267–A4269
    diabetic shoes, A5500–A5513
    dialysis, A4653–A4928
    DME, other, A4630–A4640
    dressings, A6000–A6513
    enteral, therapy, B4000–B9999
    incontinence, A4310–A4355, A5102–A5200
    infusion, A4221, A4222, A4230–A4232,
      E0776–E0791
    needle, A4212, A4215
    needle-free device, A4210
    ostomy, A4361–A4434, A5051–A5093, A5120–A5200
    parenteral, therapy, B4000–B9999
    radiological, A4641, A4642
    refill kit, infusion pump, A4220
    respiratory, A4604–A4629
    self-administered injections, A4211
    splint, Q4051
    sterile water/saline and/or dextrose, A4216–A4218
    surgical, miscellaneous, A4649
    syringe, A4206–A4209, A4213, A4232
    syringe with needle, A4206–A4209
    urinary, external, A4356–A4360
Supply/accessory/service, A9900
Support
    arch, L3040–L3090
    cervical, L0100–L0200
    spinal, L0960
    stockings, L8100–L8239
Surgical
    arthroscopy, knee, G0289, S2112
    boot, L3208–L3211
    dressing, A6196–A6406
    procedure, noncovered, G0293, G0294
    stocking, A4490–A4510

◀ **New**   ⤶ **Revised**   ✔ **Reinstated**   ~~deleted~~ **Deleted**

Surgical *(Continued)*
  supplies, A4649
  tray, A4550
Swabs, betadine or iodine, A4247
Synvisc and Synvisc-One, J7325
Syringe, A4213
  with needle, A4206–A4209
System
  external, ambulatory insulin, A9274
  rehabilitation, jaw, motion, E1700–E1702
  transport, E1035–E1039

T

Tables, bed, E0274, E0315
Tacrolimus
  oral, J7503, J7507, J7508
  parenteral, J7525
Taliglucerase, J3060
Talimogene laheroareovec, J9325
Tape, A4450–A4452
Taxi, non emergency transportation, A0100
Team, conference, G0175, G9007, S0220, S0221
Technetium TC 99M
  Arcitumomab, A9568
  Bicisate, A9557
  Depreotide, A9536
  Disofenin, A9510
  Exametazine, A9521
  Exametazine labeled autologous white blood
    cells, A9569
  Fanolesomab, A9566
  Glucepatate, A9550
  Labeled red blood cells, A9560
  Macroaggregated albumin, A9540
  Mebrofenin, A9537
  Mertiatide, A9562
  Oxidronate, A9561
  Pentetate, A9539, A9567
  Pertechnetate, A9512
  Pyrophosphate, A9538
  Sestamibi, A9500
  Succimer, A9551
  Sulfur colloid, A9541
  Teboroxime, A9501
  Tetrofosmin, A9502
  Tilmanocept, A9520
Tedizolid phosphate, J3090
TEEV, J0900
Telavancin, J3095
Telehealth, Q3014
Telehealth transmission, T1014
Temozolomide
  injection, J9328
  oral, J8700
Temporary codes, Q0000–Q9999, S0009–S9999
Temsirolimus, J9330

Tenecteplase, J3101
Teniposide, Q2017
TENS, A4595, E0720–E0749
Tent, oxygen, E0455
Terbutaline sulfate, J3105
  inhalation solution, concentrated, J7680
  inhalation solution, unit dose, J7681
Teriparatide, J3110
Terminal devices, L6700–L6895
Test
  sensory, nerve, conduction, G0255
Testosterone
  cypionate and estradiol cypionate, J1071
  enanthate, J3121
  undecanoate, J3145
Tetanus immune globulin, human, J1670
Tetracycline, J0120
Thallous Chloride TL 201, A9505
Theophylline, J2810
Therapeutic lightbox, A4634, E0203
Therapy
  activity, G0176
  electromagnetic, G0295, G0329
  enteral, supplies, B4000–B9999
  medical, nutritional, G0270, G0271
  occupational, G0129, H5300, S9129
  occupational, health, G0152
  parenteral, supplies, B4000–B9999
  respiratory, function, procedure, G0237–S0239,
    S5180, S5181
  speech, home, G0153, S9128
  wound, negative, pressure, pump, E2402
Theraskin, Q4121
Thermometer, A4931–A4932
  dialysis, A4910
Thiamine HCl, J3411
Thiethylperazine maleate, J3280
Thiotepa, J9340
Thoracic orthosis, L0210
Thoracic-hip-knee-ankle (THKAO), L1500–L1520
Thoracic-lumbar-sacral orthosis (TLSO)
  scoliosis, L1200–L1290
  spinal, L0450–L0492
Thymol turbidity, blood, P2033
Thyrotropin Alfa, J3240
Tigecycline, J3243
Tinzarparin sodium, J1655
Tip (cane, crutch, walker) replacement, A4637
Tire, wheelchair, E2211–E2225, E2381–E2395
Tirofiban, J3246
Tisagenlecleucel, Q2040 ◀
Tissue marker, A4648
TLSO, L0450–L0492, L1200–L1290
Tobacco
  intervention, G9016
Tobramycin
  inhalation solution, unit dose, J7682, J7685
  sulfate, J3260

◀ **New** ⊋ **Revised** ✔ **Reinstated** ~~deleted~~ **Deleted**

Tocilizumab, J2362

Toe device, E1831

Toilet accessories, E0167–E0179, E0243, E0244, E0625

Tolazoline HCl, J2670

Toll, non emergency transport, A0170

Topical hyperbaric oxygen chamber, A4575

Topotecan, J8705, J9351

Torsemide, J3265

Trabectedin, J9352

Tracheostoma heat moisture exchange system, A7501–A7509

Tracheostomy
  care kit, A4629
  filter, A4481
  speaking valve, L8501
  supplies, A4623, A4629, A7523–A7524
  tube, A7520–A7522

Tracheotomy mask or collar, A7525–A7526

Traction
  cervical, E0855, E0856
  device, ambulatory, E0830
  equipment, E0840–E0948
  extremity, E0870–E0880
  pelvic, E0890, E0900, E0947

Training
  diabetes, outpatient, G0108, G0109
  home health or hospice, G0162
  services, mental, health, G0177

Transcutaneous electrical nerve stimulator (TENS), E0720–E0770

Transducer protector, dialysis, E1575

Transfer (shoe orthosis), L3600–L3640

Transfer system with seat, E1035

Transparent film (for dressing), A6257–A6259

Transplant
  islet, G0341–G0343, S2102

Transport
  chair, E1035–E1039
  system, E1035–E1039
  x-ray, R0070–R0076

Transportation
  ambulance, A0021–A0999, Q3019, Q3020
  corneal tissue, V2785
  EKG (portable), R0076
  handicapped, A0130
  non emergency, A0080–A0210, T2001–T2005
  service, including ambulance, A0021, A0999, T2006
  taxi, non emergency, A0100
  toll, non emergency, A0170
  volunteer, non emergency, A0080, A0090
  x-ray (portable), R0070, R0075, *R0076*

Transportation services
  air services, A0430, A0431, A0435, A0436
  ALS disposable supplies, A0398
  ALS mileage, A0390
  ALS specialized service, A0392, A0394, A0396
  ambulance, ALS, A0426, A0427, A0433
  ambulance, outside state, Medicaid, A0021

Transportation services (Continued)
  ambulance oxygen, A0422
  ambulance, waiting time, A0420
  ancillary, lodging, escort, A0200
  ancillary, lodging, recipient, A0180
  ancillary, meals, escort, A0210
  ancillary, meals, recipient, A0190
  ancillary, parking fees, tolls, A0170
  BLS disposable supplies, A0382
  BLS mileage, A0380
  BLS specialized service, A0384
  emergency, neonatal, one-way, A0225
  extra ambulance attendant, A0424
  ground mileage, A0425
  non-emergency, air travel, A0140
  non-emergency, bus, A0110
  non-emergency, case worker, A0160
  non-emergency, mini-bus, A0120
  non-emergency, no vested interest, A0080
  non-emergency, taxi, A0100
  non-emergency, wheelchair van, A0130
  non-emergency, with vested interest, A0090
  paramedic intercept, A0432
  response and treat, no transport, A0998
  specialty transport, A0434

Transtracheal oxygen catheter, A7018

Trapeze bar, E0910–E0912, E0940

Trauma, response, team, G0390

Tray
  insertion, A4310–A4316
  irrigation, A4320
  surgical; (see also kits), A4550
  wheelchair, E0950

Treatment
  bone, G0412–G0415
  pediculosis (lice), A9180
  services, behavioral health, H0002–H2037

Treprostinil, J3285

Triamcinolone, J3301–J3303
  acetonide, J3300, J3301
  diacetate, J3302
  hexacetonide, J3303
  inhalation solution, concentrated, J7683
  inhalation solution, unit dose, J7684

Triflupromazine HCl, J3400

Trifocal, glass or plastic, V2300–V2399
  aniseikonic, V2318
  lenticular, V2315, V2321
  specialty trifocal, by report, V2399
  sphere, plus or minus, V2300–V2302
  spherocylinder, V2303–V2314
  trifocal add-over 3.25d, V2320
  trifocal, seg width over 28 mm, V2319

Trimethobenzamide HCl, J3250

Trimetrexate glucuoronate, J3305

Trimming, nails, dystrophic, G0127

Triptorelin pamoate, J3315

Truss, L8300–L8330

Truss *(Continued)*
  addition to standard pad, scrotal pad, L8330
  addition to standard pad, water pad, L8320
  double, standard pads, L8310
  single, standard pad, L8300
Tube/Tubing
  anchoring device, A5200
  blood, A4750, A4755
  corrugated tubing, non-disposable, used with large
    volume nebulizer,10 feet, A4337
  drainage extension, A4331
  gastrostomy, B4087, B4088
  irrigation, A4355
  larynectomy, A4622
  nasogastric, B4081, B4082
  oxygen, A4616
  serum clotting time, A4771
  stomach, B4083
  suction pump, each, A7002
  tire, K0091, K0093, K0095, K0097
  tracheostomy, A4622
  urinary drainage, K0280

U

Ultrasonic nebulizer, E0575
Ultrasound, *S8055, S9024*
  paranasal sinus ultrasound, S9024
  ultrasound guidance, multifetal pregnancy reduction,
    technical component, S8055
Ultraviolet, cabinet/system, *E0691, E0694*
Ultraviolet light therapy system, A4633,
    E0691–E0694
  light therapy system in 6 foot cabinet, E0694
  replacement bulb/lamp, A4633
  therapy system panel, 4 foot, E0692
  therapy system panel, 6 foot, E0693
  treatment area 2 sq feet or less, E0691
Unclassified drug, J3490
Underpads, disposable, *A4554*
Unipuncture control system, dialysis, E1580
Upper extremity addition, locking elbow, L6693
Upper extremity fracture orthosis, L3980–L3999
Upper limb prosthesis, L6000–L7499
Urea, J3350
Ureterostomy supplies, A4454–A4590
Urethral suppository, Alprostadil, J0275
Urinal, E0325, E0326
Urinary
  catheter, A4338–A4346, A4351–A4353
    indwelling catheter, A4338–A4346
    intermittent urinary catheter, A4351–A4353
    male external catheter, A4349
  collection and retention (supplies), A4310–A4360
    bedside drainage bag, A4357
    disposable external urethral clamp, A4360
    external urethral clamp, A4356

Urinary *(Continued)*
  collection and retention (supplies) *(Continued)*
    female external urinary collection device, A4328
    insertion trays, A4310–A4316, A4354–A4355
    irrigation syringe, A4322
    irrigation tray, A4320
    male external catheter/integral collection
      chamber, A4326
    perianal fecal collection pouch, A4330
    therapeutic agent urinary catheter irrigation, A4321
    urinary drainage bag, leg/abdomen, A4358
  supplies, external, A4335, A4356–A4358
    bedside drainage bag, A4357
    external urethral clamp/compression device, A4356
    incontinence supply, A4335
    urinary drainage bag, leg or abdomen, A4358
  tract implant, collagen, L8603
  tract implant, synthetic, L8606
Urine
  sensitivity study, P7001
  tests, A4250
Urofollitropin, J3355
Urokinase, J3364, J3365
Ustekinumab, J3357, J3758 ↻
U-V lens, V2755

V

Vabra aspirator, A4480
Vaccination, administration
  flublok, Q2033
  hepatitis B, G0010
  influenza virus, G0008
  pneumococcal, G0009
Vaccine
  administration, influenza, G0008
  administration, pneumococcal, G0009
  hepatitis B, administration, G0010
Vaginal
  cancer, screening, G0101
  cytopathologist, G0123
  cytopathology, G0123, G0124, G0141–G0148
  screening, cervical/vaginal, thin-layer,
    cytopathologist, G0123
  screening, cervical/vaginal, thin-layer, physician
    interpretation, G0124
  screening cytopathology smears, automated,
    G0141–G0148
Vancomycin HCl, J3370
Vaporizer, E0605
Vascular
  catheter (appliances and supplies), A4300–A4306
    disposable drug delivery system, >50 ml/hr, A4305
    disposable drug delivery system, <50 ml/hr, A4306
    implantable access catheter, external, A4300
    implantable access total, catheter, A4301
  graft material, synthetic, L8670

◀ **New**   ↻ **Revised**   ✔ **Reinstated**   ~~deleted~~ **Deleted**

Vasoxyl, J3390
Vedolizumab, J3380
Vehicle, power-operated, K0800–K0899
Velaglucerase alfa, J3385
Venous pressure clamp, dialysis, A4918
Ventilator
    battery, A4611–A4613
    home ventilator, any type, E0465, E0466
      used with invasive interface, (e.g., tracheostomy tube), E0465
      used with non-invasive interface, (e.g., mask, chest shell), E0466
    moisture exchanger, disposable, A4483
Ventricular assist device, Q0478–Q0504, Q0506–Q0509
    battery clips, electric or electric/pneumatic, replacement, Q0497
    battery, lithium-ion, electric or electric/pneumatic, replacement, Q0506
    battery, other than lithium-ion, electric or electric/ pneumatic, replacement, Q0496
    battery, pneumatic, replacement, Q0503
    battery/power-pack charger, electric or electric/ pneumatic, replacement, Q0495
    belt/vest/bag, carry external components, replacement, Q0499
    driver, replacement, Q0480
    emergency hand pump, electric or electric/pneumatic, replacement, Q0494
    emergency power source, electric, replacement, Q0490
    emergency power source, electric/pneumatic, replacement, Q0491
    emergency power supply cable, electric, replacement, Q0492
    emergency power supply cable, electric/pneumatic, replacement, Q0493
    filters, electric or electric/pneumatic, replacement, Q0500
    holster, electric or electric/pneumatic, replacement, Q0498
    leads (pneumatic/electrical), replacement, Q0487
    microprocessor control unit, electric/pneumatic combination, replacement, Q0482
    microprocessor control unit, pneumatic, replacement, Q0481
    miscellaneous supply, external VAD, Q0507
    miscellaneous supply, implanted device, Q0508
    miscellaneous supply, implanted device, payment not made under Medicare Part A, Q0509
    mobility cart, replacement, Q0502
    monitor control cable, electric, replacement, Q0485
    monitor control cable, electric/pneumatic, Q0486
    monitor/display module, electric, replacement, Q0483
    monitor/display module, electric/electric pneumatic, replacement, Q0484
    power adapter, pneumatic, replacement, vehicle type, Q0504
    power adapter, vehicle type, Q0478
    power module, replacement, Q0479

Ventricular assist device *(Continued)*
    power-pack base, electric, replacement, Q0488
    power-pack base, electric/pneumatic, replacement, Q0489
    shower cover, electric or electric/pneumatic, replacement, Q0501
Verteporfin, J3396
Vest, safety, wheelchair, E0980
Vinblastine sulfate, J9360
Vincristine sulfate, J9370, J9371
Vinorelbine tartrate, J9390
Vision service, V2020–V2799
    bifocal, glass or plastic, V2200–V2299
    contact lenses, V2500–V2599
    frames, V2020–V2025
    intraocular lenses, V2630–V2632
    low-vision aids, V2600–V2615
    miscellaneous, V2700–V2799
    prosthetic eye, V2623–V2629
    spectacle lenses, V2100–V2199
    trifocal, glass or plastic, V2300–V2399
    variable asphericity, V2410–V2499
Visit, emergency department, G0380–G0384
Visual, function, postoperative cataract surgery, G0915–G0918
Vitamin B-12 cyanocobalamin, J3420
Vitamin K, J3430
Voice
    amplifier, L8510
    prosthesis, L8511–L8514
Von Willebrand Factor Complex, human, J7179, J7183, J7187
Voriconazole, J3465

W

Waiver, T2012–T2050
    assessment/plan of care development, T2024
    case management, per month, T2022
    day habilitation, per 15 minutes, T2021
    day habilitation, per diem, T2020
    habilitation, educational, per diem, T2012
    habilitation, educational, per hour, T2013
    habilitation, prevocational, per diem, T2014
    habilitation, prevocational, per hour, T2015
    habilitation, residential, 15 minutes, T2017
    habilitation, residential, per diem, T2016
    habilitation, supported employment, 15 minutes, T2019
    habilitation, supported employment, per diem, T2018
    targeted case management, per month, T2023
    waiver services NOS, T2025
Walker, E0130–E0149
    accessories, A4636, A4637
    attachments, E0153–E0159
    enclosed, four-sided frame, E0144
    folding (pickup), E0135
    folding, wheeled, E0143

◄ New ↻ Revised ✔ Reinstated ~~deleted~~ Deleted

Walker *(Continued)*
  heavy duty, multiple braking system, E0147
  heavy duty, wheeled, rigid or folding, E0149
  heavy duty, without wheels, E0148
  rigid (pickup), E0130
  rigid, wheeled, E0141
  with trunk support, E0140
Walking splint, L4386
Washer, Gravlee jet, *A4470*
Water
  dextrose, J7042, J7060, J7070
  distilled (for nebulizer), A7018
  pressure pad/mattress, E0187, E0198
  purification system (ESRD), E1610, E1615
  softening system (ESRD), E1625
  sterile, A4714
WBC/CBC, *G0306*
Wedges, shoe, L3340–L3420
Wellness visit; annual, *G0438, G0439*
Wet mount, Q0111
Wheel attachment, rigid pickup walker, E0155
Wheelchair, E0950–E1298, K0001–K0108,
  K0801–K0899
  accessories, E0192, E0950–E1030, E1065–E1069,
    E2211–E2230, E2300–E2399, *E2626–E2633*
  amputee, E1170–E1200
  back, fully reclining, manual, E1226
  component or accessory, not otherwise
    specified, K0108
  cushions, E2601–E2625
  custom manual wheelchair base, K0008
  custom motorized/power base, K0013
  foot box, E0954 ◀
  heavy duty, E1280–E1298, K0006, K0007,
    K0801–K0886
  lateral thigh or knee support, E0953 ◀
  lightweight, E1087–E1090, E1240–E1270
  narrowing device, E0969
  power add-on, E0983–E0984
  reclining, fully, E1014, E1050–E1070, E1100–E1110
  semi-reclining, E1100–E1110
  shock absorber, E1015–E1018
  specially sized, E1220, E1230
  standard, E1130, K0001
  stump support system, K0551
  tire, E0999
  transfer board or device, E0705
  tray, K0107
  van, non-emergency, A0130
  youth, E1091
WHFO with inflatable air chamber, L3807
Whirlpool equipment, E1300–E1310
WHO, wrist extension, L3914
Wig, A9282

Wipes, A4245, A4247
Wound
  cleanser, A6260
  closure, adhesive, G0168
  cover
    alginate dressing, A6196–A6198
    collagen dressing, A6020–A6024
    foam dressing, A6209–A6214
    hydrocolloid dressing, A6234–A6239
    hydrogel dressing, A6242–A6247
    non-contact wound warming cover, and
      accessory, E0231–E0232
    specialty absorptive dressing, A6251–A6256
  filler
    alginate dressing, A6199
    collagen based, A6010
    foam dressing, A6215
    hydrocolloid dressing, A6240–A6241
    hydrogel dressing, A6248
    not elsewhere classified, A6261–A6262
  matrix, Q4114
  pouch, A6154
  therapy, negative, pressure, pump, E2402
  wound suction, A9272, K0743
Wrapping, fabric, abdominal aneurysm, *M0301*
Wrist
  disarticulation prosthesis, L6050, L6055
  electronic wrist rotator, L7259
  hand/finger orthosis (WHFO), E1805, E1825,
    L3800–L3954

X

Xenon Xe 133, A9558
X-ray
  equipment, portable, Q0092, R0070, R0075
  single, energy, absorptiometry (SEXA), G0130
  transport, R0070–R0076
Xylocaine HCl, J2000

Y

Yttrium Y-90 ibritumomab, A9543

Z

Ziconotide, J2278
Zidovudine, J3485
Ziprasidone mesylate, J3486
Zoledronic acid, J3489

◀ New ↻ Revised ✔ Reinstated ~~deleted~~ **Deleted**

2018
TABLE OF DRUGS

IA	Intra-arterial administration
IU	International unit
IV	Intravenous administration
IM	Intramuscular administration
IT	Intrathecal
SC	Subcutaneous administration
INH	Administration by inhaled solution
VAR	Various routes of administration
OTH	Other routes of administration
ORAL	Administered orally

Intravenous administration includes all methods, such as gravity infusion, injections, and timed pushes. The "VAR" posting denotes various routes of administration and is used for drugs that are commonly administered into joints, cavities, tissues, or topical applications, in addition to other parenteral administrations. Listings posted with "OTH" indicate other administration methods, such as suppositories or catheter injections.

Blue typeface terms are added by publisher.

DRUG NAME	DOSAGE	METHOD OF ADMINISTRATION	HCPCS CODE
A			
Abatacept	10 mg	IV	J0129
Abbokinase	5,000 IU vial	IV	J3364
	250,000 IU vial	IV	J3365
Abbokinase, Open Cath	5,000 IU vial	IV	J3364
Abciximab	10 mg	IV	J0130
Abelcet	10 mg	IV	J0287-J0289
Abilify Maintena	1 mg		J0401
ABLC	50 mg	IV	J0285
AbobotulinumtoxintypeA	5 units	IM	J0586
Abraxane	1 mg		J9264
Accuneb	1 mg		J7613
Acetadote	100 mg		J0132
Acetaminophen	10 mg	IV	J0131
Acetazolamide sodium	up to 500 mg	IM, IV	J1120
Acetylcysteine			
injection	100 mg	IV	J0132
unit dose form	per gram	INH	J7604, J7608
Achromycin	up to 250 mg	IM, IV	J0120
Actemra	1 mg		J3262
ACTH	up to 40 units	IV, IM, SC	J0800
Acthar	up to 40 units	IV, IM, SC	J0800
Acthib			J3490
Acthrel	1 mcg		J0795
Actimmune	3 million units	SC	J9216
Activase	1 mg	IV	J2997

▶ New	↻ Revised	✔ Reinstated	~~deleted~~ **Deleted**

DRUG NAME	DOSAGE	METHOD OF ADMINISTRATION	HCPCS CODE
Acyclovir	5 mg		**J0133**
			J8499
Adagen	25 IU		J2504
Adalimumab	20 mg	SC	**J0135**
Adcetris	1 mg	IV	J9042
Adenocard	1 mg	IV	J0153
Adenoscan	1 mg	IV	J0153
Adenosine	1 mg	IV	**J0153**
Ado-trastuzumab Emtansine	1 mg	IV	**J9354**
Adrenalin Chloride	up to 1 ml ampule	SC, IM	J0171
Adrenalin, epinephrine	0.1 mg	SC, IM	**J0171**
Adriamycin, PFS, RDF	10 mg	IV	J9000
Adrucil	500 mg	IV	J9190
Advate	per IU		J7192
Aflibercept	1 mg	OTH	**J0178**
Agalsidase beta	1 mg	IV	**J0180**
Aggrastat	0.25 mg	IM, IV	J3246
A-hydroCort	up to 50 mg	IV, IM, SC	J1710
	up to 100 mg		J1720
Akineton	per 5 mg	IM, IV	J0190
Akynzeo	300 mg and 0.5 mg		J8655
Alatrofloxacin mesylate, injection	100 mg	IV	**J0200**
Albumin			P9041, P9045, P9046, P9047
Albuterol	0.5 mg	INH	**J7620**
concentrated form	1 mg	INH	**J7610, J7611**
unit dose form	1 mg	INH	**J7609, J7613**
Aldesleukin	per single use vial	IM, IV	**J9015**
Aldomet	up to 250 mg	IV	J0210
Aldurazyme	0.1 mg		J1931
Alefacept	0.5 mg	IM, IV	**J0215**
Alemtuzumab	1 mg		J0202
Alferon N	250,000 IU	IM	J9215
Alglucerase	per 10 units	IV	**J0205**
Alglucosidase alfa	10 mg	IV	**J0220, J0221**
Alimta	10 mg		J9305
Alkaban-AQ	1 mg	IV	J9360
Alkeran	2 mg	ORAL	J8600
	50 mg	IV	J9245
AlloDerm	per square centimeter		Q4116

▶ **New** ↻ **Revised** ✔ **Reinstated** ~~deleted~~ **Deleted**

DRUG NAME	DOSAGE	METHOD OF ADMINISTRATION	HCPCS CODE
AlloSkin	per square centimeter		Q4115
Aloxi	25 mcg		J2469
Alpha 1-proteinase inhibitor, human	10 mg	IV	J0256, J0257
Alphanate			J7186
AlphaNine SD	per IU		J7193
Alprolix	per IU		J7201
Alprostadil			
injection	1.25 mcg	OTH	J0270
urethral suppository	each	OTH	J0275
Alteplase recombinant	1 mg	IV	J2997
Alupent	per 10 mg	INH	J7667, J7668
noncompounded, unit dose	10 mg	INH	J7669
unit does	10 mg	INH	J7670
AmBisome	10 mg	IV	J0289
Amcort	per 5 mg	IM	J3302
A-methaPred	up to 40 mg	IM, IV	J2920
	up to 125 mg	IM, IV	J2930
Amgen	1 mcg	SC	J9212
Amifostine	500 mg	IV	J0207
Amikacin sulfate	100 mg	IM, IV	J0278
Aminocaproic Acid			J3490
Aminolevalinic acid HCI	unit dose (354 mg)	OTH	J7308
Aminolevulinic acid Hcl 10% Gel	10 mg	OTH	J7345
Aminolevulinate	1 g	OTH	J7309
Aminophylline/Aminophyllin	up to 250 mg	IV	J0280
Amiodarone HCI	30 mg	IV	J0282
Amitriptyline HCI	up to 20 mg	IM	J1320
Amobarbital	up to 125 mg	IM, IV	J0300
Amphadase	1 ml		J3470
Amphocin	50 mg	IV	J0285
Amphotericin B	50 mg	IV	J0285
Amphotericin B, lipid complex	10 mg	IV	J0287-J0289
Ampicillin			
sodium	up to 500 mg	IM, IV	J0290
sodium/sulbactam sodium	per 1.5 g	IM, IV	J0295
Amygdalin			J3570
Amytal	up to 125 mg	IM, IV	J0300
Anabolin LA 100	up to 50 mg	IM	J2320
Anadulafungin	1 mg	IV	J0348
Anascorp	up to 120 mg	IV	J0716

▶ **New**   ↻ **Revised**   ✔ **Reinstated**   ~~deleted~~ **Deleted**

DRUG NAME	DOSAGE	METHOD OF ADMINISTRATION	HCPCS CODE
Anastrozole	1 mg		J8999
Ancef	500 mg	IV, IM	J0690
Andrest 90-4	1 mg	IM	J3121
Andro-Cyp	1 mg		J1071
Andro-Cyp 200	1 mg		J1071
Andro L.A. 200	1 mg	IM	J3121
Andro-Estro 90-4	1 mg	IM	J3121
Andro/Fem	1 mg		J1071
Androgyn L.A.	1 mg	IM	J3121
Androlone-50	up to 50 mg		J2320
Androlone-D 100	up to 50 mg	IM	J2320
Andronaq-50	up to 50 mg	IM	J3140
Andronaq-LA	1 mg		J1071
Andronate-100	1 mg		J1071
Andronate-200	1 mg		J1071
Andropository 100	1 mg	IM	J3121
Andryl 200	1 mg	IM	J3121
Anectine	up to 20 mg	IM, IV	J0330
Anergan 25	up to 50 mg	IM, IV	J2550
	12.5 mg	ORAL	Q0169
Anergan 50	up to 50 mg	IM, IV	J2550
	12.5 mg	ORAL	Q0169
Angiomax	1 mg		J0583
Anidulafungin	1 mg	IV	J0348
Anistreplase	30 units	IV	**J0350**
Antiflex	up to 60 mg	IM, IV	J2360
Anti-Inhibitor	per IU	IV	**J7198**
Antispas	up to 20 mg	IM	J0500
Antithrombin III (human)	per IU	IV	**J7197**
Antithrombin recombinant	50 IU	IV	**J7196**
Anzemet	10 mg	IV	J1260
	50 mg	ORAL	S0174
	100 mg	ORAL	Q0180
Apidra Solostar	per 50 units		J1817
A.P.L.	per 1,000 USP units	IM	J0725
Apligraf	per square centimeter		Q4101
Apomorphine Hydrochloride	1 mg	SC	**J0364**
Aprepitant	5 mg	ORAL	J8501
Apresoline	up to 20 mg	IV, IM	J0360
Aprotinin	10,000 kiu		**J0365**

▶ **New** ↻ **Revised** ✔ **Reinstated** ~~deleted~~ **Deleted**

DRUG NAME	DOSAGE	METHOD OF ADMINISTRATION	HCPCS CODE
AquaMEPHYTON	per 1 mg	IM, SC, IV	J3430
Aralast	10 mg	IV	J0256
Aralen	up to 250 mg	IM	J0390
Aramine	per 10 mg	IV, IM, SC	J0380
Aranesp			
ESRD use	1 mcg		J0882
Non-ESRD use	1 mcg		J0881
Arbutamine	1 mg	IV	J0395
Arcalyst	1 mg		J2793
Aredia	per 30 mg	IV	J2430
Arfonad, *see* Trimethaphan camsylate			
Arformoterol tartrate	15 mcg	INH	J7605
Argatroban			
(for ESRD use)	1 mg	IV	J0884
(for non-ESRD use)	1 mg	IV	J0883
Aridol	25% in 50 ml	IV	J2150
	5 mg	INH	J7665
Arimidex			J8999
Aripiprazole	0.25 mg	IM	J0400
Aripiprazole, extended release	1 mg	IV	J0401
Aripiprazole lauroxil	1 mg	IV	J1942
Aristada	3.9 ml		J1942
Aristocort Forte	per 5 mg	IM	J3302
Aristocort Intralesional	per 5 mg	IM	J3302
Aristospan Intra-Articular	per 5 mg	VAR	J3303
Aristospan Intralesional	per 5 mg	VAR	J3303
Arixtra	per 0.5 m		J1652
Aromasin			J8999
Arranon	50 mg		J9261
Arrestin	up to 200 mg	IM	J3250
	250 mg	ORAL	Q0173
Arsenic trioxide	1 mg	IV	J9017
Arzerra	10 mg		J9302
Asparaginase	1,000 units	IV, IM	J9019
	10,000 units	IV, IM	J9020
Astagraf XL	0.1 mg		J7508
Astramorph PF	up to 10 mg	IM, IV, SC	J2270
Atezolizumab	10 mg	IV	J9022
Atgam	250 mg	IV	J7504
Ativan	2 mg	IM, IV	J2060

▶ **New**   ↻ **Revised**   ✔ **Reinstated**   ~~deleted~~ **Deleted**

DRUG NAME	DOSAGE	METHOD OF ADMINISTRATION	HCPCS CODE
Atropine			
concentrated form	per mg	INH	**J7635**
unit dose form	per mg	INH	**J7636**
sulfate	0.01 mg	IV, IM, SC	**J0461, J7636**
Atrovent	per mg	INH	J7644, J7645
ATryn	50 IU	IV	J7196
Aurothioglucose	up to 50 mg	IM	**J2910**
Autologous cultured chondrocytes implant		OTH	**J7330**
Autoplex T	per IU	IV	J7198, J7199
AUVI-Q	0.15 mg		J0171
Avastin	10 mg		J9035
Avelox	100 mg		J2280
Avelumab	10 mg	IV	**J9023**
Avonex	30 mcg	IM	J1826
	1 mcg	IM	Q3027
	1 mcg	SC	Q3028
Azacitidine	1 mg	SC	**J9025**
Azasan	50 mg		J7500
Azathioprine	50 mg	ORAL	**J7500**
Azathioprine, parenteral	100 mg	IV	**J7501**
Azithromycin, dihydrate	1 gram	ORAL	**Q0144**
Azithromycin, injection	500 mg	IV	**J0456**
B			
Baciim			J3490
Bacitracin			J3490
Baclofen	10 mg	IT	J0475
Baclofen for intrathecal trial	50 mcg	OTH	J0476
Bactocill	up to 250 mg	IM, IV	J2700
BAL in oil	per 100 mg	IM	J0470
Banflex	up to 60 mg	IV, IM	J2360
Basiliximab	20 mg	IV	J0480
BCG (Bacillus Calmette and Guerin), live	per vial	IV	**J9031**
Bebulin	per IU		J7194
Beclomethasone inhalation solution, unit dose form	per mg	INH	**J7622**
Belatacept	1 mg	IV	J0485
Beleodaq	10 mg		J9032
Belimumab	10 mg	IV	J0490
Belinostat	10 mg	IV	**J9032**
Bena-D 10	up to 50 mg	IV, IM	J1200
Bena-D 50	up to 50 mg	IV, IM	J1200

▶ **New**   ⤺ **Revised**   ✔ **Reinstated**   ~~deleted~~ **Deleted**

DRUG NAME	DOSAGE	METHOD OF ADMINISTRATION	HCPCS CODE	
Benadryl	up to 50 mg	IV, IM	J1200	
Benahist 10	up to 50 mg	IV, IM	J1200	
Benahist 50	up to 50 mg	IV, IM	J1200	
Ben-Allergin-50	up to 50 mg	IV, IM	J1200	
	50 mg	ORAL	Q0163	
Bendamustine HCl				↻
Bendeka	1 mg	IV	J9034	◀
Treanda	1 mg	IV	J9033	◀
Benefix	per IU	IV	J7195	
Benlysta	10 mg		J0490	
Benoject-10	up to 50 mg	IV, IM	J1200	
Benoject-50	up to 50 mg	IV, IM	J1200	
Bentyl	up to 20 mg	IM	J0500	
Benzocaine			J3490	
Benztropine mesylate	per 1 mg	IM, IV	J0515	
Berinert	10 units		J0597	
Berubigen	up to 1,000 mcg	IM, SC	J3420	
Beta amyloid	per study dose	OTH	A9599	
Betalin 12	up to 1,000 mcg	IM, SC	J3420	
Betameth	per 3 mg	IM, IV	J0702	
Betamethasone Acetate			J3490	
Betamethasone Acetate & Betamethasone Sodium Phosphate	per 3 mg	IM	J0702	
Betamethasone inhalation solution, unit dose form	per mg	INH	J7624	
Betaseron	0.25 mg	SC	J1830	
Bethanechol chloride	up to 5 mg	SC	J0520	
Bethkis	300 mg		J7682	
Bevacizumab	10 mg	IV	J9035	
Bezlotoxumab	10 mg	IV	J0565	◀
Bicillin C-R	100,000 units		J0558	
Bicillin C-R 900/300	100,000 units	IM	J0558, J0561	
Bicillin L-A	100,000 units	IM	J0561	
BiCNU	100 mg	IV	J9050	
Biperiden lactate	per 5 mg	IM, IV	J0190	
Bitolterol mesylate				
concentrated form	per mg	INH	J7628	
unit dose form	per mg	INH	J7629	
Bivalirudin	1 mg	IV	J0583	
Blenoxane	15 units	IM, IV, SC	J9040	
Bleomycin sulfate	15 units	IM, IV, SC	J9040	
Blinatumomab	1 microgram	IV	J9039	

▶ New   ↻ Revised   ✔ Reinstated   ~~deleted~~ Deleted

DRUG NAME	DOSAGE	METHOD OF ADMINISTRATION	HCPCS CODE
Blincyto	1 mcg		J9039
Boniva	1 mg		J1740
Bortezomib	0.1 mg	IV	J9041
Botox	1 unit		J0585
Bravelle	75 IU		J3355
Brentuximab Vedotin	1 mg	IV	J9042
Brethine			
concentrated form	per 1 mg	INH	J7680
unit dose	per 1 mg	INH	J7681
	up to 1 mg	SC, IV	J3105
Bricanyl Subcutaneous	up to 1 mg	SC, IV	J3105
Brompheniramine maleate	per 10 mg	IM, SC, IV	J0945
Bronkephrine, *see* Ethylnorepinephrine HCl			
Bronkosol			
concentrated form	per mg	INH	J7647, J7648
unit dose form	per mg	INH	J7649, J7650
Brovana			J7605
Budesonide inhalation solution			
concentrated form	0.25 mg	INH	J7633, J7634
unit dose form	0.5 mg	INH	J7626, J7627
Bumetanide			J3490
Bupivacaine			J3490
Buprenex	0.3 mg		J0592
Buprenorphine Hydrochloride	0.1 mg	IM	J0592
Buprenorphine/Naloxone	1 mg	ORAL	J0571
	< = 3 mg	ORAL	J0572
	> 3 mg but < = 6 mg	ORAL	J0573
	> 6 mg but < = 10 mg	ORAL	J0574
	> 10 mg	ORAL	J0575
Busulfan	1 mg	IV	J0594
	2 mg	ORAL	J8510
Butorphanol tartrate	1 mg		J0595
C			
C1 Esterase Inhibitor	10 units	IV	J0596-J0598
Cabazitaxel	1 mg	IV	J9043
Cabergoline	0.25 mg	ORAL	J8515
Cafcit	5 mg	IV	J0706
Caffeine citrate	5 mg	IV	J0706
Caine-1	10 mg	IV	J2001
Caine-2	10 mg	IV	J2001

▶ **New**   ↻ **Revised**   ✔ **Reinstated**   ~~deleted~~ **Deleted**

DRUG NAME	DOSAGE	METHOD OF ADMINISTRATION	HCPCS CODE
Calcijex	0.1 mcg	IM	J0636
Calcimar	up to 400 units	SC, IM	J0630
Calcitonin-salmon	up to 400 units	SC, IM	J0630
Calcitriol	0.1 mcg	IM	J0636
Calcitrol			J8499
Calcium Disodium Versenate	up to 1,000 mg	IV, SC, IM	J0600
Calcium gluconate	per 10 ml	IV	J0610
Calcium glycerophosphate and calcium lactate	per 10 ml	IM, SC	J0620
Caldolor	100 mg	IV	J1741
Calphosan	per 10 ml	IM, SC	J0620
Camptosar	20 mg	IV	J9206
Canakinumab	1 mg	SC	J0638
Cancidas	5 mg		J0637
Capecitabine	150 mg	ORAL	J8520
	500 mg	ORAL	J8521
Capsaicin patch	per sq cm	OTH	J7336
Carbidopa 5 mg/levodopa 20 mg enteral suspension		IV	J7340
Carbocaine	per 10 ml	VAR	J0670
Carbocaine with Neo-Cobefrin	per 10 ml	VAR	J0670
Carboplatin	50 mg	IV	J9045
Carfilzomib	1 mg	IV	J9047
Carimune	500 mg		J1566
Carmustine	100 mg	IV	J9050
Carnitor	per 1 g	IV	J1955
Carticel			J7330
Caspofungin acetate	5 mg	IV	J0637
Cathflo Activase	1 mg		J2997
Caverject	per 1.25 mcg		J0270
Cayston	500 mg		S0073
Cefadyl	up to 1 g	IV, IM	J0710
Cefazolin sodium	500 mg	IV, IM	J0690
Cefepime hydrochloride	500 mg	IV	J0692
Cefizox	per 500 mg	IM, IV	J0715
Cefotaxime sodium	per 1 g	IV, IM	J0698
Cefotetan			J3490
Cefoxitin sodium	1 g	IV, IM	J0694
Ceftaroline fosamil	1 mg		J0712
Ceftazidime	per 500 mg	IM, IV	J0713
Ceftazidime and avibactam	0.5 g/0.125 g	IV	J0714
Ceftizoxime sodium	per 500 mg	IV, IM	J0715

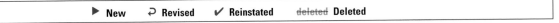

▶ New   ↻ Revised   ✔ Reinstated   ~~deleted~~ Deleted

DRUG NAME	DOSAGE	METHOD OF ADMINISTRATION	HCPCS CODE
Ceftolozane 50 mg and Tazobactam 25 mg		IV	J0695
Ceftriaxone sodium	per 250 mg	IV, IM	J0696
Cefuroxime sodium, sterile	per 750 mg	IM, IV	J0697
Celestone Soluspan	per 3 mg	IM	J0702
CellCept	250 mg	ORAL	J7517
Cel-U-Jec	per 4 mg	IM, IV	Q0511
Cenacort A-40	1 mg		J3300
	per 10 mg	IM	J3301
Cenacort Forte	per 5 mg	IM	J3302
Centruroides Immune F(ab)	up to 120 mg	IV	J0716
Cephalothin sodium	up to 1 g	IM, IV	J1890
Cephapirin sodium	up to 1 g	IV, IM	J0710
Ceprotin	10 IU		J2724
Ceredase	per 10 units	IV	J0205
Cerezyme	10 units		J1786
Certolizumab pegol	1 mg	SC	J0717
Cerubidine	10 mg	IV	J9150
Cetuximab	10 mg	IV	J9055
Chealamide	per 150 mg	IV	J3520
Chirhostim	1 mcg	IV	J2850
Chloramphenicol Sodium Succinate	up to 1 g	IV	J0720
Chlordiazepoxide HCl	up to 100 mg	IM, IV	J1990
Chloromycetin Sodium Succinate	up to 1 g	IV	J0720
Chloroprocaine HCl	per 30 ml	VAR	J2400
Chloroquine HCl	up to 250 mg	IM	J0390
Chlorothiazide sodium	per 500 mg	IV	J1205
Chlorpromazine	5 mg	ORAL	Q0161
Chlorpromazine HCl	up to 50 mg	IM, IV	J3230
Cholografin Meglumine	per ml		Q9961
Chorex-5	per 1,000 USP units	IM	J0725
Chorex-10	per 1,000 USP units	IM	J0725
Chorignon	per 1,000 USP units	IM	J0725
Chorionic Gonadotropin	per 1,000 USP units	IM	J0725
Choron 10	per 1,000 USP units	IM	J0725
Cidofovir	375 mg	IV	J0740
Cilastatin sodium, imipenem	per 250 mg	IV, IM	J0743
Cimzia	1 mg	SC	J0717
Cinacalcet		ORAL	J0604
Cinryze	10 units		J0598
Cipro IV	200 mg	IV	J0706

▶ **New**   ↻ **Revised**   ✔ **Reinstated**   ~~deleted~~ **Deleted**

DRUG NAME	DOSAGE	METHOD OF ADMINISTRATION	HCPCS CODE
Ciprofloxacin	200 mg	IV	**J0706**
octic suspension	6 mg	OTH	**J7342**
			J3490
Cisplatin, powder or solution	per 10 mg	IV	**J9060**
Cladribine	per mg	IV	**J9065**
Claforan	per 1 gm	IM, IV	J0698
Cleocin Phosphate			J3490
Clindamycin			J3490
Clofarabine	1 mg	IV	**J9027**
Clolar	1 mg		J9027
Clonidine Hydrochloride	1 mg	Epidural	**J0735**
Cobex	up to 1,000 mcg	IM, SC	J3420
Codeine phosphate	per 30 mg	IM, IV, SC	**J0745**
Codimal-A	per 10 mg	IM, SC, IV	J0945
Cogentin	per 1 mg	IM, IV	J0515
Colistimethate sodium	up to 150 mg	IM, IV	**J0770**
Collagenase, Clostridium Histolyticum	0.01 mg	OTH	**J0775**
Coly-Mycin M	up to 150 mg	IM, IV	J0770
Compa-Z	up to 10 mg	IM, IV	J0780
Compazine	up to 10 mg	IM, IV	J0780
	5 mg	ORAL	Q0164
			J8498
Compounded drug, not otherwise classified			**J7999**
Compro			J8498
Conray	per ml		Q9961
Conray 30	per ml		Q9958
Conray 43	per ml		Q9960
Copaxone	20 mg		J1595
Cophene-B	per 10 mg	IM, SC, IV	J0945
Copper contraceptive, intrauterine		OTH	**J7300**
Cordarone	30 mg	IV	J0282
Corgonject-5	per 1,000 USP units	IM	J0725
Corifact	1 IU		J7180
Corticorelin ovine triflutate	1 mcg		**J0795**
Corticotropin	up to 40 units	IV, IM, SC	**J0800**
Cortisone Acetate Micronized			J3490
Cortrosyn	per 0.25 mg	IM, IV	J0835
Corvert	1 mg		J1742
Cosmegen	0.5 mg	IV	J9120
Cosyntropin	per 0.25 mg	IM, IV	**J0833, J0834**

▶ New	↻ Revised	✔ Reinstated	~~deleted~~ Deleted

DRUG NAME	DOSAGE	METHOD OF ADMINISTRATION	HCPCS CODE
Cotranzine	up to 10 mg	IM, IV	J0780
Crofab	up to 1 gram		J0840
Cromolyn Sodium			J8499
Cromolyn sodium, unit dose form	per 10 mg	INH	J7631, J7632
Crotalidae Polyvalent Immune Fab	up to 1 gram	IV	J0840
Crysticillin 300 A.S.	up to 600,000 units	IM, IV	J2510
Crysticillin 600 A.S.	up to 600,000 units	IM, IV	J2510
Cubicin	1 mg		J0878
Cuvitru			J7799
Cyclophosphamide	100 mg	IV	J9070
oral	25 mg	ORAL	J8530
Cyclosporine	25 mg	ORAL	J7515
	100 mg	ORAL	J7502
parenteral	250 mg	IV	J7516
Cymetra	1 cc		Q4112
Cyramza	5 mg		J9308
Cysto-Cornray II	per ml		Q9958
Cystografin	per ml		Q9958
Cytarabine	100 mg	SC, IV	J9100
Cytarabine liposome	10 mg	IT	J9098
CytoGam	per vial		J0850
Cytomegalovirus immune globulin intravenous (human)	per vial	IV	J0850
Cytosar-U	100 mg	SC, IV	J9100
Cytovene	500 mg	IV	J1570
Cytoxan	100 mg	IV	J8530, J9070
D			
D-5-W, infusion	1000 cc	IV	J7070
Dacarbazine	100 mg	IV	J9130
Daclizumab	25 mg	IV	J7513
Dacogen	1 mg		J0894
Dactinomycin	0.5 mg	IV	J9120
Dalalone	1 mg	IM, IV, OTH	J1100
Dalalone L.A.	1 mg	IM	J1094
Dalbavancin	5 mg	IV	J0875
Dalteparin sodium	per 2500 IU	SC	J1645
Daptomycin	1 mg	IV	J0878
Daratumumab	10 mg	IV	J9145
Darbepoetin Alfa	1 mcg	IV, SC	J0881, J0882
Darzalex	10 mg		J9145
Daunorubicin citrate, liposomal formulation	10 mg	IV	J9151

▶ **New**   ⟲ **Revised**   ✔ **Reinstated**   ~~deleted~~ **Deleted**

DRUG NAME	DOSAGE	METHOD OF ADMINISTRATION	HCPCS CODE
Daunorubicin HCl	10 mg	IV	**J9150**
Daunoxome	10 mg	IV	J9151
DDAVP	1 mcg	IV, SC	J2597
Decadron	1 mg	IM, IV, OTH	J1100
	0.25 mg		J8540
Decadron Phosphate	1 mg	IM, IV, OTH	J1100
Decadron-LA	1 mg	IM	J1094
Deca-Durabolin	up to 50 mg	IM	J2320
Decaject	1 mg	IM, IV, OTH	J1100
Decaject-L.A.	1 mg	IM	J1094
Decitabine	1 mg	IV	**J0894**
Decolone-50	up to 50 mg	IM	J2320
Decolone-100	up to 50 mg	IM	J2320
De-Comberol	1 mg		J1071
Deferoxamine mesylate	500 mg	IM, SC, IV	**J0895**
Definity	per ml		J3490, Q9957
Degarelix	1 mg	SC	**J9155**
Dehist	per 10 mg	IM, SC, IV	J0945
Deladumone	1 mg	IM	J3121
Deladumone OB	1 mg	IM	J3121
Delatest	1 mg	IM	J3121
Delatestadiol	1 mg	IM	J3121
Delatestryl	1 mg	IM	J3121
Delestrogen	up to 10 mg	IM	J1380
Delta-Cortef	5 mg	ORAL	J7510
Demadex	10 mg/ml	IV	J3265
Demerol HCl	per 100 mg	IM, IV, SC	J2175
Denileukin diftitox	300 mcg	IV	**J9160**
Denosumab	1 mg	SC	**J0897**
DepAndro 100	1 mg		J1071
DepAndro 200	1 mg		J1071
DepAndrogyn	1 mg		J1071
DepGynogen	up to 5 mg	IM	J1000
DepMedalone 40	20 mg	IM	J1020
	40 mg	IM	J1030
	80 mg	IM	J1040
DepMedalone 80	20 mg	IM	J1020
	40 mg	IM	J1030
	80 mg	IM	J1040
DepoCyt	10 mg		J9098

▶ **New**   ↻ **Revised**   ✔ **Reinstated**   ~~deleted~~ **Deleted**

DRUG NAME	DOSAGE	METHOD OF ADMINISTRATION	HCPCS CODE
Depo-estradiol cypionate	up to 5 mg	IM	J1000
Depogen	up to 5 mg	IM	J1000
Depoject	20 mg	IM	J1020
	40 mg	IM	J1030
	80 mg	IM	J1040
Depo-Medrol	20 mg	IM	J1020
	40 mg	IM	J1030
	80 mg	IM	J1040
Depopred-40	20 mg	IM	J1020
	40 mg	IM	J1030
	80 mg	IM	J1040
Depopred-80	20 mg	IM	J1020
	40 mg	IM	J1030
	80 mg	IM	J1040
Depo-Provera Contraceptive	1 mg		J1050
Depotest	1 mg		J1071
Depo-Testadiol	1 mg		J1071
Depo-Testosterone	1 mg		J1071
Depotestrogen	1 mg		J1071
Dermagraft	per square centimeter		Q4106
Desferal Mesylate	500 mg	IM, SC, IV	J0895
Desmopressin acetate	1 mcg	IV, SC	J2597
Dexacen-4	1 mg	IM, IV, OTH	J1100
Dexacen LA-8	1 mg	IM	J1094
Dexamethasone			
concentrated form	per mg	INH	J7637
intravitreal implant	0.1 mg	OTH	J7312
unit form	per mg	INH	J7638
oral	0.25 mg	ORAL	J8540
acetate	1 mg	IM	J1094
sodium phosphate	1 mg	IM, IV, OTH	J1100
Dexasone	1 mg	IM, IV, OTH	J1100
Dexasone L.A.	1 mg	IM	J1094
Dexferrum	50 mg		J1750
Dexone	0.25 mg	ORAL	J8540
	1 mg	IM, IV, OTH	J1100
Dexone LA	1 mg	IM	J1094
Dexpak	0.25 mg	ORAL	J8540
Dexrazoxane hydrochloride	250 mg	IV	J1190
Dextran 40	500 ml	IV	J7100

▶ **New**   ⟳ **Revised**   ✔ **Reinstated**   ~~deleted~~ **Deleted**

DRUG NAME	DOSAGE	METHOD OF ADMINISTRATION	HCPCS CODE
Dextran 75	500 ml	IV	**J7110**
Dextrose 5%/normal saline solution	500 ml = 1 unit	IV	**J7042**
Dextrose/water (5%)	500 ml = 1 unit	IV	**J7060**
D.H.E. 45	per 1 mg		**J1110**
Diamox	up to 500 mg	IM, IV	**J1120**
Diazepam	up to 5 mg	IM, IV	**J3360**
Diazoxide	up to 300 mg	IV	**J1730**
Dibent	up to 20 mg	IM	**J0500**
Diclofenac sodium	37.5	IV	**J1130**
Dicyclomine HCl	up to 20 mg	IM	**J0500**
Didronel	per 300 mg	IV	**J1436**
Diethylstilbestrol diphosphate	250 mg	IV	**J9165**
Diflucan	200 mg	IV	**J1450**
DigiFab	per vial		**J1162**
Digoxin	up to 0.5 mg	IM, IV	**J1160**
Digoxin immune fab (ovine)	per vial		**J1162**
Dihydrex	up to 50 mg	IV, IM	**J1200**
	50 mg	ORAL	**Q0163**
Dihydroergotamine mesylate	per 1 mg	IM, IV	**J1110**
Dilantin	per 50 mg	IM, IV	**J1165**
Dilaudid	up to 4 mg	SC, IM, IV	**J1170**
	250 mg	OTH	**S0092**
Dilocaine	10 mg	IV	**J2001**
Dilomine	up to 20 mg	IM	**J0500**
Dilor	up to 500 mg	IM	**J1180**
Dimenhydrinate	up to 50 mg	IM, IV	**J1240**
Dimercaprol	per 100 mg	IM	**J0470**
Dimethyl sulfoxide	50%, 50 ml	OTH	**J1212**
Dinate	up to 50 mg	IM, IV	**J1240**
Dioval	up to 10 mg	IM	**J1380**
Dioval 40	up to 10 mg	IM	**J1380**
Dioval XX	up to 10 mg	IM	**J1380**
Diphenacen-50	up to 50 mg	IV, IM	**J1200**
	50 mg	ORAL	**Q0163**
Diphenhydramine HCl			
injection	up to 50 mg	IV, IM	**J1200**
oral	50 mg	ORAL	**Q0163**
Diprivan	10 mg		**J2704**
			J3490
Dipyridamole	per 10 mg	IV	**J1245**

▶ **New**   ↻ **Revised**   ✔ **Reinstated**   ~~deleted~~ **Deleted**

DRUG NAME	DOSAGE	METHOD OF ADMINISTRATION	HCPCS CODE
Disotate	per 150 mg	IV	J3520
Di-Spaz	up to 20 mg	IM	J0500
Ditate-DS	1 mg	IM	J3121
Diuril Sodium	per 500 mg	IV	J1205
D-Med 80	20 mg	IM	J1020
	40 mg	IM	J1030
	80 mg	IM	J1040
DMSO, Dimethyl sulfoxide 50%	50 ml	OTH	J1212
Dobutamine HCl	per 250 mg	IV	J1250
Dobutrex	per 250 mg	IV	J1250
Docefrez	1 mg		J9171
Docetaxel	20 mg	IV	J9170
Dolasetron mesylate			
injection	10 mg	IV	J1260
tablets	100 mg	ORAL	Q0180
Dolophine HCl	up to 10 mg	IM, SC	J1230
Dommanate	up to 50 mg	IM, IV	J1240
Donbax	10 mg		J1267
Dopamine	40 mg		J1265
Dopamine HCl	40 mg		J1265
Doribax	10 mg		J1267
Doripenem	10 mg	IV	J1267
Dornase alpha, unit dose form	per mg	INH	J7639
Dotarem	0.1 ml		A9575
Doxercalciferol	1 mcg	IV	J1270
Doxil	10 mg	IV	J9000, Q2050
Doxorubicin HCL	10 mg	IV	J9000
Doxy	100 mg		J3490
Dramamine	up to 50 mg	IM, IV	J1240
Dramanate	up to 50 mg	IM, IV	J1240
Dramilin	up to 50 mg	IM, IV	J1240
Dramocen	up to 50 mg	IM, IV	J1240
Dramoject	up to 50 mg	IM, IV	J1240
Dronabinol	2.5 mg	ORAL	Q0167
Droperidol	up to 5 mg	IM, IV	J1790
Droperidol and fentanyl citrate	up to 2 ml ampule	IM, IV	J1810
Droxia		ORAL	J8999
Drug administered through a metered dose inhaler		INH	J3535
DTIC-Dome	100 mg	IV	J9130
Dua-Gen L.A.	1 mg	IM	J3121

▶ **New**   ↻ **Revised**   ✔ **Reinstated**   deleted **Deleted**

DRUG NAME	DOSAGE	METHOD OF ADMINISTRATION	HCPCS CODE
DuoNeb	up to 2.5 mg		J7620
Duopa	20 ml		J7340
Duoval P.A.	1 mg	IM	J3121
Durabolin	up to 50 mg	IM	J2320
Duracillin A.S.	up to 600,000 units	IM, IV	J2510
Duraclon	1 mg	Epidural	J0735
Dura-Estrin	up to 5 mg	IM	J1000
Duragen-10	up to 10 mg	IM	J1380
Duragen-20	up to 10 mg	IM	J1380
Duragen-40	up to 10 mg	IM	J1380
Duralone-40	20 mg	IM	J1020
	40 mg	IM	J1030
	80 mg	IM	J1040
Duralone-80	20 mg	IM	J1020
	40 mg	IM	J1030
	80 mg	IM	J1040
Duralutin, *see* Hydroxyprogesterone Caproate			
Duramorph	up to 10 mg	IM, IV, SC	J2270, J2274
Duratest-100	1 mg		J1071
Duratest-200	1 mg		J1071
Duratestrin	1 mg		J1071
Durathate-200	1 mg	IM	J3121
Dymenate	up to 50 mg	IM, IV	J1240
Dyphylline	up to 500 mg	IM	J1180
Dysport	5 units		J0586
Dalvance	5 mg		J0875
E			
Ecallantide	1 mg	SC	J1290
Eculizumab	10 mg	IV	J1300
Edetate calcium disodium	up to 1,000 mg	IV, SC, IM	J0600
Edetate disodium	per 150 mg	IV	J3520
Elaprase	1 mg		J1743
Elavil	up to 20 mg	IM	J1320
Elelyso	10 units		J3060
Eligard	7.5 mg		J9217
Elitek	0.5 mg		J2783
Ellence	2 mg		J9178
Elliotts B solution	1 ml	OTH	J9175
Eloctate	per IU		J7205
Elosulfase alfa	1 mg	IV	J1322

▶ **New**   ↻ **Revised**   ✔ **Reinstated**   ~~deleted~~ **Deleted**

DRUG NAME	DOSAGE	METHOD OF ADMINISTRATION	HCPCS CODE
Elotuzumab	1 mg	IV	**J9176**
Eloxatin	0.5 mg		J9263
Elspar	10,000 units	IV, IM	J9020
Emend			J1453, J8501
Emete-Con, *see* Benzquinamide			
Eminase	30 units	IV	J0350
Empliciti	1 mg		J9176
Enbrel	25 mg	IM, IV	J1438
Endrate ethylenediamine-tetra-acetic acid	per 150 mg	IV	J3520
Enfuvirtide	1 mg	SC	**J1324**
Engerix-B			J3490
Enovil	up to 20 mg	IM	J1320
Enoxaparin sodium	10 mg	SC	**J1650**
Entyvio			J3380
Eovist	1 ml		A9581
Epinephrine			J7799
Epinephrine, adrenalin	0.1 mg	SC, IM	**J0171**
Epirubicin hydrochloride	2 mg		**J9178**
Epoetin alfa	100 units	IV, SC	Q4081
Epoetin alfa, non-ESRD use	1000 units	IV	**J0885**
Epoetin beta, ESRD use	1 mcg	IV	**J0887**
Epoetin beta, non-ESRD use	1 mcg	IV	**J0888**
Epogen	1,000 units		J0885
			Q4081
Epoprostenol	0.5 mg	IV	**J1325**
Eptifibatide, injection	5 mg	IM, IV	**J1327**
Eraxis	1 mg	IV	J0348
Erbitux	10 mg		J9055
Ergonovine maleate	up to 0.2 mg	IM, IV	**J1330**
Eribulin mesylate	0.1 mg	IV	**J9179**
Erivedge	150 mg		J8999
Ertapenem sodium	500 mg	IM, IV	**J1335**
Erwinase	1,000 units	IV, IM	J9019
	10,000 units	IV, IM	J9020
Erythromycin lactobionate	500 mg	IV	**J1364**
Estra-D	up to 5 mg	IM	J1000
Estradiol			
L.A.	up to 10 mg	IM	J1380
L.A. 20	up to 10 mg	IM	J1380
L.A. 40	up to 10 mg	IM	J1380

▶ **New**   ↻ **Revised**   ✔ **Reinstated**   ~~deleted~~ **Deleted**

DRUG NAME	DOSAGE	METHOD OF ADMINISTRATION	HCPCS CODE
Estradiol Cypionate	up to 5 mg	IM	J1000
Estradiol valerate	up to 10 mg	IM	J1380
Estra-L 20	up to 10 mg	IM	J1380
Estra-L 40	up to 10 mg	IM	J1380
Estra-Testrin	1 mg	IM	J3121
Estro-Cyp	up to 5 mg	IM	J1000
Estrogen, conjugated	per 25 mg	IV, IM	J1410
Estroject L.A.	up to 5 mg	IM	J1000
Estrone	per 1 mg	IM	J1435
Estrone 5	per 1 mg	IM	J1435
Estrone Aqueous	per 1 mg	IM	J1435
Estronol	per 1 mg	IM	J1435
Estronol-L.A.	up to 5 mg	IM	J1000
Etanercept, injection	25 mg	IM, IV	J1438
Etelcalcetide	0.1 mg	IV	J0606 ◀
Eteplirsen	10 mg	IV	J1428 ◀
Ethamolin	100 mg		J1430
Ethanolamine	100 mg		J1430, J3490
Ethyol	500 mg	IV	J0207
Etidronate disodium	per 300 mg	IV	J1436
Etonogestrel implant			J7307
Etopophos	10 mg	IV	J9181
Etoposide	10 mg	IV	J9181
oral	50 mg	ORAL	J8560
Euflexxa	per dose	OTH	J7323
Everolimus	0.25 mg	ORAL	J7527
Everone	1 mg	IM	J3121
Evomela	50 mg		J9245
Eylea	1 mg	OTH	J0178
F			
Fabrazyme	1 mg	IV	J0180
Factor IX			
anti-hemophilic factor, purified, non-recombinant	per IU	IV	J7193
anti-hemophilic factor, recombinant	per IU	IV	J7195, J7200-J7202
complex	per IU	IV	J7194
Factor VIIa (coagulation factor, recombinant)	1 mcg	IV	J7189

▶ **New**   ↻ **Revised**   ✔ **Reinstated**   ~~deleted~~ **Deleted**

DRUG NAME	DOSAGE	METHOD OF ADMINISTRATION	HCPCS CODE
Factor VIII (anti-hemophilic factor)			
human	per IU	IV	J7190
porcine	per IU	IV	J7191
recombinant	per IU	IV	J7182, J7185, J7192, J7188
Factor VIII (anti-hemophilic factor recombinant)			
(Afstyla)	per IU	IV	J7210
(Kovaltry)	per IU	IV	J7211
Factor VIII Fc fusion (recombinant)	per IU	IV	J7205, J7207, J7209
Factor X (human)	per IU	IV	J7175
Factor XIII A-subunit (recombinant)	per IU	IV	J7181
Factors, other hemophilia clotting	per IU	IV	J7196
Factrel	per 100 mcg	SC, IV	J1620
Famotidine			J3490
Faslodex	25 mg		J9395
Feiba NF			J7198
Feiba VH Immuno	per IU	IV	J7196
Fentanyl citrate	0.1 mg	IM, IV	J3010
Feraheme	1 mg		Q0138, Q0139
Ferric carboxymaltose	1 mg	IV	J1439
Ferric pyrophosphate citrate solution	0.1 mg of iron	IV	J1443
Ferrlecit	12.5 mg		J2916
Ferumoxytol	1 mg		Q0138, Q0139
Filgrastim			
(G-CSF)	1 mcg	SC, IV	J1442, Q5101
(TBO)	1 mcg	IV	J1447
Firazyr	1 mg	SC	J1744
Firmagon	1 mg		J9155
Flebogamma	500 mg	IV	J1572
	1 cc		J1460
Flexoject	up to 60 mg	IV, IM	J2360
Flexon	up to 60 mg	IV, IM	J2360
Flolan	0.5 mg	IV	J1325
Flo-Pred	5 mg		J7510
Florbetaben f18, diagnostic	per study dose	IV	Q9983
Floxuridine	500 mg	IV	J9200
Fluconazole	200 mg	IV	J1450
Fludara	1 mg	ORAL	J8562
	50 mg	IV	J9185

► **New**   ⏎ **Revised**   ✔ **Reinstated**   ~~deleted~~ **Deleted**

DRUG NAME	DOSAGE	METHOD OF ADMINISTRATION	HCPCS CODE
Fludarabine phosphate	1 mg	ORAL	J8562
	50 mg	IV	J9185
Flunisolide inhalation solution, unit dose form	per mg	INH	J7641
Fluocinolone		OTH	J7311, J7313
Fluorouracil	500 mg	IV	J9190
Fluphenazine decanoate	up to 25 mg		J2680
Flutamide			J8999
Flutemetamol f18, diagnostic	per study dose	IV	Q9982
Folex	5 mg	IA, IM, IT, IV	J9250
	50 mg	IA, IM, IT, IV	J9260
Folex PFS	5 mg	IA, IM, IT, IV	J9250
	50 mg	IA, IM, IT, IV	J9260
Follutein	per 1,000 USP units	IM	J0725
Folotyn	1 mg		J9307
Fomepizole	15 mg		J1451
Fomivirsen sodium	1.65 mg	Intraocular	J1452
Fondaparinux sodium	0.5 mg	SC	J1652
Formoterol	12 mcg	INH	J7640
Formoterol fumarate	20 mcg	INH	J7606
Fortaz	per 500 mg	IM, IV	J0713
Fosaprepitant	1 mg	IV	J1453
Foscarnet sodium	per 1,000 mg	IV	J1455
Foscavir	per 1,000 mg	IV	J1455
Fosphenytoin	50 mg	IV	Q2009
Fragmin	per 2,500 IU		J1645
FUDR	500 mg	IV	J9200
Fulvestrant	25 mg	IM	J9395
Fungizone intravenous	50 mg	IV	J0285
Furomide M.D.	up to 20 mg	IM, IV	J1940
Furosemide	up to 20 mg	IM, IV	J1940
G			
Gablofen	10 mg		J0475
	50 mcg		J0476
Gadavist	0.1 ml		A9585
Gadoxetate disodium	1 ml	IV	A9581
Gallium nitrate	1 mg	IV	J1457
Galsulfase	1 mg	IV	J1458
Gamastan	1 cc	IM	J1460
	over 10 cc	IM	J1560

▶ **New**   ↻ **Revised**   ✔ **Reinstated**   ~~deleted~~ **Deleted**

DRUG NAME	DOSAGE	METHOD OF ADMINISTRATION	HCPCS CODE
Gamma globulin	1 cc	IM	J1460
	over 10 cc	IM	J1560
Gammagard Liquid	500 mg	IV	J1569
Gammagard S/D			J1566
GammaGraft	per square centimeter		Q4111
Gammaplex	500 mg	IV	J1557
Gammar	1 cc	IM	J1460
	over 10 cc	IM	J1560
Gammar-IV, *see* Immune globin intravenous (human)			
Gamulin RH			
immune globulin, human	100 IU		J2791
	1 dose package, 300 mcg	IM	J2790
immune globulin, human, solvent detergent	100 IU	IV	J2792
Gamunex	500 mg	IV	J1561
Ganciclovir, implant	4.5 mg	OTH	J7310
Ganciclovir sodium	500 mg	IV	J1570
Ganirelix			J3490
Garamycin, gentamicin	up to 80 mg	IM, IV	J1580
Gastrografin	per ml		Q9963
Gatifloxacin	10 mg	IV	J1590
Gazyva	10 mg		J9301
Gefitinib	250 mg	ORAL	J8565
Gel-One	per dose	OTH	J7326
Gemcitabine HCl	200 mg	IV	J9201
Gemsar	200 mg	IV	J9201
Gemtuzumab ozogamicin	0.1 mg	IV	J9203
Gengraf	100 mg		J7502
	25 mg	ORAL	J7515
Genotropin	1 mg		J2941
Gentamicin Sulfate	up to 80 mg	IM, IV	J1580, J7699
Gentran	500 ml	IV	J7100
Gentran 75	500 ml	IV	J7110
Geodon	10 mg		J3486
Gesterol 50	per 50 mg		J2675
Glassia	10 mg	IV	J0257
Glatiramer Acetate	20 mg	SC	J1595
Gleevec (Film-Coated)	400 mg		J8999
GlucaGen	per 1 mg		J1610
Glucagon HCl	per 1 mg	SC, IM, IV	J1610

▶ New   ↻ Revised   ✔ Reinstated   ~~deleted~~ Deleted

DRUG NAME	DOSAGE	METHOD OF ADMINISTRATION	HCPCS CODE
Glukor	per 1,000 USP units	IM	J0725
Glycopyrrolate			
concentrated form	per 1 mg	INH	J7642
unit dose form	per 1 mg	INH	J7643
Gold sodium thiomalate	up to 50 mg	IM	J1600
Golimumab	1 mg	IV	J1602
Gonadorelin HCl	per 100 mcg	SC, IV	J1620
Gonal-F			J3490
Gonic	per 1,000 USP units	IM	J0725
Goserelin acetate implant	per 3.6 mg	SC	J9202
Graftjacket	per square centimeter		Q4107
Graftjacket Xpress	1 cc		Q4113
Granisetron HCl			
extended release	0.1 mg	IV	J1627
injection	100 mcg	IV	J1626
oral	1 mg	ORAL	Q0166
Gynogen L.A. A10	up to 10 mg	IM	J1380
Gynogen L.A. A20	up to 10 mg	IM	J1380
Gynogen L.A. A40	up to 10 mg	IM	J1380
H			
Halaven	0.1 mg		J9179
Haldol	up to 5 mg	IM, IV	J1630
Haloperidol	up to 5 mg	IM, IV	J1630
Haloperidol decanoate	per 50 mg	IM	J1631
Haloperidol Lactate	up to 5 mg		J1630
Hectoral	1 mcg	IV	J1270
Helixate FS	per IU		J7192
Hemin	1 mg		J1640
Hemofil M	per IU	IV	J7190
Hemophilia clotting factors (e.g., anti-inhibitors)	per IU	IV	J7198
NOC	per IU	IV	J7199
Hepagam B	0.5 ml	IM	J1571
	0.5 ml	IV	J1573
Heparin sodium	1,000 units	IV, SC	J1644
Heparin sodium (heparin lock flush)	10 units	IV	J1642
Heparin Sodium (Procine)	per 1,000 units		J1644
Hep-Lock	10 units	IV	J1642
Hep-Lock U/P	10 units	IV	J1642
Herceptin	10 mg	IV	J9355
Hexabrix 320	per ml		Q9967

▶ **New** ↻ **Revised** ✔ **Reinstated** ~~deleted~~ **Deleted**

DRUG NAME	DOSAGE	METHOD OF ADMINISTRATION	HCPCS CODE
Hexadrol Phosphate	1 mg	IM, IV, OTH	J1100
Histaject	per 10 mg	IM, SC, IV	J0945
Histerone 50	up to 50 mg	IM	J3140
Histerone 100	up to 50 mg	IM	J3140
Histrelin			
acetate	10 mcg		J1675
implant	50 mg	OTH	J9225, J9226
Hizentra, *see* Immune globulin			
Humalog	per 5 units		J1815
	per 50 units		J1817
Human fibrinogen concentrate	100 mg	IV	J7178
Humate-P	per IU		J7187
Humatrope	1 mg		J2941
Humira	20 mg		J0135
Humulin	per 5 units		J1815
	per 50 units		J1817
Hyalgan, Spurtaz or VISCO-3		IA	J7321
Hyaluronan or derivative	per dose	IV	J7327
Gel-Syn	0.1 mg	IA	J7328
Gelsyn-3	0.1 mg	IV	J7328
Gen Visc 850	1 mg	IA	J7320
Hymovis	1 mg	IA	J7322
Hyaluronic Acid			J3490
Hyaluronidase	up to 150 units	SC, IV	J3470
Hyaluronidase			
ovine	up to 999 units	VAR	J3471
ovine	per 1000 units	VAR	J3472
recombinant	1 usp	SC	J3473
Hyate:C	per IU	IV	J7191
Hybolin Decanoate	up to 50 mg	IM	J2320
Hybolin Improved, *see* Nandrolone phenpropionate			
Hycamtin	0.25 mg	ORAL	J8705
	4 mg	IV	J9351
Hydralazine HCl	up to 20 mg	IV, IM	J0360
Hydrate	up to 50 mg	IM, IV	J1240
Hydrea			J8999
Hydrocortisone acetate	up to 25 mg	IV, IM, SC	J1700
Hydrocortisone sodium phosphate	up to 50 mg	IV, IM, SC	J1710
Hydrocortisone succinate sodium	up to 100 mg	IV, IM, SC	J1720
Hydrocortone Acetate	up to 25 mg	IV, IM, SC	J1700

▶ **New**   ↻ **Revised**   ✔ **Reinstated**   ~~deleted~~ **Deleted**

DRUG NAME	DOSAGE	METHOD OF ADMINISTRATION	HCPCS CODE
Hydrocortone Phosphate	up to 50 mg	IM, IV, SC	J1710
Hydromorphone HCl	up to 4 mg	SC, IM, IV	J1170
Hydroxyprogesterone Caproate	1 mg	IM	J1725
(Makena)	10 mg	IV	J1726 ◄
NOS	10 mg	IV	J1729 ◄
Hydroxyurea			J8999
Hydroxyzine HCl	up to 25 mg	IM	J3410
Hydroxyzine Pamoate	25 mg	ORAL	Q0177
Hylan G-F 20		OTH	J7322
Hylenex	1 USP unit		J3473
Hyoscyamine sulfate	up to 0.25 mg	SC, IM, IV	J1980
Hyperrho S/D	300 mcg		J2790
	100 IU		J2792
Hyperstat IV	up to 300 mg	IV	J1730
Hyper-Tet	up to 250 units	IM	J1670
HypRho-D	300 mcg	IM	J2790
			J2791
	50 mcg		J2788
Hyrexin-50	up to 50 mg	IV, IM	J1200
Hyzine-50	up to 25 mg	IM	J3410
I			
Ibandronate sodium	1 mg	IV	J1740
Ibuprofen	100 mg	IV	J1741
Ibutilide fumarate	1 mg	IV	J1742
Icatibant	1 mg	SC	J1744
Idamycin	5 mg	IV	J9211
Idarubicin HCl	5 mg	IV	J9211
Idursulfase	1 mg	IV	J1743
Ifex	1 g	IV	J9208
Ifosfamide	1 g	IV	J9208
Ilaris	1 mg		J0638
Iloprost	20 mcg	INH	Q4074
Ilotycin, *see* Erythromycin gluceptate			
Iluvien	0.01 mg		J7313
Imferon	50 mg		J1750
Imiglucerase	10 units	IV	J1786
Imitrex	6 mg	SC	J3030
Imlygic	per 1 million plaque forming units		J9325, J9999

▶ **New**   ⤾ **Revised**   ✔ **Reinstated**   ~~deleted~~ **Deleted**

DRUG NAME	DOSAGE	METHOD OF ADMINISTRATION	HCPCS CODE
Immune globulin			
Bivigam	500 mg	IV	J1556
Cuvitru	100 mg	IV	J1555
Flebogamma	500 mg	IV	J1572
Gammagard Liquid	500 mg	IV	J1569
Gammaplex	500 mg	IV	J1557
Gamunex	500 mg	IV	J1561
HepaGam B	0.5 ml	IM	J1571
	0.5 ml	IV	J1573
Hizentra	100 mg	SC	J1559
Hyaluronidase, (HYQVIA)	100 mg	IV	J1575
NOS	500 mg	IV	J1566, J1599
Octagam	500 mg	IV	J1568
Privigen	500 mg	IV	J1459
Rhophylac	100 IU	IM	J2791
Subcutaneous	100 mg	SC	J1562
Immunosuppressive drug, not otherwise classified			J7599
Imuran	50 mg	ORAL	J7500
	100 mg	IV	J7501
Inapsine	up to 5 mg	IM, IV	J1790
Incobotulinumtoxin type A	1 unit	IM	J0588
Increlex	1 mg		J2170
Inderal	up to 1 mg	IV	J1800
Infed	50 mg		J1750
Infergen	1 mcg	SC	J9212
Inflectra			Q5102
Infliximab, injection	10 mg	IM, IV	J1745, Q5102
Infumorph	10 mg		J2274
Injectafer	1 mg		J1439
Injection sulfur hexafluoride lipid microspheres	per ml	IV	Q9950
Innohep	1,000 iu	SC	J1655
Innovar	up to 2 ml ampule	IM, IV	J1810
Insulin	5 units	SC	J1815
Insulin-Humalog	per 50 units		J1817
Insulin lispro	50 units	SC	J1817
Intal	per 10 mg	INH	J7631, J7632

▶ New   ↻ Revised   ✔ Reinstated   deleted **Deleted**

DRUG NAME	DOSAGE	METHOD OF ADMINISTRATION	HCPCS CODE
Integra			
Bilayer Matrix Wound Dressing (BMWD)	per square centimeter		Q4104
Dermal Regeneration Template (DRT)	per square centimeter		Q4105
Flowable Wound Matrix	1 cc		Q4114
Matrix	per square centimeter		Q4108
Integrilin	5 mg	IM, IV	J1327
Interferon alfa-2a, recombinant	3 million units	SC, IM	J9213
Interferon alfa-2b, recombinant	1 million units	SC, IM	J9214
Interferon alfa-n3 (human leukocyte derived)	250,000 IU	IM	J9215
Interferon alphacon-1, recombinant	1 mcg	SC	J9212
Interferon beta-1a	30 mcg	IM	J1826
	1 mcg	IM	Q3027
	1 mcg	SC	Q3028
Interferon beta-1b	0.25 mg	SC	J1830
Interferon gamma-1b	3 million units	SC	J9216
Intrauterine copper contraceptive		OTH	J7300
Intron-A	1 million units		J9214
Invanz	500 mg		J1335
Invega Sustenna	1 mg		J2426
Ipilimumab	1 mg	IV	J9228
Ipratropium bromide, unit dose form	per mg	INH	J3535, J7620, J7644, J7645
Iressa	250 mg		J8565
Irinotecan	20 mg	IV	J9206, J9205
Iron dextran	50 mg	IV, IM	J1750
Iron sucrose	1 mg	IV	J1756
Irrigation solution for Tx of bladder calculi	per 50 ml	OTH	Q2004
Isavuconazonium	1 mg	IV	J1833
Isocaine HCl	per 10 ml	VAR	J0670
Isoetharine HCl			
concentrated form	per mg	INH	J7647, J7648
unit dose form	per mg	INH	J7649, J7650
Isoproterenol HCl			
concentrated form	per mg	INH	J7657, J7658
unit dose form	per mg	INH	J7659, J7660
Isovue	per ml		Q9966, Q9967
Istodax	1 mg		J9315
Isuprel			
concentrated form	per mg	INH	J7657, J7658
unit dose form	per mg	INH	J7659, J7660

▶ **New**   ⮌ **Revised**   ✔ **Reinstated**   ~~deleted~~ **Deleted**

DRUG NAME	DOSAGE	METHOD OF ADMINISTRATION	HCPCS CODE
Itraconazole	50 mg	IV	**J1835**
Ixabepilone	1 mg	IV	**J9207**
Ixempra	1 mg		J9207
J			
Jenamicin	up to 80 mg	IM, IV	J1580
Jetrea	0.125 mg		J7316
Jevtana	1 mg		J9043
K			
Kabikinase	per 250,000 IU	IV	J2995
Kadcyla	1 mg		J9354
Kalbitor	1 mg		J1290
Kaleinate	per 10 ml	IV	J0610
Kanamycin sulfate	up to 75 mg	IM, IV	**J1850**
	up to 500 mg	IM, IV	**J1840**
Kantrex	up to 75 mg	IM, IV	J1850
	up to 500 mg	IM, IV	J1840
Keflin	up to 1 g	IM, IV	J1890
Kefurox	per 750 mg		J0697
Kefzol	500 mg	IV, IM	J0690
Kenaject-40	1 mg		J3300
	per 10 mg	IM	J3301
Kenalog-10	1 mg		J3300
	per 10 mg	IM	J3301
Kenalog-40	1 mg		J3300
	per 10 mg	IM	J3301
Kepivance	50 mcg		J2425
Keppra	10 mg		J1953
Kestrone 5	per 1 mg	IM	J1435
Ketorolac tromethamine	per 15 mg	IM, IV	**J1885**
Key-Pred 25	up to 1 ml	IM	J2650
Key-Pred 50	up to 1 ml	IM	J2650
Key-Pred-SP, *see* Prednisolone sodium phosphate			
Keytruda	1 mg		J9271
K-Flex	up to 60 mg	IV, IM	J2360
Kinevac	5 mcg	IV	J2805
Kitabis PAK	per 300 mg		J7682
Klebcil	up to 75 mg	IM, IV	J1850
	up to 500 mg	IM, IV	J1840

▶ **New** ↻ **Revised** ✔ **Reinstated** ~~deleted~~ **Deleted**

DRUG NAME	DOSAGE	METHOD OF ADMINISTRATION	HCPCS CODE
Koate-HP (anti-hemophilic factor)			
human	per IU	IV	J7190
porcine	per IU	IV	J7191
recombinant	per IU	IV	J7192
Kogenate			
human	per IU	IV	J7190
porcine	per IU	IV	J7191
recombinant	per IU	IV	J7192
Konakion	per 1 mg	IM, SC, IV	J3430
Konyne-80	per IU	IV	J7194
Krystexxa	1 mg		J2507
Kyleena	19.5 mg		J7296
Kyprolis	1 mg		J9047
Kytril	1 mg	ORAL	Q0166
	1 mg	IV	S0091
	100 mcg	IV	J1626
L			
L.A.E. 20	up to 10 mg	IM	J1380
Laetrile, Amygdalin, vitamin B-17			J3570
Lanoxin	up to 0.5 mg	IM, IV	J1160
Lanreotide	1 mg	SC	J1930
Lantus	per 5 units		J1815
Largon, *see* Propiomazine HCl			
Laronidase	0.1 mg	IV	J1931
Lasix	up to 20 mg	IM, IV	J1940
L-Caine	10 mg	IV	J2001
Lemtrada	1 mg		J0202
Lepirudin	50 mg		J1945
Leucovorin calcium	per 50 mg	IM, IV	J0640
Leukeran			J8999
Leukine	50mcg	IV	J2820
Leuprolide acetate	per 1 mg	IM	J9218
Leuprolide acetate (for depot suspension)	per 3.75 mg	IM	J1950
	7.5 mg	IM	J9217
Leuprolide acetate implant	65 mg	OTH	J9219
Leustatin	per mg	IV	J9065
Levalbuterol HCl			
concentrated form	0.5 mg	INH	J7607, J7612
unit dose form	0.5 mg	INH	J7614, J7615

▶ **New** ↻ **Revised** ✔ **Reinstated** ~~deleted~~ **Deleted**

DRUG NAME	DOSAGE	METHOD OF ADMINISTRATION	HCPCS CODE
Levaquin I.U.	250 mg	IV	J1956
Levetiracetam	10 mg	IV	J1953
Levocarnitine	per 1 gm	IV	J1955
Levo-Dromoran	up to 2 mg	SC, IV	J1960
Levofloxacin	250 mg	IV	J1956
Levoleucovorin calcium	0.5 mg	IV	J0641
Levonorgestrel implant		OTH	J7306
Levonorgestrel-releasing intrauterine contraceptive system	52 mg	OTH	J7297, J7298
Kyleena	19.5 mg	OTH	J7296
Levorphanol tartrate	up to 2 mg	SC, IV	J1960
Levsin	up to 0.25 mg	SC, IM, IV	J1980
Levulan Kerastick	unit dose (354 mg)	OTH	J7308
Lexiscan	0.1 mg		J2785
Librium	up to 100 mg	IM, IV	J1990
Lidocaine HCl	10 mg	IV	J2001
Lidoject-1	10 mg	IV	J2001
Lidoject-2	10 mg	IV	J2001
Liletta	52 mg	OTH	J7297
Lincocin	up to 300 mg	IV	J2010
Lincomycin HCl	up to 300 mg	IV	J2010
Linezolid	200 mg	IV	J2020
Lioresal	10 mg	IT	J0475
			J0476
Liquaemin Sodium	1,000 units	IV, SC	J1644
LMD (10%)	500 ml	IV	J7100
Locort	1.5 mg		J8540
Lorazepam	2 mg	IM, IV	J2060
Lovenox	10 mg	SC	J1650
Lucentis	0.1 mg		J2778
Lufyllin	up to 500 mg	IM	J1180
Lumason	per ml		Q9950
Luminal Sodium	up to 120 mg	IM, IV	J2560
Lumizyme	10 mg		J0221
Lupon Depot	7.5 mg		J9217
	3.75 mg		J1950
Lupron	per 1 mg	IM	J9218
	per 3.75 mg	IM	J1950
	7.5 mg	IM	J9217
Lyophilized, *see* Cyclophosphamide, lyophilized			

▶ **New**   ↺ **Revised**   ✔ **Reinstated**   ~~deleted~~ **Deleted**

DRUG NAME	DOSAGE	METHOD OF ADMINISTRATION	HCPCS CODE
M			
Macugen	0.3 mg		J2503
Magnesium sulfate	500 mg		**J3475**
Magnevist	per ml		**A9579**
Makena	1 mg		**J1725**
Mannitol	25% in 50 ml	IV	**J2150**
	5 mg	INH	**J7665**
Marcaine			**J3490**
Marinol	2.5 mg	ORAL	Q0167
Marmine	up to 50 mg	IM, IV	J1240
Matulane	50 mg		J8999
Maxipime	500 mg	IV	J0692
MD-76R	per ml		Q9963
MD Gastroview	per ml		Q9963
Mecasermin	1 mg	SC	**J2170**
Mechlorethamine HCl (nitrogen mustard), HN2	10 mg	IV	**J9230**
Medralone 40	20 mg	IM	J1020
	40 mg	IM	J1030
	80 mg	IM	J1040
Medralone 80	20 mg	IM	J1020
	40 mg	IM	J1030
	80 mg	IM	J1040
Medrol	per 4 mg	ORAL	**J7509**
Medroxyprogesterone acetate	1 mg*	IM	**J1050**
Mefoxin	1 g	IV, IM	J0694
Megestrol Acetate			J8999
Melphalan HCl	50 mg	IV	J9245
Melphalan, oral	2 mg	ORAL	J8600
Menoject LA	1 mg		J1071
Mepergan injection	up to 50 mg	IM, IV	J2180
Meperidine and promethazine HCl	up to 50 mg	IM, IV	**J2180**
Meperidine HCl	per 100 mg	IM, IV, SC	**J2175**
Mepivacaine HCl	per 10 ml	VAR	J0670
Mepolizumab	1 mg	IV	**J2182**
Mercaptopurine			J8999
Meropenem	100 mg	IV	**J2185**
Merrem	100 mg		J2185
Mesna	200 mg	IV	**J9209**
Mesnex	200 mg	IV	J9209

▶ **New**   ⮌ **Revised**   ✔ **Reinstated**   ~~deleted~~ **Deleted**

DRUG NAME	DOSAGE	METHOD OF ADMINISTRATION	HCPCS CODE
Metaprel			
concentrated form	per 10 mg	INH	J7667, J7668
unit dose form	per 10 mg	INH	J7669, J7670
Metaproterenol sulfate			
concentrated form	per 10 mg	INH	J7667, J7668
unit dose form	per 10 mg	INH	J7669, J7670
Metaraminol bitartrate	per 10 mg	IV, IM, SC	J0380
Metastron	per millicurie		A9600
Methacholine chloride	1 mg	INH	J7674
Methadone HCl	up to 10 mg	IM, SC	J1230
Methergine	up to 0.2 mg		J2210
Methocarbamol	up to 10 ml	IV, IM	J2800
Methotrexate LPF	5mg	IV, IM, IT, IA	J9250
	50 mg	IV, IM, IT, IA	J9260
Methotrexate, oral	2.5 mg	ORAL	J8610
Methotrexate sodium	5 mg	IV, IM, IT, IA	J9250
	50 mg	IV, IM, IT, IA	J9260
Methyldopate HCl	up to 250 mg	IV	J0210
Methylergonovine maleate	up to 0.2 mg		J2210
Methylnaltrexone	0.1 mg	SC	J2212
Methylprednisolone acetate	20 mg	IM	J1020
	40 mg	IM	J1030
	80 mg	IM	J1040
Methylprednisolone, oral	per 4 mg	ORAL	J7509
Methylprednisolone sodium succinate	up to 40 mg	IM, IV	J2920
	up to 125 mg	IM, IV	J2930
Metoclopramide HCl	up to 10 mg	IV	J2765
Metrodin	75 IU		J3355
Metronidazole			J3490
Metvixia	1 g	OTH	J7309
Miacalcin	up to 400 units	SC, IM	J0630
Micafungin sodium	1 mg		J2248
MicRhoGAM	50 mcg		J2788
Midazolam HCl	per 1 mg	IM, IV	J2250
Milrinone lactate	5 mg	IV	J2260
Minocine	1 mg		J2265
Minocycline Hydrochloride	1 mg	IV	J2265
Mircera	1 mcg		J0887, J0888
Mirena	52 mg	OTH	J7297, J7298
Mithracin	2,500 mcg	IV	J9270

▶ **New**   ↻ **Revised**   ✔ **Reinstated**   ~~deleted~~ **Deleted**

DRUG NAME	DOSAGE	METHOD OF ADMINISTRATION	HCPCS CODE
Mitomycin	0.2 mg	Ophthalmic	J7315
	5 mg	IV	J9280
Mitosol	0.2 mg	Ophthalmic	J7315
	5 mg	IV	J9280
Mitoxantrone HCl	per 5 mg	IV	J9293
Monocid, *see* Cefonicic sodium			
Monoclate-P			
human	per IU	IV	J7190
porcine	per IU	IV	J7191
Monoclonal antibodies, parenteral	5 mg	IV	J7505
Mononine	per IU	IV	J7193
Monovisc			J7327
Morphine sulfate	up to 10 mg	IM, IV, SC	J2270
preservative-free	10 mg	SC, IM, IV	J2274
Moxifloxacin	100 mg	IV	J2280
Mozobil	1 mg		J2562
M-Prednisol-40	20 mg	IM	J1020
	40 mg	IM	J1030
	80 mg	IM	J1040
M-Prednisol-80	20 mg	IM	J1020
	40 mg	IM	J1030
	80 mg	IM	J1040
Mucomyst			
unit dose form	per gram	INH	J7604, J7608
Mucosol			
injection	100 mg	IV	J0132
unit dose	per gram	INH	J7604, J7608
MultiHance	per ml		A9577
MultiHance Multipack	per ml		A9578
Muromonab-CD3	5 mg	IV	J7505
Muse		OTH	J0275
	1.25 mcg	OTH	J0270
Mustargen	10 mg	IV	J9230
Mutamycin			
	0.2 mg	Ophthalmic	J7315
	5 mg	IV	J9280
Mycamine	1 mg		J2248
Mycophenolate Mofetil	250 mg	ORAL	J7517
Mycophenolic acid	180 mg	ORAL	J7518
Myfortic	180 mg		J7518

▶ **New**   ↻ **Revised**   ✔ **Reinstated**   ~~deleted~~ **Deleted**

DRUG NAME	DOSAGE	METHOD OF ADMINISTRATION	HCPCS CODE
Myleran	1 mg		J0594
	2 mg	ORAL	J8510
Mylotarg	5mg	IV	J9300
Myobloc	per 100 units	IM	J0587
Myochrysine	up to 50 mg	IM	J1600
Myolin	up to 60 mg	IV, IM	J2360
N			
Nabilone	1 mg	ORAL	**J8650**
Nafcillin			J3490
Naglazyme	1 mg		J1458
Nalbuphine HCl	per 10 mg	IM, IV, SC	**J2300**
Naloxone HCl	per 1 mg	IM, IV, SC	**J2310, J3490**
Naltrexone			J3490
Naltrexone, depot form	1 mg	IM	**J2315**
Nandrobolic L.A.	up to 50 mg	IM	**J2320**
Nandrolone decanoate	up to 50 mg	IM	**J2320**
Narcan	1 mg	IM, IV, SC	J2310
Naropin	1 mg		J2795
Nasahist B	per 10mg	IM, SC, IV	**J0945**
Nasal vaccine inhalation		INH	**J3530**
Natalizumab	1 mg	IV	**J2323**
Natrecor	0.1 mg		J2325
Navane, *see* Thiothixene			
Navelbine	per 10 mg	IV	J9390
ND Stat	per 10 mg	IM, SC, IV	J0945
Nebcin	up to 80 mg	IM, IV	J3260
NebuPent	per 300 mg	INH	J2545, J7676
Necitumumab	1 mg	IV	**J9295**
Nelarabine	50 mg	IV	**J9261**
Nembutal Sodium Solution	per 50 mg	IM, IV, OTH	J2515
Neocyten	up to 60 mg	IV, IM	J2360
Neo-Durabolic	up to 50 mg	IM	J2320
Neoquess	up to 20 mg	IM	J0500
Neoral	100 mg		J7502
	25 mg		J7515
Neosar	100 mg	IV	J9070
Neostigmine methylsulfate	up to 0.5 mg	IM, IV, SC	**J2710**
Neo-Synephrine	up to 1 ml	SC, IM, IV	J2370
Nervocaine 1%	10 mg	IV	**J2001**
Nervocaine 2%	10 mg	IV	**J2001**

▶ **New**   ⤺ **Revised**   ✔ **Reinstated**   ~~deleted~~ **Deleted**

DRUG NAME	DOSAGE	METHOD OF ADMINISTRATION	HCPCS CODE
Nesacaine	per 30 ml	VAR	J2400
Nesacaine-MPF	per 30 ml	VAR	J2400
Nesiritide	0.1 mg	IV	J2325
Netupitant 300 mg and palonosetron 0.5 mg		ORAL	J8655
Neulasta	6 mg		J2505
Neumega	5 mg	SC	J2355
Neupogen			
(G-CSF)	1 mcg	SC, IV	J1442
Neutrexin	per 25 mg	IV	J3305
Nipent	per 10 mg	IV	J9268
Nivolumab	1 mg	IV	J9299
Nolvadex			J8999
Nordryl	up to 50mg	IV, IM	J1200
	50mg	ORAL	Q0163
Norflex	up to 60 mg	IV, IM	J2360
Norzine	up to 10 mg	IM	J3280
Not otherwise classified drugs			J3490
other than inhalation solution administered thru DME			J7799
inhalation solution administered thru DME			J7699
anti-neoplastic			J9999
chemotherapeutic		ORAL	J8999
immunosuppressive			J7599
nonchemotherapeutic		ORAL	J8499
Novantrone	per 5 mg	IV	J9293
Novarel	per 1,000 USP Units		J0725
Novolin	per 5 units		J1815
	per 50 units		J1817
Novolog	per 5 units		J1815
	per 50 units		J1817
Novo Seven	1 mcg	IV	J7189
Novoeight			J7182
NPH	5 units	SC	J1815
Nplate	100 units		J0587
	10 mcg		J2796
Nubain	per 10 mg	IM, IV, SC	J2300
Nulecit	12.5 mg		J2916
Nulicaine	10 mg	IV	J2001
Nulojix	1 mg	IV	J0485
Numorphan	up to 1 mg	IV, SC, IM	J2410
Numorphan H.P.	up to 1 mg	IV, SC, IM	J2410

▶ **New**   ↻ **Revised**   ✔ **Reinstated**   ~~deleted~~ **Deleted**

DRUG NAME	DOSAGE	METHOD OF ADMINISTRATION	HCPCS CODE	
Nusinersen	0.1 mg	IV	J2326	◀
Nutropin	1 mg		J2941	
O				
Oasis Burn Matrix	per square centimeter		Q4103	
Oasis Wound Matrix	per square centimeter		Q4102	
Obinutuzumab	10 mg		J9301	
Ocriplasmin	0.125 mg	IV	J7316	
Ocrelizumab	1 mg	IV	J2350	◀
Octagam	500 mg	IV	J1568	
Octreotide Acetate, injection	1 mg	IM	J2353	
	25 mcg	IV, SQ	J2354	
Oculinum	per unit	IM	J0585	
Ofatumumab	10 mg	IV	J9302	
Ofev			J8499	
Ofirmev	10 mg	IV	J0131	
O-Flex	up to 60 mg	IV, IM	J2360	
Oforta	10 mg		J8562	
Olanzapine	1 mg	IM	J2358	
Olaratumab	10 mg	IV	J9285	◀
Omacetaxine Mepesuccinate	0.01 mg	IV	J9262	
Omalizumab	5 mg	SC	J2357	
Omnipaque	per ml		Q9965, Q9966, Q9967	
Omnipen-N	up to 500 mg	IM, IV	J0290	
	per 1.5 gm	IM, IV	J0295	
Omniscan	per ml		A9579	
Omnitrope	1 mg		J2941	
Omontys	0.1 mg	IV, SC	J0890	
OnabotulinumtoxinA	1 unit	IM	J0585	
Oncaspar	per single dose vial	IM, IV	J9266	
Oncovin	1 mg	IV	J9370	
Ondansetron HCl	1 mg	IV	J2405	
	1 mg	ORAL	Q0162	
Onivyde	1 mg		J9205	
Opana	up to 1 mg		J2410	
Opdivo	1 mg		J9299	
Oprelvekin	5 mg	SC	J2355	
Optimark	per ml		A9579	
Optiray	per ml		Q9966, Q9967	
Optison	per ml		Q9956	

▶ **New**　↩ **Revised**　✔ **Reinstated**　~~deleted~~ **Deleted**

DRUG NAME	DOSAGE	METHOD OF ADMINISTRATION	HCPCS CODE
Oraminic II	per10mg	IM, SC, IV	J0945
Orapred	per 5 mg	ORAL	J7510
Orbactiv	10 mg		J2407
Orencia	10 mg		J0129
Oritavancin	10 mg	IV	J2407
Ormazine	up to 50 mg	IM, IV	J3230
Orphenadrine citrate	up to 60 mg	IV, IM	J2360
Orphenate	up to 60 mg	IV, IM	J2360
Orthovisc		OTH	J7324
Or-Tyl	up to 20 mg	IM	J0500
Osmitrol			J7799
Ovidrel			J3490
Oxacillin sodium	up to 250 mg	IM, IV	J2700
Oxaliplatin	0.5 mg	IV	J9263
Oxilan	per ml		Q9967
Oxymorphone HCl	up to 1 mg	IV, SC, IM	J2410
Oxytetracycline HCl	up to 50 mg	IM	J2460
Oxytocin	up to 10 units	IV, IM	J2590
Ozurdex	0.1 mg		J7312
P			
Paclitaxel	1 mg	IV	J9267
Paclitaxel protein-bound particles	1 mg	IV	J9264
Palifermin	50 mcg	IV	J2425
Paliperidone Palmitate	1 mg	IM	J2426
Palonosetron HCl	25 mcg	IV	J2469
Netupitant 300 mg and palonosetron 0.5 mg		ORAL	J8655
Pamidronate disodium	per 30 mg	IV	J2430
Panhematin	1 mg		J1640
Panitumumab	10 mg	IV	J9303
Papaverine HCl	up to 60 mg	IV, IM	J2440
Paragard T 380 A		OTH	J7300
Paraplatin	50 mg	IV	J9045
Paricalcitol, injection	1 mcg	IV, IM	J2501
Pasireotide, long acting	1 mg	IV	J2502
Pathogen(s) test for platelets		OTH	P9100
Peforomist	20 mcg		J7606
Pegademase bovine	25 IU		J2504
Pegaptinib	0.3 mg	OTH	J2503
Pegaspargase	per single dose vial	IM, IV	J9266
Pegasys			J3490

▶ **New**　⟳ **Revised**　✔ **Reinstated**　~~deleted~~ **Deleted**

DRUG NAME	DOSAGE	METHOD OF ADMINISTRATION	HCPCS CODE
Pegfilgrastim	6 mg	SC	J2505
Peginesatide	0.1 mg	IV, SC	J0890
Peg-Intron			J3490
Pegloticase	1 mg	IV	J2507
Pembrolizumab	1 mg	IV	J9271
Pemetrexed	10 mg	IV	J9305
Penicillin G Benzathine	100,000 units	IM	J0561
Penicillin G Benzathine and Penicillin G Procaine	100,000 units	IM	J0558
Penicillin G potassium	up to 600,000 units	IM, IV	J2540
Penicillin G procaine, aqueous	up to 600,000 units	IM, IV	J2510
Penicillin G Sodium			J3490
Pentam	per 300 mg		J7676
Pentamidine isethionate	per 300 mg	INH, IM	J2545, J7676
Pentastarch, 10%	100 ml		J2513
Pentazocine HCl	30 mg	IM, SC, IV	J3070
Pentobarbital sodium	per 50 mg	IM, IV, OTH	J2515
Pentostatin	per 10 mg	IV	J9268
Peramivir	1 mg	IV	J2547
Perjeta	1 mg		J9306
Permapen	up to 600,000	IM	J0561
Perphenazine			
Injection	up to 5 mg	IM, IV	J3310
tablets	4 mg	ORAL	Q0175
Persantine IV	per 10 mg	IV	J1245
Pertuzumab	1 mg	IV	J9306
Pet Imaging			
Fluciclovine F-18, diagnostic	1 millcurie	IV	A9588
Gallium Ga-68, dotatate, diagnostic	0.1 millicurie	IV	A9587
Pfizerpen	up to 600,000 units	IM, IV	J2540
Pfizerpen A.S.	up to 600,000 units	IM, IV	J2510
Phenadoz			J8498
Phenazine 25	up to 50 mg	IM, IV	J2550
	12.5 mg	ORAL	Q0169
Phenazine 50	up to 50 mg	IM, IV	J2550
	12.5 mg	ORAL	Q0169
Phenergan	12.5 mg	ORAL	Q0169
	up to 50 mg	IM, IV	J2550
			J8498
Phenobarbital sodium	up to 120 mg	IM, IV	J2560
Phentolamine mesylate	up to 5 mg	IM, IV	J2760

▶ **New**   ↻ **Revised**   ✔ **Reinstated**   ~~deleted~~ **Deleted**

DRUG NAME	DOSAGE	METHOD OF ADMINISTRATION	HCPCS CODE
Phenylephrine HCl	up to 1 ml	SC, IM, IV	J2370, J7799
Phenytoin sodium	per 50 mg	IM, IV	J1165
Photofrin	75 mg	IV	J9600
Phytonadione (Vitamin K)	per 1 mg	IM, SC, IV	J3430
Piperacillin/Tazobactam Sodium, injection	1.125 g	IV	J2543
Pitocin	up to 10 units	IV, IM	J2590
Plantinol AQ	10 mg	IV	J9060
Plasma			
cryoprecipitate reduced	each unit	IV	P9044
pooled multiple donor, frozen	each unit	IV	P9023, P9070
(single donor), pathogen reduced, frozen	each unit	IV	P9071
Plas+SD	each unit	IV	P9023
Platelets, pheresis, pathogen reduced	each unit	IV	P9073
Pathogen(s) test for platelets		OTH	P9100
Platinol	10 mg	IV, IM	J9060
Plerixafor	1 mg	SC	J2562
Plicamycin	2,500 mcg	IV	J9270
Polocaine	per 10 ml	VAR	J0670
Polycillin-N	up to 500 mg	IM, IV	J0290
	per 1.5 gm	IM, IV	J0295
Polygam	500 mg		J1566
Porfimer Sodium	75 mg	IV	J9600
Portrazza	1 mg		J9295
Positron emission tomography radiopharmaceutical, diagnostic			
for non-tumor identification, NOC		IV	A9598
for tumor identification, NOC		IV	A9597
Potassium chloride	per 2 mEq	IV	J3480
Potassium Chloride	up to 1,000 cc		J7120
Pralatrexate	1 mg	IV	J9307
Pralidoxime chloride	up to 1 g	IV, IM, SC	J2730
Predalone-50	up to 1 ml	IM	J2650
Predcor-25	up to 1 ml	IM	J2650
Predcor-50	up to 1 ml	IM	J2650
Predicort-50	up to 1 ml	IM	J2650
Prednisolone acetate	up to 1 ml	IM	J2650
Prednisolone, oral	5 mg	ORAL	J7510
Prednisone, immediate release or delayed release	1 mg	ORAL	J7512
Predoject-50	up to 1 ml	IM	J2650
Pregnyl	per 1,000 USP units	IM	J0725
Premarin Intravenous	per 25 mg	IV, IM	J1410

▶ **New**　　↻ **Revised**　　✔ **Reinstated**　　~~deleted~~ **Deleted**

DRUG NAME	DOSAGE	METHOD OF ADMINISTRATION	HCPCS CODE
Prescription, chemotherapeutic, not otherwise specified		ORAL	**J8999**
Prescription, nonchemotherapeutic, not otherwise specified		ORAL	**J8499**
Prialt	1 mcg		J2278
Primacor	5 mg	IV	J2260
Primatrix	per square centimeter		Q4110
Primaxin	per 250 mg	IV, IM	J0743
Priscoline HCl	up to 25 mg	IV	J2670
Privigen	500 mg	IV	**J1459**
Probuphine System Kit			J0570
Procainamide HCl	up to 1 g	IM, IV	**J2690**
Prochlorperazine	up to 10 mg	IM, IV	**J0780**
			J8498
Prochlorperazine maleate	5 mg	ORAL	**Q0164**
	5 mg		S0183
Procrit			J0885
			Q4081
Pro-Depo, *see* Hydroxyprogesterone Caproate			
Profasi HP	per 1,000 USP units	IM	J0725
Profilnine Heat-Treated			
non-recombinant	per IU	IV	J7193
recombinant	per IU	IU	J7195, J7200- J7202
complex	per IU	IV	J7194
Profonol	10 mg/ml		J3490
Progestaject	per 50 mg		J2675
Progesterone	per 50 mg	IM	**J2675**
Prograf			
oral	1 mg	ORAL	J7507
parenteral	5mg		J7525
Prohance Multipack	per ml		A9576
Prokine	50 mcg	IV	J2820
Prolastin	10 mg	IV	J0256
Proleukin	per single use vial	IM, IV	J9015
Prolia	1 mg		J0897
Prolixin Decanoate	up to 25 mg	IM, SC	J2680
Promazine HCl	up to 25 mg	IM	**J2950**
Promethazine			J8498
Promethazine HCl			
injection	up to 50 mg	IM, IV	**J2550**
oral	12.5 mg	ORAL	**Q0169**

▶ **New**   ⤺ **Revised**   ✔ **Reinstated**   ~~deleted~~ **Deleted**

DRUG NAME	DOSAGE	METHOD OF ADMINISTRATION	HCPCS CODE
Promethegan			J8498
Pronestyl	up to 1 g	IM, IV	J2690
Proplex SX-T			
non-recombinant	per IU	IV	J7193
recombinant	per IU		J7195, J7200-J7202
complex	per IU	IV	J7194
Proplex T			
non-recombinant	per IU	IV	J7193
recombinant	per IU		J7195, J7200-J7202
complex	per IU	IV	J7194
Propofol	10 mg	IV	J2704
Propranolol HCl	up to 1 mg	IV	J1800
Prorex-25			
	up to 50 mg	IM, IV	J2550
	12.5 mg	ORAL	Q0169
Prorex-50	up to 50 mg	IM, IV	J2550
	12.5 mg	ORAL	Q0169
Prostaglandin E1	per 1.25 mcg		J0270
Prostaphlin	up to 1 g	IM, IV	J2690
Prostigmin	up to 0.5 mg	IM, IV, SC	J2710
Prostin VR Pediatric	0.5 mg		J0270
Protamine sulfate	per 10 mg	IV	J2720
Protein C Concentrate	10 IU	IV	J2724
Prothazine	up to 50 mg	IM, IV	J2550
	12.5 mg	ORAL	Q0169
Protirelin	per 250 mcg	IV	J2725
Protonix			J3490
Protopam Chloride	up to 1 g	IV, IM, SC	J2730
Provenge			Q2043
Proventil			
concentrated form	1 mg	INH	J7610, J7611
unit dose form	1 mg	INH	J7609, J7613
Provocholine	per 1 mg		J7674
Prozine-50	up to 25 mg	IM	J2950
Pulmicort Respules			
concentrated form	0.25 mg	INH	J7633, J7634
unit does	0.5 mg	INH	J7626, J7627
Pulmozyme	per mg		J7639
Pyridoxine HCl	100 mg		J3415

▶ **New**   ↻ **Revised**   ✔ **Reinstated**   ~~deleted~~ **Deleted**

DRUG NAME	DOSAGE	METHOD OF ADMINISTRATION	HCPCS CODE
Q			
Quelicin	up to 20 mg	IV, IM	J0330
Quinupristin/dalfopristin	500 mg (150/350)	IV	J2770
Qutenza	per square cm		J7336
R			
Ramucirumab	5 mg	IV	J9308
Ranibizumab	0.1 mg	OTH	J2778
Ranitidine HCl, injection	25 mg	IV, IM	J2780
Rapamune	1 mg	ORAL	J7520
Rasburicase	0.5 mg	IV	J2783
Rebif	11 mcg		Q3026
Reclast	1 mg		J3489
Recombinate			
human	per IU	IV	J7190
porcine	per IU	IV	J7191
recombinant	per IU	IV	J7192
Recombivax			J3490
Redisol	up to 1,000 mcg	IM, SC	J3420
Regadenoson	0.1 mg	IV	J2785
Regitine	up to 5 mg	IM, IV	J2760
Reglan	up to 10 mg	IV	J2765
Regular	5 units	SC	J1815
Relefact TRH	per 250 mcg	IV	J2725
Relistor	0.1 mg	SC	J2212
Remicade	10 mg	IM, IV	J1745
Remodulin	1 mg		J3285
Renflexis			Q5102
ReoPro	10 mg	IV	J0130
Rep-Pred 40	20 mg	IM	J1020
	40 mg	IM	J1030
	80 mg	IM	J1040
Rep-Pred 80	20 mg	IM	J1020
	40 mg	IM	J1030
	80 mg	IM	J1040
Resectisol			J7799
Reslizumab	1 mg	IV	J2786
Retavase	18.1 mg	IV	J2993
Reteplase	18.8 mg	IV	J2993
Retisert			J7311
Retrovir	10 mg	IV	J3485

▶ **New**   ↻ **Revised**   ✔ **Reinstated**   ~~deleted~~ **Deleted**

DRUG NAME	DOSAGE	METHOD OF ADMINISTRATION	HCPCS CODE
Rheomacrodex	500 ml	IV	J7100
Rhesonativ	300 mcg	IM	J2790
	50 mg		J2788
Rheumatrex Dose Pack	2.5 mg	ORAL	J8610
Rho(D)			
immune globulin		IM, IV	J2791
immune globulin, human	1 dose package/ 300 mcg	IM	J2790
	50 mg	IM	J2788
immune globulin, human, solvent detergent	100	IV, IU	J2792
RhoGAM	300 mcg	IM	J2790
	50 mg		J2788
Rhophylac	100 IU	IM, IV	J2791
Riastap	100 mg		J7178
Rifadin			J3490
Rifampin			J3490
Rilonacept	1 mg	SC	J2793
RimabotulinumtoxinB	100 units	IM	J0587
Rimso-50	50 ml		J1212
Ringers lactate infusion	up to 1,000 cc	IV	J7120, J7121
Risperdal Costa	0.5 mg		J2794
Risperidone	0.5 mg	IM	J2794
Rituxan	100 mg	IV	J9310
Rituximab	100 mg	IV	J9310
Rixubis			J7200
Robaxin	up to 10 ml	IV, IM	J2800
Rocephin	per 250 mg	IV, IM	J0696
Roferon-A	3 million units	SC, IM	J9213
Rolapitant, oral, 1 mg	1 mg	ORAL	J8670
Romidepsin	1 mg	IV	J9315
Romiplostim	10 mcg	SC	J2796
Ropivacaine Hydrochloride	1 mg	OTH	J2795
Rubex	10 mg	IV	J9000
Rubramin PC	up to 1,000 mcg	IM, SC	J3420

▶ **New** ↻ **Revised** ✔ **Reinstated** ~~deleted~~ **Deleted**

DRUG NAME	DOSAGE	METHOD OF ADMINISTRATION	HCPCS CODE
S			
Saizen	1 mg		**J2941**
Saline solution	10 ml		**A4216**
5% dextrose	500 ml	IV	**J7042**
infusion	250 cc	IV	**J7050**
	1,000 cc	IV	**J7030**
sterile	500 ml = 1 unit	IV, OTH	**J7040**
Sandimmune	25 mg	ORAL	**J7515**
	100 mg	ORAL	**J7502**
	250 mg	OTH	**J7516**
Sandoglobulin, *see* Immune globin intravenous (human)			
Sandostatin, Lar Depot	25 mcg		**J2354**
	1 mg	IM	**J2353**
Sargramostim (GM-CSF)	50 mcg	IV	**J2820**
Sculptra	0.5 mg	IV	**Q2028**
Sebelelipase alfa	1 mg	IV	**J2840**
Selestoject	per 4 mg	IM, IV	**J0702**
Sermorelin acetate	1 mcg	SC	**Q0515**
Serostim	1 mg		**J2941**
Signifor LAR	20 ml		**J2502**
Siltuximab	10 mg	IV	**J2860**
Simponi Aria	1 mg		**J1602**
Simulect	20 mg		**J0480**
Sincalide	5 mcg	IV	**J2805**
Sinografin	per ml		**Q9963**
Sinusol-B	per 10 mg	IM, SC, IV	**J0945**
Sirolimus	1 mg	ORAL	**J7520**
Sivextro	1 mg		**J3090**
Skyla	13.5 mg	OTH	**J7301**
Smz-TMP			**J3490**
Sodium Chloride	1,000 cc		**J7030**
	500 ml = 1 unit		**J7040**
	500 ml		**A4217**
	250 cc		**J7050**
Bacteriostatic	10 ml		**A4216**
Sodium Chloride Concentrate			**J7799**
Sodium ferricgluconate in sucrose	12.5 mg		**J2916**

▶ **New**   ⮌ **Revised**   ✔ **Reinstated**   ~~deleted~~ **Deleted**

DRUG NAME	DOSAGE	METHOD OF ADMINISTRATION	HCPCS CODE
Sodium Hyaluronate			J3490
Euflexxa			**J7323**
Hyalgan, Spurtaz, Visco-3			**J7321**
Orthovisc			**J7324**
Solganal	up to 50 mg	IM	J2910
Soliris	10 mg		J1300
Solu-Cortef	up to 50 mg	IV, IM, SC	J1710
	100 mg		J1720
Solu-Medrol	up to 40 mg	IM, IV	J2920
	up to 125 mg	IM, IV	J2930
Solurex	1 mg	IM, IV, OTH	J1100
Solurex LA	1 mg	IM	J1094
Somatrem	1 mg	SC	**J2940**
Somatropin	1 mg	SC	**J2941**
Somatulin Depot	1 mg		J1930
Sparine	up to 25 mg	IM	J2950
Spasmoject	up to 20 mg	IM	J0500
Spectinomycin HCl	up to 2 g	IM	**J3320**
Sporanox	50 mg	IV	J1835
Staphcillin, *see* Methicillin sodium			
Stelara	1 mg		J3357
Stilphostrol	250 mg	IV	J9165
Streptase	250,000 IU	IV	J2995
Streptokinase	per 250,000	IU, IV	**J2995**
Streptomycin	up to 1 g	IM	**J3000**
Streptomycin Sulfate	up to 1 g	IM	**J3000**
Streptozocin	1 gm	IV	**J9320**
Strontium-89 chloride	per millicurie		**A9600**
Sublimaze	0.1 mg	IM, IV	J3010
Succinylcholine chloride	up to 20 mg	IV, IM	**J0330**
Sufentanil Citrate			J3490
Sumarel Dosepro	6 mg		J3030
Sumatriptan succinate	6 mg	SC	**J3030**
Supartz		OTH	**J7321**
Supprelin LA	50 mg		J9226
Surostrin	up to 20 mg	IV, IM	**J0330**
Sus-Phrine	up to 1 ml ampule	SC, IM	J0171
Synercid	500 mg (150/350)	IV	J2770
Synkavite	per 1 mg	IM, SC, IV	J3430
Synribo	0.01 mg		J9262

▶ **New** ↻ **Revised** ✔ **Reinstated** ~~deleted~~ **Deleted**

DRUG NAME	DOSAGE	METHOD OF ADMINISTRATION	HCPCS CODE
Syntocinon	up to 10 units	IV, IM	J2590
Synvisc and Synvisc-One	1 mg	OTH	J7325
Syrex	10 ml		A4216
Sytobex	1,000 mcg	IM, SC	J3420
T			
Tacrolimus			
(Envarsus XR)	0.25 mg	ORAL	J7503
oral, extended release	0.1 mg	ORAL	J7508
oral, immediate release	1 mg	ORAL	J7507
parenteral	5 mg	IV	J7525
Taliglucerase Alfa	10 units	IV	J3060
Talimogene laherparepvec	per 1 million plaque forming units	IV	J9325
Talwin	30 mg	IM, SC, IV	J3070
Tamoxifen Citrate			J8999
Taractan, *see* Chlorprothixene			
Taxol	1 mg	IV	J9267
Taxotere	20mg	IV	J9171
Tazicef	per 500 mg		J0713
Tazidime, *see* Ceftazidime Technetium TC Sestambi	per dose		A9500
			J0713
Tedizolid phosphate	1 mg	IV	J3090
TEEV	1 mg	IM	J3121
Teflaro	1 mg		J0712
Telavancin	10 mg	IV	J3095
Temodar	5 mg	ORAL	J8700, J9328
Temozolomide	1 mg	IV	J9328
	5 mg	ORAL	J8700
Temsirolimus	1 mg	IV	J9330
Tenecteplase	1 mg	IV	J3101
Teniposide	50 mg		Q2017
Tepadina	15 mg		J9340
Tequin	10 mg	IV	J1590
Terbutaline sulfate	up to 1 mg	SC, IV	J3105
concentrated form	per 1 mg	INH	J7680
unit dose form	per 1 mg	INH	J7681
Teriparatide	10 mcg	SC	J3110
Terramycin IM	up to 50 mg	IM	J2460
Testa-C	1 mg		J1071
Testadiate	1 mg	IM	J3121

▶ New   ↻ Revised   ✔ Reinstated   ~~deleted~~ Deleted

DRUG NAME	DOSAGE	METHOD OF ADMINISTRATION	HCPCS CODE
Testadiate-Depo	1 mg		J1071
Testaject-LA	1 mg		J1071
Testaqua	up to 50 mg	IM	J3140
Test-Estro Cypionates	1 mg		J1071
Test-Estro-C	1 mg		J1071
Testex	up to 100 mg	IM	J3150
Testo AQ	up to 50 mg		J3140
Testoject-50	up to 50 mg	IM	J3140
Testoject-LA	1 mg		J1071
Testone			
LA 100	1 mg	IM	J3121
LA 200	1 mg	IM	J3121
Testopel Pellets			J3490
Testosterone Aqueous	up to 50 mg	IM	J3140
Testosterone cypionate	1 mg	IM	J1071
Testosterone enanthate	1 mg	IM	J3121
Testosterone undecanoate	1 mg	IM	J3145
Testradiol 90/4	1 mg	IM	J3121
Testrin PA	1 mg	IM	J3121
Testro AQ	up to 50 mg		J3140
Tetanus immune globulin, human	up to 250 units	IM	J1670
Tetracycline	up to 250 mg	IM, IV	J0120
Thallous Chloride TI-201	per MCI		A9505
Theelin Aqueous	per 1 mg	IM	J1435
Theophylline	per 40 mg	IV	J2810
TheraCys	per vial	IV	J9031
Thiamine HCl	100 mg		J3411
Thiethylperazine maleate			
injection	up to 10 mg	IM	J3280
oral	10 mg	ORAL	Q0174
Thiotepa	15 mg	IV	J9340
Thorazine	up to 50 mg	IM, IV	J3230
Thrombate III	per IU		J7197
Thymoglobulin (*see also* Immune globin)			
anti-thymocyte globulin, equine	250 mg	IV	J7504
anti-thymocyte globulin, rabbit	25 mg	IV	J7511
Thypinone	per 250 mcg	IV	J2725
Thyrogen	0.9 mg	IM, SC	J3240
Thyrotropin Alfa, injection	0.9 mg	IM, SC	J3240
Tice BCG	per vial	IV	J9031

▶ **New**   ↻ **Revised**   ✔ **Reinstated**   ~~deleted~~ **Deleted**

DRUG NAME	DOSAGE	METHOD OF ADMINISTRATION	HCPCS CODE
Ticon			
injection	up to 200 mg	IM	J3250
oral	250 mg	ORAL	Q0173
Tigan			
injection	up to 200 mg	IM	J3250
oral	250 mg	ORAL	Q0173
Tigecycline	1 mg	IV	J3243
Tiject-20			
injection	up to 200 mg	IM	J3250
oral	250 mg	ORAL	Q0173
Tinzaparin	1,000 IU	SC	J1655
Tirofiban Hydrochloride, injection	0.25 mg	IM, IV	J3246
TNKase	1 mg	IV	J3101
Tobi	300 mg	INH	J7682, J7685
Tobramycin, inhalation solution	300 mg	INH	J7682, J7685
Tobramycin sulfate	up to 80 mg	IM, IV	J3260
Tocilizumab	1 mg	IV	J3262
Tofranil, *see* Imipramine HCl			
Tolazoline HCl	up to 25 mg	IV	J2670
Toposar	10 mg		J9181
Topotecan	0.25 mg	ORAL	J8705
	0.1 mg	IV	J9351
Toradol	per 15 mg	IM, IV	J1885
Torecan			
injection	up to 10 mg	IM	J3280
oral	10 mg	ORAL	Q0174
Torisel	1 mg		J9330
Tornalate			
concentrated form	per mg	INH	J7628
unit dose	per mg	INH	J7629
Torsemide	10 mg/ml	IV	J3265
Totacillin-N	up to 500 mg	IM, IV	J0290
	per 1.5 gm	IM, IV	J0295
Trabectedin	0.1 mg	IV	J9352
Trastuzumab	10 mg	IV	J9355
Treanda	1 mg	IV	J3490, J9033
Trelstar	3.75 mg		J3315
Treprostinil	1 mg		J3285, J7686
Trexall	2.5 mg	ORAL	J8610

▶ **New**   ↻ **Revised**   ✔ **Reinstated**   ~~deleted~~ **Deleted**

DRUG NAME	DOSAGE	METHOD OF ADMINISTRATION	HCPCS CODE
Triam-A	1 mg		J3300
	per 10 mg	IM	J3301
Triamcinolone			
concentrated form	per 1 mg	INH	J7683
unit dose	per 1 mg	INH	J7684
Triamcinolone acetonide	1 mg		J3300
	per 10 mg	IM	J3301
Triamcinolone diacetate	per 5 mg	IM	J3302
Triamcinolone hexacetonide	per 5 mg	VAR	J3303
Triesence	1 mg		J3300
	per 10 mg	IM	J3301
Triethylene thio Phosphoramide/T	15 mg		J9340
Triflupromazine HCl	up to 20 mg	IM, IV	J3400
Tri-Kort	1 mg		J3300
	per 10 mg	IM	J3301
Trilafon	4 mg	ORAL	Q0175
	up to 5 mg	IM, IV	J3310
Trilog	1 mg		J3300
	per 10 mg	IM	J3301
Trilone	per 5 mg		J3302
Trimethobenzamide HCl			
injection	up to 200 mg	IM	J3250
oral	250 mg	ORAL	Q0173
Trimetrexate glucuronate	per 25 mg	IV	J3305
Triptorelin Pamoate	3.75 mg	SC	J3315
Trisenox	1 mg	IV	J9017
Trobicin	up to 2 g	IM	J3320
Trovan	100 mg	IV	J0200
Tysabri	1 mg		J2323
Tyvaso	1.74 mg		J7686
U			
Ultravist 240	per ml		Q9966
Ultravist 300	per ml		Q9967
Ultravist 370	per ml		Q9967
Ultrazine-10	up to 10 mg	IM, IV	J0780
Unasyn	per 1.5 gm	IM, IV	J0295
Unclassified drugs (*see also* Not elsewhere classified)			J3490
Unspecified oral antiemetic			Q0181
Urea	up to 40 g	IV	J3350

▶ **New**   ↻ **Revised**   ✔ **Reinstated**   ~~deleted~~ **Deleted**

DRUG NAME	DOSAGE	METHOD OF ADMINISTRATION	HCPCS CODE
Ureaphil	up to 40 g	IV	J3350
Urecholine	up to 5 mg	SC	J0520
Urofollitropin	75 IU		J3355
Urokinase	5,000 IU vial	IV	J3364
	250,000 IU vial	IV	J3365
Ustekinumab	1 mg	SC	J3357
	1 mg	IV	J3358
V			
Valcyte			J3490
Valergen 10	10 mg	IM	J1380
Valergen 20	10 mg	IM	J1380
Valergen 40	up to 10 mg	IM	J1380
Valertest No. 1	1 mg	IM	J3121
Valertest No. 2	1 mg	IM	J3121
Valganciclovir HCL			J8499
Valium	up to 5 mg	IM, IV	J3360
Valrubicin, intravesical	200 mg	OTH	J9357
Valstar	200 mg	OTH	J9357
Vancocin	500 mg	IV, IM	J3370
Vancoled	500 mg	IV, IM	J3370
Vancomycin HCl	500 mg	IV, IM	J3370
Vantas	50 mg		J9226, J9225
Varubi	90 mg		J8670
Vasceze	per 10 mg		J1642
Vasoxyl, *see* Methoxamine HCl			
Vectibix	10 mg		J9303
Vedolizumab	1 mg	IV	J3380
Velaglucerase alfa	100 units	IV	J3385
Velban	1 mg	IV	J9360
Velcade	0.1 mg		J9041
Veletri	0.5 mg		J1325
Velsar	1 mg	IV	J9360
Venofer	1 mg	IV	J1756
Ventavis	20 mcg		Q4074
Ventolin	0.5 mg	INH	J7620
concentrated form	1 mg	INH	J7610, J7611
unit dose form	1 mg	INH	J7609, J7613
VePesid	50 mg	ORAL	J8560
Veritas Collagen Matrix			J3490

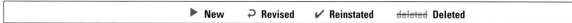

▶ **New**   ⟳ **Revised**   ✔ **Reinstated**   ~~deleted~~ **Deleted**

DRUG NAME	DOSAGE	METHOD OF ADMINISTRATION	HCPCS CODE
Versed	per 1 mg	IM, IV	J2250
Verteporfin	0.1 mg	IV	**J3396**
Vesprin	up to 20 mg	IM, IV	J3400
VFEND IV	10 mg	IV	J3465
V-Gan 25	up to 50 mg	IM, IV	J2550
	12.5 mg	ORAL	Q0169
V-Gan 50	up to 50 mg	IM, IV	J2550
	12.5 mg	ORAL	Q0169
Viadur	65 mg	OTH	J9219
Vibativ	10 mg		J3095
Vinblastine sulfate	1 mg	IV	**J9360**
Vincasar PFS	1 mg	IV	J9370
Vincristine sulfate	1 mg	IV	**J9370**
Vincristine sulfate Liposome	1 mg	IV	**J9371**
Vinorelbine tartrate	per 10 mg	IV	**J9390**
Vispaque	per ml		Q9966, Q9967
Vistaject-25	up to 25 mg	IM	J3410
Vistaril	up to 25 mg	IM	J3410
	25mg	ORAL	Q0177
Vistide	375 mg	IV	J0740
Visudyne	0.1 mg	IV	J3396
Vitamin B-12 cyanocobalamin	up to 1,000 mcg	IM, SC	**J3420**
Vitamin K, phytonadione, menadione, menadiol sodium diphosphate	per 1 mg	IM, SC, IV	**J3430**
Vitrase	per 1 USP unit		J3471
Vivaglobin	100 mg		J1562
Vivitrol	1 mg		J2315
Von Willebrand Factor Complex, human	per IU VWF:RCo	IV	**J7187**
Wilate	per IU VWF	IV	**J7183**
Vonvendi	per IU VWF	IV	**J7179**
Voriconazole	10 mg	IV	**J3465**
Vpriv	100 units		J3385
W			
Wehamine	up to 50 mg	IM, IV	J1240
Wehdryl	up to 50 mg	IM, IV	J1200
	50 mg	ORAL	Q0163
Wellcovorin	per 50 mg	IM, IV	J0640
Wilate	per IU	IV	J7183
Win Rho SD	100 IU	IV	J2792
Wyamine Sulfate, *see* Mephentermine sulfate			

▶ **New**   ↻ **Revised**   ✔ **Reinstated**   ~~deleted~~ **Deleted**

DRUG NAME	DOSAGE	METHOD OF ADMINISTRATION	HCPCS CODE
Wycillin	up to 600,000 units	IM, IV	J2510
Wydase	up to 150 units	SC, IV	J3470
X			
Xeloda	150 mg	ORAL	J8520
	500 mg	ORAL	J8521
Xeomin	1 unit		J0588
Xgera	1 mg		J0987
Xgeva	1 mg		J0897
Xiaflex	0.01 mg		J0775
Xolair	5 mg		J2357
Xopenex	0.5 mg	INH	J7620
concentrated form	1 mg	INH	J7610, J7611, J7612
unit dose form	1 mg	INH	J7609, J7613, J7614
Xylocaine HCl	10 mg	IV	J2001
Xyntha	per IU	IV	J7185, J7192, J7182, J7188
Y			
Yervoy	1 mg		J9228
Yondelis	0.1 mg		J9352, J9999
Z			
Zaltrap	1 mg		J9400
Zanosar	1 g	IV	J9320
Zantac	25 mg	IV, IM	J2780
Zarxio	1 mcg		Q5101
Zemaira	10 mg	IV	J0256
Zemplar	1 mcg	IM, IV	J2501
Zenapax	25 mg	IV	J7513
Zerbaxa	1 gm		J0695
Zetran	up to 5 mg	IM, IV	J3360
Ziconotide	1 mcg	OTH	J2278
Zidovudine	10 mg	IV	J3485
Zinacef	per 750 mg	IM, IV	J0697
Zinecard	per 250 mg		J1190
Ziprasidone Mesylate	10 mg	IM	J3486
Zithromax	1 gm	ORAL	Q0144
Injection	500 mg	IV	J0456
Ziv-Aflibercept	1 mg	IV	J9400
Zmax	1 g		Q0144

▶ New   ↻ Revised   ✔ Reinstated   ~~deleted~~ Deleted

DRUG NAME	DOSAGE	METHOD OF ADMINISTRATION	HCPCS CODE
Zofran	1 mg	IV	J2405
	1 mg	ORAL	Q0162
Zoladex	per 3.6 mg	SC	J9202
Zoledronic Acid	1 mg	IV	**J3489**
Zolicef	500 mg	IV, IM	J0690
Zometra	1 mg		J3489
Zorbtive	1 mg		J2941
Zortress	0.25 mg	ORAL	J7527
Zosyn	1.125 g	IV	J2543
Zovirax	5 mg		J8499
Zyprexa Relprevv	1 mg		J2358
Zyvox	200 mg	IV	J2020

▶ New   ↻ Revised   ✔ Reinstated   ~~deleted~~ Deleted

HCPCS 2018 LEVEL II NATIONAL CODES

2018 HCPCS quarterly updates available on the companion website at: http://www.codingupdates.com

DISCLAIMER

Every effort has been made to make this text complete and accurate, but no guarantee, warranty, or representation is made for its accuracy or completeness. This text is based on the Centers for Medicare and Medicaid Services Healthcare Common Procedure Coding System (HCPCS).

Do not report HCPCS modifiers with PQRI CPT Category II codes, rather use Category II modifiers (i.e., 1P, 2P, 3P, or 8P) or the claim may be returned or denied.

LEVEL II NATIONAL MODIFIERS

✳ **A1** Dressing for one wound

✳ **A2** Dressing for two wounds

✳ **A3** Dressing for three wounds

✳ **A4** Dressing for four wounds

✳ **A5** Dressing for five wounds

✳ **A6** Dressing for six wounds

✳ **A7** Dressing for seven wounds

✳ **A8** Dressing for eight wounds

✳ **A9** Dressing for nine or more wounds

✪ **AA** Anesthesia services performed personally by anesthesiologist

   IOM: 100-04, 12, 90.4

✪ **AD** Medical supervision by a physician: more than four concurrent anesthesia procedures

   IOM: 100-04, 12, 90.4

✳ **AE** Registered dietician

✳ **AF** Specialty physician

✳ **AG** Primary physician

✪ **AH** Clinical psychologist

   IOM: 100-04, 12, 170

✳ **AI** Principal physician of record

✪ **AJ** Clinical social worker

   IOM: 100-04, 12, 170; 100-04, 12, 150

✳ **AK** Nonparticipating physician

✪ **AM** Physician, team member service

   Not assigned for Medicare

   Cross Reference QM

✳ **AO** Alternate payment method declined by provider of service

✳ **AP** Determination of refractive state was not performed in the course of diagnostic ophthalmological examination

✳ **AQ** Physician providing a service in an unlisted health professional shortage area (HPSA)

✳ **AR** Physician provider services in a physician scarcity area

✳ **AS** Physician assistant, nurse practitioner, or clinical nurse specialist services for assistant at surgery

✳ **AT** Acute treatment (this modifier should be used when reporting service 98940, 98941, 98942)

✳ **AU** Item furnished in conjunction with a urological, ostomy, or tracheostomy supply

✳ **AV** Item furnished in conjunction with a prosthetic device, prosthetic or orthotic

✳ **AW** Item furnished in conjunction with a surgical dressing

✳ **AX** Item furnished in conjunction with dialysis services

✳ **AY** Item or service furnished to an ESRD patient that is not for the treatment of ESRD

⊘ **AZ** Physician providing a service in a dental health professional shortage area for the purpose of an electronic health record incentive payment

✳ **BA** Item furnished in conjunction with parenteral enteral nutrition (PEN) services

✳ **BL** Special acquisition of blood and blood products

✳ **BO** Orally administered nutrition, not by feeding tube

✳ **BP** The beneficiary has been informed of the purchase and rental options and has elected to purchase the item

✳ **BR** The beneficiary has been informed of the purchase and rental options and has elected to rent the item

✳ **BU** The beneficiary has been informed of the purchase and rental options and after 30 days has not informed the supplier of his/her decision

✳ **CA** Procedure payable only in the inpatient setting when performed emergently on an outpatient who expires prior to admission

✳ **CB** Service ordered by a renal dialysis facility (RDF) physician as part of the ESRD beneficiary's dialysis benefit, is not part of the composite rate, and is separately reimbursable

✳ **CC** Procedure code change (Use CC when the procedure code submitted was changed either for administrative reasons or because an incorrect code was filed)

✪ **CD** AMCC test has been ordered by an ESRD facility or MCP physician that is part of the composite rate and is not separately billable

---

▶ New   ↻ Revised   ✔ Reinstated   ~~deleted~~ Deleted   ⊘ Not covered or valid by Medicare

✪ Special coverage instructions   ✳ Carrier discretion   Ⓑ Bill Part B MAC   Ⓑ Bill DME MAC

⊘ **CE** AMCC test has been ordered by an ESRD facility or MCP physician that is a composite rate test but is beyond the normal frequency covered under the rate and is separately reimbursable based on medical necessity

⊘ **CF** AMCC test has been ordered by an ESRD facility or MCP physician that is not part of the composite rate and is separately billable

✳ **CG** Policy criteria applied

⊘ **CH** 0 percent impaired, limited or restricted

⊘ **CI** At least 1 percent but less than 20 percent impaired, limited or restricted

⊘ **CJ** At least 20 percent but less than 40 percent impaired, limited or restricted

⊘ **CK** At least 40 percent but less than 60 percent impaired, limited or restricted

⊘ **CL** At least 60 percent but less than 80 percent impaired, limited or restricted

⊘ **CM** At least 80 percent but less than 100 percent impaired, limited or restricted

⊘ **CN** 100 percent impaired, limited or restricted

~~CP~~ ~~Adjunctive service related to a procedure assigned to a comprehensive ambulatory payment classification (C-APC) procedure, but reported on a different claim~~ ✖

✳ **CR** Catastrophe/Disaster related

✳ **CS** Item or service related, in whole or in part, to an illness, injury, or condition that was caused by or exacerbated by the effects, direct or indirect, of the 2010 oil spill in the Gulf of Mexico, including but not limited to subsequent clean-up activities

✳ **CT** Computed tomography services furnished using equipment that does not meet each of the attributes of the national electrical manufacturers association (NEMA) XR-29-2013 standard

✳ **DA** Oral health assessment by a licensed health professional other than a dentist

✳ **E1** Upper left, eyelid

✳ **E2** Lower left, eyelid

✳ **E3** Upper right, eyelid

✳ **E4** Lower right, eyelid

⊘ **EA** Erythropoetic stimulating agent (ESA) administered to treat anemia due to anti-cancer chemotherapy

CMS requires claims for non-ESRD ESAs (J0881 and J0885) to include one of three modifiers: EA, EB, EC.

⊘ **EB** Erythropoetic stimulating agent (ESA) administered to treat anemia due to anti-cancer radiotherapy

CMS requires claims for non-ESRD ESAs (J0881 and J0885) to include one of three modifiers: EA, EB, EC.

⊘ **EC** Erythropoetic stimulating agent (ESA) administered to treat anemia not due to anti-cancer radiotherapy or anti-cancer chemotherapy

CMS requires claims for non-ESRD ESAs (J0881 and J0885) to include one of three modifiers: EA, EB, EC.

⊘ **ED** Hematocrit level has exceeded 39% (or hemoglobin level has exceeded 13.0 g/dl) for 3 or more consecutive billing cycles immediately prior to and including the current cycle

⊘ **EE** Hematocrit level has not exceeded 39% (or hemoglobin level has not exceeded 13.0 g/dl) for 3 or more consecutive billing cycles immediately prior to and including the current cycle

⊘ **EJ** Subsequent claims for a defined course of therapy, e.g., EPO, sodium hyaluronate, infliximab

⊘ **EM** Emergency reserve supply (for ESRD benefit only)

✳ **EP** Service provided as part of Medicaid early periodic screening diagnosis and treatment (EPSDT) program

✳ **ET** Emergency services

✳ **EX** Expatriate beneficiary

✳ **EY** No physician or other licensed health care provider order for this item or service

Items billed before a signed and dated order has been received by the supplier must be submitted with an EY modifier added to each related HCPCS code.

✳ **F1** Left hand, second digit

✳ **F2** Left hand, third digit

✳ **F3** Left hand, fourth digit

✳ **F4** Left hand, fifth digit

✳ **F5** Right hand, thumb

✳ **F6** Right hand, second digit

✳ **F7** Right hand, third digit

▶ **New**   ⟲ **Revised**   ✔ **Reinstated**   ~~deleted~~ **Deleted**   ⊘ **Not covered or valid by Medicare**
⊛ **Special coverage instructions**   ✳ **Carrier discretion**   Ⓑ **Bill Part B MAC**   Ⓑ **Bill DME MAC**

✳ **F8** Right hand, fourth digit

✳ **F9** Right hand, fifth digit

✳ **FA** Left hand, thumb

⊘ **FB** Item provided without cost to provider, supplier or practitioner, or full credit received for replaced device (examples, but not limited to, covered under warranty, replaced due to defect, free samples)

✿ **FC** Partial credit received for replaced device

✳ **FP** Service provided as part of family planning program

✳ **FX** X-ray taken using film

▶ ✳ **FY** X-ray taken using computed radiography technology/cassette-based imaging

✳ **G1** Most recent URR reading of less than 60

IOM: 100-04, 8, 50.9

✳ **G2** Most recent URR reading of 60 to 64.9

IOM: 100-04, 8, 50.9

✳ **G3** Most recent URR reading of 65 to 69.9

IOM: 100-04, 8, 50.9

✳ **G4** Most recent URR reading of 70 to 74.9

IOM: 100-04, 8, 50.9

✳ **G5** Most recent URR reading of 75 or greater

IOM: 100-04, 8, 50.9

✳ **G6** ESRD patient for whom less than six dialysis sessions have been provided in a month

IOM: 100-04, 8, 50.9

✿ **G7** Pregnancy resulted from rape or incest or pregnancy certified by physician as life threatening

IOM: 100-02, 15, 20.1; 100-03, 3, 170.3

✳ **G8** Monitored anesthesia care (MAC) for deep complex, complicated, or markedly invasive surgical procedure

✳ **G9** Monitored anesthesia care for patient who has history of severe cardiopulmonary condition

✳ **GA** Waiver of liability statement issued as required by payer policy, individual case

An item/service is expected to be denied as not reasonable and necessary and an ABN is on file. Modifier GA can be used on either a specific or a miscellaneous HCPCS code. Modifiers GA and GY should never be reported together on the same line for the same HCPCS code.

✳ **GB** Claim being resubmitted for payment because it is no longer covered under a global payment demonstration

✿ **GC** This service has been performed in part by a resident under the direction of a teaching physician.

IOM: 100-04, 12, 90.4, 100

✳ **GD** Units of service exceeds medically unlikely edit value and represents reasonable and necessary services

✿ **GE** This service has been performed by a resident without the presence of a teaching physician under the primary care exception

✳ **GF** Non-physician (e.g., nurse practitioner (NP), certified registered nurse anesthetist (CRNA), certified registered nurse (CRN), clinical nurse specialist (CNS), physician assistant (PA)) services in a critical access hospital

✳ **GG** Performance and payment of a screening mammogram and diagnostic mammogram on the same patient, same day

✳ **GH** Diagnostic mammogram converted from screening mammogram on same day

✳ **GJ** "Opt out" physician or practitioner emergency or urgent service

✳ **GK** Reasonable and necessary item/service associated with a GA or GZ modifier

An upgrade is defined as an item that goes beyond what is medically necessary under Medicare's coverage requirements. An item can be considered an upgrade even if the physician has signed an order for it. When suppliers know that an item will not be paid in full because it does not meet the coverage criteria stated in the LCD, the supplier can still obtain partial payment at the time of initial determination if the claim is billed using one of the upgrade modifiers (GK or GL). (https://www.cms.gov/manuals/downloads/clm104c01.pdf)

▶ **New**	↻ **Revised**	✔ **Reinstated**	~~deleted~~ **Deleted**	⊘ **Not covered or valid by Medicare**
✿ **Special coverage instructions**		✳ **Carrier discretion**	Ⓟ **Bill Part B MAC**	Ⓓ **Bill DME MAC**

✳ **GL**   Medically unnecessary upgrade provided instead of non-upgraded item, no charge, no Advance Beneficiary Notice (ABN)

✳ **GM**   Multiple patients on one ambulance trip

✳ **GN**   Services delivered under an outpatient speech language pathology plan of care

✳ **GO**   Services delivered under an outpatient occupational therapy plan of care

✳ **GP**   Services delivered under an outpatient physical therapy plan of care

✳ **GQ**   Via asynchronous telecommunications system

✳ **GR**   This service was performed in whole or in part by a resident in a department of Veterans Affairs medical center or clinic, supervised in accordance with VA policy

⊛ **GS**   Dosage of erythropoietin-stimulating agent has been reduced and maintained in response to hematocrit or hemoglobin level

⊛ **GT**   Via interactive audio and video telecommunication systems

✳ **GU**   Waiver of liability statement issued as required by payer policy, routine notice

⊛ **GV**   Attending physician not employed or paid under arrangement by the patient's hospice provider

⊛ **GW**   Service not related to the hospice patient's terminal condition

✳ **GX**   Notice of liability issued, voluntary under payer policy

GX modifier must be submitted with non-covered charges only. This modifier differentiates from the required uses in conjunction with ABN. (https://www.cms.gov/manuals/downloads/clm104c01.pdf)

⊘ **GY**   Item or service statutorily excluded, does not meet the definition of any Medicare benefit or, for non-Medicare insurers, is not a contract benefit

Examples of "statutorily excluded" include: Infusion drug not administered using a durable infusion pump, a wheelchair that is for use for mobility outside the home or hearing aids. GA and GY should never be coded together on the same line for the same HCPCS code. (https://www.cms.gov/manuals/downloads/clm104c01.pdf)

⊘ **GZ**   Item or service expected to be denied as not reasonable or necessary

Used when an ABN is not on file and can be used on either a specific or a miscellaneous HCPCS code. It would never be correct to place any combination of GY, GZ or GA modifiers on the same claim line and will result in rejected or denied claim for invalid coding. (https://www.cms.gov/manuals/downloads/clm104c01.pdf)

⊘ **H9**   Court-ordered

⊘ **HA**   Child/adolescent program

⊘ **HB**   Adult program, nongeriatric

⊘ **HC**   Adult program, geriatric

⊘ **HD**   Pregnant/parenting women's program

⊘ **HE**   Mental health program

⊘ **HF**   Substance abuse program

⊘ **HG**   Opioid addiction treatment program

⊘ **HH**   Integrated mental health/substance abuse program

⊘ **HI**   Integrated mental health and intellectual disability/developmental disabilities program

⊘ **HJ**   Employee assistance program

⊘ **HK**   Specialized mental health programs for high-risk populations

⊘ **HL**   Intern

⊘ **HM**   Less than bachelor degree level

⊘ **HN**   Bachelors degree level

⊘ **HO**   Masters degree level

⊘ **HP**   Doctoral level

⊘ **HQ**   Group setting

⊘ **HR**   Family/couple with client present

⊘ **HS**   Family/couple without client present

⊘ **HT**   Multi-disciplinary team

⊘ **HU**   Funded by child welfare agency

⊘ **HV**   Funded by state addictions agency

⊘ **HW**   Funded by state mental health agency

⊘ **HX**   Funded by county/local agency

⊘ **HY**   Funded by juvenile justice agency

⊘ **HZ**   Funded by criminal justice agency

✳ **J1**   Competitive acquisition program no-pay submission for a prescription number

✳ **J2**   Competitive acquisition program, restocking of emergency drugs after emergency administration

▶ **New**   ↻ **Revised**   ✔ **Reinstated**   ~~deleted~~ **Deleted**   ⊘ **Not covered or valid by Medicare**

⊛ **Special coverage instructions**   ✳ **Carrier discretion**   ⊚ **Bill Part B MAC**   ⊚ **Bill DME MAC**

* **J3** Competitive acquisition program (CAP), drug not available through CAP as written, reimbursed under average sales price methodology

* **J4** DMEPOS item subject to DMEPOS competitive bidding program that is furnished by a hospital upon discharge

* **JA** Administered intravenously

This modifier is informational only (not a payment modifier) and may be submitted with all injection codes. According to Medicare, reporting this modifier is voluntary. (CMS Pub. 100-04, chapter 8, section 60.2.3.1 and Pub. 100-04, chapter 17, section 80.11)

* **JB** Administered subcutaneously

* **JC** Skin substitute used as a graft

* **JD** Skin substitute not used as a graft

* **JE** Administered via dialysate

▶ * **JG** Drug or biological acquired with 340B drug pricing program discount

* **JW** Drug amount discarded/not administered to any patient

Use JW to identify unused drugs or biologicals from single use vial/package that are appropriately discarded. Bill on separate line for payment of discarded drug/biological.

IOM: 100-4, 17, 40

* **K0** Lower extremity prosthesis functional Level 0 - does not have the ability or potential to ambulate or transfer safely with or without assistance and a prosthesis does not enhance their quality of life or mobility.

* **K1** Lower extremity prosthesis functional Level 1 - has the ability or potential to use a prosthesis for transfers or ambulation on level surfaces at fixed cadence. Typical of the limited and unlimited household ambulator.

* **K2** Lower extremity prosthesis functional Level 2 - has the ability or potential for ambulation with the ability to traverse low level environmental barriers such as curbs, stairs or uneven surfaces. Typical of the limited community ambulator.

* **K3** Lower extremity prosthesis functional Level 3 - has the ability or potential for ambulation with variable cadence. Typical of the community ambulator who has the ability to traverse most environmental barriers and may have vocational, therapeutic, or exercise activity that demands prosthetic utilization beyond simple locomotion.

* **K4** Lower extremity prosthesis functional Level 4 - has the ability or potential for prosthetic ambulation that exceeds the basic ambulation skills, exhibiting high impact, stress, or energy levels, typical of the prosthetic demands of the child, active adult, or athlete.

* **KA** Add on option/accessory for wheelchair

* **KB** Beneficiary requested upgrade for ABN, more than 4 modifiers identified on claim

* **KC** Replacement of special power wheelchair interface

* **KD** Drug or biological infused through DME

* **KE** Bid under round one of the DMEPOS competitive bidding program for use with non-competitive bid base equipment

* **KF** Item designated by FDA as Class III device

* **KG** DMEPOS item subject to DMEPOS competitive bidding program number 1

* **KH** DMEPOS item, initial claim, purchase or first month rental

* **KI** DMEPOS item, second or third month rental

* **KJ** DMEPOS item, parenteral enteral nutrition (PEN) pump or capped rental, months four to fifteen

* **KK** DMEPOS item subject to DMEPOS competitive bidding program number 2

* **KL** DMEPOS item delivered via mail

* **KM** Replacement of facial prosthesis including new impression/moulage

* **KN** Replacement of facial prosthesis using previous master model

* **KO** Single drug unit dose formulation

* **KP** First drug of a multiple drug unit dose formulation

* **KQ** Second or subsequent drug of a multiple drug unit dose formulation

* **KR** Rental item, billing for partial month

⊘ **KS** Glucose monitor supply for diabetic beneficiary not treated with insulin

* **KT** Beneficiary resides in a competitive bidding area and travels outside that competitive bidding area and receives a competitive bid item

* **KU** DMEPOS item subject to DMEPOS competitive bidding program number 3

✳ **KV** DMEPOS item subject to DMEPOS competitive bidding program that is furnished as part of a professional service

✳ **KW** DMEPOS item subject to DMEPOS competitive bidding program number 4

✳ **KX** Requirements specified in the medical policy have been met

Used for physical, occupational, or speech-language therapy to request an exception to therapy payment caps and indicate the services are reasonable and necessary and that there is documentation of medical necessity in the patient's medical record. (Pub 100-04 Attachment - Business Requirements Centers for Medicare and Medicaid Services, Transmittal 2457, April 27, 2012)

Medicare requires modifier KX for implanted permanent cardiac pacemakers, single chamber or duel chamber, for one of the following CPT codes: 33206, 33207, 33208.

✳ **KY** DMEPOS item subject to DMEPOS competitive bidding program number 5

✳ **KZ** New coverage not implemented by managed care

✳ **LC** Left circumflex coronary artery

✳ **LD** Left anterior descending coronary artery

✳ **LL** Lease/rental (use the LL modifier when DME equipment rental is to be applied against the purchase price)

✳ **LM** Left main coronary artery

✳ **LR** Laboratory round trip

⊛ **LS** FDA-monitored intraocular lens implant

✳ **LT** Left side (used to identify procedures performed on the left side of the body)

Modifiers LT and RT identify procedures which can be performed on paired organs. Used for procedures performed on one side only. Should also be used when the procedures are similar but not identical and are performed on paired body parts.

✳ **M2** Medicare secondary payer (MSP)

✳ **MS** Six month maintenance and servicing fee for reasonable and necessary parts and labor which are not covered under any manufacturer or supplier warranty

✳ **NB** Nebulizer system, any type, FDA-cleared for use with specific drug

✳ **NR** New when rented (use the NR modifier when DME which was new at the time of rental is subsequently purchased)

✳ **NU** New equipment

✳ **P1** A normal healthy patient

✳ **P2** A patient with mild systemic disease

✳ **P3** A patient with severe systemic disease

✳ **P4** A patient with severe systemic disease that is a constant threat to life

✳ **P5** A moribund patient who is not expected to survive without the operation

✳ **P6** A declared brain-dead patient whose organs are being removed for donor purposes

⊘ **PA** Surgical or other invasive procedure on wrong body part

⊘ **PB** Surgical or other invasive procedure on wrong patient

⊘ **PC** Wrong surgery or other invasive procedure on patient

✳ **PD** Diagnostic or related non diagnostic item or service provided in a wholly owned or operated entity to a patient who is admitted as an inpatient within 3 days

✳ **PI** Positron emission tomography (PET) or PET/computed tomography (CT) to inform the initial treatment strategy of tumors that are biopsy proven or strongly suspected of being cancerous based on other diagnostic testing

✳ **PL** Progressive addition lenses

✳ **PM** Post mortem

✳ **PN** Non-excepted service provided at an off-campus, outpatient, provider-based department of a hospital

✳ **PO** Expected services provided at off-campus, outpatient, provider-based department of a hospital

✳ **PS** Positron emission tomography (PET) or PET/computed tomography (CT) to inform the subsequent treatment strategy of cancerous tumors when the beneficiary's treating physician determines that the PET study is needed to inform subsequent anti-tumor strategy

---

▶ **New**   ↻ **Revised**   ✔ **Reinstated**   ~~deleted~~ **Deleted**   ⊘ **Not covered or valid by Medicare**

⊛ **Special coverage instructions**   ✳ **Carrier discretion**   Ⓑ **Bill Part B MAC**   Ⓔ **Bill DME MAC**

✳ **PT** Colorectal cancer screening test; converted to diagnostic text or other procedure

Assign this modifier with the appropriate CPT procedure code for colonoscopy, flexible sigmoidoscopy, or barium enema when the service is initiated as a colorectal cancer screening service but then becomes a diagnostic service. (MLN Matters article MM7012 (PDF, 75 KB) Reference Medicare Transmittal 3232 April 3, 2015.

⊙ **Q0** Investigational clinical service provided in a clinical research study that is in an approved clinical research study

⊙ **Q1** Routine clinical service provided in a clinical research study that is in an approved clinical research study

✳ **Q2** Demonstration procedure/service

✳ **Q3** Live kidney donor surgery and related services

✳ **Q4** Service for ordering/referring physician qualifies as a service exemption

↻ ⊙ **Q5** Service furnished under a reciprocal billing arrangementby a substitute physician or by a substitute physical therapist furnishing outpatient physical therapy services in a health professional shortage area, a medically underserved area, or a rural area

IOM: 100-04, 1, 30.2.10

↻ ⊙ **Q6** Service furnished under a fee-for-time compensation arrangement by a substitute physician or by a substitute physical therapist furnishing outpatient physical therapy services in a health professional shortage area, a medically underserved area, or a rural area

IOM: 100-04, 1, 30.2.11

✳ **Q7** One Class A finding

✳ **Q8** Two Class B findings

✳ **Q9** One Class B and two Class C findings

✳ **QC** Single channel monitoring

✳ **QD** Recording and storage in solid state memory by a digital recorder

✳ **QE** Prescribed amount of oxygen is less than 1 liter per minute (LPM)

✳ **QF** Prescribed amount of oxygen exceeds 4 liters per minute (LPM) and portable oxygen is prescribed

✳ **QG** Prescribed amount of oxygen is greater than 4 liters per minute (LPM)

✳ **QH** Oxygen conserving device is being used with an oxygen delivery system

⊙ **QJ** Services/items provided to a prisoner or patient in state or local custody, however, the state or local government, as applicable, meets the requirements in 42 CFR 411.4 (B)

⊙ **QK** Medical direction of two, three, or four concurrent anesthesia procedures involving qualified individuals

IOM: 100-04, 12, 50K, 90

✳ **QL** Patient pronounced dead after ambulance called

✳ **QM** Ambulance service provided under arrangement by a provider of services

✳ **QN** Ambulance service furnished directly by a provider of services

⊙ **QP** Documentation is on file showing that the laboratory test(s) was ordered individually or ordered as a CPT-recognized panel other than automated profile codes 80002-80019, G0058, G0059, and G0060.

▶ ✳ **QQ** Ordering professional consulted a qualified clinical decision support mechanism for this service and the related data was provided to the furnishing professional

⊙ **QS** Monitored anesthesia care service

IOM: 100-04, 12, 30.6, 501

✳ **QT** Recording and storage on tape by an analog tape recorder

✳ **QW** CLIA-waived test

✳ **QX** CRNA service: with medical direction by a physician

⊙ **QY** Medical direction of one certified registered nurse anesthetist (CRNA) by an anesthesiologist

IOM: 100-04, 12, 50K, 90

✳ **QZ** CRNA service: without medical direction by a physician

---

▶ **New**   ↻ **Revised**   ✔ **Reinstated**   ~~deleted~~ **Deleted**   ⊘ **Not covered or valid by Medicare**

⊙ **Special coverage instructions**   ✳ **Carrier discretion**   ⑧ **Bill Part B MAC**   ⑧ **Bill DME MAC**

✳ **RA** Replacement of a DME, orthotic or prosthetic item

Contractors will deny claims for replacement parts when furnished in conjunction with the repair of a capped rental item and billed with modifier RB, including claims for parts submitted using code E1399, that are billed during the capped rental period (i.e., the last day of the 13th month of continuous use or before). Repair includes all maintenance, servicing, and repair of capped rental DME because it is included in the allowed rental payment amounts. (Pub 100-20 One-Time Notification Centers for Medicare & Medicaid Services, Transmittal: 901, May 13, 2011)

✳ **RB** Replacement of a part of a DME, orthotic or prosthetic item furnished as part of a repair

✳ **RC** Right coronary artery

✳ **RD** Drug provided to beneficiary, but not administered "incident-to"

✳ **RE** Furnished in full compliance with FDA-mandated risk evaluation and mitigation strategy (REMS)

✳ **RI** Ramus intermedius coronary artery

✳ **RR** Rental (use the "RR" modifier when DME is to be rented)

✳ **RT** Right side (used to identify procedures performed on the right side of the body)

Modifiers LT and RT identify procedures which can be performed on paired organs. Used for procedures performed on one side only. Should also be used when the procedures are similar but not identical and are performed on paired body parts.

⊘ **SA** Nurse practitioner rendering service in collaboration with a physician

⊘ **SB** Nurse midwife

✳ **SC** Medically necessary service or supply

⊘ **SD** Services provided by registered nurse with specialized, highly technical home infusion training

⊘ **SE** State and/or federally funded programs/services

✳ **SF** Second opinion ordered by a professional review organization (PRO) per Section 9401, P.L. 99-272 (100% reimbursement — no Medicare deductible or coinsurance)

✳ **SG** Ambulatory surgical center (ASC) facility service

Only valid for surgical codes. After 1/1/08 not required for ASC facility charges.

⊘ **SH** Second concurrently administered infusion therapy

⊘ **SJ** Third or more concurrently administered infusion therapy

⊘ **SK** Member of high risk population (use only with codes for immunization)

⊘ **SL** State supplied vaccine

⊘ **SM** Second surgical opinion

⊘ **SN** Third surgical opinion

⊘ **SQ** Item ordered by home health

⊘ **SS** Home infusion services provided in the infusion suite of the IV therapy provider

⊘ **ST** Related to trauma or injury

⊘ **SU** Procedure performed in physician's office (to denote use of facility and equipment)

⊘ **SV** Pharmaceuticals delivered to patient's home but not utilized

✳ **SW** Services provided by a certified diabetic educator

⊘ **SY** Persons who are in close contact with member of high-risk population (use only with codes for immunization)

~~SZ~~ ~~Habilitative services~~ ✖

✳ **T1** Left foot, second digit

✳ **T2** Left foot, third digit

✳ **T3** Left foot, fourth digit

✳ **T4** Left foot, fifth digit

✳ **T5** Right foot, great toe

✳ **T6** Right foot, second digit

✳ **T7** Right foot, third digit

✳ **T8** Right foot, fourth digit

✳ **T9** Right foot, fifth digit

✳ **TA** Left foot, great toe

▶ ✳ **TB** Drug or biological acquired with 340B drug pricing program discount, reported for informational purposes

---

▶ New ↻ Revised ✔ Reinstated ~~deleted~~ Deleted ⊘ Not covered or valid by Medicare
✪ Special coverage instructions ✳ Carrier discretion Ⓟ Bill Part B MAC Ⓓ Bill DME MAC

⁎ **TC**   Technical component; Under certain circumstances, a charge may be made for the technical component alone; under those circumstances the technical component charge is identified by adding modifier TC to the usual procedure number; technical component charges are institutional charges and not billed separately by physicians; however, portable x-ray suppliers only bill for technical component and should utilize modifier TC; the charge data from portable x-ray suppliers will then be used to build customary and prevailing profiles.

⊘ **TD**   RN

⊘ **TE**   LPN/LVN

⊘ **TF**   Intermediate level of care

⊘ **TG**   Complex/high tech level of care

⊘ **TH**   Obstetrical treatment/services, prenatal or postpartum

⊘ **TJ**   Program group, child and/or adolescent

⊘ **TK**   Extra patient or passenger, non-ambulance

⊘ **TL**   Early intervention/individualized family service plan (IFSP)

⊘ **TM**   Individualized education program (IEP)

⊘ **TN**   Rural/outside providers' customary service area

⊘ **TP**   Medical transport, unloaded vehicle

⊘ **TQ**   Basic life support transport by a volunteer ambulance provider

⊘ **TR**   School-based individual education program (IEP) services provided outside the public school district responsible for the student

⁎ **TS**   Follow-up service

⊘ **TT**   Individualized service provided to more than one patient in same setting

⊘ **TU**   Special payment rate, overtime

⊘ **TV**   Special payment rates, holidays/weekends

⊘ **TW**   Back-up equipment

⊘ **U1**   Medicaid Level of Care 1, as defined by each State

⊘ **U2**   Medicaid Level of Care 2, as defined by each State

⊘ **U3**   Medicaid Level of Care 3, as defined by each State

⊘ **U4**   Medicaid Level of Care 4, as defined by each State

⊘ **U5**   Medicaid Level of Care 5, as defined by each State

⊘ **U6**   Medicaid Level of Care 6, as defined by each State

⊘ **U7**   Medicaid Level of Care 7, as defined by each State

⊘ **U8**   Medicaid Level of Care 8, as defined by each State

⊘ **U9**   Medicaid Level of Care 9, as defined by each State

⊘ **UA**   Medicaid Level of Care 10, as defined by each State

⊘ **UB**   Medicaid Level of Care 11, as defined by each State

⊘ **UC**   Medicaid Level of Care 12, as defined by each State

⊘ **UD**   Medicaid Level of Care 13, as defined by each State

⁎ **UE**   Used durable medical equipment

⊘ **UF**   Services provided in the morning

⊘ **UG**   Services provided in the afternoon

⊘ **UH**   Services provided in the evening

⁎ **UJ**   Services provided at night

⊘ **UK**   Services provided on behalf of the client to someone other than the client (collateral relationship)

⁎ **UN**   Two patients served

⁎ **UP**   Three patients served

⁎ **UQ**   Four patients served

⁎ **UR**   Five patients served

⁎ **US**   Six or more patients served

⁎ **V1**   Demonstration Modifier 1

⁎ **V2**   Demonstration Modifier 2

⁎ **V3**   Demonstration Modifier 3

⁎ **V5**   Vascular catheter (alone or with any other vascular access)

⁎ **V6**   Arteriovenous graft (or other vascular access not including a vascular catheter)

⁎ **V7**   Arteriovenous fistula only (in use with two needles)

▶ ⁎ **VM**   Medicare diabetes prevention program (MDPP) virtual make-up session

⁎ **VP**   Aphakic patient

▶ New   ⤴ Revised   ✔ Reinstated   ~~deleted~~ Deleted   ⊘ Not covered or valid by Medicare
✪ Special coverage instructions   ⁎ Carrier discretion   ⑧ Bill Part B MAC   ⑧ Bill DME MAC

▶ ✳ **X1** Continuous/broad services: for reporting services by clinicians, who provide the principal care for a patient, with no planned endpoint of the relationship; services in this category represent comprehensive care, dealing with the entire scope of patient problems, either directly or in a care coordination role; reporting clinician service examples include, but are not limited to: primary care, and clinicians providing comprehensive care to patients in addition to specialty care

▶ ✳ **X2** Continuous/focused services: for reporting services by clinicians whose expertise is needed for the ongoing management of a chronic disease or a condition that needs to be managed and followed with no planned endpoint to the relationship; reporting clinician service examples include but are not limited to: a rheumatologist taking care of the patient's rheumatoid arthritis longitudinally but not providing general primary care services

▶ ✳ **X3** Episodic/broad servies: for reporting services by clinicians who have broad responsibility for the comprehensive needs of the patient that is limited to a defined period and circumstance such as a hospitalization; reporting clinician service examples include but are not limited to the hospitalist's services rendered providing comprehensive and general care to a patient while admitted to the hospital

▶ ✳ **X4** Episodic/focused services: for reporting services by clinicians who provide focused care on particular types of treatment limited to a defined period and circumstance; the patient has a problem, acute or chronic, that will be treated with surgery, radiation, or some other type of generally time-limited intervention; reporting clinician service examples include but are not limited to, the orthopedic surgeon performing a knee replacement and seeing the patient through the postoperative period

▶ ✳ **X5** Diagnostic services requested by another clinician: for reporting services by a clinician who furnishes care to the patient only as requested by another clinician or subsequent and related services requested by another clinician; this modifier is reported for patient relationships that may not be adequately captured by the above alternative categories; reporting clinician service examples include but are not limited to, the radiologist's interpretation of an imaging study requested by another clinician

✳ **XE** Separate encounter, a service that is distinct because it occurred during a separate encounter

✳ **XP** Separate practitioner, a service that is distinct because it was performed by a different practitioner

✳ **XS** Separate structure, a service that is distinct because it was performed on a separate organ/structure

✳ **XU** Unusual non-overlapping service, the use of a service that is distinct because it does not overlap usual components of the main service

✳ **ZA** Novartis/Sandoz

✳ **ZB** Pfizer/Hospira

▶ ✳ **ZC** Merck/Samsung Bioepis

▶ New   ↻ Revised   ✔ Reinstated   ~~deleted~~ Deleted   ⊘ Not covered or valid by Medicare

✪ Special coverage instructions   ✳ Carrier discretion   Ⓑ Bill Part B MAC   Ⓑ Bill DME MAC

Ambulance Modifiers

Modifiers that are used on claims for ambulance services are created by combining two alpha characters. Each alpha character, with the exception of X, represents an origin (source) code or a destination code. The pair of alpha codes creates one modifier. The first position alpha-code = origin; the second position alpha-code = destination. On form CMS-1491, used to report ambulance services, Item 12 should contain the origin code and Item 13 should contain the destination code. Origin and destination codes and their descriptions are as follows:

D	Diagnostic or therapeutic site other than P or H when these are used as origin codes
E	Residential, domiciliary, custodial facility (other than an 1819 facility)
G	Hospital-based dialysis facility (hospital or hospital related)
H	Hospital
I	Site of transfer (e.g., airport or helicopter pad) between modes of ambulance transport
J	Non-hospital-based dialysis facility
N	Skilled nursing facility (SNF) (1819 facility)
P	Physician's office (includes HMO non-hospital facility, clinic, etc.)
R	Residence
S	Scene of accident or acute event
X	Destination code only. Intermediate stop at physician's office en route to the hospital (includes non-hospital facility, clinic, etc.)

TRANSPORT SERVICES INCLUDING AMBULANCE (A0000-A0999)

⊘ **A0021** Ambulance service, outside state per mile, transport (Medicaid only) Ⓑ

Cross Reference A0030

⊘ **A0080** Non-emergency transportation, per mile - vehicle provided by volunteer (individual or organization), with no vested interest Ⓑ

⊘ **A0090** Non-emergency transportation, per mile - vehicle provided by individual (family member, self, neighbor) with vested interest Ⓑ

⊘ **A0100** Non-emergency transportation; taxi Ⓑ

⊘ **A0110** Non-emergency transportation and bus, intra or inter state carrier Ⓑ

⊘ **A0120** Non-emergency transportation: mini-bus, mountain area transports, or other transportation systems Ⓑ

⊘ **A0130** Non-emergency transportation: wheelchair van Ⓑ

⊘ **A0140** Non-emergency transportation and air travel (private or commercial), intra or inter state Ⓑ

⊘ **A0160** Non-emergency transportation: per mile - caseworker or social worker Ⓑ

⊘ **A0170** Transportation: ancillary: parking fees, tolls, other Ⓑ

⊘ **A0180** Non-emergency transportation: ancillary: lodging - recipient Ⓑ

⊘ **A0190** Non-emergency transportation: ancillary: meals - recipient Ⓑ

⊘ **A0200** Non-emergency transportation: ancillary: lodging - escort Ⓑ

⊘ **A0210** Non-emergency transportation: ancillary: meals - escort Ⓑ

⊘ **A0225** Ambulance service, neonatal transport, base rate, emergency transport, one way Ⓑ

⊘ **A0380** BLS mileage (per mile) Ⓑ

Cross Reference A0425

⊘ **A0382** BLS routine disposable supplies Ⓑ

⊘ **A0384** BLS specialized service disposable supplies; defibrillation (used by ALS ambulances and BLS ambulances in jurisdictions where defibrillation is permitted in BLS ambulances) Ⓑ

⊘ **A0390** ALS mileage (per mile) Ⓑ

Cross Reference A0425

⊘ **A0392** ALS specialized service disposable supplies; defibrillation (to be used only in jurisdictions where defibrillation cannot be performed in BLS ambulances) Ⓑ

⊘ **A0394** ALS specialized service disposable supplies; IV drug therapy Ⓑ

⊘ **A0396** ALS specialized service disposable supplies; esophageal intubation Ⓑ

⊘ **A0398** ALS routine disposable supplies Ⓑ

⊘ **A0420** Ambulance waiting time (ALS or BLS), one half (½) hour increments Ⓑ

Waiting Time Table			
UNITS	TIME	UNITS	TIME
1	½ to 1 hr.	6	3 to 3½ hrs.
2	1 to 1½ hrs.	7	3½ to 4 hrs.
3	1½ to 2 hrs.	8	4 to 4½ hrs.
4	2 to 2½ hrs.	9	4½ to 5 hrs.
5	2½ to 3 hrs.	10	5 to 5½ hrs.

⊘ **A0422** Ambulance (ALS or BLS) oxygen and oxygen supplies, life sustaining situation Ⓑ

⊘ **A0424** Extra ambulance attendant, ground (ALS or BLS) or air (fixed or rotary winged); (requires medical review) Ⓑ

✳ **A0425** Ground mileage, per statute mile Ⓑ

✳ **A0426** Ambulance service, advanced life support, non-emergency transport, Level 1 (ALS 1) Ⓑ

✳ **A0427** Ambulance service, advanced life support, emergency transport, Level 1 (ALS 1-Emergency) Ⓑ

✳ **A0428** Ambulance service, basic life support, non-emergency transport (BLS) Ⓑ

✳ **A0429** Ambulance service, basic life support, emergency transport (BLS-Emergency) Ⓑ

✳ **A0430** Ambulance service, conventional air services, transport, one way (fixed wing) Ⓑ

✳ **A0431** Ambulance service, conventional air services, transport, one way (rotary wing) Ⓑ

✳ **A0432** Paramedic intercept (PI), rural area, transport furnished by a volunteer ambulance company, which is prohibited by state law from billing third party payers Ⓑ

✳ **A0433** Advanced life support, Level 2 (ALS2) Ⓑ

✳ **A0434** Specialty care transport (SCT) Ⓑ

▶ New ↻ Revised ✔ Reinstated ~~deleted~~ Deleted ⊘ Not covered or valid by Medicare
⊕ Special coverage instructions ✳ Carrier discretion Ⓑ Bill Part B MAC Ⓑ Bill DME MAC

✳ **A0435** Fixed wing air mileage, per statute mile Ⓑ

✳ **A0436** Rotary wing air mileage, per statute mile Ⓑ

⊘ **A0888** Noncovered ambulance mileage, per mile (e.g., for miles traveled beyond closest appropriate facility) Ⓑ

⊘ **A0998** Ambulance response and treatment, no transport Ⓑ

IOM: 100-02, 10, 20

❂ **A0999** Unlisted ambulance service Ⓑ

IOM: 100-02, 10, 20

MEDICAL AND SURGICAL SUPPLIES
(A4000-A8004)

Injection and Infusion

✳ **A4206** Syringe with needle, sterile 1 cc or less, each Ⓓ Ⓑ

✳ **A4207** Syringe with needle, sterile 2 cc, each Ⓓ Ⓑ

✳ **A4208** Syringe with needle, sterile 3 cc, each Ⓓ Ⓑ

✳ **A4209** Syringe with needle, sterile 5 cc or greater, each Ⓓ Ⓑ

⊘ **A4210** Needle-free injection device, each Ⓑ

IOM: 100-03, 4, 280.1

❂ **A4211** Supplies for self-administered injections Ⓓ Ⓑ

IOM: 100-02, 15, 50

✳ **A4212** Non-coring needle or stylet with or without catheter Ⓑ

✳ **A4213** Syringe, sterile, 20 cc or greater, each Ⓑ Ⓓ

✳ **A4215** Needle, sterile, any size, each Ⓓ Ⓑ

❂ **A4216** Sterile water, saline and/or dextrose diluent/flush, 10 ml Ⓓ Ⓑ

IOM: 100-02, 15, 50

❂ **A4217** Sterile water/saline, 500 ml Ⓑ Ⓓ

IOM: 100-02, 15, 50

❂ **A4218** Sterile saline or water, metered dose dispenser, 10 ml Ⓓ Ⓑ

❂ **A4220** Refill kit for implantable infusion pump Ⓓ

Do not report with 95990 or 95991 since Medicare payment for these codes includes the refill kit.

IOM: 100-03, 4, 280.1

✳ **A4221** Supplies for maintenance of non-insulin drug infusion catheter, per week (list drugs separately) Ⓑ

Includes dressings for catheter site and flush solutions not directly related to drug infusion.

✳ **A4222** Infusion supplies for external drug infusion pump, per cassette or bag (list drug separately) Ⓓ

Includes cassette or bag, diluting solutions, tubing and/or administration supplies, port cap changes, compounding charges, and preparation charges.

✳ **A4223** Infusion supplies not used with external infusion pump, per cassette or bag (list drugs separately) Ⓓ

IOM: 100-03, 4, 280.1

✳ **A4224** Supplies for maintenance of insulin infusion catheter, per week Ⓑ

❂ **A4225** Supplies for external insulin infusion pump, syringe type cartridge, sterile, each Ⓓ

IOM: 100-03, 1, 50.3

❂ **A4230** Infusion set for external insulin pump, non-needle cannula type Ⓓ

Requires prior authorization and copy of invoice.

IOM: 100-03, 4, 280.1

❂ **A4231** Infusion set for external insulin pump, needle type Ⓓ

Requires prior authorization and copy of invoice.

IOM: 100-03, 4, 280.1

⊘ **A4232** Syringe with needle for external insulin pump, sterile, 3 cc Ⓓ

Reports insulin reservoir for use with external insulin infusion pump (E0784); may be glass or plastic; includes needle for drawing up insulin. Does not include insulin for use in reservoir.

IOM: 100-03, 4, 280.1

Replacement Batteries

✳ **A4233** Replacement battery, alkaline (other than J cell), for use with medically necessary home blood glucose monitor owned by patient, each Ⓓ

✳ **A4234** Replacement battery, alkaline, J cell, for use with medically necessary home blood glucose monitor owned by patient, each Ⓓ

✳ **A4235** Replacement battery, lithium, for use with medically necessary home blood glucose monitor owned by patient, each Ⓑ

▶ New ↻ Revised ✔ Reinstated ~~deleted~~ Deleted ⊘ Not covered or valid by Medicare
❂ Special coverage instructions ✳ Carrier discretion Ⓑ Bill Part B MAC Ⓓ Bill DME MAC

✳ **A4236** Replacement battery, silver oxide, for use with medically necessary home blood glucose monitor owned by patient, each ⑨

Miscellaneous Supplies

✳ **A4244** Alcohol or peroxide, per pint ⑨ Ⓑ

✳ **A4245** Alcohol wipes, per box ⑨ Ⓑ

✳ **A4246** Betadine or pHisoHex solution, per pint ⑨ Ⓑ

✳ **A4247** Betadine or iodine swabs/wipes, per box Ⓑ Ⓑ

✳ **A4248** Chlorhexidine containing antiseptic, 1 ml ⑨ Ⓑ

⊘ **A4250** Urine test or reagent strips or tablets (100 tablets or strips) ⑨ Ⓑ

IOM: 100-02, 15, 110

⊘ **A4252** Blood ketone test or reagent strip, each ⑨

✪ **A4253** Blood glucose test or reagent strips for home blood glucose monitor, per 50 strips ⑨

Test strips (1 unit = 50 strips); non-insulin treated (every 3 months) 100 test strips (1×/day testing), 100 lancets (1×/day testing); modifier KS

IOM: 100-03, 1, 40.2

✪ **A4255** Platforms for home blood glucose monitor, 50 per box ⑨

IOM: 100-03, 1, 40.2

✪ **A4256** Normal, low and high calibrator solution/chips ⑨

IOM: 100-03, 1, 40.2

✳ **A4257** Replacement lens shield cartridge for use with laser skin piercing device, each ⑨

✪ **A4258** Spring-powered device for lancet, each ⑨

IOM: 100-03, 1, 40.2

✪ **A4259** Lancets, per box of 100 ⑨

IOM: 100-03, 1, 40.2

⊘ **A4261** Cervical cap for contraceptive use ⑨

✪ **A4262** Temporary, absorbable lacrimal duct implant, each ⑨

IOM: 100-04, 12, 20.3, 30.4

✪ **A4263** Permanent, long term, non-dissolvable lacrimal duct implant, each ⑨

Bundled with insertion if performed in physician office.

IOM: 100-04, 12, 30.4

⊘ **A4264** Permanent implantable contraceptive intratubal occlusion device(s) and delivery system ⑨

Reports the Essure device.

✪ **A4265** Paraffin, per pound ⑨ Ⓑ

IOM: 100-03, 4, 280.1

⊘ **A4266** Diaphragm for contraceptive use ⑨

⊘ **A4267** Contraceptive supply, condom, male, each ⑨

⊘ **A4268** Contraceptive supply, condom, female, each ⑨

⊘ **A4269** Contraceptive supply, spermicide (e.g., foam, gel), each ⑨

✳ **A4270** Disposable endoscope sheath, each ⑨

✳ **A4280** Adhesive skin support attachment for use with external breast prosthesis, each ⑨

✳ **A4281** Tubing for breast pump, replacement Ⓑ

✳ **A4282** Adapter for breast pump, replacement ⑨

✳ **A4283** Cap for breast pump bottle, replacement ⑨

✳ **A4284** Breast shield and splash protector for use with breast pump, replacement ⑨

✳ **A4285** Polycarbonate bottle for use with breast pump, replacement ⑨

✳ **A4286** Locking ring for breast pump, replacement ⑨

✳ **A4290** Sacral nerve stimulation test lead, each ⑨

Service not separately priced by Part B (e.g., services not covered, bundled, used by Part A only)

Implantable Catheters

✪ **A4300** Implantable access catheter, (e.g., venous, arterial, epidural subarachnoid, or peritoneal, etc.) external access ⑨

IOM: 100-02, 15, 120

✳ **A4301** Implantable access total; catheter, port/reservoir (e.g., venous, arterial, epidural, subarachnoid, peritoneal, etc.) ⑨

Disposable Drug Delivery System

✳ **A4305** Disposable drug delivery system, flow rate of 50 ml or greater per hour ⑨ Ⓑ

✳ **A4306** Disposable drug delivery system, flow rate of less than 50 ml per hour ⑨ Ⓑ

▶ New   ↩ Revised   ✔ Reinstated   ~~deleted~~ Deleted   ⊘ Not covered or valid by Medicare

✪ Special coverage instructions   ✳ Carrier discretion   ⑨ Bill Part B MAC   Ⓑ Bill DME MAC

Incontinence Appliances and Care Supplies

⊕ **A4310** Insertion tray without drainage bag and without catheter (accessories only) Ⓑ Ⓑ

IOM: 100-02, 15, 120

⊕ **A4311** Insertion tray without drainage bag with indwelling catheter, Foley type, two-way latex with coating (Teflon, silicone, silicone elastomer, or hydrophilic, etc.) Ⓑ Ⓑ

IOM: 100-02, 15, 120

⊕ **A4312** Insertion tray without drainage bag with indwelling catheter, Foley type, two-way, all silicone Ⓑ Ⓑ

Must meet criteria for indwelling catheter and medical record must justify need for:

• Recurrent encrustation

• Inability to pass a straight catheter

• Sensitivity to latex

Must be medically necessary.

IOM: 100-02, 15, 120

⊕ **A4313** Insertion tray without drainage bag with indwelling catheter, Foley type, three-way, for continuous irrigation Ⓑ Ⓑ

Must meet criteria for indwelling catheter and medical record must justify need for:

• Recurrent encrustation

• Inability to pass a straight catheter

• Sensitivity to latex

Must be medically necessary.

IOM: 100-02, 15, 120

⊕ **A4314** Insertion tray with drainage bag with indwelling catheter, Foley type, two-way latex with coating (Teflon, silicone, silicone elastomer or hydrophilic, etc.) Ⓑ Ⓑ

IOM: 100-02, 15, 120

⊕ **A4315** Insertion tray with drainage bag with indwelling catheter, Foley type, two-way, all silicone Ⓑ Ⓑ

IOM: 100-02, 15, 120

⊕ **A4316** Insertion tray with drainage bag with indwelling catheter, Foley type, three-way, for continuous irrigation Ⓑ Ⓑ

IOM: 100-02, 15, 120

⊕ **A4320** Irrigation tray with bulb or piston syringe, any purpose Ⓑ Ⓑ

IOM: 100-02, 15, 120

⊕ **A4321** Therapeutic agent for urinary catheter irrigation Ⓑ Ⓑ

IOM: 100-02, 15, 120

⊕ **A4322** Irrigation syringe, bulb, or piston, each Ⓑ Ⓑ

IOM: 100-02, 15, 120

⊕ **A4326** Male external catheter with integral collection chamber, any type, each Ⓑ Ⓑ

IOM: 100-02, 15, 120

⊕ **A4327** Female external urinary collection device; meatal cup, each Ⓑ Ⓑ

IOM: 100-02, 15, 120

⊕ **A4328** Female external urinary collection device; pouch, each Ⓑ Ⓑ

IOM: 100-02, 15, 120

⊕ **A4330** Perianal fecal collection pouch with adhesive, each Ⓑ Ⓑ

IOM: 100-02, 15, 120

⊕ **A4331** Extension drainage tubing, any type, any length, with connector/adaptor, for use with urinary leg bag or urostomy pouch, each Ⓑ Ⓑ

IOM: 100-02, 15, 120

⊕ **A4332** Lubricant, individual sterile packet, each Ⓑ Ⓑ

IOM: 100-02, 15, 120

⊕ **A4333** Urinary catheter anchoring device, adhesive skin attachment, each Ⓑ Ⓑ

IOM: 100-02, 15, 120

⊕ **A4334** Urinary catheter anchoring device, leg strap, each Ⓑ Ⓑ

IOM: 100-02, 15, 120

⊕ **A4335** Incontinence supply; miscellaneous Ⓑ Ⓑ

IOM: 100-02, 15, 120

⊕ **A4336** Incontinence supply, urethral insert, any type, each Ⓑ Ⓑ

IOM: 100-02, 15, 120

⊕ **A4337** Incontinence supply, rectal insert, any type, each Ⓑ Ⓑ

IOM: 100-02, 15, 120

⊕ **A4338** Indwelling catheter; Foley type, two-way latex with coating (Teflon, silicone, silicone elastomer, or hydrophilic, etc.), each Ⓑ Ⓑ

IOM: 100-02, 15, 120

▶ **New**   ↻ **Revised**   ✔ **Reinstated**   ~~deleted~~ **Deleted**   ⊘ **Not covered or valid by Medicare**

⊕ **Special coverage instructions**   ✱ **Carrier discretion**   Ⓑ **Bill Part B MAC**   Ⓑ **Bill DME MAC**

✪ **A4340** Indwelling catheter; specialty type (e.g., coude, mushroom, wing, etc.), each Ⓠ Ⓑ

Must meet criteria for indwelling catheter and medical record must justify need for:

• Recurrent encrustation

• Inability to pass a straight catheter

• Sensitivity to latex

Must be medically necessary.

IOM: 100-02, 15, 120

✪ **A4344** Indwelling catheter, Foley type, two-way, all silicone, each Ⓑ Ⓑ

Must meet criteria for indwelling catheter and medical record must justify need for:

• Recurrent encrustation

• Inability to pass a straight catheter

• Sensitivity to latex

Must be medically necessary.

IOM: 100-02, 15, 120

✪ **A4346** Indwelling catheter; Foley type, three way for continuous irrigation, each Ⓠ Ⓑ

IOM: 100-02, 15, 120

✪ **A4349** Male external catheter, with or without adhesive, disposable, each Ⓑ Ⓑ

IOM: 100-02, 15, 120

✪ **A4351** Intermittent urinary catheter; straight tip, with or without coating (Teflon, silicone, silicone elastomer, or hydrophilic, etc.), each Ⓑ Ⓑ

IOM: 100-02, 15, 120

✪ **A4352** Intermittent urinary catheter; coude (curved) tip, with or without coating (Teflon, silicone, silicone elastomeric, or hydrophilic, etc.), each Ⓠ Ⓑ

IOM: 100-02, 15, 120

✪ **A4353** Intermittent urinary catheter, with insertion supplies Ⓠ Ⓑ

IOM: 100-02, 15, 120

✪ **A4354** Insertion tray with drainage bag but without catheter Ⓠ Ⓑ

IOM: 100-02, 15, 120

✪ **A4355** Irrigation tubing set for continuous bladder irrigation through a three-way indwelling Foley catheter, each Ⓑ Ⓑ

IOM: 100-02, 15, 120

External Urinary Supplies

✪ **A4356** External urethral clamp or compression device (not to be used for catheter clamp), each Ⓠ Ⓑ

IOM: 100-02, 15, 120

✪ **A4357** Bedside drainage bag, day or night, with or without anti-reflux device, with or without tube, each Ⓠ Ⓑ

IOM: 100-02, 15, 120

✪ **A4358** Urinary drainage bag, leg or abdomen, vinyl, with or without tube, with straps, each Ⓠ Ⓑ

IOM: 100-02, 15, 120

✪ **A4360** Disposable external urethral clamp or compression device, with pad and/or pouch, each Ⓠ Ⓑ

Ostomy Supplies

✪ **A4361** Ostomy faceplate, each Ⓠ Ⓑ

IOM: 100-02, 15, 120

✪ **A4362** Skin barrier; solid, 4 × 4 or equivalent; each Ⓠ Ⓑ

IOM: 100-02, 15, 120

✪ **A4363** Ostomy clamp, any type, replacement only, each Ⓠ Ⓑ

✪ **A4364** Adhesive, liquid or equal, any type, per oz Ⓠ Ⓑ

Fee schedule category: Ostomy, tracheostomy, and urologicals items.

IOM: 100-02, 15, 120

✳ **A4366** Ostomy vent, any type, each Ⓠ Ⓑ

✪ **A4367** Ostomy belt, each Ⓠ Ⓑ

IOM: 100-02, 15, 120

✳ **A4368** Ostomy filter, any type, each Ⓠ Ⓑ

✪ **A4369** Ostomy skin barrier, liquid (spray, brush, etc.), per oz Ⓠ Ⓑ

IOM: 100-02, 15, 120

✪ **A4371** Ostomy skin barrier, powder, per oz Ⓠ Ⓑ

IOM: 100-02, 15, 120

✪ **A4372** Ostomy skin barrier, solid 4 × 4 or equivalent, standard wear, with built-in convexity, each Ⓠ Ⓑ

IOM: 100-02, 15, 120

✪ **A4373** Ostomy skin barrier, with flange (solid, flexible, or accordion), with built-in convexity, any size, each Ⓠ Ⓑ

IOM: 100-02, 15, 120

▶ **New**   ⟳ **Revised**   ✔ **Reinstated**   ~~deleted~~ **Deleted**   ⊘ **Not covered or valid by Medicare**

✪ **Special coverage instructions**   ✳ **Carrier discretion**   Ⓠ **Bill Part B MAC**   Ⓑ **Bill DME MAC**

⊕ **A4375** Ostomy pouch, drainable, with faceplate attached, plastic, each Ⓑ Ⓓ

IOM: 100-02, 15, 120

⊕ **A4376** Ostomy pouch, drainable, with faceplate attached, rubber, each Ⓑ Ⓓ

IOM: 100-02, 15, 120

⊕ **A4377** Ostomy pouch, drainable, for use on faceplate, plastic, each Ⓑ Ⓓ

IOM: 100-02, 15, 120

⊕ **A4378** Ostomy pouch, drainable, for use on faceplate, rubber, each Ⓑ Ⓓ

IOM: 100-02, 15, 120

⊕ **A4379** Ostomy pouch, urinary, with faceplate attached, plastic, each Ⓑ Ⓓ

IOM: 100-02, 15, 120

⊕ **A4380** Ostomy pouch, urinary, with faceplate attached, rubber, each Ⓑ Ⓓ

IOM: 100-02, 15, 120

⊕ **A4381** Ostomy pouch, urinary, for use on faceplate, plastic, each Ⓑ Ⓓ

IOM: 100-02, 15, 120

⊕ **A4382** Ostomy pouch, urinary, for use on faceplate, heavy plastic, each Ⓑ Ⓓ

IOM: 100-02, 15, 120

⊕ **A4383** Ostomy pouch, urinary, for use on faceplate, rubber, each Ⓑ Ⓓ

IOM: 100-02, 15, 120

⊕ **A4384** Ostomy faceplate equivalent, silicone ring, each Ⓑ Ⓓ

IOM: 100-02, 15, 120

⊕ **A4385** Ostomy skin barrier, solid 4 × 4 or equivalent, extended wear, without built-in convexity, each Ⓑ Ⓓ

IOM: 100-02, 15, 120

⊕ **A4387** Ostomy pouch closed, with barrier attached, with built-in convexity (1 piece), each Ⓑ Ⓓ

IOM: 100-02, 15, 120

⊕ **A4388** Ostomy pouch, drainable, with extended wear barrier attached (1 piece), each Ⓑ Ⓓ

IOM: 100-02, 15, 120

⊕ **A4389** Ostomy pouch, drainable, with barrier attached, with built-in convexity (1 piece), each Ⓑ Ⓓ

IOM: 100-02, 15, 120

⊕ **A4390** Ostomy pouch, drainable, with extended wear barrier attached, with built-in convexity (1 piece), each Ⓑ Ⓓ

IOM: 100-02, 15, 120

⊕ **A4391** Ostomy pouch, urinary, with extended wear barrier attached (1 piece), each Ⓑ Ⓓ

IOM: 100-02, 15, 120

⊕ **A4392** Ostomy pouch, urinary, with standard wear barrier attached, with built-in convexity (1 piece), each Ⓑ Ⓓ

IOM: 100-02, 15, 120

⊕ **A4393** Ostomy pouch, urinary, with extended wear barrier attached, with built-in convexity (1 piece), each Ⓑ Ⓓ

IOM: 100-02, 15, 120

⊕ **A4394** Ostomy deodorant, with or without lubricant, for use in ostomy pouch, per fluid ounce Ⓑ Ⓓ

IOM: 100-02, 15, 20

⊕ **A4395** Ostomy deodorant for use in ostomy pouch, solid, per tablet Ⓑ Ⓓ

IOM: 100-02, 15, 20

⊕ **A4396** Ostomy belt with peristomal hernia support Ⓑ Ⓓ

IOM: 100-02, 15, 120

⊕ **A4397** Irrigation supply; sleeve, each Ⓑ Ⓓ

IOM: 100-02, 15, 120

⊕ **A4398** Ostomy irrigation supply; bag, each Ⓑ Ⓓ

IOM: 100-02, 15, 120

⊕ **A4399** Ostomy irrigation supply; cone/catheter, with or without brush Ⓑ Ⓓ

IOM: 100-02, 15, 120

⊕ **A4400** Ostomy irrigation set Ⓑ Ⓓ

IOM: 100-02, 15, 120

⊕ **A4402** Lubricant, per ounce Ⓑ Ⓓ

IOM: 100-02, 15, 120

⊕ **A4404** Ostomy ring, each Ⓑ Ⓓ

IOM: 100-02, 15, 120

⊕ **A4405** Ostomy skin barrier, non-pectin based, paste, per ounce Ⓑ Ⓓ

IOM: 100-02, 15, 120

⊕ **A4406** Ostomy skin barrier, pectin-based, paste, per ounce Ⓑ Ⓓ

IOM: 100-02, 15, 120

⊕ **A4407** Ostomy skin barrier, with flange (solid, flexible, or accordion), extended wear, with built-in convexity, 4 × 4 inches or smaller, each Ⓑ Ⓓ

IOM: 100-02, 15, 120

▶ New ↻ Revised ✔ Reinstated ~~deleted~~ Deleted ⊘ Not covered or valid by Medicare
⊕ Special coverage instructions ✳ Carrier discretion Ⓑ Bill Part B MAC Ⓓ Bill DME MAC

✪ **A4408** Ostomy skin barrier, with flange (solid, flexible, or accordion), extended wear, with built-in convexity, larger than 4 × 4 inches, each Ⓑ Ⓓ

IOM: 100-02, 15, 120

✪ **A4409** Ostomy skin barrier, with flange (solid, flexible, or accordion), extended wear, without built-in convexity, 4 × 4 inches or smaller, each Ⓑ Ⓓ

IOM: 100-02, 15, 120

✪ **A4410** Ostomy skin barrier, with flange (solid, flexible, or accordion), extended wear, without built-in convexity, larger than 4 × 4 inches, each Ⓑ Ⓓ

IOM: 100-02, 15, 120

✪ **A4411** Ostomy skin barrier, solid 4 × 4 or equivalent, extended wear, with built-in convexity, each Ⓑ Ⓓ

✪ **A4412** Ostomy pouch, drainable, high output, for use on a barrier with flange (2 piece system), without filter, each Ⓑ Ⓓ

IOM: 100-02, 15, 120

✪ **A4413** Ostomy pouch, drainable, high output, for use on a barrier with flange (2 piece system), with filter, each Ⓑ Ⓓ

IOM: 100-02, 15, 120

✪ **A4414** Ostomy skin barrier, with flange (solid, flexible, or accordion), without built-in convexity, 4 × 4 inches or smaller, each Ⓑ Ⓓ

IOM: 100-02, 15, 120

✪ **A4415** Ostomy skin barrier, with flange (solid, flexible, or accordion), without built-in convexity, larger than 4 × 4 inches, each Ⓑ Ⓓ

IOM: 100-02, 15, 120

✳ **A4416** Ostomy pouch, closed, with barrier attached, with filter (1 piece), each Ⓑ Ⓓ

✳ **A4417** Ostomy pouch, closed, with barrier attached, with built-in convexity, with filter (1 piece), each Ⓑ Ⓓ

✳ **A4418** Ostomy pouch, closed; without barrier attached, with filter (1 piece), each Ⓑ Ⓓ

✳ **A4419** Ostomy pouch, closed; for use on barrier with non-locking flange, with filter (2 piece), each Ⓑ Ⓓ

✳ **A4420** Ostomy pouch, closed; for use on barrier with locking flange (2 piece), each Ⓑ Ⓓ

↻ ✳ **A4421** Ostomy supply; miscellaneous Ⓑ Ⓓ

✪ **A4422** Ostomy absorbent material (sheet/pad/crystal packet) for use in ostomy pouch to thicken liquid stomal output, each Ⓑ Ⓓ

IOM: 100-02, 15, 120

✳ **A4423** Ostomy pouch, closed; for use on barrier with locking flange, with filter (2 piece), each Ⓑ Ⓓ

✳ **A4424** Ostomy pouch, drainable, with barrier attached, with filter (1 piece), each Ⓑ Ⓓ

✳ **A4425** Ostomy pouch, drainable; for use on barrier with non-locking flange, with filter (2 piece system), each Ⓑ Ⓓ

✳ **A4426** Ostomy pouch, drainable; for use on barrier with locking flange (2 piece system), each Ⓑ Ⓓ

✳ **A4427** Ostomy pouch, drainable; for use on barrier with locking flange, with filter (2 piece system), each Ⓑ Ⓓ

✳ **A4428** Ostomy pouch, urinary, with extended wear barrier attached, with faucet-type tap with valve (1 piece), each Ⓑ Ⓓ

✳ **A4429** Ostomy pouch, urinary, with barrier attached, with built-in convexity, with faucet-type tap with valve (1 piece), each Ⓑ Ⓓ

✳ **A4430** Ostomy pouch, urinary, with extended wear barrier attached, with built-in convexity, with faucet-type tap with valve (1 piece), each Ⓑ Ⓓ

✳ **A4431** Ostomy pouch, urinary; with barrier attached, with faucet-type tap with valve (1 piece), each Ⓑ Ⓓ

✳ **A4432** Ostomy pouch, urinary; for use on barrier with non-locking flange, with faucet-type tap with valve (2 piece), each Ⓑ Ⓓ

✳ **A4433** Ostomy pouch, urinary; for use on barrier with locking flange (2 piece), each Ⓑ Ⓓ

✳ **A4434** Ostomy pouch, urinary; for use on barrier with locking flange, with faucet-type tap with valve (2 piece), each Ⓑ Ⓓ

✳ **A4435** Ostomy pouch, drainable, high output, with extended wear barrier (one-piece system), with or without filter, each Ⓑ Ⓓ

▶ New　↻ Revised　✔ Reinstated　~~deleted~~ Deleted　⊘ Not covered or valid by Medicare
✪ Special coverage instructions　✳ Carrier discretion　Ⓑ Bill Part B MAC　Ⓓ Bill DME MAC

Miscellaneous Supplies

✿ **A4450** Tape, non-waterproof, per 18 square inches Ⓑ Ⓑ

If used with surgical dressings, billed with AW modifier (in addition to appropriate A1-A9 modifier).

IOM: 100-02, 15, 120

✿ **A4452** Tape, waterproof, per 18 square inches Ⓑ Ⓑ

If used with surgical dressings, billed with AW modifier (in addition to appropriate A1-A9 modifier).

IOM: 100-02, 15, 120

✿ **A4455** Adhesive remover or solvent (for tape, cement or other adhesive), per ounce Ⓑ Ⓑ

IOM: 100-02, 15, 120

✿ **A4456** Adhesive remover, wipes, any type, each Ⓑ Ⓑ

May be reimbursed for male or female clients to home health DME providers and DME medical suppliers in the home setting.

IOM: 100-02, 15, 120

✳ **A4458** Enema bag with tubing, reusable Ⓑ

✳ **A4459** Manual pump-operated enema system, includes balloon, catheter and all accessories, reusable, any type Ⓑ

✳ **A4461** Surgical dressing holder, non-reusable, each Ⓑ Ⓑ

✳ **A4463** Surgical dressing holder, reusable, each Ⓑ Ⓑ

✳ **A4465** Non-elastic binder for extremity Ⓑ

⊘ **A4467** Belt, strap, sleeve, garment, or covering, any type Ⓖ

✿ **A4470** Gravlee jet washer Ⓖ

Symptoms suggestive of endometrial disease must be present for this disposable diagnostic tool to be covered.

IOM: 100-02, 16, 90; 100-03, 4, 230.5

✿ **A4480** VABRA aspirator Ⓖ

Symptoms suggestive of endometrial disease must be present for this disposable diagnostic tool to be covered.

IOM: 100-02, 16, 90; 100-03, 4, 230.6

✿ **A4481** Tracheostoma filter, any type, any size, each Ⓑ Ⓖ

IOM: 100-02, 15, 120

✿ **A4483** Moisture exchanger, disposable, for use with invasive mechanical ventilation Ⓑ

IOM: 100-02, 15, 120

⊘ **A4490** Surgical stockings above knee length, each Ⓑ

IOM: 100-02, 15, 100; 100-02, 15, 110; 100-03, 4, 280.1

⊘ **A4495** Surgical stockings thigh length, each Ⓑ

IOM: 100-02, 15, 100; 100-02, 15, 110; 100-03, 4, 280.1

⊘ **A4500** Surgical stockings below knee length, each Ⓑ

IOM: 100-02, 15, 100; 100-02, 15, 110; 100-03, 4, 280.1

⊘ **A4510** Surgical stockings full length, each Ⓑ

IOM: 100-02, 15, 100; 100-02, 15, 110; 100-03, 4, 280.1

⊘ **A4520** Incontinence garment, any type (e.g., brief, diaper), each Ⓖ

IOM: 100-03, 4, 280.1

✿ **A4550** Surgical trays Ⓖ

No longer payable by Medicare; included in practice expense for procedures. Some private payers may pay, most private payers follow Medicare guidelines.

IOM: 100-04, 12, 20.3, 30.4

⊘ **A4553** Non-disposable underpads, all sizes Ⓖ

IOM: 100-03, 4, 280.1

⊘ **A4554** Disposable underpads, all sizes Ⓖ

IOM: 100-03, 4, 280.1

⊘ **A4555** Electrode/transducer for use with electrical stimulation device used for cancer treatment, replacement only Ⓑ Ⓑ

✳ **A4556** Electrodes, (e.g., apnea monitor), per pair Ⓑ Ⓑ

✳ **A4557** Lead wires, (e.g., apnea monitor), per pair Ⓑ Ⓑ

✳ **A4558** Conductive gel or paste, for use with electrical device (e.g., TENS, NMES), per oz Ⓑ Ⓑ

✳ **A4559** Coupling gel or paste, for use with ultrasound device, per oz Ⓑ Ⓑ

✳ **A4561** Pessary, rubber, any type Ⓖ

✳ **A4562** Pessary, non-rubber, any type Ⓑ

✳ **A4565** Slings Ⓖ

▶ New　↩ Revised　✔ Reinstated　deleted Deleted　⊘ Not covered or valid by Medicare
✿ Special coverage instructions　✳ Carrier discretion　Ⓑ Bill Part B MAC　Ⓑ Bill DME MAC

⊘ **A4566** Shoulder sling or vest design, abduction restrainer, with or without swathe control, prefabricated, includes fitting and adjustment Ⓑ

⊘ **A4570** Splint Ⓑ

IOM: 100-02, 6, 10; 100-02, 15, 100; 100-04, 4, 240

↻ ✳ **A4575** Topical hyperbaric oxygen chamber, disposable Ⓑ

⊘ **A4580** Cast supplies (e.g., plaster) Ⓑ

IOM: 100-02, 6, 10; 100-02, 15, 100; 100-04, 4, 240

⊘ **A4590** Special casting material (e.g., fiberglass) Ⓑ

IOM: 100-02, 6, 10; 100-02, 15, 100; 100-04, 4, 240

✿ **A4595** Electrical stimulator supplies, 2 lead, per month (e.g., TENS, NMES) Ⓑ Ⓑ

IOM: 100-03, 2, 160.13

✳ **A4600** Sleeve for intermittent limb compression device, replacement only, each Ⓑ

✳ **A4601** Lithium ion battery, rechargeable, for non-prosthetic use, replacement Ⓑ

✳ **A4602** Replacement battery for external infusion pump owned by patient, lithium, 1.5 volt, each Ⓑ

✳ **A4604** Tubing with integrated heating element for use with positive airway pressure device Ⓑ

✳ **A4605** Tracheal suction catheter, closed system, each Ⓑ

✳ **A4606** Oxygen probe for use with oximeter device, replacement Ⓑ

✳ **A4608** Transtracheal oxygen catheter, each Ⓑ

Supplies for Respiratory and Oxygen Equipment

⊘ **A4611** Battery, heavy duty; replacement for patient owned ventilator Ⓑ

⊘ **A4612** Battery cables; replacement for patient-owned ventilator Ⓑ

⊘ **A4613** Battery charger; replacement for patient-owned ventilator Ⓑ

✳ **A4614** Peak expiratory flow rate meter, hand held Ⓑ Ⓑ

✿ **A4615** Cannula, nasal Ⓑ Ⓑ

✿ **A4616** Tubing (oxygen), per foot Ⓑ Ⓑ

IOM: 100-03, 2, 160.6; 100-04, 20, 100.2

✿ **A4617** Mouth piece Ⓑ Ⓑ

IOM: 100-03, 2, 160.6; 100-04, 20, 100.2

✿ **A4618** Breathing circuits Ⓑ Ⓑ

IOM: 100-03, 2, 160.6; 100-04, 20, 100.2

✿ **A4619** Face tent Ⓑ Ⓑ

IOM: 100-03, 2, 160.6; 100-04, 20, 100.2

✿ **A4620** Variable concentration mask Ⓑ Ⓑ

IOM: 100-03, 2, 160.6; 100-04, 20, 100.2

✿ **A4623** Tracheostomy, inner cannula Ⓑ Ⓑ

IOM: 100-02, 15, 120; 100-03, 1, 20.9

✳ **A4624** Tracheal suction catheter, any type, other than closed system, each Ⓑ Ⓑ

Sterile suction catheters are medically necessary only for tracheostomy suctioning. Limitations include three suction catheters per day when covered for medically necessary tracheostomy suctioning. Assign DX V44.0 or V55.0 on the claim form. (CMS Manual System, Pub. 100-3, NCD manual, Chapter 1, Section 280-1)

✿ **A4625** Tracheostomy care kit for new tracheostomy Ⓑ Ⓑ

Dressings used with tracheostomies are included in the allowance for the code. This starter kit is covered after a surgical tracheostomy. (https://www .noridianmedicare.com/dme/coverage/docs/lcds/current_lcds/tracheostomy_care_supplies.htm)

IOM: 100-02, 15, 120

✿ **A4626** Tracheostomy cleaning brush, each Ⓑ Ⓑ

IOM: 100-02, 15, 120

⊘ **A4627** Spacer, bag, or reservoir, with or without mask, for use with metered dose inhaler Ⓑ Ⓑ

IOM: 100-02, 15, 110

✳ **A4628** Oropharyngeal suction catheter, each Ⓑ Ⓑ

No more than three catheters per week are covered for medically necessary oropharyngeal suctioning because the catheters can be reused if cleansed and disinfected. (MS Manual System, Pub. 100-3, NCD manual, Chapter 1, Section 280-1)

✿ **A4629** Tracheostomy care kit for established tracheostomy Ⓑ Ⓑ

IOM: 100-02, 15, 120

▶ **New**   ↻ **Revised**   ✔ **Reinstated**   ~~deleted~~ **Deleted**   ⊘ **Not covered or valid by Medicare**
✿ **Special coverage instructions**   ✳ **Carrier discretion**   Ⓑ **Bill Part B MAC**   Ⓑ **Bill DME MAC**

Replacement Parts

⊗ **A4630** Replacement batteries, medically necessary, transcutaneous electrical stimulator, owned by patient Ⓑ

IOM: 100-03, 3, 160.7

✳ **A4633** Replacement bulb/lamp for ultraviolet light therapy system, each Ⓑ

✳ **A4634** Replacement bulb for therapeutic light box, tabletop model Ⓑ

⊗ **A4635** Underarm pad, crutch, replacement, each Ⓑ

IOM: 100-03, 4, 280.1

⊗ **A4636** Replacement, handgrip, cane, crutch, or walker, each Ⓑ

IOM: 100-03, 4, 280.1

⊗ **A4637** Replacement, tip, cane, crutch, walker, each Ⓑ

IOM: 100-03, 4, 280.1

✳ **A4638** Replacement battery for patient-owned ear pulse generator, each Ⓑ

✳ **A4639** Replacement pad for infrared heating pad system, each Ⓑ

⊗ **A4640** Replacement pad for use with medically necessary alternating pressure pad owned by patient Ⓑ

IOM: 100-03, 4, 280.1; 100-08, 5, 5.2.3

Supplies for Radiological Procedures

✳ **A4641** Radiopharmaceutical, diagnostic, not otherwise classified Ⓑ

Is not an applicable tracer for PET scans

✳ **A4642** Indium In-111 satumomab pendetide, diagnostic, per study dose, up to 6 millicuries Ⓟ

Miscellaneous Supplies

✳ **A4648** Tissue marker, implantable, any type, each Ⓟ

✳ **A4649** Surgical supply miscellaneous Ⓟ Ⓑ

✳ **A4650** Implantable radiation dosimeter, each Ⓟ

⊗ **A4651** Calibrated microcapillary tube, each Ⓓ

IOM: 100-04, 3, 40.3

⊗ **A4652** Microcapillary tube sealant Ⓑ

IOM: 100-04, 3, 40.3

Supplies for Dialysis

✳ **A4653** Peritoneal dialysis catheter anchoring device, belt, each Ⓑ

⊗ **A4657** Syringe, with or without needle, each Ⓑ

IOM: 100-04, 8, 90.3.2

⊗ **A4660** Sphygmomanometer/blood pressure apparatus with cuff and stethoscope Ⓑ

IOM: 100-04, 8, 90.3.2

⊗ **A4663** Blood pressure cuff only Ⓓ

IOM: 100-04, 8, 90.3.2

⊘ **A4670** Automatic blood pressure monitor Ⓓ

IOM: 100-04, 8, 90.3.2

⊗ **A4671** Disposable cycler set used with cycler dialysis machine, each Ⓓ

IOM: 100-04, 8, 90.3.2

⊗ **A4672** Drainage extension line, sterile, for dialysis, each Ⓑ

IOM: 100-04, 8, 90.3.2

⊗ **A4673** Extension line with easy lock connectors, used with dialysis Ⓓ

IOM: 100-04, 8, 90.3.2

⊗ **A4674** Chemicals/antiseptics solution used to clean/sterilize dialysis equipment, per 8 oz Ⓑ

IOM: 100-04, 8, 90.3.2

⊗ **A4680** Activated carbon filters for hemodialysis, each Ⓓ

IOM: 100-04, 8, 90.3.2

⊗ **A4690** Dialyzers (artificial kidneys), all types, all sizes, for hemodialysis, each Ⓑ

IOM: 100-04, 8, 90.3.2

⊗ **A4706** Bicarbonate concentrate, solution, for hemodialysis, per gallon Ⓑ

IOM: 100-04, 8, 90.3.2

⊗ **A4707** Bicarbonate concentrate, powder, for hemodialysis, per packet Ⓑ

IOM: 100-04, 8, 90.3.2

⊗ **A4708** Acetate concentrate solution, for hemodialysis, per gallon Ⓑ

IOM: 100-04, 8, 90.3.2

⊗ **A4709** Acid concentrate, solution, for hemodialysis, per gallon Ⓑ

IOM: 100-04, 8, 90.3.2

⊗ **A4714** Treated water (deionized, distilled, or reverse osmosis) for peritoneal dialysis, per gallon Ⓑ

IOM: 100-03, 4, 230.7; 100-04, 3, 40.3

▶ **New** ↻ **Revised** ✔ **Reinstated** ~~deleted~~ **Deleted** ⊘ **Not covered or valid by Medicare**
⊗ **Special coverage instructions** ✳ **Carrier discretion** Ⓟ **Bill Part B MAC** Ⓓ **Bill DME MAC**

✪ **A4719** "Y set" tubing for peritoneal dialysis ⑧

IOM: 100-04, 8, 90.3.2

✪ **A4720** Dialysate solution, any concentration of dextrose, fluid volume greater than 249 cc, but less than or equal to 999 cc, for peritoneal dialysis ⑧

Do not use AX modifier.

IOM: 100-04, 8, 90.3.2

✪ **A4721** Dialysate solution, any concentration of dextrose, fluid volume greater than 999 cc but less than or equal to 1999 cc, for peritoneal dialysis ⑧

IOM: 100-04, 8, 90.3.2

✪ **A4722** Dialysate solution, any concentration of dextrose, fluid volume greater than 1999 cc but less than or equal to 2999 cc, for peritoneal dialysis ⑧

IOM: 100-04, 8, 90.3.2

✪ **A4723** Dialysate solution, any concentration of dextrose, fluid volume greater than 2999 cc but less than or equal to 3999 cc, for peritoneal dialysis ⑧

IOM: 100-04, 8, 90.3.2

✪ **A4724** Dialysate solution, any concentration of dextrose, fluid volume greater than 3999 cc but less than or equal to 4999 cc for peritoneal dialysis ⑧

IOM: 100-04, 8, 90.3.2

✪ **A4725** Dialysate solution, any concentration of dextrose, fluid volume greater than 4999 cc but less than or equal to 5999 cc, for peritoneal dialysis ⑧

IOM: 100-04, 8, 90.3.2

✪ **A4726** Dialysate solution, any concentration of dextrose, fluid volume greater than 5999 cc, for peritoneal dialysis ⑧

IOM: 100-04, 8, 90.3.2

✳ **A4728** Dialysate solution, non-dextrose containing, 500 ml ⑧

✪ **A4730** Fistula cannulation set for hemodialysis, each ⑧

IOM: 100-04, 8, 90.3.2

✪ **A4736** Topical anesthetic, for dialysis, per gram ⑧

IOM: 100-04, 8, 90.3.2

✪ **A4737** Injectable anesthetic, for dialysis, per 10 ml ⑧

IOM: 100-04, 8, 90.3.2

✪ **A4740** Shunt accessory, for hemodialysis, any type, each ⑧

IOM: 100-04, 8, 90.3.2

✪ **A4750** Blood tubing, arterial or venous, for hemodialysis, each ⑧

IOM: 100-04, 8, 90.3.2

✪ **A4755** Blood tubing, arterial and venous combined, for hemodialysis, each ⑧

IOM: 100-04, 8, 90.3.2

✪ **A4760** Dialysate solution test kit, for peritoneal dialysis, any type, each ⑧

IOM: 100-04, 8, 90.3.2

✪ **A4765** Dialysate concentrate, powder, additive for peritoneal dialysis, per packet ⑧

IOM: 100-04, 8, 90.3.2

✪ **A4766** Dialysate concentrate, solution, additive for peritoneal dialysis, per 10 ml ⑧

IOM: 100-04, 8, 90.3.2

✪ **A4770** Blood collection tube, vacuum, for dialysis, per 50 ⑧

IOM: 100-04, 8, 90.3.2

✪ **A4771** Serum clotting time tube, for dialysis, per 50 ⑧

IOM: 100-04, 8, 90.3.2

✪ **A4772** Blood glucose test strips, for dialysis, per 50 ⑧

IOM: 100-04, 8, 90.3.2

✪ **A4773** Occult blood test strips, for dialysis, per 50 ⑧

IOM: 100-04, 8, 90.3.2

✪ **A4774** Ammonia test strips, for dialysis, per 50 ⑧

IOM: 100-04, 8, 90.3.2

✪ **A4802** Protamine sulfate, for hemodialysis, per 50 mg ⑧

IOM: 100-04, 8, 90.3.2

✪ **A4860** Disposable catheter tips for peritoneal dialysis, per 10 ⑧

IOM: 100-04, 8, 90.3.2

✪ **A4870** Plumbing and/or electrical work for home hemodialysis equipment ⑧

IOM: 100-04, 8, 90.3.2

✪ **A4890** Contracts, repair and maintenance, for hemodialysis equipment ⑧

IOM: 100-02, 15, 110.2

✪ **A4911** Drain bag/bottle, for dialysis, each ⑧

✪ **A4913** Miscellaneous dialysis supplies, not otherwise specified ⑧

Items not related to dialysis must not be billed with the miscellaneous codes A4913 or E1699.

▶ New   ↻ Revised   ✔ Reinstated   ~~deleted~~ Deleted   ⊘ Not covered or valid by Medicare

✪ Special coverage instructions   ✳ Carrier discretion   ⑨ Bill Part B MAC   ⑧ Bill DME MAC

⊘ **A4918** Venous pressure clamp, for hemodialysis, each Ⓑ

⊘ **A4927** Gloves, non-sterile, per 100 Ⓖ

⊘ **A4928** Surgical mask, per 20 Ⓖ

⊘ **A4929** Tourniquet for dialysis, each Ⓑ

⊘ **A4930** Gloves, sterile, per pair Ⓖ

✳ **A4931** Oral thermometer, reusable, any type, each Ⓖ

✳ **A4932** Rectal thermometer, reusable, any type, each Ⓖ

Additional Ostomy Supplies

⊘ **A5051** Ostomy pouch, closed; with barrier attached (1 piece), each Ⓑ Ⓑ

IOM: 100-02, 15, 120

⊘ **A5052** Ostomy pouch, closed; without barrier attached (1 piece), each Ⓑ Ⓑ

IOM: 100-02, 15, 120

⊘ **A5053** Ostomy pouch, closed; for use on faceplate, each Ⓑ Ⓖ

IOM: 100-02, 15, 120

⊘ **A5054** Ostomy pouch, closed; for use on barrier with flange (2 piece), each Ⓑ Ⓑ

IOM: 100-02, 15, 120

⊘ **A5055** Stoma cap Ⓑ Ⓑ

IOM: 100-02, 15, 120

⊘ **A5056** Ostomy pouch, drainable, with extended wear barrier attached, with filter, (1 piece), each Ⓑ Ⓖ

IOM: 100-02, 15, 120

⊘ **A5057** Ostomy pouch, drainable, with extended wear barrier attached, with built in convexity, with filter, (1 piece), each Ⓑ Ⓑ

IOM: 100-02, 15, 120

✳ **A5061** Ostomy pouch, drainable; with barrier attached, (1 piece), each Ⓑ Ⓑ

IOM: 100-02, 15, 120

⊘ **A5062** Ostomy pouch, drainable; without barrier attached (1 piece), each Ⓑ Ⓑ

IOM: 100-02, 15, 120

⊘ **A5063** Ostomy pouch, drainable; for use on barrier with flange (2 piece system), each Ⓑ Ⓖ

IOM: 100-02, 15, 120

⊘ **A5071** Ostomy pouch, urinary; with barrier attached (1 piece), each Ⓑ Ⓑ

IOM: 100-02, 15, 120

⊘ **A5072** Ostomy pouch, urinary; without barrier attached (1 piece), each Ⓑ Ⓑ

IOM: 100-02, 15, 120

⊘ **A5073** Ostomy pouch, urinary; for use on barrier with flange (2 piece), each Ⓑ Ⓑ

IOM: 100-02, 15, 120

⊘ **A5081** Stoma plug or seal, any type Ⓑ Ⓑ

IOM: 100-02, 15, 120

⊘ **A5082** Continent device; catheter for continent stoma Ⓑ Ⓑ

IOM: 100-02, 15, 120

✳ **A5083** Continent device, stoma absorptive cover for continent stoma Ⓑ Ⓑ

⊘ **A5093** Ostomy accessory; convex insert Ⓑ Ⓑ

IOM: 100-02, 15, 120

Additional Incontinence and Ostomy Supplies

⊘ **A5102** Bedside drainage bottle with or without tubing, rigid or expandable, each Ⓑ Ⓑ

IOM: 100-02, 15, 120

⊘ **A5105** Urinary suspensory, with leg bag, with or without tube, each Ⓑ Ⓑ

IOM: 100-02, 15, 120

⊘ **A5112** Urinary drainage bag, leg bag, leg or abdomen, latex, with or without tube, with straps, each Ⓑ Ⓖ

IOM: 100-02, 15, 120

⊘ **A5113** Leg strap; latex, replacement only, per set Ⓑ Ⓑ

IOM: 100-02, 15, 120

⊘ **A5114** Leg strap; foam or fabric, replacement only, per set Ⓑ Ⓑ

IOM: 100-02, 15, 120

⊘ **A5120** Skin barrier, wipes or swabs, each Ⓑ Ⓑ

IOM: 100-02, 15, 120

⊘ **A5121** Skin barrier; solid, 6 × 6 or equivalent, each Ⓑ Ⓑ

IOM: 100-02, 15, 120

⊘ **A5122** Skin barrier; solid, 8 × 8 or equivalent, each Ⓑ Ⓖ

IOM: 100-02, 15, 120

⊘ **A5126** Adhesive or non-adhesive; disk or foam pad Ⓑ Ⓑ

IOM: 100-02, 15, 120

⊘ **A5131** Appliance cleaner, incontinence and ostomy appliances, per 16 oz Ⓑ Ⓑ

IOM: 100-02, 15, 120

▶ **New**   ↻ **Revised**   ✔ **Reinstated**   ~~deleted~~ **Deleted**   ⊘ **Not covered or valid by Medicare**

⊘ **Special coverage instructions**   ✳ **Carrier discretion**   Ⓑ **Bill Part B MAC**   Ⓖ **Bill DME MAC**

✿ **A5200** Percutaneous catheter/tube anchoring device, adhesive skin attachment Ⓟ Ⓑ

IOM: 100-02, 15, 120

Diabetic Shoes, Fitting, and Modifications

✿ **A5500** For diabetics only, fitting (including follow-up), custom preparation and supply of off-the-shelf depth-inlay shoe manufactured to accommodate multi-density insert(s), per shoe Ⓑ

IOM: 100-02, 15, 140

✿ **A5501** For diabetics only, fitting (including follow-up), custom preparation and supply of shoe molded from cast(s) of patient's foot (custom-molded shoe), per shoe Ⓑ

The diabetic patient must have at least one of the following conditions: peripheral neuropathy with evidence of callus formation, pre-ulcerative calluses, previous ulceration, foot deformity, previous amputation or poor circulation.

IOM: 100-02, 15, 140

✿ **A5503** For diabetics only, modification (including fitting) of off-the-shelf depth-inlay shoe or custom-molded shoe with roller or rigid rocker bottom, per shoe Ⓑ

IOM: 100-02, 15, 140

✿ **A5504** For diabetics only, modification (including fitting) of off-the-shelf depth-inlay shoe or custom-molded shoe with wedge(s), per shoe Ⓑ

IOM: 100-02, 15, 140

✿ **A5505** For diabetics only, modification (including fitting) of off-the-shelf depth-inlay shoe or custom-molded shoe with metatarsal bar, per shoe Ⓑ

IOM: 100-02, 15, 140

✿ **A5506** For diabetics only, modification (including fitting) of off-the-shelf depth-inlay shoe or custom-molded shoe with off-set heel(s), per shoe Ⓑ

IOM: 100-02, 15, 140

✿ **A5507** For diabetics only, not otherwise specified modification (including fitting) of off-the-shelf depth-inlay shoe or custom-molded shoe, per shoe Ⓑ

Only used for not otherwise specified therapeutic modifications to shoe or for repairs to a diabetic shoe(s)

IOM: 100-02, 15, 140

✿ **A5508** For diabetics only, deluxe feature of off-the-shelf depth-inlay shoe or custom-molded shoe, per shoe Ⓑ

IOM: 100-02, 15, 40

✿ **A5510** For diabetics only, direct formed, compression molded to patient's foot without external heat source, multiple-density insert(s) prefabricated, per shoe Ⓑ

IOM: 100-02, 15, 140

✳ **A5512** For diabetics only, multiple density insert, direct formed, molded to foot after external heat source of 230 degrees Fahrenheit or higher, total contact with patient's foot, including arch, base layer minimum of 1/4 inch material of shore a 35 durometer or 3/16 inch material of shore a 40 durometer (or higher), prefabricated, each Ⓑ

✳ **A5513** For diabetics only, multiple density insert, custom molded from model of patient's foot, total contact with patient's foot, including arch, base layer minimum of 3/16 inch material of shore a 35 durometer (or higher), includes arch filler and other shaping material, custom fabricated, each Ⓑ

Dressings

⊘ **A6000** Non-contact wound warming wound cover for use with the non-contact wound warming device and warming card Ⓑ

IOM: 100-02, 16, 20

✿ **A6010** Collagen based wound filler, dry form, sterile, per gram of collagen Ⓟ Ⓑ

IOM: 100-02, 15, 100

✿ **A6011** Collagen based wound filler, gel/paste, per gram of collagen Ⓟ Ⓑ

IOM: 100-02, 15, 100

✿ **A6021** Collagen dressing, sterile, size 16 sq. in. or less, each Ⓟ Ⓑ

IOM: 100-02, 15, 100

✿ **A6022** Collagen dressing, sterile, size more than 16 sq. in. but less than or equal to 48 sq. in., each Ⓟ Ⓑ

IOM: 100-02, 15, 100

✿ **A6023** Collagen dressing, sterile, size more than 48 sq. in., each Ⓟ Ⓑ

IOM: 100-02, 15, 100

▶ **New**   ↻ **Revised**   ✔ **Reinstated**   ~~deleted~~ **Deleted**   ⊘ **Not covered or valid by Medicare**
✿ **Special coverage instructions**   ✳ **Carrier discretion**   Ⓟ **Bill Part B MAC**   Ⓑ **Bill DME MAC**

✪ **A6024**   Collagen dressing wound filler, sterile, per 6 inches Ⓑ Ⓑ

IOM: 100-02, 15, 100

✱ **A6025**   Gel sheet for dermal or epidermal application, (e.g., silicone, hydrogel, other), each Ⓑ Ⓑ

If used for the treatment of keloids or other scars, a silicone gel sheet will not meet the definition of the surgical dressing benefit and will be denied as noncovered.

✪ **A6154**   Wound pouch, each Ⓑ Ⓑ

Waterproof collection device with drainable port that adheres to skin around wound. Usual dressing change is up to 3 times per week.

IOM: 100-02, 15, 100

✪ **A6196**   Alginate or other fiber gelling dressing, wound cover, sterile, pad size 16 sq. in. or less, each dressing Ⓑ Ⓑ

IOM: 100-02, 15, 100

✪ **A6197**   Alginate or other fiber gelling dressing, wound cover, sterile, pad size more than 16 sq. in., but less than or equal to 48 sq. in., each dressing Ⓑ Ⓑ

IOM: 100-02, 15, 100

✪ **A6198**   Alginate or other fiber gelling dressing, wound cover, sterile, pad size more than 48 sq. in., each dressing Ⓑ Ⓑ

IOM: 100-02, 15, 100

✪ **A6199**   Alginate or other fiber gelling dressing, wound filler, sterile, per 6 inches Ⓑ Ⓑ

IOM: 100-02, 15, 100

✪ **A6203**   Composite dressing, sterile, pad size 16 sq. in. or less, with any size adhesive border, each dressing Ⓑ Ⓑ

Usual composite dressing change is up to 3 times per week, one wound cover per dressing change.

IOM: 100-02, 15, 100

✪ **A6204**   Composite dressing, sterile, pad size more than 16 sq. in. but less than or equal to 48 sq. in., with any size adhesive border, each dressing Ⓑ Ⓑ

Usual composite dressing change is up to 3 times per week, one wound cover per dressing change.

IOM: 100-02, 15, 100

✪ **A6205**   Composite dressing, sterile, pad size more than 48 sq. in., with any size adhesive border, each dressing Ⓑ Ⓑ

Usual composite dressing change is up to 3 times per week, one wound cover per dressing change.

IOM: 100-02, 15, 100

✪ **A6206**   Contact layer, sterile, 16 sq. in. or less, each dressing Ⓑ Ⓑ

Contact layers are porous to allow wound fluid to pass through for absorption by separate overlying dressing and are not intended to be changed with each dressing change. Usual dressing change is up to once per week.

IOM: 100-02, 15, 100

✪ **A6207**   Contact layer, sterile, more than 16 sq. in. but less than or equal to 48 sq. in., each dressing Ⓑ Ⓑ

Contact layer dressings are used to line the entire wound; they are not intended to be changed with each dressing change. Usual dressing change is up to once per week.

IOM: 100-02, 15, 100

✪ **A6208**   Contact layer, sterile, more than 48 sq. in., each dressing Ⓑ Ⓑ

Contact layer dressings are used to line the entire wound; they are not intended to be changed with each dressing change. Usual dressing change is up to once per week.

IOM: 100-02, 15, 100

✪ **A6209**   Foam dressing, wound cover, sterile, pad size 16 sq. in. or less, without adhesive border, each dressing Ⓑ Ⓑ

Made of open cell, medical grade expanded polymer; with nonadherent property over wound site

IOM: 100-02, 15, 100

⊗ **A6210** Foam dressing, wound cover, sterile, pad size more than 16 sq. in. but less than or equal to 48 sq. in., without adhesive border, each dressing Ⓑ Ⓑ

Foam dressings are covered items when used on full thickness wounds (e.g., stage III or IV ulcers) with moderate to heavy exudates. Usual dressing change for a foam wound cover when used as primary dressing is up to 3 times per week. When foam wound cover is used as a secondary dressing for wounds with very heavy exudates, dressing change may be up to 3 times per week. Usual dressing change for foam wound fillers is up to once per day (A6209-A6215).

IOM: 100-02, 15, 100

⊗ **A6211** Foam dressing, wound cover, sterile, pad size more than 48 sq. in., without adhesive border, each dressing Ⓑ Ⓑ

IOM: 100-02, 15, 100

⊗ **A6212** Foam dressing, wound cover, sterile, pad size 16 sq. in. or less, with any size adhesive border, each dressing Ⓑ Ⓑ

IOM: 100-02, 15, 100

⊗ **A6213** Foam dressing, wound cover, sterile, pad size more than 16 sq. in. but less than or equal to 48 sq. in., with any size adhesive border, each dressing Ⓑ Ⓑ

IOM: 100-02, 15, 100

⊗ **A6214** Foam dressing, wound cover, sterile, pad size more than 48 sq. in., with any size adhesive border, each dressing Ⓑ Ⓑ

IOM: 100-02, 15, 100

⊗ **A6215** Foam dressing, wound filler, sterile, per gram Ⓑ Ⓑ

IOM: 100-02, 15, 100

⊗ **A6216** Gauze, non-impregnated, non-sterile, pad size 16 sq. in. or less, without adhesive border, each dressing Ⓑ Ⓑ

IOM: 100-02, 15, 100

⊗ **A6217** Gauze, non-impregnated, non-sterile, pad size more than 16 sq. in. but less than or equal to 48 sq. in., without adhesive border, each dressing Ⓑ Ⓑ

IOM: 100-02, 15, 100

⊗ **A6218** Gauze, non-impregnated, non-sterile, pad size more than 48 sq. in., without adhesive border, each dressing Ⓑ Ⓑ

IOM: 100-02, 15, 100

⊗ **A6219** Gauze, non-impregnated, sterile, pad size 16 sq. in. or less, with any size adhesive border, each dressing Ⓑ Ⓑ

IOM: 100-02, 15, 100

⊗ **A6220** Gauze, non-impregnated, sterile, pad size more than 16 sq. in. but less than or equal to 48 sq. in., with any size adhesive border, each dressing Ⓑ Ⓑ

IOM: 100-02, 15, 100

⊗ **A6221** Gauze, non-impregnated, sterile, pad size more than 48 sq. in., with any size adhesive border, each dressing Ⓑ Ⓑ

IOM: 100-02, 15, 100

⊗ **A6222** Gauze, impregnated with other than water, normal saline, or hydrogel, sterile, pad size 16 sq. in. or less, without adhesive border, each dressing Ⓑ Ⓑ

Substances may have been incorporated into dressing material (i.e., iodinated agents, petrolatum, zinc paste, crystalline sodium chloride, chlorhexadine gluconate [CHG], bismuth tribromophenate [BTP], water, aqueous saline, hydrogel, or agents).

IOM: 100-02, 15, 100

⊗ **A6223** Gauze, impregnated with other than water, normal saline, or hydrogel, sterile, pad size more than 16 sq. in. but less than or equal to 48 sq. in., without adhesive border, each dressing Ⓑ Ⓑ

IOM: 100-02, 15, 100

⊗ **A6224** Gauze, impregnated with other than water, normal saline, or hydrogel, sterile, pad size more than 48 square inches, without adhesive border, each dressing Ⓑ Ⓑ

IOM: 100-02, 15, 100

⊗ **A6228** Gauze, impregnated, water or normal saline, sterile, pad size 16 sq. in. or less, without adhesive border, each dressing Ⓑ Ⓑ

IOM: 100-02, 15, 100

⊗ **A6229** Gauze, impregnated, water or normal saline, sterile, pad size more than 16 sq. in. but less than or equal to 48 sq. in., without adhesive border, each dressing Ⓑ Ⓑ

IOM: 100-02, 15, 100

⊗ **A6230** Gauze, impregnated, water or normal saline, sterile, pad size more than 48 sq. in., without adhesive border, each dressing Ⓑ Ⓑ

IOM: 100-02, 15, 100

▶ New ↻ Revised ✔ Reinstated ~~deleted~~ Deleted ⊘ Not covered or valid by Medicare ⊗ Special coverage instructions ✳ Carrier discretion Ⓑ Bill Part B MAC Ⓑ Bill DME MAC

MEDICAL AND SURGICAL SUPPLIES A6210 — A6230

121

⊕ **A6231** Gauze, impregnated, hydrogel, for direct wound contact, sterile, pad size 16 sq. in. or less, each dressing ⑨ Ⓑ

IOM: 100-02, 15, 100

⊕ **A6232** Gauze, impregnated, hydrogel, for direct wound contact, sterile, pad size greater than 16 sq. in., but less than or equal to 48 sq. in., each dressing Ⓑ Ⓑ

IOM: 100-02, 15, 100

⊕ **A6233** Gauze, impregnated, hydrogel, for direct wound contact, sterile, pad size more than 48 sq. in., each dressing Ⓑ Ⓑ

IOM: 100-02, 15, 100

⊕ **A6234** Hydrocolloid dressing, wound cover, sterile, pad size 16 sq. in. or less, without adhesive border, each dressing ⑨ Ⓑ

This type of dressing is usually used on wounds with light to moderate exudate with an average of three dressing changes per week.

IOM: 100-02, 15, 100

⊕ **A6235** Hydrocolloid dressing, wound cover, sterile, pad size more than 16 sq. in. but less than or equal to 48 sq. in., without adhesive border, each dressing ⑨ Ⓑ

IOM: 100-02, 15, 100

⊕ **A6236** Hydrocolloid dressing, wound cover, sterile, pad size more than 48 sq. in., without adhesive border, each dressing ⑨ Ⓑ

IOM: 100-02, 15, 100

⊕ **A6237** Hydrocolloid dressing, wound cover, sterile, pad size 16 sq. in. or less, with any size adhesive border, each dressing Ⓑ Ⓑ

IOM: 100-02, 15, 100

⊕ **A6238** Hydrocolloid dressing, wound cover, sterile, pad size more than 16 sq. in. but less than or equal to 48 sq. in., with any size adhesive border, each dressing Ⓑ Ⓑ

IOM: 100-02, 15, 100

⊕ **A6239** Hydrocolloid dressing, wound cover, sterile, pad size more than 48 sq. in., with any size adhesive border, each dressing ⑨ Ⓑ

IOM: 100-02, 15, 100

⊕ **A6240** Hydrocolloid dressing, wound filler, paste, sterile, per ounce Ⓑ Ⓑ

IOM: 100-02, 15, 100

⊕ **A6241** Hydrocolloid dressing, wound filler, dry form, sterile, per gram ⑨ Ⓑ

IOM: 100-02, 15, 100

⊕ **A6242** Hydrogel dressing, wound cover, sterile, pad size 16 sq. in. or less, without adhesive border, each dressing Ⓑ Ⓑ

Considered medically necessary when used on full thickness wounds with minimal or no exudate (e.g., stage III or IV ulcers)

Usually up to one dressing change per day is considered medically necessary, but if well documented and medically necessary, the payer may allow more frequent dressing changes.

IOM: 100-02, 15, 100

⊕ **A6243** Hydrogel dressing, wound cover, sterile, pad size more than 16 sq. in. but less than or equal to 48 sq. in., without adhesive border, each dressing ⑨ Ⓑ

IOM: 100-02, 15, 100

⊕ **A6244** Hydrogel dressing, wound cover, sterile, pad size more than 48 sq. in., without adhesive border, each dressing ⑨ Ⓑ

IOM: 100-02, 15, 100

⊕ **A6245** Hydrogel dressing, wound cover, sterile, pad size 16 sq. in. or less, with any size adhesive border, each dressing ⑨ Ⓑ

Coverage of a non-elastic gradient compression wrap is limited to one per 6 months per leg.

IOM: 100-02, 15, 100

⊕ **A6246** Hydrogel dressing, wound cover, sterile, pad size more than 16 sq. in. but less than or equal to 48 sq. in., with any size adhesive border, each dressing ⑨ Ⓑ

IOM: 100-02, 15, 100

⊕ **A6247** Hydrogel dressing, wound cover, sterile, pad size more than 48 sq. in., with any size adhesive border, each dressing ⑨ Ⓑ

IOM: 100-02, 15, 100

⊕ **A6248** Hydrogel dressing, wound filler, gel, per fluid ounce ⑨ Ⓑ

IOM: 100-02, 15, 100

⊕ **A6250** Skin sealants, protectants, moisturizers, ointments, any type, any size ⑨ Ⓑ

IOM: 100-02, 15, 100

▶ **New**   ↺ **Revised**   ✔ **Reinstated**   ~~deleted~~ **Deleted**   ⊘ **Not covered or valid by Medicare**

⊕ **Special coverage instructions**   ✳ **Carrier discretion**   ⑨ **Bill Part B MAC**   Ⓑ **Bill DME MAC**

⊗ **A6251** Specialty absorptive dressing, wound cover, sterile, pad size 16 sq. in. or less, without adhesive border, each dressing ⓑ ⓓ

IOM: 100-02, 15, 100

⊗ **A6252** Specialty absorptive dressing, wound cover, sterile, pad size more than 16 sq. in. but less than or equal to 48 sq. in., without adhesive border, each dressing ⓑ ⓓ

IOM: 100-02, 15, 100

⊗ **A6253** Specialty absorptive dressing, wound cover, sterile, pad size more than 48 sq. in., without adhesive border, each dressing ⓑ ⓓ

IOM: 100-02, 15, 100

⊗ **A6254** Specialty absorptive dressing, wound cover, sterile, pad size 16 sq. in. or less, with any size adhesive border, each dressing ⓑ ⓓ

IOM: 100-02, 15, 100

⊗ **A6255** Specialty absorptive dressing, wound cover, sterile, pad size more than 16 sq. in. but less than or equal to 48 sq. in., with any size adhesive border, each dressing ⓑ ⓓ

IOM: 100-02, 15, 100

⊗ **A6256** Specialty absorptive dressing, wound cover, sterile, pad size more than 48 sq. in., with any size adhesive border, each dressing ⓑ ⓓ

Considered medically necessary when used for moderately or highly exudative wounds (e.g., stage III or IV ulcers)

IOM: 100-02, 15, 100

⊗ **A6257** Transparent film, sterile, 16 sq. in. or less, each dressing ⓑ ⓓ

Considered medically necessary when used on open partial thickness wounds with minimal exudate or closed wounds

IOM: 100-02, 15, 100

⊗ **A6258** Transparent film, sterile, more than 16 sq. in. but less than or equal to 48 sq. in., each dressing ⓑ ⓓ

IOM: 100-02, 15, 100

⊗ **A6259** Transparent film, sterile, more than 48 sq. in., each dressing ⓑ ⓓ

IOM: 100-02, 15, 100

⊗ **A6260** Wound cleansers, any type, any size ⓑ ⓓ

IOM: 100-02, 15, 100

⊗ **A6261** Wound filler, gel/paste, per fluid ounce, not otherwise specified ⓑ ⓓ

Units of service for wound fillers are 1 gram, 1 fluid ounce, 6 inch length, or 1 yard depending on product.

IOM: 100-02, 15, 100

⊗ **A6262** Wound filler, dry form, per gram, not otherwise specified ⓑ ⓓ

Dry forms (e.g., powder, granules, beads) are used to eliminate dead space in an open wound.

IOM: 100-02, 15, 100

⊗ **A6266** Gauze, impregnated, other than water, normal saline, or zinc paste, sterile, any width, per linear yard ⓑ ⓓ

IOM: 100-02, 15, 100

⊗ **A6402** Gauze, non-impregnated, sterile, pad size 16 sq. in. or less, without adhesive border, each dressing ⓑ ⓓ

IOM: 100-02, 15, 100

⊗ **A6403** Gauze, non-impregnated, sterile, pad size more than 16 sq. in., less than or equal to 48 sq. in., without adhesive border, each dressing ⓑ ⓓ

IOM: 100-02, 15, 100

⊗ **A6404** Gauze, non-impregnated, sterile, pad size more than 48 sq. in., without adhesive border, each dressing ⓑ ⓓ

IOM: 100-02, 15, 100

✳ **A6407** Packing strips, non-impregnated, sterile, up to 2 inches in width, per linear yard ⓑ ⓓ

IOM: 100-02, 15, 100

⊗ **A6410** Eye pad, sterile, each ⓑ ⓓ

IOM: 100-02, 15, 100

⊗ **A6411** Eye pad, non-sterile, each ⓑ ⓓ

IOM: 100-02, 15, 100

✳ **A6412** Eye patch, occlusive, each ⓑ ⓓ

Bandages

⊘ **A6413** Adhesive bandage, first-aid type, any size, each ⓑ ⓓ

First aid type bandage is a wound cover with a pad size of less than 4 square inches. Does not meet the definition of the surgical dressing benefit and will be denied as non-covered.

▶ New   ↻ Revised   ✔ Reinstated   ~~deleted~~ Deleted   ⊘ Not covered or valid by Medicare
⊗ Special coverage instructions   ✳ Carrier discretion   ⓑ Bill Part B MAC   ⓓ Bill DME MAC

* **A6441** Padding bandage, non-elastic, non-woven/non-knitted, width greater than or equal to three inches and less than five inches, per yard Ⓑ Ⓑ

* **A6442** Conforming bandage, non-elastic, knitted/woven, non-sterile, width less than three inches, per yard Ⓑ Ⓑ

Non-elastic, moderate or high compression that is typically sustained for one week

* **A6443** Conforming bandage, non-elastic, knitted/woven, non-sterile, width greater than or equal to three inches and less than five inches, per yard Ⓑ Ⓑ

* **A6444** Conforming bandage, non-elastic, knitted/woven, non-sterile, width greater than or equal to five inches, per yard Ⓑ Ⓑ

* **A6445** Conforming bandage, non-elastic, knitted/woven, sterile, width less than three inches, per yard Ⓑ Ⓑ

* **A6446** Conforming bandage, non-elastic, knitted/woven, sterile, width greater than or equal to three inches and less than five inches, per yard Ⓑ Ⓑ

* **A6447** Conforming bandage, non-elastic, knitted/woven, sterile, width greater than or equal to five inches, per yard Ⓑ Ⓑ

* **A6448** Light compression bandage, elastic, knitted/woven, width less than three inches, per yard Ⓑ Ⓑ

Used to hold wound cover dressings in place over a wound. Example is an ACE type elastic bandage.

* **A6449** Light compression bandage, elastic, knitted/woven, width greater than or equal to three inches and less than five inches, per yard Ⓑ Ⓑ

* **A6450** Light compression bandage, elastic, knitted/woven, width greater than or equal to five inches, per yard Ⓑ Ⓑ

* **A6451** Moderate compression bandage, elastic, knitted/woven, load resistance of 1.25 to 1.34 foot pounds at 50% maximum stretch, width greater than or equal to three inches and less than five inches, per yard Ⓑ Ⓑ

Elastic bandages that produce moderate compression that is typically sustained for one week

Medicare considers coverage if part of a multi-layer compression bandage system for the treatment of a venous stasis ulcer. Do not assign for strains or sprains.

* **A6452** High compression bandage, elastic, knitted/woven, load resistance greater than or equal to 1.35 foot pounds at 50% maximum stretch, width greater than or equal to three inches and less than five inches, per yard Ⓑ Ⓑ

Elastic bandages that produce high compression that is typically sustained for one week

* **A6453** Self-adherent bandage, elastic, non-knitted/non-woven, width less than three inches, per yard Ⓑ Ⓑ

* **A6454** Self-adherent bandage, elastic, non-knitted/non-woven, width greater than or equal to three inches and less than five inches, per yard Ⓑ Ⓑ

* **A6455** Self-adherent bandage, elastic, non-knitted/non-woven, width greater than or equal to five inches, per yard Ⓑ Ⓑ

* **A6456** Zinc paste impregnated bandage, non-elastic, knitted/woven, width greater than or equal to three inches and less than five inches, per yard Ⓑ Ⓑ

* **A6457** Tubular dressing with or without elastic, any width, per linear yard Ⓑ Ⓑ

Compression Garments

✿ **A6501** Compression burn garment, bodysuit (head to foot), custom fabricated Ⓑ Ⓑ

Garments used to reduce hypertrophic scarring and joint contractures following burn injury

IOM: 100-02, 15, 100

✿ **A6502** Compression burn garment, chin strap, custom fabricated Ⓑ Ⓑ

IOM: 100-02, 15, 100

✿ **A6503** Compression burn garment, facial hood, custom fabricated Ⓑ Ⓑ

IOM: 100-02, 15, 100

✿ **A6504** Compression burn garment, glove to wrist, custom fabricated Ⓑ Ⓑ

IOM: 100-02, 15, 100

✿ **A6505** Compression burn garment, glove to elbow, custom fabricated Ⓑ Ⓑ

IOM: 100-02, 15, 100

✿ **A6506** Compression burn garment, glove to axilla, custom fabricated Ⓑ Ⓑ

IOM: 100-02, 15, 100

✿ **A6507** Compression burn garment, foot to knee length, custom fabricated Ⓑ Ⓑ

IOM: 100-02, 15, 100

▶ New   ↻ Revised   ✔ Reinstated   ~~deleted~~ Deleted   ⊘ Not covered or valid by Medicare
✿ Special coverage instructions   * Carrier discretion   Ⓑ Bill Part B MAC   Ⓑ Bill DME MAC

✿ **A6508** Compression burn garment, foot to thigh length, custom fabricated ⑨ Ⓑ

IOM: 100-02, 15, 100

✿ **A6509** Compression burn garment, upper trunk to waist including arm openings (vest), custom fabricated ⑨ Ⓑ

IOM: 100-02, 15, 100

✿ **A6510** Compression burn garment, trunk, including arms down to leg openings (leotard), custom fabricated Ⓑ Ⓑ

IOM: 100-02, 15, 100

✿ **A6511** Compression burn garment, lower trunk including leg openings (panty), custom fabricated ⑨ Ⓑ

IOM: 100-02, 15, 100

✿ **A6512** Compression burn garment, not otherwise classified Ⓑ Ⓑ

IOM: 100-02, 15, 100

✳ **A6513** Compression burn mask, face and/or neck, plastic or equal, custom fabricated Ⓑ

⊘ **A6530** Gradient compression stocking, below knee, 18-30 mmHg, each Ⓑ

IOM: 100-03, 4, 280.1

✿ **A6531** Gradient compression stocking, below knee, 30-40 mmHg, each Ⓑ

Covered when used in treatment of open venous stasis ulcer. Modifiers A1-A9 are not assigned. Must be billed with AW, RT, or LT.

IOM: 100-02, 15, 100

✿ **A6532** Gradient compression stocking, below knee, 40-50 mmHg, each Ⓑ

Covered when used in treatment of open venous stasis ulcer. Modifiers A1-A9 are not assigned. Must be billed with AW, RT, or LT.

IOM: 100-02, 15, 100

⊘ **A6533** Gradient compression stocking, thigh length, 18-30 mmHg, each Ⓑ

IOM: 100-02, 15, 130; 100-03, 4, 280.1

⊘ **A6534** Gradient compression stocking, thigh length, 30-40 mmHg, each Ⓑ

IOM: 100-02, 15, 130; 100-03, 4, 280.1

⊘ **A6535** Gradient compression stocking, thigh length, 40-50 mmHg, each ⑨

IOM: 100-02, 15, 130; 100-03, 4, 280.1

⊘ **A6536** Gradient compression stocking, full length/chap style, 18-30 mmHg, each Ⓑ

IOM: 100-02, 15, 130; 100-03, 4, 280.1

⊘ **A6537** Gradient compression stocking, full length/chap style, 30-40 mmHg, each Ⓑ

IOM: 100-02, 15, 130; 100-03, 4, 280.1

⊘ **A6538** Gradient compression stocking, full length/chap style, 40-50 mmHg, each ⑨

IOM: 100-02, 15, 130; 100-03, 4, 280.1

⊘ **A6539** Gradient compression stocking, waist length, 18-30 mmHg, each ⑨

IOM: 100-02, 15, 130; 100-03, 4, 280.1

⊘ **A6540** Gradient compression stocking, waist length, 30-40 mmHg, each ⑨

IOM: 100-02, 15, 130; 100-03, 4, 280.1

⊘ **A6541** Gradient compression stocking, waist length, 40-50 mmHg, each Ⓑ

IOM: 100-02, 15, 130; 100-03, 4, 280.1

⊘ **A6544** Gradient compression stocking, garter belt Ⓑ

IOM: 100-02, 15, 130; 100-03, 4, 280.1

✿ **A6545** Gradient compression wrap, non-elastic, below knee, 30-50 mm hg, each Ⓑ

Modifiers RT and/or LT must be appended. When assigned for bilateral items (left/right) on the same date of service, bill both items on the same claim line using RT/LT modifiers and 2 units of service.

IOM: 10-02, 15, 100

⊘ **A6549** Gradient compression stocking/sleeve, not otherwise specified ⑨

IOM: 100-02, 15, 130; 100-03, 4, 280.1

Wound Care

✳ **A6550** Wound care set, for negative pressure wound therapy electrical pump, includes all supplies and accessories ⑨

Respiratory Supplies

✳ **A7000** Canister, disposable, used with suction pump, each Ⓑ

✳ **A7001** Canister, non-disposable, used with suction pump, each Ⓑ

✳ **A7002** Tubing, used with suction pump, each Ⓑ

✳ **A7003** Administration set, with small volume nonfiltered pneumatic nebulizer, disposable Ⓑ

✳ **A7004** Small volume nonfiltered pneumatic nebulizer, disposable Ⓑ

▶ **New** ↻ **Revised** ✔ **Reinstated** ~~deleted~~ **Deleted** ⊘ **Not covered or valid by Medicare**

✿ **Special coverage instructions** ✳ **Carrier discretion** ⑨ **Bill Part B MAC** Ⓑ **Bill DME MAC**

✳ **A7005** Administration set, with small volume nonfiltered pneumatic nebulizer, non-disposable Ⓑ

✳ **A7006** Administration set, with small volume filtered pneumatic nebulizer Ⓑ

✳ **A7007** Large volume nebulizer, disposable, unfilled, used with aerosol compressor Ⓑ

✳ **A7008** Large volume nebulizer, disposable, prefilled, used with aerosol compressor Ⓑ

✳ **A7009** Reservoir bottle, nondisposable, used with large volume ultrasonic nebulizer Ⓑ

✳ **A7010** Corrugated tubing, disposable, used with large volume nebulizer, 100 feet Ⓑ

✳ **A7012** Water collection device, used with large volume nebulizer Ⓑ

✳ **A7013** Filter, disposable, used with aerosol compressor or ultrasonic generator Ⓑ

✳ **A7014** Filter, non-disposable, used with aerosol compressor or ultrasonic generator Ⓑ

✳ **A7015** Aerosol mask, used with DME nebulizer Ⓑ

✳ **A7016** Dome and mouthpiece, used with small volume ultrasonic nebulizer Ⓑ

☼ **A7017** Nebulizer, durable, glass or autoclavable plastic, bottle type, not used with oxygen Ⓑ

IOM: 100-03, 4, 280.1

✳ **A7018** Water, distilled, used with large volume nebulizer, 1000 ml Ⓑ

✳ **A7020** Interface for cough stimulating device, includes all components, replacement only Ⓑ

✳ **A7025** High frequency chest wall oscillation system vest, replacement for use with patient owned equipment, each Ⓑ

✳ **A7026** High frequency chest wall oscillation system hose, replacement for use with patient owned equipment, each Ⓑ

✳ **A7027** Combination oral/nasal mask, used with continuous positive airway pressure device, each Ⓑ

✳ **A7028** Oral cushion for combination oral/nasal mask, replacement only, each Ⓑ

✳ **A7029** Nasal pillows for combination oral/nasal mask, replacement only, pair Ⓑ

✳ **A7030** Full face mask used with positive airway pressure device, each Ⓑ

✳ **A7031** Face mask interface, replacement for full face mask, each Ⓑ

✳ **A7032** Cushion for use on nasal mask interface, replacement only, each Ⓑ

✳ **A7033** Pillow for use on nasal cannula type interface, replacement only, pair Ⓑ

✳ **A7034** Nasal interface (mask or cannula type) used with positive airway pressure device, with or without head strap Ⓑ

✳ **A7035** Headgear used with positive airway pressure device Ⓑ

✳ **A7036** Chinstrap used with positive airway pressure device Ⓑ

✳ **A7037** Tubing used with positive airway pressure device Ⓑ

✳ **A7038** Filter, disposable, used with positive airway pressure device Ⓑ

✳ **A7039** Filter, non disposable, used with positive airway pressure device Ⓑ

✳ **A7040** One way chest drain valve Ⓖ

✳ **A7041** Water seal drainage container and tubing for use with implanted chest tube Ⓑ

✳ **A7044** Oral interface used with positive airway pressure device, each Ⓑ

☼ **A7045** Exhalation port with or without swivel used with accessories for positive airway devices, replacement only Ⓖ

IOM: 100-03, 4, 230.17

☼ **A7046** Water chamber for humidifier, used with positive airway pressure device, replacement, each Ⓑ

IOM: 100-03, 4, 230.17

✳ **A7047** Oral interface used with respiratory suction pump, each Ⓑ

✳ **A7048** Vacuum drainage collection unit and tubing kit, including all supplies needed for collection unit change, for use with implanted catheter, each Ⓖ

Tracheostomy Supplies

☼ **A7501** Tracheostoma valve, including diaphragm, each Ⓑ

IOM: 100-02, 15, 120

☼ **A7502** Replacement diaphragm/faceplate for tracheostoma valve, each Ⓑ

IOM: 100-02, 15, 120

☼ **A7503** Filter holder or filter cap, reusable, for use in a tracheostoma heat and moisture exchange system, each Ⓑ

IOM: 100-02, 15, 120

▶ **New** ↻ **Revised** ✔ **Reinstated** ~~deleted~~ **Deleted** ⊘ **Not covered or valid by Medicare**
☼ **Special coverage instructions** ✳ **Carrier discretion** Ⓑ **Bill Part B MAC** Ⓓ **Bill DME MAC**

✪ **A7504**   Filter for use in a tracheostoma heat and moisture exchange system, each Ⓑ

IOM: 100-02, 15, 120

✪ **A7505**   Housing, reusable without adhesive, for use in a heat and moisture exchange system and/or with a tracheostoma valve, each Ⓑ

IOM: 100-02, 15, 120

✪ **A7506**   Adhesive disc for use in a heat and moisture exchange system and/or with tracheostoma valve, any type, each Ⓑ

IOM: 100-02, 15, 120

✪ **A7507**   Filter holder and integrated filter without adhesive, for use in a tracheostoma heat and moisture exchange system, each Ⓑ

IOM: 100-02, 15, 120

✪ **A7508**   Housing and integrated adhesive, for use in a tracheostoma heat and moisture exchange system and/or with a tracheostoma valve, each Ⓑ

IOM: 100-02, 15, 120

✪ **A7509**   Filter holder and integrated filter housing, and adhesive, for use as a tracheostoma heat and moisture exchange system, each Ⓑ

IOM: 100-02, 15, 120

✳ **A7520**   Tracheostomy/laryngectomy tube, non-cuffed, polyvinylchloride (PVC), silicone or equal, each Ⓑ

✳ **A7521**   Tracheostomy/laryngectomy tube, cuffed, polyvinylchloride (PVC), silicone or equal, each Ⓑ

✳ **A7522**   Tracheostomy/laryngectomy tube, stainless steel or equal (sterilizable and reusable), each Ⓑ

✳ **A7523**   Tracheostomy shower protector, each Ⓑ

✳ **A7524**   Tracheostoma stent/stud/button, each Ⓑ

✳ **A7525**   Tracheostomy mask, each Ⓑ

✳ **A7526**   Tracheostomy tube collar/holder, each Ⓑ

✳ **A7527**   Tracheostomy/laryngectomy tube plug/stop, each Ⓑ

Helmets

✳ **A8000**   Helmet, protective, soft, prefabricated, includes all components and accessories Ⓑ

✳ **A8001**   Helmet, protective, hard, prefabricated, includes all components and accessories Ⓑ

✳ **A8002**   Helmet, protective, soft, custom fabricated, includes all components and accessories Ⓑ

✳ **A8003**   Helmet, protective, hard, custom fabricated, includes all components and accessories Ⓑ

✳ **A8004**   Soft interface for helmet, replacement only Ⓑ

ADMINISTRATIVE, MISCELLANEOUS, AND INVESTIGATIONAL (A9000-A9999)

NOTE: The following codes do not imply that codes in other sections are necessarily covered.

Miscellaneous Supplies

✪ **A9150**   Non-prescription drugs Ⓑ

IOM: 100-02, 15, 50

⊘ **A9152**   Single vitamin/mineral/trace element, oral, per dose, not otherwise specified Ⓑ

⊘ **A9153**   Multiple vitamins, with or without minerals and trace elements, oral, per dose, not otherwise specified Ⓑ

✳ **A9155**   Artificial saliva, 30 ml Ⓑ

⊘ **A9180**   Pediculosis (lice infestation) treatment, topical, for administration by patient/caretaker Ⓑ

⊘ **A9270**   Non-covered item or service Ⓑ

IOM: 100-02, 16, 20

⊘ **A9272**   Wound suction, disposable, includes dressing, all accessories and components, any type, each Ⓑ

⊘ **A9273**   Hot water bottle, ice cap or collar, heat and/or cold wrap, any type Ⓑ

⊘ **A9274**   External ambulatory insulin delivery system, disposable, each, includes all supplies and accessories Ⓑ

⊘ **A9275**   Home glucose disposable monitor, includes test strips Ⓑ

⊘ **A9276**   Sensor; invasive (e.g., subcutaneous), disposable, for use with interstitial continuous glucose monitoring system, one unit = 1 day supply Ⓑ

⊘ **A9277**   Transmitter; external, for use with interstitial continuous glucose monitoring system Ⓑ

▶ New   ⟲ Revised   ✔ Reinstated   ~~deleted~~ Deleted   ⊘ Not covered or valid by Medicare
✪ Special coverage instructions   ✳ Carrier discretion   Ⓑ Bill Part B MAC   Ⓑ Bill DME MAC

⊘ **A9278** Receiver (monitor); external, for use with interstitial continuous glucose monitoring system Ⓑ

⊘ **A9279** Monitoring feature/device, stand-alone or integrated, any type, includes all accessories, components and electronics, not otherwise classified Ⓖ

⊘ **A9280** Alert or alarm device, not otherwise classified Ⓖ

⊘ **A9281** Reaching/grabbing device, any type, any length, each Ⓖ

⊘ **A9282** Wig, any type, each Ⓖ

⊘ **A9283** Foot pressure off loading/supportive device, any type, each Ⓖ

❂ **A9284** Spirometer, non-electronic, includes all accessories Ⓑ

✳ **A9285** Inversion/eversion correction device Ⓖ

⊘ **A9286** Hygienic item or device, disposable or non-disposable, any type, each Ⓑ

⊘ **A9300** Exercise equipment Ⓖ

IOM: 100-02, 15, 110.1; 100-03, 4, 280.1

Supplies for Radiology Procedures (Radiopharmaceuticals)

✳ **A9500** Technetium Tc-99m sestamibi, diagnostic, per study dose Ⓑ

Should be filed on same claim as procedure code reporting radiopharmaceutical. Verify with payer definition of a "study."

✳ **A9501** Technetium Tc-99m teboroxime, diagnostic, per study dose Ⓑ

✳ **A9502** Technetium Tc-99m tetrofosmin, diagnostic, per study dose Ⓑ

✳ **A9503** Technetium Tc-99m medronate, diagnostic, per study dose, up to 30 millicuries Ⓑ

✳ **A9504** Technetium Tc-99m apcitide, diagnostic, per study dose, up to 20 millicuries Ⓑ

✳ **A9505** Thallium Tl-201 thallous chloride, diagnostic, per millicurie Ⓑ

✳ **A9507** Indium In-111 capromab pendetide, diagnostic, per study dose, up to 10 millicuries Ⓑ

✳ **A9508** Iodine I-131 iobenguane sulfate, diagnostic, per 0.5 millicurie Ⓑ

✳ **A9509** Iodine I-123 sodium iodide, diagnostic, per millicurie Ⓑ

✳ **A9510** Technetium Tc-99m disofenin, diagnostic, per study dose, up to 15 millicuries Ⓑ

✳ **A9512** Technetium Tc-99m pertechnetate, diagnostic, per millicurie Ⓑ

✳ **A9515** Choline C-11, diagnostic, per study dose up to 20 millicuries

✳ **A9516** Iodine I-123 sodium iodide, diagnostic, per 100 microcuries, up to 999 microcuries Ⓑ

✳ **A9517** Iodine I-131 sodium iodide capsule(s), therapeutic, per millicurie Ⓑ

✳ **A9520** Technetium Tc-99m tilmanocept, diagnostic, up to 0.5 millicuries Ⓖ

✳ **A9521** Technetium Tc-99m exametazime, diagnostic, per study dose, up to 25 millicuries Ⓑ

✳ **A9524** Iodine I-131 iodinated serum albumin, diagnostic, per 5 microcuries Ⓑ

✳ **A9526** Nitrogen N-13 ammonia, diagnostic, per study dose, up to 40 millicuries Ⓑ

✳ **A9527** Iodine I-125, sodium iodide solution, therapeutic, per millicurie Ⓑ

✳ **A9528** Iodine I-131 sodium iodide capsule(s), diagnostic, per millicurie Ⓖ

✳ **A9529** Iodine I-131 sodium iodide solution, diagnostic, per millicurie Ⓑ

✳ **A9530** Iodine I-131 sodium iodide solution, therapeutic, per millicurie Ⓑ

✳ **A9531** Iodine I-131 sodium iodide, diagnostic, per microcurie (up to 100 microcuries) Ⓑ

✳ **A9532** Iodine I-125 serum albumin, diagnostic, per 5 microcuries Ⓑ

✳ **A9536** Technetium Tc-99m depreotide, diagnostic, per study dose, up to 35 millicuries Ⓑ

✳ **A9537** Technetium Tc-99m mebrofenin, diagnostic, per study dose, up to 15 millicuries Ⓑ

✳ **A9538** Technetium Tc-99m pyrophosphate, diagnostic, per study dose, up to 25 millicuries Ⓑ

✳ **A9539** Technetium Tc-99m pentetate, diagnostic, per study dose, up to 25 millicuries Ⓑ

✳ **A9540** Technetium Tc-99m macroaggregated albumin, diagnostic, per study dose, up to 10 millicuries Ⓖ

✳ **A9541** Technetium Tc-99m sulfur colloid, diagnostic, per study dose, up to 20 millicuries Ⓑ

▶ **New** ↻ **Revised** ✔ **Reinstated** ~~deleted~~ **Deleted** ⊘ **Not covered or valid by Medicare**
❂ **Special coverage instructions** ✳ **Carrier discretion** Ⓑ **Bill Part B MAC** Ⓖ **Bill DME MAC**

✳ **A9542** Indium In-111 ibritumomab tiuxetan, diagnostic, per study dose, up to 5 millicuries ⓑ

Specifically for diagnostic use.

✳ **A9543** Yttrium Y-90 ibritumomab tiuxetan, therapeutic, per treatment dose, up to 40 millicuries ⓑ

Specifically for therapeutic use.

✳ **A9546** Cobalt Co-57/58, cyanocobalamin, diagnostic, per study dose, up to 1 microcurie ⓑ

✳ **A9547** Indium In-111 oxyquinoline, diagnostic, per 0.5 millicurie ⓑ

✳ **A9548** Indium In-111 pentetate, diagnostic, per 0.5 millicurie ⓑ

✳ **A9550** Technetium Tc-99m sodium gluceptate, diagnostic, per study dose, up to 25 millicuries ⓑ

✳ **A9551** Technetium Tc-99m succimer, diagnostic, per study dose, up to 10 millicuries ⓑ

✳ **A9552** Fluorodeoxyglucose F-18 FDG, diagnostic, per study dose, up to 45 millicuries ⓑ

✳ **A9553** Chromium Cr-51 sodium chromate, diagnostic, per study dose, up to 250 microcuries ⓑ

✳ **A9554** Iodine I-125 sodium Iothalamate, diagnostic, per study dose, up to 10 microcuries ⓑ

✳ **A9555** Rubidium Rb-82, diagnostic, per study dose, up to 60 millicuries ⓑ

✳ **A9556** Gallium Ga-67 citrate, diagnostic, per millicurie ⓑ

✳ **A9557** Technetium Tc-99m bicisate, diagnostic, per study dose, up to 25 millicuries ⓑ

✳ **A9558** Xenon Xe-133 gas, diagnostic, per 10 millicuries ⓑ

✳ **A9559** Cobalt Co-57 cyanocobalamin, oral, diagnostic, per study dose, up to 1 microcurie ⓑ

✳ **A9560** Technetium Tc-99m labeled red blood cells, diagnostic, per study dose, up to 30 millicuries ⓑ

✳ **A9561** Technetium Tc-99m oxidronate, diagnostic, per study dose, up to 30 millicuries ⓑ

✳ **A9562** Technetium Tc-99m mertiatide, diagnostic, per study dose, up to 15 millicuries ⓑ

✳ **A9563** Sodium phosphate P-32, therapeutic, per millicurie ⓑ

✳ **A9564** Chromic phosphate P-32 suspension, therapeutic, per millicurie ⓑ

✳ **A9566** Technetium Tc-99m fanolesomab, diagnostic, per study dose, up to 25 millicuries ⓑ

✳ **A9567** Technetium Tc-99m pentetate, diagnostic, aerosol, per study dose, up to 75 millicuries ⓑ

✳ **A9568** Technetium TC-99m arcitumomab, diagnostic, per study dose, up to 45 millicuries ⓑ

✳ **A9569** Technetium Tc-99m exametazime labeled autologous white blood cells, diagnostic, per study dose ⓑ

✳ **A9570** Indium In-111 labeled autologous white blood cells, diagnostic, per study dose ⓑ

✳ **A9571** Indium In-111 labeled autologous platelets, diagnostic, per study dose ⓑ

✳ **A9572** Indium In-111 pentetreotide, diagnostic, per study dose, up to 6 millicuries ⓑ

✳ **A9575** Injection, gadoterate meglumine, 0.1 ml ⓑ

✳ **A9576** Injection, gadoteridol, (ProHance Multipack), per ml ⓑ

✳ **A9577** Injection, gadobenate dimeglumine (MultiHance), per ml ⓑ

✳ **A9578** Injection, gadobenate dimeglumine (MultiHance Multipack), per ml ⓑ

✳ **A9579** Injection, gadolinium-based magnetic resonance contrast agent, not otherwise specified (NOS), per ml ⓑ

✳ **A9580** Sodium fluoride F-18, diagnostic, per study dose, up to 30 millicuries ⓑ

✳ **A9581** Injection, gadoxetate disodium, 1 ml ⓑ

Local Medicare contractors may require the use of modifier JW to identify unused product from single-dose vials that are appropriately discarded.

✳ **A9582** Iodine I-123 iobenguane, diagnostic, per study dose, up to 15 millicuries ⓑ

Molecular imaging agent that assists in the identification of rare neuroendocrine tumors.

✳ **A9583** Injection, gadofosveset trisodium, 1 ml ⓑ

✳ **A9584** Iodine 1-123 ioflupane, diagnostic, per study dose, up to 5 millicuries ⓑ

✳ **A9585** Injection, gadobutrol, 0.1 ml ⓑ

↻ ✪ **A9586** Florbetapir F18, diagnostic, per study dose, up to 10 millicuries ⓑ

✳ **A9587** Gallium Ga-68, dotatate, diagnostic, 0.1 millicurie

▶ New	↻ Revised	✔ Reinstated	~~deleted~~ Deleted	⊘ Not covered or valid by Medicare
✪ Special coverage instructions	✳ Carrier discretion	ⓑ Bill Part B MAC	ⓓ Bill DME MAC	

✳ **A9588**   Fluciclovine F-18, diagnostic,
1 millicurie

✳ **A9597**   Positron emission tomography
radiopharmaceutical, diagnostic, for
tumor identification, not otherwise
classified

✳ **A9598**   Positron emission tomography
radiopharmaceutical, diagnostic, for
non-tumor identification, not otherwise
classified

~~A9599~~   ~~Radiopharmaceutical, diagnostic, for~~ ✖
~~beta-amyloid positron emission~~
~~tomography (PET) imaging, per study~~
~~dose, not otherwise specified~~

✳ **A9600**   Strontium Sr-89 chloride, therapeutic,
per millicurie Ⓑ

✳ **A9604**   Samarium SM-153 lexidronam,
therapeutic, per treatment dose, up to
150 millicuries Ⓑ

↺ ✳ **A9606**   Radium Ra-223 dichloride, therapeutic,
per microcurie

⊗ **A9698**   Non-radioactive contrast imaging
material, not otherwise classified, per
study Ⓑ

IOM: 100-04, 12, 70; 100-04, 13, 20

✳ **A9699**   Radiopharmaceutical, therapeutic, not
otherwise classified Ⓑ

⊗ **A9700**   Supply of injectable contrast material
for use in echocardiography, per
study Ⓠ

IOM: 100-04, 12, 30.4

Miscellaneous Service Component

✳ **A9900**   Miscellaneous DME supply, accessory,
and/or service component of another
HCPCS code Ⓠ Ⓑ

On DMEPOS fee schedule as a payable
replacement for miscellaneous
implanted or non-implanted items.

✳ **A9901**   DME delivery, set up, and/or dispensing
service component of another HCPCS
code Ⓑ

✳ **A9999**   Miscellaneous DME supply or
accessory, not otherwise specified Ⓑ Ⓑ

On DMEPOS fee schedule as a payable
replacement for miscellaneous
implanted or non-implanted items.

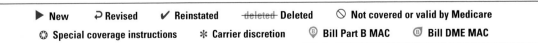

▶ New   ↺ Revised   ✔ Reinstated   ~~deleted~~ Deleted   ⊘ Not covered or valid by Medicare

⊗ Special coverage instructions   ✳ Carrier discretion   Ⓠ Bill Part B MAC   Ⓑ Bill DME MAC

ENTERAL AND PARENTERAL THERAPY
(B4000-B9999)

Enteral Feeding Supplies

⊕ **B4034** Enteral feeding supply kit; syringe fed, per day, includes but not limited to feeding/flushing syringe, administration set tubing, dressings, tape ⑧

Dressings used with gastrostomy tubes for enteral nutrition (covered under the prosthetic device benefit) are included in the payment.

IOM: 100-02, 15, 120; 100-03, 3, 180.2; 100-04, 20, 100.2.2

⊕ **B4035** Enteral feeding supply kit; pump fed, per day, includes but not limited to feeding/flushing syringe, administration set tubing, dressings, tape ⑧

IOM: 100-02, 15, 120; 100-03, 3, 180.2; 100-04, 20, 100.2.2

⊕ **B4036** Enteral feeding supply kit; gravity fed, per day, includes but not limited to feeding/flushing syringe, administration set tubing, dressings, tape ⑧

IOM: 100-02, 15, 120; 100-03, 3, 180.2; 100-04, 20, 100.2.2

⊕ **B4081** Nasogastric tubing with stylet ⑧

More than 3 nasogastric tubes (B4081-B4083), or 1 gastrostomy/jejunostomy tube (B4087-B4088) every three months is rarely medically necessary.

IOM: 100-02, 15, 120; 100-03, 3, 180.2; 100-04, 20, 100.2.2

⊕ **B4082** Nasogastric tubing without stylet ⑧

IOM: 100-02, 15, 120; 100-03, 3, 180.2; 100-04, 20, 100.2.2

⊕ **B4083** Stomach tube - Levine type ⑧

IOM: 100-02, 15, 120; 100-03, 3, 180.2; 100-04, 20, 100.2.2

✳ **B4087** Gastrostomy/jejunostomy tube, standard, any material, any type, each ⑧

✳ **B4088** Gastrostomy/jejunostomy tube, low-profile, any material, any type, each ⑧

Enteral Formulas and Additives

⊘ **B4100** Food thickener, administered orally, per ounce ⑧

⊕ **B4102** Enteral formula, for adults, used to replace fluids and electrolytes (e.g., clear liquids), 500 ml = 1 unit ⑧

IOM: 100-03, 3, 180.2

⊕ **B4103** Enteral formula, for pediatrics, used to replace fluids and electrolytes (e.g., clear liquids), 500 ml = 1 unit ⑧

IOM: 100-03, 3, 180.2

⊕ **B4104** Additive for enteral formula (e.g., fiber) ⑧

IOM: 100-03, 3, 180.2

⊕ **B4149** Enteral formula, manufactured blenderized natural foods with intact nutrients, includes proteins, fats, carbohydrates, vitamins and minerals, may include fiber, administered through an enteral feeding tube, 100 calories = 1 unit ⑧

Produced to meet unique nutrient needs for specific disease conditions; medical record must document specific condition and need for special nutrient.

IOM: 100-02, 15, 120; 100-03, 3, 180.2; 100-04, 20, 100.2.2

⊕ **B4150** Enteral formulae, nutritionally complete with intact nutrients, includes proteins, fats, carbohydrates, vitamins, and minerals, may include fiber, administered through an enteral feeding tube, 100 calories = 1 unit ⑧

IOM: 100-02, 15, 120; 100-03, 3, 180.2; 100-04, 20, 100.2.2

⊕ **B4152** Enteral formula, nutritionally complete, calorically dense (equal to or greater than 1.5 kcal/ml) with intact nutrients, includes proteins, fats, carbohydrates, vitamins and minerals, may include fiber, administered through an enteral feeding tube, 100 calories = 1 unit ⑧

IOM: 100-02, 15, 120; 100-03, 3, 180.2; 100-04, 20, 100.2.2

▶ New   ↻ Revised   ✔ Reinstated   ~~deleted~~ Deleted   ⊘ Not covered or valid by Medicare

⊕ Special coverage instructions   ✳ Carrier discretion   ⑧ Bill Part B MAC   ⑧ Bill DME MAC

⊛ **B4153**   Enteral formula, nutritionally complete, hydrolyzed proteins (amino acids and peptide chain), includes fats, carbohydrates, vitamins and minerals, may include fiber, administered through an enteral feeding tube, 100 calories = 1 unit ⑧

If 2 enteral nutrition products described by same HCPCS code and provided at same time billed on single claim line with units of service reflecting total calories of both nutrients

IOM: 100-02, 15, 120; 100-03, 3, 180.2; 100-04, 20, 100.2.2

⊛ **B4154**   Enteral formula, nutritionally complete, for special metabolic needs, excludes inherited disease of metabolism, includes altered composition of proteins, fats, carbohydrates, vitamins and/or minerals, may include fiber, administered through an enteral feeding tube, 100 calories = 1 unit ⑧

IOM: 100-02, 15, 120; 100-03, 3, 180.2; 100-04, 20, 100.2.2

⊛ **B4155**   Enteral formula, nutritionally incomplete/modular nutrients, includes specific nutrients, carbohydrates (e.g., glucose polymers), proteins/amino acids (e.g., glutamine, arginine), fat (e.g., medium chain triglycerides) or combination, administered through an enteral feeding tube, 100 calories = 1 unit ⑧

IOM: 100-02, 15, 120; 100-03, 3, 180.2; 100-04, 20, 100.2.2

⊛ **B4157**   Enteral formula, nutritionally complete, for special metabolic needs for inherited disease of metabolism, includes proteins, fats, carbohydrates, vitamins and minerals, may include fiber, administered through an enteral feeding tube, 100 calories = 1 unit ⑧

IOM: 100-03, 3, 180.2

⊛ **B4158**   Enteral formula, for pediatrics, nutritionally complete with intact nutrients, includes proteins, fats, carbohydrates, vitamins and minerals, may include fiber and/or iron, administered through an enteral feeding tube, 100 calories = 1 unit ⑧

IOM: 100-03, 3, 180.2

⊛ **B4159**   Enteral formula, for pediatrics, nutritionally complete soy based with intact nutrients, includes proteins, fats, carbohydrates, vitamins and minerals, may include fiber and/or iron, administered through an enteral feeding tube, 100 calories = 1 unit ⑧

IOM: 100-03, 3, 180.2

⊛ **B4160**   Enteral formula, for pediatrics, nutritionally complete calorically dense (equal to or greater than 0.7 kcal/ml) with intact nutrients, includes proteins, fats, carbohydrates, vitamins and minerals, may include fiber, administered through an enteral feeding tube, 100 calories = 1 unit ⑧

IOM: 100-03, 3, 180.2

⊛ **B4161**   Enteral formula, for pediatrics, hydrolyzed/amino acids and peptide chain proteins, includes fats, carbohydrates, vitamins and minerals, may include fiber, administered through an enteral feeding tube, 100 calories = 1 unit ⑧

IOM: 100-03, 3, 180.2

⊛ **B4162**   Enteral formula, for pediatrics, special metabolic needs for inherited disease of metabolism, includes proteins, fats, carbohydrates, vitamins and minerals, may include fiber, administered through an enteral feeding tube, 100 calories = 1 unit ⑧

IOM: 100-03, 3, 180.2

Parenteral Nutritional Solutions and Supplies

⊛ **B4164**   Parenteral nutrition solution: carbohydrates (dextrose), 50% or less (500 ml = 1 unit) - home mix ⑧

IOM: 100-02, 15, 120; 100-03, 3, 180.2; 100-04, 20, 100.2.2

⊛ **B4168**   Parenteral nutrition solution; amino acid, 3.5%, (500 ml = 1 unit) - home mix ⑧

IOM: 100-02, 15, 120; 100-03, 3, 180.2; 100-04, 20, 100.2.2

⊛ **B4172**   Parenteral nutrition solution; amino acid, 5.5% through 7%, (500 ml = 1 unit) - home mix ⑧

IOM: 100-02, 15, 120; 100-03, 3, 180.2; 100-04, 20, 100.2.2

⊛ **B4176**   Parenteral nutrition solution; amino acid, 7% through 8.5%, (500 ml = 1 unit) - home mix ⑧

IOM: 100-02, 15, 120; 100-03, 3, 180.2; 100-04, 20, 100.2.2

⊛ **B4178**   Parenteral nutrition solution: amino acid, greater than 8.5% (500 ml = 1 unit) - home mix ⑧

IOM: 100-02, 15, 120; 100-03, 3, 180.2; 100-04, 20, 100.2.2

⊛ **B4180**   Parenteral nutrition solution; carbohydrates (dextrose), greater than 50% (500 ml = 1 unit) - home mix ⑧

IOM: 100-02, 15, 120; 100-03, 3, 180.2; 100-04, 20, 100.2.2

▶ New	⟳ Revised	✔ Reinstated	~~deleted~~ Deleted	⊘ Not covered or valid by Medicare
⊛ Special coverage instructions		✳ Carrier discretion	⑧ Bill Part B MAC	⑧ Bill DME MAC

⊛ **B4185** Parenteral nutrition solution, per 10 grams lipids Ⓑ

⊛ **B4189** Parenteral nutrition solution; compounded amino acid and carbohydrates with electrolytes, trace elements, and vitamins, including preparation, any strength, 10 to 51 grams of protein - premix Ⓑ

IOM: 100-02, 15, 120; 100-03, 3, 180.2; 100-04, 20, 100.2.2

⊛ **B4193** Parenteral nutrition solution; compounded amino acid and carbohydrates with electrolytes, trace elements, and vitamins, including preparation, any strength, 52 to 73 grams of protein - premix Ⓑ

IOM: 100-02, 15, 120; 100-03, 3, 180.2; 100-04, 20, 100.2.2

⊛ **B4197** Parenteral nutrition solution; compounded amino acid and carbohydrates with electrolytes, trace elements and vitamins, including preparation, any strength, 74 to 100 grams of protein - premix Ⓑ

IOM: 100-02, 15, 120; 100-03, 3, 180.2; 100-04, 20, 100.2.2

⊛ **B4199** Parenteral nutrition solution; compounded amino acid and carbohydrates with electrolytes, trace elements and vitamins, including preparation, any strength, over 100 grams of protein - premix Ⓑ

IOM: 100-02, 15, 120; 100-03, 3, 180.2; 100-04, 20, 100.2.2

⊛ **B4216** Parenteral nutrition; additives (vitamins, trace elements, heparin, electrolytes) home mix per day Ⓑ

IOM: 100-02, 15, 120; 100-03, 3, 180.2; 100-04, 20, 100.2.2

⊛ **B4220** Parenteral nutrition supply kit; premix, per day Ⓑ

IOM: 100-02, 15, 120; 100-03, 3, 180.2; 100-04, 20, 100.2.2

⊛ **B4222** Parenteral nutrition supply kit; home mix, per day Ⓖ

IOM: 100-02, 15, 120; 100-03, 3, 180.2; 100-04, 20, 100.2.2

⊛ **B4224** Parenteral nutrition administration kit, per day Ⓑ

Dressings used with parenteral nutrition (covered under the prosthetic device benefit) are included in the payment. (www.cms.gov/medicare-coverage-database/)

IOM: 100-02, 15, 120; 100-03, 3, 180.2; 100-04, 20, 100.2.2

⊛ **B5000** Parenteral nutrition solution compounded amino acid and carbohydrates with electrolytes, trace elements, and vitamins, including preparation, any strength, renal - Aminosyn-RF, NephrAmine, RenAmine - premix Ⓑ

IOM: 100-02, 15, 120; 100-03, 3, 180.2; 100-04, 20, 100.2.2

⊛ **B5100** Parenteral nutrition solution compounded amino acid and carbohydrates with electrolytes, trace elements, and vitamins, including preparation, any strength, hepatic, HepatAmine - premix Ⓑ

IOM: 100-02, 15, 120; 100-03, 3, 180.2; 100-04, 20, 100.2.2

⊛ **B5200** Parenteral nutrition solution compounded amino acid and carbohydrates with electrolytes, trace elements, and vitamins, including preparation, any strength, stress-branch chain amino acids-FreAmine-HBC - premix Ⓑ

IOM: 100-02, 15, 120; 100-03, 3, 180.2; 100-04, 20, 100.2.2

Enteral and Parenteral Pumps

⊛ **B9002** Enteral nutrition infusion pump, any type Ⓑ

IOM: 100-02, 15, 120; 100-03, 3, 180.2; 100-04, 20, 100.2.2

⊛ **B9004** Parenteral nutrition infusion pump, portable Ⓑ

IOM: 100-02, 15, 120; 100-03, 3, 180.2; 100-04, 20, 100.2.2

⊛ **B9006** Parenteral nutrition infusion pump, stationary Ⓑ

IOM: 100-02, 15, 120; 100-03, 3, 180.2; 100-04, 20, 100.2.2

⊛ **B9998** NOC for enteral supplies Ⓖ

IOM: 100-02, 15, 120; 100-03, 3, 180.2; 100-04, 20, 100.2.2

⊛ **B9999** NOC for parenteral supplies Ⓑ

Determine if an alternative HCPCS Level II or a CPT code better describes the service being reported. This code should be reported only if a more specific code is unavailable.

IOM: 100-02, 15, 120; 100-03, 3, 180.2; 100-04, 20, 100.2.2

▶ New   ↻ Revised   ✔ Reinstated   deleted Deleted   ⊘ Not covered or valid by Medicare
⊛ Special coverage instructions   ✳ Carrier discretion   Ⓑ Bill Part B MAC   Ⓖ Bill DME MAC

CMS HOSPITAL OUTPATIENT PAYMENT SYSTEM (C1000-C9999)

NOTE: C-codes are used on Medicare Ambulatory Surgical Center (ASC) and Hospital Outpatient Prospective Payment System (OPPS) claims, but may also be recognized on claims from other providers or by other payment systems. As of 10/01/2006, the following non-OPPS providers have been able to bill Medicare using the C-codes, or an appropriate CPT code on Types of Bill (TOBs) 12X, 13X, or 85X:

- Critical Access Hospitals (CAHs);
- Indian Health Service Hospitals (IHS);
- Hospitals located in American Samoa, Guam, Saipan or the Virgin Islands; and
- Maryland waiver hospitals.

The billing of C-codes by Method I and Method II Critical Access Hospitals (CAHs) is limited to the billing for facility (technical) services. The C-codes shall not be billed by Method II CAHs for professional services with revenue codes (RCs) 96X, 97X, or 98X.

C codes are updated quarterly by the Centers for Medicare and Medicaid Services (CMS).

Devices and Supplies

⊛ **C1713** Anchor/Screw for opposing bone-to-bone or soft tissue-to-bone (implantable)

⊛ **C1714** Catheter, transluminal atherectomy, directional

⊛ **C1715** Brachytherapy needle

Brachytherapy Sources

⊛ **C1716** Brachytherapy source, non-stranded, gold-198, per source

⊛ **C1717** Brachytherapy source, non-stranded, high dose rate iridium 192, per source

⊛ **C1719** Brachytherapy source, non-stranded, non-high dose rate iridium-192, per source

Cardioverter-Defibrilators

⊛ **C1721** Cardioverter-defibrillator, dual chamber (implantable)
Related CPT codes: 33224, 33240, 33249.

⊛ **C1722** Cardioverter-defibrillator, single chamber (implantable)
Related CPT codes: 33240, 33249.

Catheters

⊛ **C1724** Catheter, transluminal atherectomy, rotational

⊛ **C1725** Catheter, transluminal angioplasty, non-laser (may include guidance, infusion/perfusion capability)

⊛ **C1726** Catheter, balloon dilatation, non-vascular

⊛ **C1727** Catheter, balloon tissue dissector, non-vascular (insertable)

⊛ **C1728** Catheter, brachytherapy seed administration

⊛ **C1729** Catheter, drainage

⊛ **C1730** Catheter, electrophysiology, diagnostic, other than 3D mapping (19 or fewer electrodes)

⊛ **C1731** Catheter, electrophysiology, diagnostic, other than 3D mapping (20 or more electrodes)

⊛ **C1732** Catheter, electrophysiology, diagnostic/ablation, 3D or vector mapping

⊛ **C1733** Catheter, electrophysiology, diagnostic/ablation, other than 3D or vector mapping, other than cool-tip

⊛ **C1749** Endoscope, retrograde imaging/illumination colonoscope device (implantable)

⊛ **C1750** Catheter, hemodialysis/peritoneal, long-term

⊛ **C1751** Catheter, infusion, inserted peripherally, centrally, or midline (other than hemodialysis)

⊛ **C1752** Catheter, hemodialysis/peritoneal, short-term

⊛ **C1753** Catheter, intravascular ultrasound

⊛ **C1754** Catheter, intradiscal

⊛ **C1755** Catheter, instraspinal

⊛ **C1756** Catheter, pacing, transesophageal

⊛ **C1757** Catheter, thrombectomy/embolectomy

⊛ **C1758** Catheter, ureteral

⊛ **C1759** Catheter, intracardiac echocardiography

Devices

- ⊕ **C1760** Closure device, vascular (implantable/insertable)
- ⊕ **C1762** Connective tissue, human (includes fascia lata)
- ⊕ **C1763** Connective tissue, non-human (includes synthetic)
- ⊕ **C1764** Event recorder, cardiac (implantable)
- ⊕ **C1765** Adhesion barrier
- ⊕ **C1766** Introducer/sheath, guiding, intracardiac electrophysiological, steerable, other than peel-away
- ⊕ **C1767** Generator, neurostimulator (implantable), nonrechargeable

  Related CPT codes: 61885, 61886, 63685, 64590.
- ⊕ **C1768** Graft, vascular
- ⊕ **C1769** Guide wire
- ⊕ **C1770** Imaging coil, magnetic reasonance (insertable)
- ⊕ **C1771** Repair device, urinary, incontinence, with sling graft
- ⊕ **C1772** Infusion pump, programmable (implantable)
- ⊕ **C1773** Retrieval device, insertable (used to retrieve fractured medical devices)
- ⊕ **C1776** Joint device (implantable)
- ⊕ **C1777** Lead, cardioverter-defibrillator, endocardial single coil (implantable)

  Related CPT codes: 33216, 33217, 33249.
- ⊕ **C1778** Lead, neurostimulator (implantable)

  Related CPT codes: 43647, 63650, 63655, 63663, 63664, 64553, 64555, 64560, 64561, 64565, 64573, 64575, 64577, 64580, 64581.
- ⊕ **C1779** Lead, pacemaker, trasvenous VDD single pass

  Related CPT codes: 33206, 33207, 33208, 33210, 33211, 33214, 33216, 33217, 33249.
- ⊕ **C1780** Lens, intraocular (new technology)
- ⊕ **C1781** Mesh (implantable)
- ⊕ **C1782** Morcellator
- ⊕ **C1783** Ocular implant, aqueous drainage assist device
- ⊕ **C1784** Ocular device, intraoperative, detached retina

- ⊕ **C1785** Pacemaker, dual chamber, rate-responsive (implantable)

  Related CPT codes: 33206, 33207, 33208, 33213, 33214, 33224.
- ⊕ **C1786** Pacemaker, single chamber, rate-responsive (implantable)

  Related CPT codes: 33206, 33207, 33212.
- ⊕ **C1787** Patient programmer, neurostimulator
- ⊕ **C1788** Port, indwelling (implantable)
- ⊕ **C1789** Prosthesis, breast (implantable)
- ⊕ **C1813** Prosthesis, penile, inflatable
- ⊕ **C1814** Retinal tamponade device, silicone oil
- ⊕ **C1815** Prosthesis, urinary sphincter (implantable)
- ⊕ **C1816** Receiver and/or transmitter, neurostimulator (implantable)
- ⊕ **C1817** Septal defect implant system, intracardiac
- ⊕ **C1818** Integrated keratoprosthesic
- ⊕ **C1819** Surgical tissue localization and excision device (implantable)
- ⊕ **C1820** Generator, neurostimulator (implantable), with rechargeable battery and charging system

  Related CPT codes: 61885, 61886, 63685, 64590.
- ⊕ **C1821** Interspinous process distraction device (implantable)
- ↻ ⊕ **C1822** Generator, neurostimulator (implantable), high frequency, with rechargeable battery and charging system
- ⊕ **C1830** Powered bone marrow biopsy needle
- ⊕ **C1840** Lens, intraocular (telescopic)
- ⊕ **C1841** Retinal prosthesis, includes all internal and external components
- ⊕ **C1842** Retinal prosthesis, includes all internal and external components; add-on to C1841
- ⊕ **C1874** Stent, coated/covered, with delivery system
- ⊕ **C1875** Stent, coated/covered, without delivery system
- ⊕ **C1876** Stent, non-coated/non-covered, with delivery system
- ⊕ **C1877** Stent, non-coated/non-covered, without delivery system
- ⊕ **C1878** Material for vocal cord medialization, synthetic (implantable)
- ⊕ **C1880** Vena cava filter
- ⊕ **C1881** Dialysis access system (implantable)

▶ New   ↻ Revised   ✔ Reinstated   ~~deleted~~ Deleted   ⊘ Not covered or valid by Medicare
⊕ Special coverage instructions   ✳ Carrier discretion   Ⓑ Bill Part B MAC   Ⓓ Bill DME MAC

⊛ **C1882** Cardioverter-defibrillator, other than single or dual chamber (implantable)

Related CPT codes: 33224, 33240, 33249.

⊛ **C1883** Adapter/Extension, pacing lead or neurostimulator lead (implantable)

⊛ **C1884** Embolization protective system

⊛ **C1885** Catheter, transluminal angioplasty, laser

⊛ **C1886** Catheter, extravascular tissue ablation, any modality (insertable)

⊛ **C1887** Catheter, guiding (may include infusion/perfusion capability)

⊛ **C1888** Catheter, ablation, non-cardiac, endovascular (implantable)

⊛ **C1889** Implantable/insertable device for device intensive procedure, not otherwise classified

⊛ **C1891** Infusion pump, non-programmable, permanent (implantable)

⊛ **C1892** Introducer/sheath, guiding, intracardiac electrophysiological, fixed-curve, peel-away

⊛ **C1893** Introducer/sheath, guiding, intracardiac electrophysiological, fixed-curve, other than peel-away

⊛ **C1894** Introducer/sheath, other than guiding, other than intracardiac electrophysiological, non-laser

⊛ **C1895** Lead, cardioverter-defibrillator, endocardial dual coil (implantable)

Related CPT codes: 33216, 33217, 33249.

⊛ **C1896** Lead, cardioverter-defibrillator, other than endocardial single or dual coil (implantable)

Related CPT codes: 33216, 33217, 33249.

⊛ **C1897** Lead, neurostimulator test kit (implantable)

Related CPT codes: 43647, 63650, 63655, 63663, 63664, 64553, 64555, 64560, 64561, 64565, 64575, 64577, 64580, 64581.

⊛ **C1898** Lead, pacemaker, other than transvenous VDD single pass

Related CPT codes: 33206, 33207, 33208, 33210, 33211, 33214, 33216, 33217, 33249.

⊛ **C1899** Lead, pacemaker/cardioverter-defibrillator combination (implantable)

Related CPT codes: 33216, 33217, 33249.

⊛ **C1900** Lead, left ventricular coronary venous system

Related CPT codes: 33224, 33225.

↻ ⊛ **C2613** Lung biopsy plug with delivery system

⊛ **C2614** Probe, percutaneous lumbar discectomy

⊛ **C2615** Sealant, pulmonary, liquid

Brachytherapy Source

⊛ **C2616** Brachytherapy source, non-stranded, yttrium-90, per source

Cardiovascular and Genitourinary Devices

⊛ **C2617** Stent, non-coronary, temporary, without delivery system

⊛ **C2618** Probe/needle, cryoablation

⊛ **C2619** Pacemaker, dual chamber, non rate-responsive (implantable)

Related CPT codes: 33206, 33207, 33208, 33213, 33214, 33224.

⊛ **C2620** Pacemaker, single chamber, non rate-responsive (implantable)

Related CPT codes: 33206, 33207, 33212, 33224.

⊛ **C2621** Pacemaker, other than single or dual chamber (implantable)

Related CPT codes: 33206, 33207, 33208, 33212, 33213, 33214, 33224.

⊛ **C2622** Prosthesis, penile, non-inflatable

↻ ⊛ **C2623** Catheter, transluminal angioplasty, drug-coated, non-laser

↻ ⊛ **C2624** Implantable wireless pulmonary artery pressure sensor with delivery catheter, including all system components

⊛ **C2625** Stent, non-coronary, temporary, with delivery system

⊛ **C2626** Infusion pump, non-programmable, temporary (implantable)

⊛ **C2627** Catheter, suprapubic/cystoscopic

⊛ **C2628** Catheter, occlusion

⊛ **C2629** Introducer/Sheath, other than guiding, other than intracardiac electrophysiological, laser

⊛ **C2630** Catheter, electrophysiology, diagnostic/ablation, other than 3D or vector mapping, cool-tip

⊛ **C2631** Repair device, urinary, incontinence, without sling graft

---

▶ **New** ↻ **Revised** ✔ **Reinstated** ~~deleted~~ **Deleted** ⊘ **Not covered or valid by Medicare**

⊛ **Special coverage instructions** ✳ **Carrier discretion** Ⓟ **Bill Part B MAC** Ⓓ **Bill DME MAC**

Brachytherapy Sources

⊛ **C2634** Brachytherapy source, non-stranded, high activity, iodine-125, greater than 1.01 mci (NIST), per source

⊛ **C2635** Brachytherapy source, non-stranded, high activity, palladium-103, greater than 2.2 mci (NIST), per source

⊛ **C2636** Brachytherapy linear source, non-stranded, palladium-103, per 1 mm

⊛ **C2637** Brachytherapy source, non-stranded, Ytterbium-169, per source

⊛ **C2638** Brachytherapy source, stranded, iodine-125, per source

⊛ **C2639** Brachytherapy source, non-stranded, iodine-125, per source

⊛ **C2640** Brachytherapy source, stranded, palladium-103, per source

⊛ **C2641** Brachytherapy source, non-stranded, palladium-103, per source

⊛ **C2642** Brachytherapy source, stranded, cesium-131, per source

⊛ **C2643** Brachytherapy source, non-stranded, cesium-131, per source

⊛ **C2644** Brachytherapy source, Cesium-131 chloride solution, per millicurie

⊛ **C2645** Brachytherapy planar source, palladium-103, per square millimeter

⊛ **C2698** Brachytherapy source, stranded, not otherwise specified, per source

⊛ **C2699** Brachytherapy source, non-stranded, not otherwise specified, per source

Skin Substitute Graft Application

⊛ **C5271** Application of low cost skin substitute graft to trunk, arms, legs, total wound surface area up to 100 sq cm; first 25 sq cm or less wound surface area

⊛ **C5272** Application of low cost skin substitute graft to trunk, arms, legs, total wound surface area up to 100 sq cm; each additional 25 sq cm wound surface area, or part thereof (list separately in addition to code for primary procedure)

⊛ **C5273** Application of low cost skin substitute graft to trunk, arms, legs, total wound surface area greater than or equal to 100 sq cm; first 100 sq cm wound surface area, or 1% of body area of infants and children

⊛ **C5274** Application of low cost skin substitute graft to trunk, arms, legs, total wound surface area greater than or equal to 100 sq cm; each additional 100 sq cm wound surface area, or part thereof, or each additional 1% of body area of infants and children, or part thereof (list separately in addition to code for primary procedure)

⊛ **C5275** Application of low cost skin substitute graft to face, scalp, eyelids, mouth, neck, ears, orbits, genitalia, hands, feet, and/or multiple digits, total wound surface area up to 100 sq cm; first 25 sq cm or less wound surface area

⊛ **C5276** Application of low cost skin substitute graft to face, scalp, eyelids, mouth, neck, ears, orbits, genitalia, hands, feet, and/or multiple digits, total wound surface area up to 100 sq cm; each additional 25 sq cm wound surface area, or part thereof (list separately in addition to code for primary procedure)

⊛ **C5277** Application of low cost skin substitute graft to face, scalp, eyelids, mouth, neck, ears, orbits, genitalia, hands, feet, and/or multiple digits, total wound surface area greater than or equal to 100 sq cm; first 100 sq cm wound surface area, or 1% of body area of infants and children

⊛ **C5278** Application of low cost skin substitute graft to face, scalp, eyelids, mouth, neck, ears, orbits, genitalia, hands, feet, and/or multiple digits, total wound surface area greater than or equal to 100 sq cm; each additional 100 sq cm wound surface area, or part thereof, or each additional 1% of body area of infants and children, or part thereof (list separately in addition to code for primary procedure)

Magnetic Resonance Angiography: Trunk and Lower Extremities

⊛ **C8900** Magnetic resonance angiography with contrast, abdomen

⊛ **C8901** Magnetic resonance angiography without contrast, abdomen

⊛ **C8902** Magnetic resonance angiography without contrast followed by with contrast, abdomen

⊛ **C8903** Magnetic resonance imaging with contrast, breast; unilateral

⊛ **C8904** Magnetic resonance imaging without contrast, breast; unilateral

---

▶ New   ↻ Revised   ✔ Reinstated   ~~deleted~~ Deleted   ⊘ Not covered or valid by Medicare
⊛ Special coverage instructions   ✳ Carrier discretion   ⑨ Bill Part B MAC   ⑧ Bill DME MAC

⊛ **C8905** Magnetic resonance imaging without contrast followed by with contrast, breast; unilateral

⊛ **C8906** Magnetic resonance imaging with contrast, breast; bilateral

⊛ **C8907** Magnetic resonance imaging without contrast, breast; bilateral

⊛ **C8908** Magnetic resonance imaging without contrast followed by with contrast, breast; bilateral

⊛ **C8909** Magnetic resonance angiography with contrast, chest (excluding myocardium)

⊛ **C8910** Magnetic resonance angiography without contrast, chest (excluding myocardium)

⊛ **C8911** Magnetic resonance angiography without contrast followed by with contrast, chest (excluding myocardium)

⊛ **C8912** Magnetic resonance angiography with contrast, lower extremity

⊛ **C8913** Magnetic resonance angiography without contrast, lower extremity

⊛ **C8914** Magnetic resonance angiography without contrast followed by with contrast, lower extremity

⊛ **C8918** Magnetic resonance angiography with contrast, pelvis

⊛ **C8919** Magnetic resonance angiography without contrast, pelvis

⊛ **C8920** Magnetic resonance angiography without contrast followed by with contrast, pelvis

Transthoracic and Transesophageal Echocardiography

⊛ **C8921** Transthoracic echocardiography with contrast, or without contrast followed by with contrast, for congenital cardiac anomalies; complete

⊛ **C8922** Transthoracic echocardiography with contrast, or without contrast followed by with contrast, for congenital cardiac anomalies; follow-up or limited study

⊛ **C8923** Transthoracic echocardiography with contrast, or without contrast followed by with contrast, real-time with image documentation (2D), includes M-mode recording, when performed, complete, without spectral or color Doppler echocardiography

⊛ **C8924** Transthoracic echocardiography with contrast, or without contrast followed by with contrast, real-time with image documentation (2D), includes M-mode recording, when performed, follow-up or limited study

⊛ **C8925** Transesophageal echocardiography (TEE) with contrast, or without contrast followed by with contrast, real time with image documentation (2D) (with or without M-mode recording); including probe placement, image acquisition, interpretation and report

⊛ **C8926** Transesophageal echocardiography (TEE) with contrast, or without contrast followed by with contrast, for congenital cardiac anomalies; including probe placement, image acquisition, interpretation and report

⊛ **C8927** Transesophageal echocardiography (TEE) with contrast, or without contrast followed by with contrast, for monitoring purposes, including probe placement, real time 2-dimensional image acquisition and interpretation leading to ongoing (continuous) assessment of (dynamically changing) cardiac pumping function and to therapeutic measures on an immediate time basis

⊛ **C8928** Transthoracic echocardiography with contrast, or without contrast followed by with contrast, real-time with image documentation (2D), includes M-mode recording, when performed, during rest and cardiovascular stress test using treadmill, bicycle exercise and/or pharmacologically induced stress, with interpretation and report

⊛ **C8929** Transthoracic echocardiography with contrast, or without contrast followed by with contrast, real-time with image documentation (2D), includes M-mode recording, when performed, complete, with spectral Doppler echocardiography, and with color flow Doppler echocardiography

⊛ **C8930** Transthoracic echocardiography, with contrast, or without contrast followed by with contrast, real-time with image documentation (2D), includes M-mode recording, when performed, during rest and cardiovascular stress test using treadmill, bicycle exercise and/or pharmacologically induced stress, with interpretation and report; including performance of continuous electrocardiographic monitoring, with physician supervision

▶ **New**   ↻ **Revised**   ✔ **Reinstated**   ~~deleted~~ **Deleted**   ⊘ **Not covered or valid by Medicare**
⊛ **Special coverage instructions**   ✳ **Carrier discretion**   ⑧ **Bill Part B MAC**   ⑧ **Bill DME MAC**

Magnetic Resonance Angiography: Spine and Upper Extremities

⊛ **C8931** Magnetic resonance angiography with contrast, spinal canal and contents

⊛ **C8932** Magnetic resonance angiography without contrast, spinal canal and contents

⊛ **C8933** Magnetic resonance angiography without contrast followed by with contrast, spinal canal and contents

⊛ **C8934** Magnetic resonance angiography with contrast, upper extremity

⊛ **C8935** Magnetic resonance angiography without contrast, upper extremity

⊛ **C8936** Magnetic resonance angiography without contrast followed by with contrast, upper extremity

Drugs and Biologicals

⊛ **C8957** Intravenous infusion for therapy/diagnosis; initiation of prolonged infusion (more than 8 hours), requiring use of portable or implantable pump

▶ ⊛ **C9014** Injection, cerliponase alfa, 1 mg

▶ ⊛ **C9015** Injection, C-1 esterase inhibitor (human), haegarda, 10 units

▶ ⊛ **C9016** Injection, triptorelin extended release, 3.75 mg

▶ ⊛ **C9024** Injection, liposomal, 1 mg daunorubicin and 2.27 mg cytarabine

▶ ⊛ **C9028** Injection, inotuzumab ozogamicin, 0.1 mg

▶ ⊛ **C9029** Injection, guselkumab, 1 mg

⊛ **C9113** Injection, pantoprazole sodium, per vial

⊛ **C9132** Prothrombin complex concentrate (human), Kcentra, per i.u. of Factor IX activity

~~C9140~~ ~~Injection, factor VIII (antihemophilic factor, recombinant) (afstyla), 1 i.u.~~ ✖
Cross Reference J7210

↻ ⊛ **C9248** Injection, clevidipine butyrate, 1 mg

⊛ **C9250** Human plasma fibrin sealant, vapor-heated, solvent-detergent (ARTISS), 2 ml
Example of diagnosis codes to be reported with C9250: T20.00-T25.799.

⊛ **C9254** Injection, lacosamide, 1 mg

⊛ **C9257** injection, bevacizumab, 0.25 mg

⊛ **C9275** Injection, hexaminolevulinate hydrochloride, 100 mg, per study dose

⊛ **C9285** Lidocaine 70 mg/tetracaine 70 mg, per patch

⊛ **C9290** Injection, bupivacine liposome, 1 mg

⊛ **C9293** Injection, glucarpidase, 10 units

⊛ **C9352** Microporous collagen implantable tube (NeuraGen Nerve Guide), per centimeter length

⊛ **C9353** Microporous collagen implantable slit tube (NeuraWrap Nerve Protector), per centimeter length

⊛ **C9354** Acellular pericardial tissue matrix of non-human origin (Veritas), per square centimeter

⊛ **C9355** Collagen nerve cuff (NeuroMatrix), per 0.5 centimeter length

⊛ **C9356** Tendon, porous matrix of cross-linked collagen and glycosaminoglycan matrix (TenoGlide Tendon Protector Sheet), per square centimeter

⊛ **C9358** Dermal substitute, native, non-denatured collagen, fetal bovine origin (SurgiMend Collagen Matrix), per 0.5 square centimeters

⊛ **C9359** Porous purified collagen matrix bone void filler (Integra Mozaik Osteoconductive Scaffold Putty, Integra OS Osteoconductive Scaffold Putty), per 0.5 cc

⊛ **C9360** Dermal substitute, native, non-denatured collagen, neonatal bovine origin (SurgiMend Collagen Matrix), per 0.5 square centimeters

⊛ **C9361** Collagen matrix nerve wrap (NeuroMend Collagen Nerve Wrap), per 0.5 centimeter length

⊛ **C9362** Porous purified collagen matrix bone void filler (Integra Mozaik Osteoconductive Scaffold Strip), per 0.5 cc

⊛ **C9363** Skin substitute, Integra Meshed Bilayer Wound Matrix, per square centimeter

⊛ **C9364** Porcine implant, Permacol, per square centimeter

⊛ **C9399** Unclassified drugs or biologicals

↻ ⊛ **C9447** Injection, phenylephrine and ketorolac, 4 ml vial

⊛ **C9460** Injection, cangrelor, 1 mg

⊛ **C9482** Injection, sotalol hydrochloride, 1 mg

~~C9483~~ ~~Injection, atezolizumab, 10 mg~~ ✖
Cross Reference J9022

~~C9484~~ ~~Injection, eteplirsen, 10 mg~~ ✖
Cross Reference J1428

▶ New ↻ Revised ✔ Reinstated ~~deleted~~ Deleted ⊘ Not covered or valid by Medicare ⊛ Special coverage instructions ✱ Carrier discretion Ⓑ Bill Part B MAC Ⓓ Bill DME MAC

CMS HOSPITAL OUTPATIENT PAYMENT SYSTEM C8931 — C9484

139

~~C9485~~ ~~Injection, olaratumab, 10 mg~~ ✖

Cross Reference J9285

~~C9486~~ ~~Injection, granisetron extended release, 0.1 mg~~ ✖

Cross Reference J1627

~~C9487~~ ~~Ustekinumab, for intravenous injection, 1 mg~~ ✖

Cross Reference Q9989

▶ ⊗ **C9488** Injection, conivaptan hydrochloride, 1 mg

~~C9489~~ ~~Injection, nusinersen, 0.1 mg~~ ✖

Cross Reference J2326

~~C9490~~ ~~Injection, bezlotoxumab, 10 mg~~ ✖

Cross Reference J0565

~~C9491~~ ~~Injection, avelumab, 10 mg~~ ✖

Cross Reference J9023

▶ ⊗ **C9492** Injection, durvalumab, 10 mg

▶ ⊗ **C9493** Injection, edaravone, 1 mg

~~C9494~~ ~~Injection, ocrelizumab, 1 mg~~ ✖

Cross Reference J2350

⊗ **C9497** Loxapine, inhalation powder, 10 mg

Percutaneous Transcatheter and Transluminal Coronary Procedures

⊗ **C9600** Percutaneous transcatheter placement of drug eluting intracoronary stent(s), with coronary angioplasty when performed; a single major coronary artery or branch

⊗ **C9601** Percutaneous transcatheter placement of drug-eluting intracoronary stent(s), with coronary angioplasty when performed; each additional branch of a major coronary artery (list separately in addition to code for primary procedure)

⊗ **C9602** Percutaneous transluminal coronary atherectomy, with drug eluting intracoronary stent, with coronary angioplasty when performed; a single major coronary artery or branch

⊗ **C9603** Percutaneous transluminal coronary atherectomy, with drug-eluting intracoronary stent, with coronary angioplasty when performed; each additional branch of a major coronary artery (list separately in addition to code for primary procedure)

⊗ **C9604** Percutaneous transluminal revascularization of or through coronary artery bypass graft (internal mammary, free arterial, venous), any combination of drug-eluting intracoronary stent, atherectomy and angioplasty, including distal protection when performed; a single vessel

⊗ **C9605** Percutaneous transluminal revascularization of or through coronary artery bypass graft (internal mammary, free arterial, venous), any combination of drug-eluting intracoronary stent, atherectomy and angioplasty, including distal protection when performed; each additional branch subtended by the bypass graft (list separately in addition to code for primary procedure)

⊗ **C9606** Percutaneous transluminal revascularization of acute total/subtotal occlusion during acute myocardial infarction, coronary artery or coronary artery bypass graft, any combination of drug-eluting intracoronary stent, atherectomy and angioplasty, including aspiration thrombectomy when performed, single vessel

⊗ **C9607** Percutaneous transluminal revascularization of chronic total occlusion, coronary artery, coronary artery branch, or coronary artery bypass graft, any combination of drug-eluting intracoronary stent, atherectomy and angioplasty; single vessel

⊗ **C9608** Percutaneous transluminal revascularization of chronic total occlusion, coronary artery, coronary artery branch, or coronary artery bypass graft, any combination of drug-eluting intracoronary stent, atherectomy and angioplasty; each additional coronary artery, coronary artery branch, or bypass graft (list separately in addition to code for primary procedure)

Therapeutic Services and Supplies

⊗ **C9725** Placement of endorectal intracavitary applicator for high intensity brachytherapy

⊗ **C9726** Placement and removal (if performed) of applicator into breast for intraoperative radiation therapy, add-on to primary breast procedure

⊗ **C9727** Insertion of implants into the soft palate; minimum of three implants

---

▶ **New**   ↻ **Revised**   ✔ **Reinstated**   ~~deleted~~ **Deleted**   ⊘ **Not covered or valid by Medicare**

⊗ **Special coverage instructions**   ✳ **Carrier discretion**   Ⓑ **Bill Part B MAC**   Ⓓ **Bill DME MAC**

⊛ **C9728** Placement of interstitial device(s) for radiation therapy/surgery guidance (e.g., fiducial markers, dosimeter), for other than the following sites (any approach): abdomen, pelvis, prostate, retroperitoneum, thorax, single or multiple

⊛ **C9733** Non-ophthalmic fluorescent vascular angiography

⊛ **C9734** Focused ultrasound ablation/ therapeutic intervention, other than uterine leiomyomata, with magnetic resonance (MR) guidance

▶ ⊛ **C9738** Adjunctive blue light cystoscopy with fluorescent imaging agent (list separately in addition to code for primary procedure)

⊛ **C9739** Cystourethroscopy, with insertion of transprostatic implant; 1 to 3 implants

⊛ **C9740** Cystourethroscopy, with insertion of transprostatic implant; 4 or more implants

⊛ **C9741** Right heart catheterization with implantation of wireless pressure sensor in the pulmonary artery, including any type of measurement, angiography, imaging supervision, interpretation, and report

⊛ **C9744** Ultrasound, abdominal, with contrast

▶ ⊛ **C9745** Nasal endoscopy, surgical; balloon dilation of eustachian tube

▶ ⊛ **C9746** Transperineal implantation of permanent adjustable balloon continence device, with cystourethroscopy, when performed and/or fluoroscopy, when performed

▶ ⊛ **C9747** Ablation of prostate, transrectal, high intensity focused ultrasound (HIFU), including imaging guidance

▶ ⊛ **C9748** Transurethral destruction of prostate tissue; by radiofrequency water vapor (steam) thermal therapy

⊛ **C9898** Radiolabeled product provided during a hospital inpatient stay

⊛ **C9899** Implanted prosthetic device, payable only for inpatients who do not have inpatient coverage

---

▶ **New** ⤺ **Revised** ✔ **Reinstated** deleted **Deleted** ⊘ **Not covered or valid by Medicare**
⊛ **Special coverage instructions** ✳ **Carrier discretion** Ⓑ **Bill Part B MAC** Ⓓ **Bill DME MAC**

DURABLE MEDICAL EQUIPMENT (E0100-E8002)

Canes

⊕ **E0100** Cane, includes canes of all materials, adjustable or fixed, with tip Ⓑ

IOM: 100-02, 15, 110.1; 100-03, 4, 280.1; 100-03, 4, 280.2

⊕ **E0105** Cane, quad or three prong, includes canes of all materials, adjustable or fixed, with tips Ⓑ

IOM: 100-02, 15, 110.1; 100-03, 4, 280.1; 100-03, 4, 280.2

Crutches

⊕ **E0110** Crutches, forearm, includes crutches of various materials, adjustable or fixed, pair, complete with tips and handgrips Ⓑ

Crutches are covered when prescribed for a patient who is normally ambulatory but suffers from a condition that impairs ambulation. Provides minimal to moderate weight support while ambulating.

IOM: 100-02, 15, 110.1; 100-03, 4, 280.1

⊕ **E0111** Crutch forearm, includes crutches of various materials, adjustable or fixed, each, with tips and handgrips Ⓑ

IOM: 100-02, 15, 110.1; 100-03, 4, 280.1

⊕ **E0112** Crutches, underarm, wood, adjustable or fixed, pair, with pads, tips, and handgrips Ⓑ

IOM: 100-02, 15, 110.1; 100-03, 4, 280.1

⊕ **E0113** Crutch underarm, wood, adjustable or fixed, each, with pad, tip, and handgrip Ⓑ

IOM: 100-02, 15, 110.1; 100-03, 4, 280.1

⊕ **E0114** Crutches, underarm, other than wood, adjustable or fixed, pair, with pads, tips and handgrips Ⓑ

IOM: 100-02, 15, 110.1; 100-03, 4, 280.1

⊕ **E0116** Crutch, underarm, other than wood, adjustable or fixed, with pad, tip, handgrip, with or without shock absorber, each Ⓑ

IOM: 100-02, 15, 110.1; 100-03, 4, 280.1

⊕ **E0117** Crutch, underarm, articulating, spring assisted, each Ⓑ

IOM: 100-02, 15, 110.1

✳ **E0118** Crutch substitute, lower leg platform, with or without wheels, each Ⓑ

Walkers

⊕ **E0130** Walker, rigid (pickup), adjustable or fixed height Ⓑ

Standard walker criteria for payment: Individual has a mobility limitation that significantly impairs ability to participate in mobility-related activities of daily living that cannot be adequately or safely addressed by a cane. The patient is able to use the walker safely; the functional mobility deficit can be resolved with use of a standard walker.

IOM: 100-02, 15, 110.1; 100-03, 4, 280.1

⊕ **E0135** Walker, folding (pickup), adjustable or fixed height Ⓑ

IOM: 100-02, 15, 110.1; 100-03, 4, 280.1

⊕ **E0140** Walker, with trunk support, adjustable or fixed height, any type Ⓑ

IOM: 100-02, 15, 110.1; 100-03, 4, 280.1

⊕ **E0141** Walker, rigid, wheeled, adjustable or fixed height Ⓑ

IOM: 100-02, 15, 110.1; 100-03, 4, 280.1

⊕ **E0143** Walker, folding, wheeled, adjustable or fixed height Ⓑ

IOM: 100-02, 15, 110.1; 100-03, 4, 280.1

⊕ **E0144** Walker, enclosed, four sided framed, rigid or folding, wheeled, with posterior seat Ⓑ

IOM: 100-02, 15, 110.1; 100-03, 4, 280.1

⊕ **E0147** Walker, heavy duty, multiple braking system, variable wheel resistance Ⓑ

Heavy-duty walker is labeled as capable of supporting more than 300 pounds

IOM: 100-02, 15, 110.1; 100-03, 4, 280.1

✳ **E0148** Walker, heavy duty, without wheels, rigid or folding, any type, each Ⓑ

Heavy-duty walker is labeled as capable of supporting more than 300 pounds

✳ **E0149** Walker, heavy duty, wheeled, rigid or folding, any type Ⓑ

Heavy-duty walker is labeled as capable of supporting more than 300 pounds

---

▶ **New**   ↻ **Revised**   ✔ **Reinstated**   ~~deleted~~ **Deleted**   ⊘ **Not covered or valid by Medicare**

⊕ **Special coverage instructions**   ✳ **Carrier discretion**   Ⓑ **Bill Part B MAC**   Ⓓ **Bill DME MAC**

✳ **E0153** Platform attachment, forearm crutch, each ⑧

✳ **E0154** Platform attachment, walker, each ⑧

✳ **E0155** Wheel attachment, rigid pick-up walker, per pair ⑧

Attachments

✳ **E0156** Seat attachment, walker ⑧

✳ **E0157** Crutch attachment, walker, each ⑧

✳ **E0158** Leg extensions for walker, per set of four (4) ⑧

Leg extensions are considered medically necessary DME for patients 6 feet tall or more.

✳ **E0159** Brake attachment for wheeled walker, replacement, each ⑧

Sitz Bath/Equipment

✺ **E0160** Sitz type bath or equipment, portable, used with or without commode ⑧

IOM: 100-03, 4, 280.1

✺ **E0161** Sitz type bath or equipment, portable, used with or without commode, with faucet attachment/s ⑧

IOM: 100-03, 4, 280.1

✺ **E0162** Sitz bath chair ⑧

IOM: 100-03, 4, 280.1

Commodes

✺ **E0163** Commode chair, mobile or stationary, with fixed arms ⑧

IOM: 100-02, 15, 110.1; 100-03, 4, 280.1

✺ **E0165** Commode chair, mobile or stationary, with detachable arms ⑧

IOM: 100-02, 15, 110.1; 100-03, 4, 280.1

✺ **E0167** Pail or pan for use with commode chair, replacement only ⑧

IOM: 100-03, 4, 280.1

✳ **E0168** Commode chair, extra wide and/or heavy duty, stationary or mobile, with or without arms, any type, each ⑧

Extra-wide or heavy duty commode chair is labeled as capable of supporting more than 300 pounds

✳ **E0170** Commode chair with integrated seat lift mechanism, electric, any type ⑧

✳ **E0171** Commode chair with integrated seat lift mechanism, non-electric, any type ⑧

⊘ **E0172** Seat lift mechanism placed over or on top of toilet, any type ⑧

✳ **E0175** Foot rest, for use with commode chair, each ⑧

Decubitus Care Equipment

✺ **E0181** Powered pressure reducing mattress overlay/pad, alternating, with pump, includes heavy duty ⑧

Requires the provider to determine medical necessity compliance. To demonstrate the requirements in the medical policy were met, attach KX.

IOM: 100-03, 4, 280.1; 100-08, 5, 5.2.3

✺ **E0182** Pump for alternating pressure pad, for replacement only ⑧

IOM: 100-03, 4, 280.1; 100-08, 5, 5.2.3

✺ **E0184** Dry pressure mattress ⑧

IOM: 100-03, 4, 280.1; 100-08, 5, 5.2.3

✺ **E0185** Gel or gel-like pressure pad for mattress, standard mattress length and width ⑧

IOM: 100-03, 4, 280.1; 100-08, 5, 5.2.3

✺ **E0186** Air pressure mattress ⑧

IOM: 100-03, 4, 280.1

✺ **E0187** Water pressure mattress ⑧

IOM: 100-03, 4, 280.1

✺ **E0188** Synthetic sheepskin pad ⑧

IOM: 100-03, 4, 280.1; 100-08, 5, 5.2.3

✺ **E0189** Lambswool sheepskin pad, any size ⑧

IOM: 100-03, 4, 280.1; 100-08, 5, 5.2.3

✺ **E0190** Positioning cushion/pillow/wedge, any shape or size, includes all components and accessories ⑧

IOM: 100-02, 15, 110.1

✳ **E0191** Heel or elbow protector, each ⑧

✳ **E0193** Powered air flotation bed (low air loss therapy) ⑧

✺ **E0194** Air fluidized bed ⑧

IOM: 100-03, 4, 280.1

✺ **E0196** Gel pressure mattress ⑧

IOM: 100-03, 4, 280.1

▶ **New**　↻ **Revised**　✔ **Reinstated**　~~deleted~~ **Deleted**　⊘ **Not covered or valid by Medicare**
✺ **Special coverage instructions**　✳ **Carrier discretion**　Ⓟ **Bill Part B MAC**　Ⓑ **Bill DME MAC**

DURABLE MEDICAL EQUIPMENT　E0153 — E0196

143

⊗ **E0197**   Air pressure pad for mattress, standard mattress length and width Ⓑ

IOM: 100-03, 4, 280.1

⊗ **E0198**   Water pressure pad for mattress, standard mattress length and width Ⓑ

IOM: 100-03, 4, 280.1

⊗ **E0199**   Dry pressure pad for mattress, standard mattress length and width Ⓑ

IOM: 100-03, 4, 280.1

Heat/Cold Application

⊗ **E0200**   Heat lamp, without stand (table model), includes bulb, or infrared element Ⓑ

Covered when medical review determines patient's medical condition is one for which application of heat by heat lamp is therapeutically effective

IOM: 100-02, 15, 110.1; 100-03, 4, 280.1

✳ **E0202**   Phototherapy (bilirubin) light with photometer Ⓑ

⊘ **E0203**   Therapeutic lightbox, minimum 10,000 lux, table top model Ⓑ

IOM: 100-03, 4, 280.1

⊗ **E0205**   Heat lamp, with stand, includes bulb, or infrared element Ⓑ

IOM: 100-02, 15, 110.1; 100-03, 4, 280.1

⊗ **E0210**   Electric heat pad, standard Ⓑ

Flexible device containing electric resistive elements producing heat; has fabric cover to prevent burns; with or without timing devices for automatic shut-off

IOM: 100-03, 4, 280.1

⊗ **E0215**   Electric heat pad, moist Ⓑ

Flexible device containing electric resistive elements producing heat. Must have component that will absorb and retain liquid (water).

IOM: 100-03, 4, 280.1

⊗ **E0217**   Water circulating heat pad with pump Ⓑ

Consists of flexible pad containing series of channels through which water is circulated by means of electrical pumping mechanism and heated in external reservoir

IOM: 100-03, 4, 280.1

⊗ **E0218**   Water circulating cold pad with pump Ⓑ

IOM: 100-03, 4, 280.1

✳ **E0221**   Infrared heating pad system Ⓑ

⊗ **E0225**   Hydrocollator unit, includes pads Ⓑ

IOM: 100-02, 15, 230; 100-03, 4, 280.1

⊘ **E0231**   Non-contact wound warming device (temperature control unit, AC adapter and power cord) for use with warming card and wound cover Ⓑ

IOM: 100-02, 16, 20

⊘ **E0232**   Warming card for use with the non-contact wound warming device and non-contact wound warming wound cover Ⓑ

IOM: 100-02, 16, 20

⊗ **E0235**   Paraffin bath unit, portable, (see medical supply code A4265 for paraffin) Ⓑ

Ordered by physician and patient's condition expected to be relieved by long term use of modality

IOM: 100-02, 15, 230; 100-03, 4, 280.1

⊗ **E0236**   Pump for water circulating pad Ⓑ

IOM: 100-03, 4, 280.1

⊗ **E0239**   Hydrocollator unit, portable Ⓑ

IOM: 100-02, 15, 230; 100-03, 4, 280.1

Bath and Toilet Aids

⊘ **E0240**   Bath/shower chair, with or without wheels, any size Ⓑ

IOM: 100-03, 4, 280.1

⊘ **E0241**   Bath tub wall rail, each Ⓑ

IOM: 100-02, 15, 110.1; 100-03, 4, 280.1

⊘ **E0242**   Bath tub rail, floor base Ⓑ

IOM: 100-02, 15, 110.1; 100-03, 4, 280.1

⊘ **E0243**   Toilet rail, each Ⓑ

IOM: 100-02, 15, 110.1; 100-03, 4, 280.1

⊘ **E0244**   Raised toilet seat Ⓑ

IOM: 100-03, 4, 280.1

⊘ **E0245**   Tub stool or bench Ⓑ

IOM: 100-03, 4, 280.1

✳ **E0246**   Transfer tub rail attachment Ⓑ

⊗ **E0247**   Transfer bench for tub or toilet with or without commode opening Ⓑ

IOM: 100-03, 4, 280.1

▶ **New**   ↻ **Revised**   ✔ **Reinstated**   ~~deleted~~ **Deleted**   ⊘ **Not covered or valid by Medicare**

⊗ **Special coverage instructions**   ✳ **Carrier discretion**   Ⓟ **Bill Part B MAC**   Ⓑ **Bill DME MAC**

⊛ **E0248**   Transfer bench, heavy duty, for tub or toilet with or without commode opening Ⓑ

Heavy duty transfer bench is labeled as capable of supporting more than 300 pounds

IOM: 100-03, 4, 280.1

Pad for Heating Unit

⊛ **E0249**   Pad for water circulating heat unit, for replacement only Ⓖ

Describes durable replacement pad used with water circulating heat pump system

IOM: 100-03, 4, 280.1

Hospital Beds and Accessories

⊛ **E0250**   Hospital bed, fixed height, with any type side rails, with mattress Ⓖ

IOM: 100-02, 15, 110.1; 100-03, 4, 280.7

⊛ **E0251**   Hospital bed, fixed height, with any type side rails, without mattress Ⓖ

IOM: 100-02, 15, 110.1; 100-03, 4, 280.7

⊛ **E0255**   Hospital bed, variable height, hi-lo, with any type side rails, with mattress Ⓖ

IOM: 100-02, 15, 110.1; 100-03, 4, 280.7

⊛ **E0256**   Hospital bed, variable height, hi-lo, with any type side rails, without mattress Ⓖ

IOM: 100-02, 15, 110.1; 100-03, 4, 280.7

⊛ **E0260**   Hospital bed, semi-electric (head and foot adjustment), with any type side rails, with mattress Ⓖ

IOM: 100-02, 15, 110.1; 100-03, 4, 280.7

⊛ **E0261**   Hospital bed, semi-electric (head and foot adjustment), with any type side rails, without mattress Ⓖ

IOM: 100-02, 15, 110.1; 100-03, 4, 280.7

⊛ **E0265**   Hospital bed, total electric (head, foot and height adjustments), with any type side rails, with mattress Ⓖ

IOM: 100-02, 15, 110.1; 100-03, 4, 280.7

⊛ **E0266**   Hospital bed, total electric (head, foot and height adjustments), with any type side rails, without mattress Ⓖ

IOM: 100-02, 15, 110.1; 100-03, 4, 280.7

⊘ **E0270**   Hospital bed, institutional type includes: oscillating, circulating and Stryker frame, with mattress Ⓑ

IOM: 100-03, 4, 280.1

⊛ **E0271**   Mattress, innerspring Ⓖ

IOM: 100-03, 4, 280.1; 100-03, 4, 280.7

⊛ **E0272**   Mattress, foam rubber Ⓖ

IOM: 100-03, 4, 280.1; 100-03, 4, 280.7

⊘ **E0273**   Bed board Ⓑ

IOM: 100-03, 4, 280.1

⊘ **E0274**   Over-bed table Ⓑ

IOM: 100-03, 4, 280.1

⊛ **E0275**   Bed pan, standard, metal or plastic Ⓑ

IOM: 100-03, 4, 280.1

⊛ **E0276**   Bed pan, fracture, metal or plastic Ⓑ

IOM: 100-03, 4, 280.1

⊛ **E0277**   Powered pressure-reducing air mattress Ⓖ

IOM: 100-03, 4, 280.1

✳ **E0280**   Bed cradle, any type Ⓑ

⊛ **E0290**   Hospital bed, fixed height, without side rails, with mattress Ⓖ

IOM: 100-02, 15, 110.1; 100-03, 4, 280.7

⊛ **E0291**   Hospital bed, fixed height, without side rails, without mattress Ⓖ

IOM: 100-02, 15, 110.1; 100-03, 4, 280.7

⊛ **E0292**   Hospital bed, variable height, hi-lo, without side rails, with mattress Ⓖ

IOM: 100-02, 15, 110.1; 100-03, 4, 280.7

⊛ **E0293**   Hospital bed, variable height, hi-lo, without side rails, without mattress Ⓖ

IOM: 100-02, 15, 110.1; 100-03, 4, 280.7

⊛ **E0294**   Hospital bed, semi-electric (head and foot adjustment), without side rails, with mattress Ⓖ

IOM: 100-02, 15, 110.1; 100-03, 4, 280.7

⊛ **E0295**   Hospital bed, semi-electric (head and foot adjustment), without side rails, without mattress Ⓖ

IOM: 100-02, 15, 110.1; 100-03, 4, 280.7

⊛ **E0296**   Hospital bed, total electric (head, foot and height adjustments), without side rails, with mattress Ⓖ

IOM: 100-02, 15, 110.1; 100-03, 4, 280.7

⊛ **E0297**   Hospital bed, total electric (head, foot and height adjustments), without side rails, without mattress Ⓖ

IOM: 100-02, 15, 110.1; 100-03, 4, 280.7

▶ New	↻ Revised	✔ Reinstated	~~deleted~~ Deleted	⊘ Not covered or valid by Medicare
⊛ Special coverage instructions		✳ Carrier discretion	Ⓑ Bill Part B MAC	Ⓖ Bill DME MAC

✱ **E0300** Pediatric crib, hospital grade, fully enclosed, with or without top enclosure ⑧

✪ **E0301** Hospital bed, heavy duty, extra wide, with weight capacity greater than 350 pounds, but less than or equal to 600 pounds, with any type side rails, without mattress ⑧

IOM: 100-03, 4, 280.7

✪ **E0302** Hospital bed, extra heavy duty, extra wide, with weight capacity greater than 600 pounds, with any type side rails, without mattress ⑧

IOM: 100-03, 4, 280.7

✪ **E0303** Hospital bed, heavy duty, extra wide, with weight capacity greater than 350 pounds, but less than or equal to 600 pounds, with any type side rails, with mattress ⑧

IOM: 100-03, 4, 280.7

✪ **E0304** Hospital bed, extra heavy duty, extra wide, with weight capacity greater than 600 pounds, with any type side rails, with mattress ⑧

IOM: 100-03, 4, 280.7

✪ **E0305** Bed side rails, half length ⑧

IOM: 100-03, 4, 280.7

✪ **E0310** Bed side rails, full length ⑧

IOM: 100-03, 4, 280.7

⊘ **E0315** Bed accessory: board, table, or support device, any type ⑧

IOM: 100-03, 4, 280.1

✱ **E0316** Safety enclosure frame/canopy for use with hospital bed, any type ⑧

✪ **E0325** Urinal; male, jug-type, any material ⑧

IOM: 100-03, 4, 280.1

✪ **E0326** Urinal; female, jug-type, any material ⑧

IOM: 100-03, 4, 280.1

✱ **E0328** Hospital bed, pediatric, manual, 360 degree side enclosures, top of headboard, footboard and side rails up to 24 inches above the spring, includes mattress ⑧

✱ **E0329** Hospital bed, pediatric, electric or semi-electric, 360 degree side enclosures, top of headboard, footboard and side rails up to 24 inches above the spring, includes mattress ⑧

✱ **E0350** Control unit for electronic bowel irrigation/evacuation system ⑧

Pulsed Irrigation Enhanced Evacuation (PIEE) is pulsed irrigation of severely impacted fecal material and may be necessary for patients who have not responded to traditional bowel program.

✱ **E0352** Disposable pack (water reservoir bag, speculum, valving mechanism and collection bag/box) for use with the electronic bowel irrigation/evacuation system ⑧

Therapy kit includes 1 B-Valve circuit, 2 containment bags, 1 lubricating jelly, 1 bed pad, 1 tray liner-waste disposable bag, and 2 hose clamps

✱ **E0370** Air pressure elevator for heel ⑧

✱ **E0371** Non powered advanced pressure reducing overlay for mattress, standard mattress length and width ⑧

Patient has at least one large Stage III or Stage IV pressure sore (greater than 2 × 2 cm.) on trunk, with only two turning surfaces on which to lie

✱ **E0372** Powered air overlay for mattress, standard mattress length and width ⑧

✱ **E0373** Non powered advanced pressure reducing mattress ⑧

Oxygen and Related Respiratory Equipment

✪ **E0424** Stationary compressed gaseous oxygen system, rental; includes container, contents, regulator, flowmeter, humidifier, nebulizer, cannula or mask, and tubing ⑧

IOM: 100-03, 4, 280.1; 100-04, 20, 30.6

✪ **E0425** Stationary compressed gas system, purchase; includes regulator, flowmeter, humidifier, nebulizer, cannula or mask, and tubing ⑧

IOM: 100-03, 4, 280.1; 100-04, 20, 30.6

✪ **E0430** Portable gaseous oxygen system, purchase; includes regulator, flowmeter, humidifier, cannula or mask, and tubing ⑧

IOM: 100-03, 4, 280.1; 100-04, 20, 30.6

✪ **E0431** Portable gaseous oxygen system, rental; includes portable container, regulator, flowmeter, humidifier, cannula or mask, and tubing ⑧

IOM: 100-03, 4, 280.1; 100-04, 20, 30.6

▶ New	⟲ Revised	✔ Reinstated	deleted Deleted	⊘ Not covered or valid by Medicare
✪ Special coverage instructions		✱ Carrier discretion	⑨ Bill Part B MAC	⑧ Bill DME MAC

✳ **E0433** Portable liquid oxygen system, rental; home liquefier used to fill portable liquid oxygen containers, includes portable containers, regulator, flowmeter, humidifier, cannula or mask and tubing, with or without supply reservoir and contents gauge Ⓑ

⊛ **E0434** Portable liquid oxygen system, rental; includes portable container, supply reservoir, humidifier, flowmeter, refill adaptor, contents gauge, cannula or mask, and tubing Ⓑ

Fee schedule payments for stationary oxygen system rentals are all-inclusive and represent monthly allowance for beneficiary. Non-Medicare payers may rent device to beneficiaries, or arrange for purchase of device.

IOM: 100-03, 4, 280.1; 100-04, 20, 30.6

⊛ **E0435** Portable liquid oxygen system, purchase; includes portable container, supply reservoir, flowmeter, humidifier, contents gauge, cannula or mask, tubing and refill adaptor Ⓑ

IOM: 100-03, 4, 280.1; 100-04, 20, 30.6

⊛ **E0439** Stationary liquid oxygen system, rental; includes container, contents, regulator, flowmeter, humidifier, nebulizer, cannula or mask, & tubing Ⓑ

This allowance includes payment for equipment, contents, and accessories furnished during rental month

IOM: 100-03, 4, 280.1; 100-04, 20, 30.6

⊛ **E0440** Stationary liquid oxygen system, purchase; includes use of reservoir, contents indicator, regulator, flowmeter, humidifier, nebulizer, cannula or mask, and tubing Ⓑ

IOM: 100-03, 4, 280.1; 100-04, 20, 30.6

⊛ **E0441** Stationary oxygen contents, gaseous, 1 month's supply = 1 unit Ⓑ

IOM: 100-03, 4, 280.1; 100-04, 20, 30.6

⊛ **E0442** Stationary oxygen contents, liquid, 1 month's supply = 1 unit Ⓑ

IOM: 100-03, 4, 280.1; 100-04, 20, 30.6

⊛ **E0443** Portable oxygen contents, gaseous, 1 month's supply = 1 unit Ⓑ

IOM: 100-03, 4, 280.1; 100-04, 20, 30.6

⊛ **E0444** Portable oxygen contents, liquid, 1 month's supply = 1 unit Ⓑ

IOM: 100-03, 4, 280.1; 100-04, 20, 30.6

✳ **E0445** Oximeter device for measuring blood oxygen levels non-invasively Ⓑ

↻✳ **E0446** Topical oxygen delivery system, not otherwise specified, includes all supplies and accessories Ⓑ

⊛ **E0455** Oxygen tent, excluding croup or pediatric tents Ⓑ

IOM: 100-03, 4, 280.1; 100-04, 20, 30.6

⊘ **E0457** Chest shell (cuirass) Ⓑ

⊘ **E0459** Chest wrap Ⓑ

✳ **E0462** Rocking bed with or without side rails Ⓑ

⊛ **E0465** Home ventilator, any type, used with invasive interface, (e.g., tracheostomy tube) Ⓑ

IOM: 100-03, 4, 280.1

⊛ **E0466** Home ventilator, any type, used with non-invasive interface, (e.g., mask, chest shell) Ⓑ

IOM: 100-03, 4, 280.1

⊛ **E0470** Respiratory assist device, bi-level pressure capability, without backup rate feature, used with noninvasive interface, e.g., nasal or facial mask (intermittent assist device with continuous positive airway pressure device) Ⓑ

IOM: 100-03, 4, 240.2

⊛ **E0471** Respiratory assist device, bi-level pressure capability, with back-up rate feature, used with noninvasive interface, e.g., nasal or facial mask (intermittent assist device with continuous positive airway pressure device) Ⓑ

IOM: 100-03, 4, 240.2

⊛ **E0472** Respiratory assist device, bi-level pressure capability, with backup rate feature, used with invasive interface, e.g., tracheostomy tube (intermittent assist device with continuous positive airway pressure device) Ⓑ

IOM: 100-03, 4, 240.2

⊛ **E0480** Percussor, electric or pneumatic, home model Ⓑ

IOM: 100-03, 4, 240.2

⊘ **E0481** Intrapulmonary percussive ventilation system and related accessories Ⓑ

IOM: 100-03, 4, 240.2

✳ **E0482** Cough stimulating device, alternating positive and negative airway pressure Ⓑ

✳ **E0483** High frequency chest wall oscillation air-pulse generator system, (includes hoses and vest), each Ⓑ

▶ New ↻ Revised ✔ Reinstated deleted Deleted ⊘ Not covered or valid by Medicare
⊛ Special coverage instructions ✳ Carrier discretion Ⓟ Bill Part B MAC Ⓑ Bill DME MAC

* **E0484** Oscillatory positive expiratory pressure device, non-electric, any type, each ⑧

* **E0485** Oral device/appliance used to reduce upper airway collapsibility, adjustable or non-adjustable, prefabricated, includes fitting and adjustment ⑧

* **E0486** Oral device/appliance used to reduce upper airway collapsibility, adjustable or non-adjustable, custom fabricated, includes fitting and adjustment ⑧

⊛ **E0487** Spirometer, electronic, includes all accessories ⑧

IPPB Machines

⊛ **E0500** IPPB machine, all types, with built-in nebulization; manual or automatic valves; internal or external power source ⑧

IOM: 100-03, 4, 240.2

Humidifiers/Nebulizers/Compressors for Use with Oxygen IPPB Equipment

⊛ **E0550** Humidifier, durable for extensive supplemental humidification during IPPB treatments or oxygen delivery ⑧

IOM: 100-03, 4, 240.2

⊛ **E0555** Humidifier, durable, glass or autoclavable plastic bottle type, for use with regulator or flowmeter ⑧

IOM: 100-03, 4, 280.1; 100-04, 20, 30.6

⊛ **E0560** Humidifier, durable for supplemental humidification during IPPB treatment or oxygen delivery ⑧

IOM: 100-03, 4, 280.1

* **E0561** Humidifier, non-heated, used with positive airway pressure device ⑧

* **E0562** Humidifier, heated, used with positive airway pressure device ⑧

* **E0565** Compressor, air power source for equipment which is not self-contained or cylinder driven ⑧

⊛ **E0570** Nebulizer, with compressor ⑧

IOM: 100-03, 4, 240.2; 100-03, 4, 280.1

* **E0572** Aerosol compressor, adjustable pressure, light duty for intermittent use ⑧

* **E0574** Ultrasonic/electronic aerosol generator with small volume nebulizer ⑧

↺⊛ **E0575** Nebulizer, ultrasonic, large volume ⑧

IOM: 100-03, 4, 240.2

⊛ **E0580** Nebulizer, durable, glass or autoclavable plastic, bottle type, for use with regulator or flowmeter ⑧

IOM: 100-03, 4, 240.2; 100-03, 4, 280.1

⊛ **E0585** Nebulizer, with compressor and heater ⑧

IOM: 100-03, 4, 240.2; 100-03, 4, 280.1

Suction Pump/CPAP

⊛ **E0600** Respiratory suction pump, home model, portable or stationary, electric ⑧

IOM: 100-03, 4, 240.2

⊛ **E0601** Continuous positive airway pressure (CPAP) device ⑧

IOM: 100-03, 4, 240.4

Breast Pump

* **E0602** Breast pump, manual, any type ⑧

Bill either manual breast pump or breast pump kit

* **E0603** Breast pump, electric (AC and/or DC), any type ⑧

* **E0604** Breast pump, hospital grade, electric (AC and/or DC), any type ⑧

Other Breathing Aids

⊛ **E0605** Vaporizer, room type ⑧

IOM: 100-03, 4, 240.2

⊛ **E0606** Postural drainage board ⑧

IOM: 100-03, 4, 240.2

Monitoring Equipment

⊛ **E0607** Home blood glucose monitor ⑧

Document recipient or caregiver is competent to monitor equipment and that device is designed for home rather than clinical use

IOM: 100-03, 4, 280.1; 100-03, 1, 40.2

▶ **New**　↺ **Revised**　✔ **Reinstated**　~~deleted~~ **Deleted**　⊘ **Not covered or valid by Medicare**

⊛ **Special coverage instructions**　* **Carrier discretion**　⑨ **Bill Part B MAC**　⑧ **Bill DME MAC**

⊛ **E0610** Pacemaker monitor, self-contained, (checks battery depletion, includes audible and visible check systems) ⑧

IOM: 100-03, 1, 20.8

⊛ **E0615** Pacemaker monitor, self-contained, checks battery depletion and other pacemaker components, includes digital/visible check systems ⑧

IOM: 100-03, 1, 20.8

✳ **E0616** Implantable cardiac event recorder with memory, activator and programmer ⑧

Assign when two 30-day pre-symptom external loop recordings fail to establish a definitive diagnosis.

✳ **E0617** External defibrillator with integrated electrocardiogram analysis ⑧

✳ **E0618** Apnea monitor, without recording feature ⑧

✳ **E0619** Apnea monitor, with recording feature ⑤

✳ **E0620** Skin piercing device for collection of capillary blood, laser, each ⑧

Patient Lifts

⊛ **E0621** Sling or seat, patient lift, canvas or nylon ⑤

IOM: 100-03, 4, 240.2, 280.4

⊘ **E0625** Patient lift, bathroom or toilet, not otherwise classified ⑧

IOM: 100-03, 4, 240.2

⊛ **E0627** Seat lift mechanism, electric, any type ⑤

IOM: 100-03, 4, 280.4; 100-04, 4, 20

⊛ **E0629** Seat lift mechanism, non-electric, any type ⑤

IOM: 100-04, 4, 20

⊛ **E0630** Patient lift, hydraulic or mechanical, includes any seat, sling, strap(s) or pad(s) ⑤

IOM: 100-03, 4, 240.2

⊛ **E0635** Patient lift, electric, with seat or sling ⑤

IOM: 100-03, 4, 240.2

✳ **E0636** Multipositional patient support system, with integrated lift, patient accessible controls ⑧

⊘ **E0637** Combination sit to stand frame/table system, any size including pediatric, with seat lift feature, with or without wheels ⑧

IOM: 100-03, 4, 240.2

⊘ **E0638** Standing frame/table system, one position (e.g., upright, supine or prone stander), any size including pediatric, with or without wheels ⑤

IOM: 100-03, 4, 240.2

✳ **E0639** Patient lift, moveable from room to room with disassembly and reassembly, includes all components/accessories ⑧

✳ **E0640** Patient lift, fixed system, includes all components/accessories ⑧

⊘ **E0641** Standing frame/table system, multi-position (e.g., three-way stander), any size including pediatric, with or without wheels ⑤

IOM: 100-03, 4, 240.2

⊘ **E0642** Standing frame/table system, mobile (dynamic stander), any size including pediatric ⑤

IOM: 100-03, 4, 240.2

Pneumatic Compressor and Appliances

⊛ **E0650** Pneumatic compressor, non-segmental home model ⑧

Lymphedema pumps are classified as segmented or nonsegmented, depending on whether distinct segments of devices can be inflated sequentially.

IOM: 100-03, 4, 280.6

⊛ **E0651** Pneumatic compressor, segmental home model without calibrated gradient pressure ⑧

IOM: 100-03, 4, 280.6

⊛ **E0652** Pneumatic compressor, segmental home model with calibrated gradient pressure ⑤

IOM: 100-03, 4, 280.6

⊛ **E0655** Non-segmental pneumatic appliance for use with pneumatic compressor, half arm ⑤

IOM: 100-03, 4, 280.6

⊛ **E0656** Segmental pneumatic appliance for use with pneumatic compressor, trunk ⑧

⊛ **E0657** Segmental pneumatic appliance for use with pneumatic compressor, chest ⑤

▶ New ↻ Revised ✔ Reinstated ~~deleted~~ Deleted ⊘ Not covered or valid by Medicare
⊛ Special coverage instructions ✳ Carrier discretion ⑨ Bill Part B MAC ⑤ Bill DME MAC

⊕ **E0660**   Non-segmental pneumatic appliance for use with pneumatic compressor, full leg Ⓑ

IOM: 100-03, 4, 280.6

⊕ **E0665**   Non-segmental pneumatic appliance for use with pneumatic compressor, full arm Ⓑ

IOM: 100-03, 4, 280.6

⊕ **E0666**   Non-segmental pneumatic appliance for use with pneumatic compressor, half leg Ⓑ

IOM: 100-03, 4, 280.6

⊕ **E0667**   Segmental pneumatic appliance for use with pneumatic compressor, full leg Ⓑ

IOM: 100-03, 4, 280.6

⊕ **E0668**   Segmental pneumatic appliance for use with pneumatic compressor, full arm Ⓑ

IOM: 100-03, 4, 280.6

⊕ **E0669**   Segmental pneumatic appliance for use with pneumatic compressor, half leg Ⓑ

IOM: 100-03, 4, 280.6

⊕ **E0670**   Segmental pneumatic appliance for use with pneumatic compressor, integrated, 2 full legs and trunk Ⓑ

IOM: 100-03, 4, 280.6

⊕ **E0671**   Segmental gradient pressure pneumatic appliance, full leg Ⓑ

IOM: 100-03, 4, 280.6

⊕ **E0672**   Segmental gradient pressure pneumatic appliance, full arm Ⓑ

IOM: 100-03, 4, 280.6

⊕ **E0673**   Segmental gradient pressure pneumatic appliance, half leg Ⓑ

IOM: 100-03, 4, 280.6

∗ **E0675**   Pneumatic compression device, high pressure, rapid inflation/deflation cycle, for arterial insufficiency (unilateral or bilateral system) Ⓑ

∗ **E0676**   Intermittent limb compression device (includes all accessories), not otherwise specified Ⓑ

Ultraviolet Light Therapy Systems

∗ **E0691**   Ultraviolet light therapy system, includes bulbs/lamps, timer and eye protection; treatment area 2 square feet or less Ⓑ

∗ **E0692**   Ultraviolet light therapy system panel, includes bulbs/lamps, timer and eye protection, 4 foot panel Ⓑ

∗ **E0693**   Ultraviolet light therapy system panel, includes bulbs/lamps, timer and eye protection, 6 foot panel Ⓑ

∗ **E0694**   Ultraviolet multidirectional light therapy system in 6 foot cabinet, includes bulbs/lamps, timer and eye protection Ⓑ

Safety Equipment

∗ **E0700**   Safety equipment, device or accessory, any type Ⓑ

⊕ **E0705**   Transfer device, any type, each Ⓑ

Restraints

∗ **E0710**   Restraints, any type (body, chest, wrist or ankle) Ⓑ

Transcutaneous and/or Neuromuscular Electrical Nerve Stimulators (TENS)

⊕ **E0720**   Transcutaneous electrical nerve stimulation (TENS) device, two lead, localized stimulation Ⓑ

A Certificate of Medical Necessity (CMN) is not needed for a TENS rental, but is needed purchase.

IOM: 100-03, 2, 160.2; 100-03, 4, 280.1

⊕ **E0730**   Transcutaneous electrical nerve stimulation (TENS) device, four or more leads, for multiple nerve stimulation Ⓑ

IOM: 100-03, 2, 160.2; 100-03, 4, 280.1

⊕ **E0731**   Form fitting conductive garment for delivery of TENS or NMES (with conductive fibers separated from the patient's skin by layers of fabric) Ⓑ

IOM: 100-03, 2, 160.13

⊕ **E0740**   Non-implanted pelvic floor electrical stimulator, complete system Ⓑ

IOM: 100-03, 4, 230.8

∗ **E0744**   Neuromuscular stimulator for scoliosis Ⓑ

⊕ **E0745**   Neuromuscular stimulator, electronic shock unit Ⓑ

IOM: 100-03, 2, 160.12

⊕ **E0746**   Electromyography (EMG), biofeedback device Ⓑ

IOM: 100-03, 1, 30.1

▶ New   ⟲ Revised   ✔ Reinstated   ~~deleted~~ Deleted   ⊘ Not covered or valid by Medicare
⊕ Special coverage instructions   ∗ Carrier discretion   Ⓟ Bill Part B MAC   Ⓑ Bill DME MAC

✪ **E0747** Osteogenesis stimulator, electrical, non-invasive, other than spinal applications Ⓑ

Devices are composed of two basic parts: Coils that wrap around cast and pulse generator that produces electric current

✪ **E0748** Osteogenesis stimulator, electrical, non-invasive, spinal applications Ⓑ

Device should be applied within 30 days as adjunct to spinal fusion surgery

✪ **E0749** Osteogenesis stimulator, electrical, surgically implanted Ⓑ

✳ **E0755** Electronic salivary reflex stimulator (intra-oral/non-invasive) Ⓑ

✳ **E0760** Osteogenesis stimulator, low intensity ultrasound, non-invasive Ⓑ

Ultrasonic osteogenesis stimulator may not be used concurrently with other noninvasive stimulators

✪ **E0761** Non-thermal pulsed high frequency radiowaves, high peak power electromagnetic energy treatment device Ⓑ

✳ **E0762** Transcutaneous electrical joint stimulation device system, includes all accessories Ⓑ

✪ **E0764** Functional neuromuscular stimulator, transcutaneous stimulation of sequential muscle groups of ambulation with computer control, used for walking by spinal cord injured, entire system, after completion of training program Ⓑ

IOM: 100-03, 2, 160.12

✳ **E0765** FDA approved nerve stimulator, with replaceable batteries, for treatment of nausea and vomiting Ⓑ

✳ **E0766** Electrical stimulation device used for cancer treatment, includes all accessories, any type Ⓑ

✪ **E0769** Electrical stimulation or electromagnetic wound treatment device, not otherwise classified Ⓑ

IOM: 100-04, 32, 11.1

✪ **E0770** Functional electrical stimulator, transcutaneous stimulation of nerve and/or muscle groups, any type, complete system, not otherwise specified Ⓑ

Infusion Supplies

✳ **E0776** IV pole Ⓑ

✳ **E0779** Ambulatory infusion pump, mechanical, reusable, for infusion 8 hours or greater Ⓑ

Requires prior authorization and copy of invoice

This is a capped rental infusion pump modifier. The correct monthly modifier (KH, KI, KJ) is used to indicate which month the rental is for (i.e. KH, month 1; KI, months 2 and 3; KJ, months 4 through 13).

✳ **E0780** Ambulatory infusion pump, mechanical, reusable, for infusion less than 8 hours Ⓑ

Requires prior authorization and copy of invoice

✪ **E0781** Ambulatory infusion pump, single or multiple channels, electric or battery operated with administrative equipment, worn by patient Ⓑ

IOM: 100-03, 1, 50.3

✪ **E0782** Infusion pump, implantable, non-programmable (includes all components, e.g., pump, cathether, connectors, etc.) Ⓑ

IOM: 100-03, 1, 50.3

✪ **E0783** Infusion pump system, implantable, programmable (includes all components, e.g., pump, catheter, connectors, etc.) Ⓑ

IOM: 100-03, 1, 50.3

✪ **E0784** External ambulatory infusion pump, insulin Ⓑ

IOM: 100-03, 4, 280.14

✪ **E0785** Implantable intraspinal (epidural/intrathecal) catheter used with implantable infusion pump, replacement Ⓑ

IOM: 100-03, 1, 50.3

✪ **E0786** Implantable programmable infusion pump, replacement (excludes implantable intraspinal catheter) Ⓑ

IOM: 100-03, 1, 50.3

✪ **E0791** Parenteral infusion pump, stationary, single or multi-channel Ⓑ

IOM: 100-02, 15, 120; 100-03, 3, 180.2; 100-04, 20, 100.2.2

▶ **New**   ↻ **Revised**   ✔ **Reinstated**   ~~deleted~~ **Deleted**   ⊘ **Not covered or valid by Medicare**
✪ **Special coverage instructions**   ✳ **Carrier discretion**   Ⓑ **Bill Part B MAC**   Ⓓ **Bill DME MAC**

Traction Equipment and Orthopedic Devices

⊕ **E0830** Ambulatory traction device, all types, each ⑤

IOM: 100-03, 4, 280.1

⊕ **E0840** Traction frame, attached to headboard, cervical traction ⑧

IOM: 100-03, 4, 280.1

✳ **E0849** Traction equipment, cervical, free-standing stand/frame, pneumatic, applying traction force to other than mandible ⑧

⊕ **E0850** Traction stand, free standing, cervical traction ⑧

IOM: 100-03, 4, 280.1

✳ **E0855** Cervical traction equipment not requiring additional stand or frame ⑧

✳ **E0856** Cervical traction device, with inflatable air bladder(s) ⑧

⊕ **E0860** Traction equipment, overdoor, cervical ⑧

IOM: 100-03, 4, 280.1

⊕ **E0870** Traction frame, attached to footboard, extremity traction, (e.g., Buck's) ⑧

IOM: 100-03, 4, 280.1

⊕ **E0880** Traction stand, free standing, extremity traction, (e.g., Buck's) ⑧

IOM: 100-03, 4, 280.1

⊕ **E0890** Traction frame, attached to footboard, pelvic traction ⑧

IOM: 100-03, 4, 280.1

⊕ **E0900** Traction stand, free standing, pelvic traction, (e.g., Buck's) ⑧

IOM: 100-03, 4, 280.1

⊕ **E0910** Trapeze bars, A/K/A patient helper, attached to bed, with grab bar ⑧

IOM: 100-03, 4, 280.1

⊕ **E0911** Trapeze bar, heavy duty, for patient weight capacity greater than 250 pounds, attached to bed, with grab bar ⑧

IOM: 100-03, 4, 280.1

⊕ **E0912** Trapeze bar, heavy duty, for patient weight capacity greater than 250 pounds, free standing, complete with grab bar ⑧

IOM: 100-03, 4, 280.1

⊕ **E0920** Fracture frame, attached to bed, includes weights ⑧

IOM: 100-03, 4, 280.1

⊕ **E0930** Fracture frame, free standing, includes weights ⑧

IOM: 100-03, 4, 280.1

⊕ **E0935** Continuous passive motion exercise device for use on knee only ⑧

To qualify for coverage, use of device must commence within two days following surgery

IOM: 100-03, 4, 280.1

⊘ **E0936** Continuous passive motion exercise device for use other than knee ⑧

⊕ **E0940** Trapeze bar, free standing, complete with grab bar ⑧

IOM: 100-03, 4, 280.1

⊕ **E0941** Gravity assisted traction device, any type ⑧

IOM: 100-03, 4, 280.1

✳ **E0942** Cervical head harness/halter ⑧

✳ **E0944** Pelvic belt/harness/boot ⑧

✳ **E0945** Extremity belt/harness ⑧

⊕ **E0946** Fracture, frame, dual with cross bars, attached to bed, (e.g., Balken, 4 poster) ⑧

IOM: 100-03, 4, 280.1

⊕ **E0947** Fracture frame, attachments for complex pelvic traction ⑧

IOM: 100-03, 4, 280.1

⊕ **E0948** Fracture frame, attachments for complex cervical traction ⑧

IOM: 100-03, 4, 280.1

Wheelchair Accessories

↻⊕ **E0950** Wheelchair accessory, tray, each ⑧

IOM: 100-03, 4, 280.1

✳ **E0951** Heel loop/holder, any type, with or without ankle strap, each ⑧

⊕ **E0952** Toe loop/holder, any type, each ⑧

IOM: 100-03, 4, 280.1

▶✳ **E0953** Wheelchair accessory, lateral thigh or knee support, any type, including fixed mounting hardware, each

▶✳ **E0954** Wheelchair accessory, foot box, any type, includes attachment and mounting hardware, each foot

✳ **E0955** Wheelchair accessory, headrest, cushioned, any type, including fixed mounting hardware, each ⑧

▶ New   ↻ Revised   ✔ Reinstated   ~~deleted~~ Deleted   ⊘ Not covered or valid by Medicare
⊕ Special coverage instructions   ✳ Carrier discretion   ⑧ Bill Part B MAC   ⑤ Bill DME MAC

✳ **E0956** Wheelchair accessory, lateral trunk or hip support, any type, including fixed mounting hardware, each ⑧

✳ **E0957** Wheelchair accessory, medial thigh support, any type, including fixed mounting hardware, each ⑧

✪ **E0958** Manual wheelchair accessory, one-arm drive attachment, each ⑩

IOM: 100-03, 4, 280.1

✳ **E0959** Manual wheelchair accessory, adapter for amputee, each ⑧

IOM: 100-03, 4, 280.1

✳ **E0960** Wheelchair accessory, shoulder harness/straps or chest strap, including any type mounting hardware ⑧

✳ **E0961** Manual wheelchair accessory, wheel lock brake extension (handle), each ⑧

IOM: 100-03, 4, 280.1

✳ **E0966** Manual wheelchair accessory, headrest extension, each ⑩

IOM: 100-03, 4, 280.1

✪ **E0967** Manual wheelchair accessory, hand rim with projections, any type, replacement only, each ⑧

IOM: 100-03, 4, 280.1

✪ **E0968** Commode seat, wheelchair ⑧

IOM: 100-03, 4, 280.1

✪ **E0969** Narrowing device, wheelchair ⑧

IOM: 100-03, 4, 280.1

⊘ **E0970** No.2 footplates, except for elevating leg rest ⑧

IOM: 100-03, 4, 280.1

Cross Reference K0037, K0042

✳ **E0971** Manual wheelchair accessory, anti-tipping device, each ⑧

IOM: 100-03, 4, 280.1

Cross Reference K0021

✪ **E0973** Wheelchair accessory, adjustable height, detachable armrest, complete assembly, each ⑧

IOM: 100-03, 4, 280.1

✪ **E0974** Manual wheelchair accessory, anti-rollback device, each ⑩

IOM: 100-03, 4, 280.1

✳ **E0978** Wheelchair accessory, positioning belt/safety belt/pelvic strap, each ⑧

✳ **E0980** Safety vest, wheelchair ⑧

✳ **E0981** Wheelchair accessory, seat upholstery, replacement only, each ⑩

✳ **E0982** Wheelchair accessory, back upholstery, replacement only, each ⑧

✳ **E0983** Manual wheelchair accessory, power add-on to convert manual wheelchair to motorized wheelchair, joystick control ⑧

✳ **E0984** Manual wheelchair accessory, power add-on to convert manual wheelchair to motorized wheelchair, tiller control ⑧

✳ **E0985** Wheelchair accessory, seat lift mechanism ⑧

✳ **E0986** Manual wheelchair accessory, push-rim activated power assist system ⑧

✳ **E0988** Manual wheelchair accessory, lever-activated, wheel drive, pair ⑧

✳ **E0990** Wheelchair accessory, elevating leg rest, complete assembly, each ⑧

IOM: 100-03, 4, 280.1

✳ **E0992** Manual wheelchair accessory, solid seat insert ⑧

✪ **E0994** Arm rest, each ⑩

IOM: 100-03, 4, 280.1

✳ **E0995** Wheelchair accessory, calf rest/pad, replacement only, each ⑧

IOM: 100-03, 4, 280.1

✳ **E1002** Wheelchair accessory, power seating system, tilt only ⑩

✳ **E1003** Wheelchair accessory, power seating system, recline only, without shear reduction ⑧

✳ **E1004** Wheelchair accessory, power seating system, recline only, with mechanical shear reduction ⑧

✳ **E1005** Wheelchair accessory, power seating system, recline only, with power shear reduction ⑧

✳ **E1006** Wheelchair accessory, power seating system, combination tilt and recline, without shear reduction ⑧

✳ **E1007** Wheelchair accessory, power seating system, combination tilt and recline, with mechanical shear reduction ⑩

✳ **E1008** Wheelchair accessory, power seating system, combination tilt and recline, with power shear reduction ⑧

✳ **E1009** Wheelchair accessory, addition to power seating system, mechanically linked leg elevation system, including pushrod and leg rest, each ⑧

▶ **New**   ↻ **Revised**   ✔ **Reinstated**   ~~deleted~~ **Deleted**   ⊘ **Not covered or valid by Medicare**
✪ **Special coverage instructions**   ✳ **Carrier discretion**   ⑧ **Bill Part B MAC**   ⑩ **Bill DME MAC**

✳ **E1010** Wheelchair accessory, addition to power seating system, power leg elevation system, including leg rest, pair Ⓑ

⊛ **E1011** Modification to pediatric size wheelchair, width adjustment package (not to be dispensed with initial chair) Ⓑ

IOM: 100-03, 4, 280.1

✳ **E1012** Wheelchair accessory, addition to power seating system, center mount power elevating leg rest/platform, complete system, any type, each

⊛ **E1014** Reclining back, addition to pediatric size wheelchair Ⓑ

IOM: 100-03, 4, 280.1

⊛ **E1015** Shock absorber for manual wheelchair, each Ⓑ

IOM: 100-03, 4, 280.1

⊛ **E1016** Shock absorber for power wheelchair, each Ⓑ

IOM: 100-03, 4, 280.1

⊛ **E1017** Heavy duty shock absorber for heavy duty or extra heavy duty manual wheelchair, each Ⓑ

IOM: 100-03, 4, 280.1

⊛ **E1018** Heavy duty shock absorber for heavy duty or extra heavy duty power wheelchair, each Ⓑ

IOM: 100-03, 4, 280.1

⊛ **E1020** Residual limb support system for wheelchair, any type Ⓑ

IOM: 100-03, 3, 280.3

✳ **E1028** Wheelchair accessory, manual swing-away, retractable or removable mounting hardware for joystick, other control interface or positioning accessory Ⓑ

✳ **E1029** Wheelchair accessory, ventilator tray, fixed Ⓑ

✳ **E1030** Wheelchair accessory, ventilator tray, gimbaled Ⓑ

Rollabout Chair, Transfer System, Transport Chair

⊛ **E1031** Rollabout chair, any and all types with casters 5" or greater Ⓑ

IOM: 100-03, 4, 280.1

⊛ **E1035** Multi-positional patient transfer system, with integrated seat, operated by care giver, patient weight capacity up to and including 300 lbs Ⓑ

IOM: 100-02, 15, 110

✳ **E1036** Multi-positional patient transfer system, extra-wide, with integrated seat, operated by caregiver, patient weight capacity greater than 300 lbs Ⓑ

⊛ **E1037** Transport chair, pediatric size Ⓑ

IOM: 100-03, 4, 280.1

⊛ **E1038** Transport chair, adult size, patient weight capacity up to and including 300 pounds Ⓑ

IOM: 100-03, 4, 280.1

✳ **E1039** Transport chair, adult size, heavy duty, patient weight capacity greater than 300 pounds Ⓑ

Wheelchair: Fully Reclining

⊛ **E1050** Fully-reclining wheelchair, fixed full length arms, swing away detachable elevating leg rests Ⓑ

IOM: 100-03, 4, 280.1

⊛ **E1060** Fully-reclining wheelchair, detachable arms, desk or full length, swing away detachable elevating legrests Ⓑ

IOM: 100-03, 4, 280.1

⊛ **E1070** Fully-reclining wheelchair, detachable arms (desk or full length) swing away detachable footrests Ⓑ

IOM: 100-03, 4, 280.1

Wheelchair: Hemi

⊛ **E1083** Hemi-wheelchair, fixed full length arms, swing away detachable elevating leg rest Ⓑ

IOM: 100-03, 4, 280.1

⊛ **E1084** Hemi-wheelchair, detachable arms desk or full length arms, swing away detachable elevating leg rests Ⓑ

IOM: 100-03, 4, 280.1

⊘ **E1085** Hemi-wheelchair, fixed full length arms, swing away detachable foot rests Ⓑ

IOM: 100-03, 4, 280.1

Cross Reference K0002

▶ **New**	↻ **Revised**	✔ **Reinstated**	~~deleted~~ **Deleted**	⊘ **Not covered or valid by Medicare**
⊛ **Special coverage instructions**		✳ **Carrier discretion**	Ⓟ **Bill Part B MAC**	Ⓑ **Bill DME MAC**

⊘ **E1086** Hemi-wheelchair, detachable arms desk or full length, swing away detachable footrests ⑬

IOM: 100-03, 4, 280.1

Cross Reference K0002

Wheelchair: High-strength Lightweight

✪ **E1087** High strength lightweight wheelchair, fixed full length arms, swing away detachable elevating leg rests ⑬

IOM: 100-03, 4, 280.1

✪ **E1088** High strength lightweight wheelchair, detachable arms desk or full length, swing away detachable elevating leg rests ⑬

IOM: 100-03, 4, 280.1

⊘ **E1089** High strength lightweight wheelchair, fixed length arms, swing away detachable footrest ⑬

IOM: 100-03, 4, 280.1

Cross Reference K0004

⊘ **E1090** High strength lightweight wheelchair, detachable arms desk or full length, swing away detachable foot rests ⑬

IOM: 100-03, 4, 280.1

Cross Reference K0004

Wheelchair: Wide Heavy Duty

✪ **E1092** Wide heavy duty wheelchair, detachable arms (desk or full length) swing away detachable elevating leg rests ⑬

IOM: 100-03, 4, 280.1

✪ **E1093** Wide heavy duty wheelchair, detachable arms (desk or full length arms), swing away detachable foot rests ⑬

IOM: 100-03, 4, 280.1

Wheelchair: Semi-reclining

✪ **E1100** Semi-reclining wheelchair, fixed full length arms, swing away detachable elevating leg rests ⑬

IOM: 100-03, 4, 280.1

✪ **E1110** Semi-reclining wheelchair, detachable arms (desk or full length), elevating leg rest ⑬

IOM: 100-03, 4, 280.1

Wheelchair: Standard

⊘ **E1130** Standard wheelchair, fixed full length arms, fixed or swing away detachable footrests ⑬

IOM: 100-03, 4, 280.1

Cross Reference K0001

⊘ **E1140** Wheelchair, detachable arms, desk or full length, swing away detachable footrests ⑬

IOM: 100-03, 4, 280.1

Cross Reference K0001

✪ **E1150** Wheelchair, detachable arms, desk or full length, swing away detachable elevating legrests ⑬

IOM: 100-03, 4, 280.1

✪ **E1160** Wheelchair, fixed full length arms, swing away detachable elevating legrests ⑬

IOM: 100-03, 4, 280.1

✳ **E1161** Manual adult size wheelchair, includes tilt in space ⑬

Wheelchair: Amputee

✪ **E1170** Amputee wheelchair, fixed full length arms, swing away detachable elevating legrests ⑬

IOM: 100-03, 4, 280.1

✪ **E1171** Amputee wheelchair, fixed full length arms, without footrests or legrest ⑬

IOM: 100-03, 4, 280.1

✪ **E1172** Amputee wheelchair, detachable arms (desk or full length) without footrests or legrest ⑬

IOM: 100-03, 4, 280.1

✪ **E1180** Amputee wheelchair, detachable arms (desk or full length) swing away detachable footrests ⑬

IOM: 100-03, 4, 280.1

✪ **E1190** Amputee wheelchair, detachable arms (desk or full length), swing away detachable elevating legrests ⑬

IOM: 100-03, 4, 280.1

✪ **E1195** Heavy duty wheelchair, fixed full length arms, swing away detachable elevating legrests ⑬

IOM: 100-03, 4, 280.1

✪ **E1200** Amputee wheelchair, fixed full length arms, swing away detachable footrest ⑬

IOM: 100-03, 4, 280.1

▶ New	↩ Revised	✔ Reinstated	~~deleted~~ Deleted	⊘ Not covered or valid by Medicare
✪ Special coverage instructions		✳ Carrier discretion	⑱ Bill Part B MAC	⑬ Bill DME MAC

Wheelchair: Other and Accessories

⊗ **E1220** Wheelchair; specially sized or constructed, (indicate brand name, model number, if any) and justification Ⓖ

IOM: 100-03, 4, 280.3

⊗ **E1221** Wheelchair with fixed arm, footrests Ⓑ

IOM: 100-03, 4, 280.3

⊗ **E1222** Wheelchair with fixed arm, elevating legrests Ⓑ

IOM: 100-03, 4, 280.3

⊗ **E1223** Wheelchair with detachable arms, footrests Ⓑ

IOM: 100-03, 4, 280.3

⊗ **E1224** Wheelchair with detachable arms, elevating legrests Ⓖ

IOM: 100-03, 4, 280.3

⊗ **E1225** Wheelchair accessory, manual semi-reclining back, (recline greater than 15 degrees, but less than 80 degrees), each Ⓑ

IOM: 100-03, 4, 280.3

⊗ **E1226** Wheelchair accessory, manual fully reclining back, (recline greater than 80 degrees), each Ⓑ

IOM: 100-03, 4, 280.1

⊗ **E1227** Special height arms for wheelchair Ⓖ

IOM: 100-03, 4, 280.3

⊗ **E1228** Special back height for wheelchair Ⓑ

IOM: 100-03, 4, 280.3

Wheelchair: Pediatric

✳ **E1229** Wheelchair, pediatric size, not otherwise specified Ⓖ

⊗ **E1230** Power operated vehicle (three or four wheel non-highway), specify brand name and model number Ⓑ

Patient is unable to operate manual wheelchair; patient capable of safely operating controls for scooter; patient can transfer safely in and out of scooter

IOM: 100-08, 5, 5.2.3

⊗ **E1231** Wheelchair, pediatric size, tilt-in-space, rigid, adjustable, with seating system Ⓑ

IOM: 100-03, 4, 280.1

⊗ **E1232** Wheelchair, pediatric size, tilt-in-space, folding, adjustable, with seating system Ⓑ

IOM: 100-03, 4, 280.1

⊗ **E1233** Wheelchair, pediatric size, tilt-in-space, rigid, adjustable, without seating system Ⓑ

IOM: 100-03, 4, 280.1

⊗ **E1234** Wheelchair, pediatric size, tilt-in-space, folding, adjustable, without seating system Ⓑ

IOM: 100-03, 4, 280.1

⊗ **E1235** Wheelchair, pediatric size, rigid, adjustable, with seating system Ⓑ

IOM: 100-03, 4, 280.1

⊗ **E1236** Wheelchair, pediatric size, folding, adjustable, with seating system Ⓑ

IOM: 100-03, 4, 280.1

⊗ **E1237** Wheelchair, pediatric size, rigid, adjustable, without seating system Ⓖ

IOM: 100-03, 4, 280.1

⊗ **E1238** Wheelchair, pediatric size, folding, adjustable, without seating system Ⓖ

IOM: 100-03, 4, 280.1

✳ **E1239** Power wheelchair, pediatric size, not otherwise specified Ⓑ

Wheelchair: Lightweight

⊗ **E1240** Lightweight wheelchair, detachable arms, (desk or full length) swing away detachable, elevating leg rests Ⓑ

IOM: 100-03, 4, 280.1

⊘ **E1250** Lightweight wheelchair, fixed full length arms, swing away detachable footrest Ⓑ

IOM: 100-03, 4, 280.1

Cross Reference K0003

⊘ **E1260** Lightweight wheelchair, detachable arms (desk or full length) swing away detachable footrest Ⓑ

IOM: 100-03, 4, 280.1

Cross Reference K0003

⊗ **E1270** Lightweight wheelchair, fixed full length arms, swing away detachable elevating legrests Ⓖ

IOM: 100-03, 4, 280.1

▶ **New** ⟳ **Revised** ✔ **Reinstated** ~~deleted~~ **Deleted** ⊘ **Not covered or valid by Medicare** ⊗ **Special coverage instructions** ✳ **Carrier discretion** Ⓖ **Bill Part B MAC** Ⓑ **Bill DME MAC**

Wheelchair: Heavy Duty

⊛ **E1280** Heavy duty wheelchair, detachable arms (desk or full length), elevating legrests Ⓑ

IOM: 100-03, 4, 280.1

⊘ **E1285** Heavy duty wheelchair, fixed full length arms, swing away detachable footrest Ⓑ

IOM: 100-03, 4, 280.1

Cross Reference K0006

⊘ **E1290** Heavy duty wheelchair, detachable arms (desk or full length) swing away detachable footrest Ⓓ

IOM: 100-03, 4, 280.1

Cross Reference K0006

⊛ **E1295** Heavy duty wheelchair, fixed full length arms, elevating legrest Ⓑ

IOM: 100-03, 4, 280.1

⊛ **E1296** Special wheelchair seat height from floor Ⓑ

IOM: 100-03, 4, 280.3

⊛ **E1297** Special wheelchair seat depth, by upholstery Ⓓ

IOM: 100-03, 4, 280.3

⊛ **E1298** Special wheelchair seat depth and/or width, by construction Ⓑ

IOM: 100-03, 4, 280.3

Whirlpool Equipment

⊘ **E1300** Whirlpool, portable (overtub type) Ⓑ

IOM: 100-03, 4, 280.1

⊛ **E1310** Whirlpool, non-portable (built-in type) Ⓑ

IOM: 100-03, 4, 280.1

Additional Oxygen Related Equipment

✳ **E1352** Oxygen accessory, flow regulator capable of positive inspiratory pressure Ⓑ

⊛ **E1353** Regulator Ⓓ

IOM: 100-03, 4, 240.2

✳ **E1354** Oxygen accessory, wheeled cart for portable cylinder or portable concentrator, any type, replacement only, each Ⓓ

⊛ **E1355** Stand/rack Ⓓ

IOM: 100-03, 4, 240.2

✳ **E1356** Oxygen accessory, battery pack/cartridge for portable concentrator, any type, replacement only, each Ⓓ

✳ **E1357** Oxygen accessory, battery charger for portable concentrator, any type, replacement only, each Ⓓ

⊛ **E1358** Oxygen accessory, DC power adapter for portable concentrator, any type, replacement only, each Ⓓ

⊛ **E1372** Immersion external heater for nebulizer Ⓓ

IOM: 100-03, 4, 240.2

⊛ **E1390** Oxygen concentrator, single delivery port, capable of delivering 85 percent or greater oxygen concentration at the prescribed flow rate Ⓓ

IOM: 100-03, 4, 240.2

⊛ **E1391** Oxygen concentrator, dual delivery port, capable of delivering 85 percent or greater oxygen concentration at the prescribed flow rate, each Ⓓ

IOM: 100-03, 4, 240.2

⊛ **E1392** Portable oxygen concentrator, rental Ⓓ

IOM: 100-03, 4, 240.2

✳ **E1399** Durable medical equipment, miscellaneous Ⓑ Ⓓ

Example: Therapeutic exercise putty; rubber exercise tubing; anti-vibration gloves.

On DMEPOS fee schedule as a payable replacement for miscellaneous implanted or non-implanted items.

⊛ **E1405** Oxygen and water vapor enriching system with heated delivery Ⓓ

IOM: 100-03, 4, 240.2

⊛ **E1406** Oxygen and water vapor enriching system without heated delivery Ⓓ

IOM: 100-03, 4, 240.2

Artificial Kidney Machines and Accessories

⊛ **E1500** Centrifuge, for dialysis Ⓓ

⊛ **E1510** Kidney, dialysate delivery syst kidney machine, pump recirculating, air removal syst. flowrate meter, power off, heater and temperature control with alarm, I.V. poles, pressure gauge, concentrate container Ⓓ

⊛ **E1520** Heparin infusion pump for hemodialysis Ⓓ

⊛ **E1530** Air bubble detector for hemodialysis, each, replacement Ⓓ

▶ New	↻ Revised	✔ Reinstated	~~deleted~~ Deleted	⊘ Not covered or valid by Medicare
⊛ Special coverage instructions		✳ Carrier discretion	Ⓑ Bill Part B MAC	Ⓓ Bill DME MAC

⊛ **E1540** Pressure alarm for hemodialysis, each, replacement Ⓑ

⊛ **E1550** Bath conductivity meter for hemodialysis, each Ⓑ

⊛ **E1560** Blood leak detector for hemodialysis, each, replacement Ⓑ

⊛ **E1570** Adjustable chair, for ESRD patients Ⓑ

⊛ **E1575** Transducer protectors/fluid barriers for hemodialysis, any size, per 10 Ⓑ

⊛ **E1580** Unipuncture control system for hemodialysis Ⓑ

⊛ **E1590** Hemodialysis machine Ⓑ

⊛ **E1592** Automatic intermittent peritoneal dialysis system Ⓑ

⊛ **E1594** Cycler dialysis machine for peritoneal dialysis Ⓑ

⊛ **E1600** Delivery and/or installation charges for hemodialysis equipment Ⓑ

⊛ **E1610** Reverse osmosis water purification system, for hemodialysis Ⓑ

IOM: 100-03, 4, 230.7

⊛ **E1615** Deionizer water purification system, for hemodialysis Ⓑ

IOM: 100-03, 4, 230.7

⊛ **E1620** Blood pump for hemodialysis replacement Ⓑ

⊛ **E1625** Water softening system, for hemodialysis Ⓑ

IOM: 100-03, 4, 230.7

✳ **E1630** Reciprocating peritoneal dialysis system Ⓑ

⊛ **E1632** Wearable artificial kidney, each Ⓑ

⊛ **E1634** Peritoneal dialysis clamps, each Ⓑ

IOM: 100-04, 8, 60.4.2; 100-04, 8, 90.1; 100-04, 18, 80; 100-04, 18, 90

⊛ **E1635** Compact (portable) travel hemodialyzer system Ⓑ

⊛ **E1636** Sorbent cartridges, for hemodialysis, per 10 Ⓑ

⊛ **E1637** Hemostats, each Ⓑ

⤸⊛ **E1639** Scale, each Ⓑ

⊛ **E1699** Dialysis equipment, not otherwise specified Ⓑ

Jaw Motion Rehabilitation System

✳ **E1700** Jaw motion rehabilitation system Ⓑ

Must be prescribed by physician

✳ **E1701** Replacement cushions for jaw motion rehabilitation system, pkg. of 6 Ⓑ

✳ **E1702** Replacement measuring scales for jaw motion rehabilitation system, pkg. of 200 Ⓑ

Other Orthopedic Devices

✳ **E1800** Dynamic adjustable elbow extension/flexion device, includes soft interface material Ⓑ

✳ **E1801** Static progressive stretch elbow device, extension and/or flexion, with or without range of motion adjustment, includes all components and accessories Ⓑ

✳ **E1802** Dynamic adjustable forearm pronation/supination device, includes soft interface material Ⓑ

✳ **E1805** Dynamic adjustable wrist extension/flexion device, includes soft interface material Ⓑ

✳ **E1806** Static progressive stretch wrist device, flexion and/or extension, with or without range of motion adjustment, includes all components and accessories Ⓑ

✳ **E1810** Dynamic adjustable knee extension/flexion device, includes soft interface material Ⓑ

✳ **E1811** Static progressive stretch knee device, extension and/or flexion, with or without range of motion adjustment, includes all components and accessories Ⓑ

✳ **E1812** Dynamic knee, extension/flexion device with active resistance control Ⓑ

✳ **E1815** Dynamic adjustable ankle extension/flexion device, includes soft interface material Ⓑ

✳ **E1816** Static progressive stretch ankle device, flexion and/or extension, with or without range of motion adjustment, includes all components and accessories Ⓑ

✳ **E1818** Static progressive stretch forearm pronation/supination device with or without range of motion adjustment, includes all components and accessories Ⓑ

✳ **E1820** Replacement soft interface material, dynamic adjustable extension/flexion device Ⓑ

▶ **New**   ⤸ **Revised**   ✔ **Reinstated**   ~~deleted~~ **Deleted**   ⊘ **Not covered or valid by Medicare**
⊛ **Special coverage instructions**   ✳ **Carrier discretion**   Ⓟ **Bill Part B MAC**   Ⓑ **Bill DME MAC**

* **E1821** Replacement soft interface material/ cuffs for bi-directional static progressive stretch device Ⓑ

* **E1825** Dynamic adjustable finger extension/ flexion device, includes soft interface material Ⓑ

* **E1830** Dynamic adjustable toe extension/ flexion device, includes soft interface material Ⓑ

* **E1831** Static progressive stretch toe device, extension and/or flexion, with or without range of motion adjustment, includes all components and accessories Ⓑ

* **E1840** Dynamic adjustable shoulder flexion/ abduction/rotation device, includes soft interface material Ⓑ

* **E1841** Static progressive stretch shoulder device, with or without range of motion adjustment, includes all components and accessories Ⓑ

Miscellaneous

* **E1902** Communication board, non-electronic augmentative or alternative communication device Ⓑ

* **E2000** Gastric suction pump, home model, portable or stationary, electric Ⓑ

☼ **E2100** Blood glucose monitor with integrated voice synthesizer Ⓑ

  IOM: 100-03, 4, 230.16

☼ **E2101** Blood glucose monitor with integrated lancing/blood sample Ⓑ

  IOM: 100-03, 4, 230.16

* **E2120** Pulse generator system for tympanic treatment of inner ear endolymphatic fluid Ⓑ

Wheelchair Assessories: Manual and Power

* **E2201** Manual wheelchair accessory, nonstandard seat frame, width greater than or equal to 20 inches and less than 24 inches Ⓑ

* **E2202** Manual wheelchair accessory, nonstandard seat frame width, 24-27 inches Ⓑ

* **E2203** Manual wheelchair accessory, nonstandard seat frame depth, 20 to less than 22 inches Ⓑ

* **E2204** Manual wheelchair accessory, nonstandard seat frame depth, 22 to 25 inches Ⓑ

* **E2205** Manual wheelchair accessory, handrim without projections (includes ergonomic or contoured), any type, replacement only, each Ⓑ

* **E2206** Manual wheelchair accessory, wheel lock assembly, complete, replacement only, each Ⓑ

* **E2207** Wheelchair accessory, crutch and cane holder, each Ⓑ

* **E2208** Wheelchair accessory, cylinder tank carrier, each Ⓑ

* **E2209** Accessory arm trough, with or without hand support, each Ⓑ

* **E2210** Wheelchair accessory, bearings, any type, replacement only, each Ⓑ

* **E2211** Manual wheelchair accessory, pneumatic propulsion tire, any size, each Ⓑ

* **E2212** Manual wheelchair accessory, tube for pneumatic propulsion tire, any size, each Ⓑ

* **E2213** Manual wheelchair accessory, insert for pneumatic propulsion tire (removable), any type, any size, each Ⓑ

* **E2214** Manual wheelchair accessory, pneumatic caster tire, any size, each Ⓑ

* **E2215** Manual wheelchair accessory, tube for pneumatic caster tire, any size, each Ⓑ

* **E2216** Manual wheelchair accessory, foam filled propulsion tire, any size, each Ⓑ

* **E2217** Manual wheelchair accessory, foam filled caster tire, any size, each Ⓑ

* **E2218** Manual wheelchair accessory, foam propulsion tire, any size, each Ⓑ

* **E2219** Manual wheelchair accessory, foam caster tire, any size, each Ⓑ

* **E2220** Manual wheelchair accessory, solid (rubber/plastic) propulsion tire, any size, replacement only, each Ⓑ

* **E2221** Manual wheelchair accessory, solid (rubber/plastic) caster tire (removable), any size, replacement only, each Ⓑ

* **E2222** Manual wheelchair accessory, solid (rubber/plastic) caster tire with integrated wheel, any size, replacement only, each Ⓑ

* **E2224** Manual wheelchair accessory, propulsion wheel excludes tire, any size, replacement only, each Ⓑ

▶ New   ↻ Revised   ✔ Reinstated   ~~deleted~~ Deleted   ⊘ Not covered or valid by Medicare
☼ Special coverage instructions   ✳ Carrier discretion   Ⓟ Bill Part B MAC   Ⓑ Bill DME MAC

* **E2225** Manual wheelchair accessory, caster wheel excludes tire, any size, replacement only, each ⑧

* **E2226** Manual wheelchair accessory, caster fork, any size, replacement only, each ⑧

* **E2227** Manual wheelchair accessory, gear reduction drive wheel, each ⑧

* **E2228** Manual wheelchair accessory, wheel braking system and lock, complete, each ⑧

* **E2230** Manual wheelchair accessory, manual standing system ⑧

* **E2231** Manual wheelchair accessory, solid seat support base (replaces sling seat), includes any type mounting hardware ⑧

* **E2291** Back, planar, for pediatric size wheelchair including fixed attaching hardware ⑧

* **E2292** Seat, planar, for pediatric size wheelchair including fixed attaching hardware ⑧

* **E2293** Back, contoured, for pediatric size wheelchair including fixed attaching hardware ⑧

* **E2294** Seat, contoured, for pediatric size wheelchair including fixed attaching hardware ⑧

* **E2295** Manual wheelchair accessory, for pediatric size wheelchair, dynamic seating frame, allows coordinated movement of multiple positioning features ⑧

* **E2300** Wheelchair accessory, power seat elevation system, any type ⑧

* **E2301** Wheelchair accessory, power standing system, any type ⑧

* **E2310** Power wheelchair accessory, electronic connection between wheelchair controller and one power seating system motor, including all related electronics, indicator feature, mechanical function selection switch, and fixed mounting hardware ⑧

* **E2311** Power wheelchair accessory, electronic connection between wheelchair controller and two or more power seating system motors, including all related electronics, indicator feature, mechanical function selection switch, and fixed mounting hardware ⑧

* **E2312** Power wheelchair accessory, hand or chin control interface, mini-proportional remote joystick, proportional, including fixed mounting hardware ⑧

* **E2313** Power wheelchair accessory, harness for upgrade to expandable controller, including all fasteners, connectors and mounting hardware, each ⑧

* **E2321** Power wheelchair accessory, hand control interface, remote joystick, nonproportional, including all related electronics, mechanical stop switch, and fixed mounting hardware ⑧

* **E2322** Power wheelchair accessory, hand control interface, multiple mechanical switches, nonproportional, including all related electronics, mechanical stop switch, and fixed mounting hardware ⑧

* **E2323** Power wheelchair accessory, specialty joystick handle for hand control interface, prefabricated ⑧

* **E2324** Power wheelchair accessory, chin cup for chin control interface ⑧

* **E2325** Power wheelchair accessory, sip and puff interface, nonproportional, including all related electronics, mechanical stop switch, and manual swingaway mounting hardware ⑧

* **E2326** Power wheelchair accessory, breath tube kit for sip and puff interface ⑧

* **E2327** Power wheelchair accessory, head control interface, mechanical, proportional, including all related electronics, mechanical direction change switch, and fixed mounting hardware ⑧

* **E2328** Power wheelchair accessory, head control or extremity control interface, electronic, proportional, including all related electronics and fixed mounting hardware ⑧

* **E2329** Power wheelchair accessory, head control interface, contact switch mechanism, nonproportional, including all related electronics, mechanical stop switch, mechanical direction change switch, head array, and fixed mounting hardware ⑧

* **E2330** Power wheelchair accessory, head control interface, proximity switch mechanism, nonproportional, including all related electronics, mechanical stop switch, mechanical direction change switch, head array, and fixed mounting hardware ⑧

▶ **New**   ↻ **Revised**   ✔ **Reinstated**   ~~deleted~~ **Deleted**   ⊘ **Not covered or valid by Medicare**

⑤ **Special coverage instructions**   ✳ **Carrier discretion**   ⑨ **Bill Part B MAC**   ⑧ **Bill DME MAC**

✳ **E2331** Power wheelchair accessory, attendant control, proportional, including all related electronics and fixed mounting hardware Ⓑ

✳ **E2340** Power wheelchair accessory, nonstandard seat frame width, 20-23 inches

✳ **E2341** Power wheelchair accessory, nonstandard seat frame width, 24-27 inches Ⓑ

✳ **E2342** Power wheelchair accessory, nonstandard seat frame depth, 20 or 21 inches Ⓑ

✳ **E2343** Power wheelchair accessory, nonstandard seat frame depth, 22-25 inches Ⓑ

✳ **E2351** Power wheelchair accessory, electronic interface to operate speech generating device using power wheelchair control interface Ⓑ

✳ **E2358** Power wheelchair accessory, Group 34 non-sealed lead acid battery, each Ⓑ

✳ **E2359** Power wheelchair accessory, Group 34 sealed lead acid battery, each (e.g., gel cell, absorbed glassmat) Ⓑ

✳ **E2360** Power wheelchair accessory, 22 NF non-sealed lead acid battery, each Ⓑ

✳ **E2361** Power wheelchair accessory, 22NF sealed lead acid battery, each, (e.g., gel cell, absorbed glassmat) Ⓑ

✳ **E2362** Power wheelchair accessory, group 24 non-sealed lead acid battery, each Ⓑ

✳ **E2363** Power wheelchair accessory, group 24 sealed lead acid battery, each (e.g., gel cell, absorbed glassmat) Ⓑ

✳ **E2364** Power wheelchair accessory, U-1 non-sealed lead acid battery, each Ⓑ

✳ **E2365** Power wheelchair accessory, U-1 sealed lead acid battery, each (e.g., gel cell, absorbed glassmat) Ⓑ

✳ **E2366** Power wheelchair accessory, battery charger, single mode, for use with only one battery type, sealed or non-sealed, each Ⓑ

✳ **E2367** Power wheelchair accessory, battery charger, dual mode, for use with either battery type, sealed or non-sealed, each Ⓑ

✳ **E2368** Power wheelchair component, drive wheel motor, replacement only Ⓑ

✳ **E2369** Power wheelchair component, drive wheel gear box, replacement only Ⓑ

✳ **E2370** Power wheelchair component, integrated drive wheel motor and gear box combination, replacement only Ⓑ

✳ **E2371** Power wheelchair accessory, group 27 sealed lead acid battery, (e.g., gel cell, absorbed glass mat), each Ⓑ

✳ **E2372** Power wheelchair accessory, group 27 non-sealed lead acid battery, each Ⓑ

✳ **E2373** Power wheelchair accessory, hand or chin control interface, compact remote joystick, proportional, including fixed mounting hardware Ⓑ

✪ **E2374** Power wheelchair accessory, hand or chin control interface, standard remote joystick (not including controller), proportional, including all related electronics and fixed mounting hardware, replacement only Ⓑ

✪ **E2375** Power wheelchair accessory, non-expandable controller, including all related electronics and mounting hardware, replacement only Ⓑ

✪ **E2376** Power wheelchair accessory, expandable controller, including all related electronics and mounting hardware, replacement only Ⓑ

✪ **E2377** Power wheelchair accessory, expandable controller, including all related electronics and mounting hardware, upgrade provided at initial issue Ⓑ

✳ **E2378** Power wheelchair component, actuator, replacement only Ⓑ

✪ **E2381** Power wheelchair accessory, pneumatic drive wheel tire, any size, replacement only, each Ⓑ

✪ **E2382** Power wheelchair accessory, tube for pneumatic drive wheel tire, any size, replacement only, each Ⓑ

✪ **E2383** Power wheelchair accessory, insert for pneumatic drive wheel tire (removable), any type, any size, replacement only, each Ⓑ

✪ **E2384** Power wheelchair accessory, pneumatic caster tire, any size, replacement only, each Ⓑ

✪ **E2385** Power wheelchair accessory, tube for pneumatic caster tire, any size, replacement only, each Ⓑ

✪ **E2386** Power wheelchair accessory, foam filled drive wheel tire, any size, replacement only, each Ⓑ

✪ **E2387** Power wheelchair accessory, foam filled caster tire, any size, replacement only, each Ⓑ

✪ **E2388** Power wheelchair accessory, foam drive wheel tire, any size, replacement only, each Ⓑ

▶ New	↻ Revised	✔ Reinstated	~~deleted~~ Deleted	⊘ Not covered or valid by Medicare
✪ Special coverage instructions	✳ Carrier discretion	Ⓑ Bill Part B MAC	Ⓓ Bill DME MAC	

⊙ **E2389** Power wheelchair accessory, foam caster tire, any size, replacement only, each ⑧

⊙ **E2390** Power wheelchair accessory, solid (rubber/plastic) drive wheel tire, any size, replacement only, each ⑧

⊙ **E2391** Power wheelchair accessory, solid (rubber/plastic) caster tire (removable), any size, replacement only, each ⑤

⊙ **E2392** Power wheelchair accessory, solid (rubber/plastic) caster tire with integrated wheel, any size, replacement only, each ⑤

⊙ **E2394** Power wheelchair accessory, drive wheel excludes tire, any size, replacement only, each ⑤

⊙ **E2395** Power wheelchair accessory, caster wheel excludes tire, any size, replacement only, each ⑤

⊙ **E2396** Power wheelchair accessory, caster fork, any size, replacement only, each ⑧

✳ **E2397** Power wheelchair accessory, lithium-based battery, each ⑤

Negative Pressure

✳ **E2402** Negative pressure wound therapy electrical pump, stationary or portable ⑧

Document at least every 30 calendar days the quantitative wound characteristics, including wound surface area (length, width and depth).

Medicare coverage up to a maximum of 15 dressing kits (A6550) per wound per month unless documentation states that the wound size requires more than one dressing kit for each dressing change.

Speech Device

⊙ **E2500** Speech generating device, digitized speech, using pre-recorded messages, less than or equal to 8 minutes recording time ⑧

IOM: 100-03, 1, 50.1

⊙ **E2502** Speech generating device, digitized speech, using pre-recorded messages, greater than 8 minutes but less than or equal to 20 minutes recording time ⑧

IOM: 100-03, 1, 50.1

⊙ **E2504** Speech generating device, digitized speech, using pre-recorded messages, greater than 20 minutes but less than or equal to 40 minutes recording time ⑧

IOM: 100-03, 1, 50.1

⊙ **E2506** Speech generating device, digitized speech, using pre-recorded messages, greater than 40 minutes recording time ⑧

IOM: 100-03, 1, 50.1

⊙ **E2508** Speech generating device, synthesized speech, requiring message formulation by spelling and access by physical contact with the device ⑧

IOM: 100-03, 1, 50.1

⊙ **E2510** Speech generating device, synthesized speech, permitting multiple methods of message formulation and multiple methods of device access ⑧

IOM: 100-03, 1, 50.1

⊙ **E2511** Speech generating software program, for personal computer or personal digital assistant ⑤

IOM: 100-03, 1, 50.1

⊙ **E2512** Accessory for speech generating device, mounting system ⑧

IOM: 100-03, 1, 50.1

⊙ **E2599** Accessory for speech generating device, not otherwise classified ⑧

IOM: 100-03, 1, 50.1

Wheelchair: Cushion

✳ **E2601** General use wheelchair seat cushion, width less than 22 inches, any depth ⑧

✳ **E2602** General use wheelchair seat cushion, width 22 inches or greater, any depth ⑧

✳ **E2603** Skin protection wheelchair seat cushion, width less than 22 inches, any depth ⑧

✳ **E2604** Skin protection wheelchair seat cushion, width 22 inches or greater, any depth ⑧

✳ **E2605** Positioning wheelchair seat cushion, width less than 22 inches, any depth ⑧

✳ **E2606** Positioning wheelchair seat cushion, width 22 inches or greater, any depth ⑧

✳ **E2607** Skin protection and positioning wheelchair seat cushion, width less than 22 inches, any depth ⑧

▶ New   ↻ Revised   ✔ Reinstated   ~~deleted~~ Deleted   ⊘ Not covered or valid by Medicare
⊙ Special coverage instructions   ✳ Carrier discretion   ⑨ Bill Part B MAC   ⑧ Bill DME MAC

* **E2608** Skin protection and positioning wheelchair seat cushion, width 22 inches or greater, any depth Ⓑ

* **E2609** Custom fabricated wheelchair seat cushion, any size Ⓑ

* **E2610** Wheelchair seat cushion, powered Ⓑ

* **E2611** General use wheelchair back cushion, width less than 22 inches, any height, including any type mounting hardware Ⓑ

* **E2612** General use wheelchair back cushion, width 22 inches or greater, any height, including any type mounting hardware Ⓑ

* **E2613** Positioning wheelchair back cushion, posterior, width less than 22 inches, any height, including any type mounting hardware Ⓑ

* **E2614** Positioning wheelchair back cushion, posterior, width 22 inches or greater, any height, including any type mounting hardware Ⓑ

* **E2615** Positioning wheelchair back cushion, posterior-lateral, width less than 22 inches, any height, including any type mounting hardware Ⓑ

* **E2616** Positioning wheelchair back cushion, posterior-lateral, width 22 inches or greater, any height, including any type mounting hardware Ⓑ

* **E2617** Custom fabricated wheelchair back cushion, any size, including any type mounting hardware Ⓑ

* **E2619** Replacement cover for wheelchair seat cushion or back cushion, each Ⓑ

* **E2620** Positioning wheelchair back cushion, planar back with lateral supports, width less than 22 inches, any height, including any type mounting hardware Ⓑ

* **E2621** Positioning wheelchair back cushion, planar back with lateral supports, width 22 inches or greater, any height, including any type mounting hardware Ⓑ

Wheelchair: Skin Protection

* **E2622** Skin protection wheelchair seat cushion, adjustable, width less than 22 inches, any depth Ⓑ

* **E2623** Skin protection wheelchair seat cushion, adjustable, width 22 inches or greater, any depth Ⓑ

* **E2624** Skin protection and positioning wheelchair seat cushion, adjustable, width less than 22 inches, any depth Ⓑ

* **E2625** Skin protection and positioning wheelchair seat cushion, adjustable, width 22 inches or greater, any depth Ⓑ

Wheelchair: Arm Support

* **E2626** Wheelchair accessory, shoulder elbow, mobile arm support attached to wheelchair, balanced, adjustable Ⓑ

* **E2627** Wheelchair accessory, shoulder elbow, mobile arm support attached to wheelchair, balanced, adjustable rancho type Ⓑ

* **E2628** Wheelchair accessory, shoulder elbow, mobile arm support attached to wheelchair, balanced, reclining Ⓑ

* **E2629** Wheelchair accessory, shoulder elbow, mobile arm support attached to wheelchair, balanced, friction arm support (friction dampening to proximal and distal joints) Ⓑ

* **E2630** Wheelchair accessory, shoulder elbow, mobile arm support, monosuspension arm and hand support, overhead elbow forearm hand sling support, yoke type suspension support Ⓑ

* **E2631** Wheelchair accessory, addition to mobile arm support, elevating proximal arm Ⓑ

* **E2632** Wheelchair accessory, addition to mobile arm support, offset or lateral rocker arm with elastic balance control Ⓑ

* **E2633** Wheelchair accessory, addition to mobile arm support, supinator Ⓑ

Pediatric Gait Trainer

⊘ **E8000** Gait trainer, pediatric size, posterior support, includes all accessories and components Ⓑ

⊘ **E8001** Gait trainer, pediatric size, upright support, includes all accessories and components Ⓑ

⊘ **E8002** Gait trainer, pediatric size, anterior support, includes all accessories and components Ⓑ

▶ **New**   ↻ **Revised**   ✔ **Reinstated**   ~~deleted~~ **Deleted**   ⊘ **Not covered or valid by Medicare**
✿ **Special coverage instructions**   * **Carrier discretion**   Ⓟ **Bill Part B MAC**   Ⓑ **Bill DME MAC**

TEMPORARY PROCEDURES/PROFESSIONAL SERVICES (G0000-G9999)

NOTE: Series "G", "K", and "Q" in the Level II coding are reserved for CMS assignment. "G", "K", and "Q" codes are temporary national codes for items or services requiring uniform national coding between one year's update and the next. Sometimes "temporary" codes remain for more than one update. If "G", "K", and "Q" codes are not converted to permanent codes in Level I or Level II series in the following update, they will remain active until converted in following years or until CMS notifies contractors to delete them. All active "G", "K", and "Q" codes at the time of update will be included on the update file for contractors. In addition, deleted codes are retained on the file for informational purposes, with a deleted indicator, for four years.

Vaccine Administration

✳ **G0008** Administration of influenza virus vaccine Ⓑ

Coinsurance and deductible do not apply. If provided, report significant, separately identifiable E/M for medically necessary services (V04.81).

✳ **G0009** Administration of pneumococcal vaccine Ⓑ

Reported once in a lifetime based on risk; Medicare covers cost of vaccine and administration (V03.82)

Copayment, coinsurance, and deductible waived. (https://www.cms. gov/MLNProducts/downloads/MPS_ QuickReferenceChart_1.pdf)

✳ **G0010** Administration of hepatitis B vaccine Ⓑ

Report for other than OPPs. Coinsurance and deductible apply; Medicare covers both cost of vaccine and administration (V05.3)

Copayment/coinsurance and deductible are waived. (https://www.cms.gov/ MLNProducts/downloads/MPS_ QuickReferenceChart_1.pdf)

Semen Analysis

✳ **G0027** Semen analysis; presence and/or motility of sperm excluding Huhner Ⓑ

Screening Services

⊘ **G0101** Cervical or vaginal cancer screening; pelvic and clinical breast examination Ⓑ

Covered once every two years and annually if high risk for cervical/vaginal cancer, or if childbearing age patient has had an abnormal Pap smear in preceding three years. High risk diagnosis, V15.89

⊘ **G0102** Prostate cancer screening; digital rectal examination Ⓑ

Covered annually by Medicare (V76.44). Not separately payable with an E/M code (99201-99499).

IOM: 100-02, 6, 10; 100-04, 4, 240; 100-04, 18, 50.1

⊘ **G0103** Prostate cancer screening; prostate specific antigen test (PSA) Ⓑ

Covered annually by Medicare (V76.44)

IOM: 100-02, 6, 10; 100-04, 4, 240; 100-04, 18, 50

⊘ **G0104** Colorectal cancer screening; flexible sigmoidoscopy Ⓑ

Covered once every 48 months for beneficiaries age 50+

Co-insurance waived under Section 4104.

⊘ **G0105** Colorectal cancer screening; colonoscopy on individual at high risk Ⓑ

Screening colonoscopy covered once every 24 months for high risk for developing colorectal cancer. May use modifier 53 if appropriate (physician fee schedule).

Co-insurance waived under Section 4104.

⊘ **G0106** Colorectal cancer screening; alternative to G0104, screening sigmoidoscopy, barium enema Ⓑ

Barium enema (not high risk) (alternative to G0104). Covered once every 4 years for beneficiaries age 50+. Use modifier 26 for professional component only.

▶ New   ↻ Revised   ✔ Reinstated   ~~deleted~~ Deleted   ⊘ Not covered or valid by Medicare
⊛ Special coverage instructions   ✳ Carrier discretion   Ⓑ Bill Part B MAC   Ⓓ Bill DME MAC

Diabetes Management Training Services

✳ **G0108** Diabetes outpatient self-management training services, individual, per 30 minutes ⑧

Report for beneficiaries diagnosed with diabetes.

Effective January 2011, DSMT will be included in the list of reimbursable Medicare telehealth services.

✳ **G0109** Diabetes outpatient self-management training services, group session (2 or more) per 30 minutes ⑧

Report for beneficiaries diagnosed with diabetes.

Effective January 2011, DSMT will be included in the list of reimbursable Medicare telehealth services.

Screening Services

✳ **G0117** Glaucoma screening for high risk patients furnished by an optometrist or ophthalmologist ⑧

Covered once per year (full 11 months between screenings). Bundled with all other ophthalmic services provided on same day. Diagnosis code V80.1.

✳ **G0118** Glaucoma screening for high risk patient furnished under the direct supervision of an optometrist or ophthalmologist ⑧

Covered once per year (full 11 months between screenings). Diagnosis code V80.1.

✪ **G0120** Colorectal cancer screening; alternative to G0105, screening colonoscopy, barium enema. ⑧

Barium enema for patients with a high risk of developing colorectal. Covered once every 2 years. Used as an alternative to G0105. Use modifier 26 for professional component only.

✪ **G0121** Colorectal cancer screening; colonoscopy on individual not meeting criteria for high risk ⑧

Screening colonoscopy for patients that are not high risk. Covered once every 10 years, but not within 48 months of a G0104. For non-Medicare patients report 45378.

Co-insurance waived under Section 4104.

⊘ **G0122** Colorectal cancer screening; barium enema ⑧

Medicare: this service is denied as noncovered, because it fails to meet the requirements of the benefit. The beneficiary is liable for payment.

✪ **G0123** Screening cytopathology, cervical or vaginal (any reporting system), collected in preservative fluid, automated thin layer preparation, screening by cytotechnologist under physician supervision ⑧

Use G0123 or G0143 or G0144 or G0145 or G0147 or G0148 or P3000 for Pap smears NOT requiring physician interpretation (technical component).

IOM: 100-03, 3, 190.2; 100-04, 18, 30

✪ **G0124** Screening cytopathology, cervical or vaginal (any reporting system), collected in preservative fluid, automated thin layer preparation, requiring interpretation by physician ⑧

Report professional component for Pap smears requiring physician interpretation.

IOM: 100-03, 3, 190.2; 100-04, 18, 30

Miscellaneous Services, Diagnostic and Therapeutic

✪ **G0127** Trimming of dystrophic nails, any number ⑧

Must be used with a modifier (Q7, Q8, or Q9) to show that the foot care service is needed because the beneficiary has a systemic disease. Limit 1 unit of service.

IOM: 100-02, 15, 290

✪ **G0128** Direct (face-to-face with patient) skilled nursing services of a registered nurse provided in a comprehensive outpatient rehabilitation facility, each 10 minutes beyond the first 5 minutes ⑧

A separate nursing service that is clearly identifiable in the Plan of Treatment and not part of other services. Documentation must support this service. Examples include: Insertion of a urinary catheter, intramuscular injections, bowel disimpaction, nursing assessment, and education. Restricted coverage by Medicare.

▶ New   ↻ Revised   ✔ Reinstated   deleted Deleted   ⊘ Not covered or valid by Medicare

✪ Special coverage instructions   ✳ Carrier discretion   ⑧ Bill Part B MAC   ⑧ Bill DME MAC

* **G0129** Occupational therapy services requiring the skills of a qualified occupational therapist, furnished as a component of a partial hospitalization treatment program, per session (45 minutes or more) ⑧

☉ **G0130** Single energy x-ray absorptiometry (SEXA) bone density study, one or more sites; appendicular skeleton (peripheral) (e.g., radius, wrist, heel) ⑧

Covered every 24 months (more frequently if medically necessary). Use modifier 26 for professional component only.

Preventive service; no deductible

IOM: 100-03, 2, 150.3; 100-04, 13, 140.1

* **G0141** Screening cytopathology smears, cervical or vaginal, performed by automated system, with manual rescreening, requiring interpretation by physician ⑧

Co-insurance, copay, and deductible waived

Report professional component for Pap smears requiring physician interpretation. Refer to diagnosis of V15.89, V76.2, V76.47, or V76.49 to report appropriate risk level.

* **G0143** Screening cytopathology, cervical or vaginal (any reporting system), collected in preservative fluid, automated thin layer preparation, with manual screening and rescreening by cytotechnologist under physician supervision ⑧

Co-insurance, copay, and deductible waived

* **G0144** Screening cytopathology, cervical or vaginal (any reporting system), collected in preservative fluid, automated thin layer preparation, with screening by automated system, under physician supervision ⑧

Co-insurance, copay, and deductible waived

* **G0145** Screening cytopathology, cervical or vaginal (any reporting system), collected in preservative fluid, automated thin layer preparation, with screening by automated system and manual rescreening under physician supervision ⑧

Co-insurance, copay, and deductible waived

* **G0147** Screening cytopathology smears, cervical or vaginal; performed by automated system under physician supervision ⑧

Co-insurance, copay, and deductible waived

* **G0148** Screening cytopathology smears, cervical or vaginal; performed by automated system with manual rescreening ⑧

Co-insurance, copay, and deductible waived

* **G0151** Services performed by a qualified physical therapist in the home health or hospice setting, each 15 minutes ⑧

* **G0152** Services performed by a qualified occupational therapist in the home health or hospice setting, each 15 minutes ⑧

* **G0153** Services performed by a qualified speech-language pathologist in the home health or hospice setting, each 15 minutes ⑧

* **G0155** Services of clinical social worker in home health or hospice settings, each 15 minutes ⑧

* **G0156** Services of home health/health aide in home health or hospice settings, each 15 minutes ⑧

* **G0157** Services performed by a qualified physical therapist assistant in the home health or hospice setting, each 15 minutes ⑧

* **G0158** Services performed by a qualified occupational therapist assistant in the home health or hospice setting, each 15 minutes ⑧

* **G0159** Services performed by a qualified physical therapist, in the home health setting, in the establishment or delivery of a safe and effective physical therapy maintenance program, each 15 minutes ⑧

* **G0160** Services performed by a qualified occupational therapist, in the home health setting, in the establishment or delivery of a safe and effective occupational therapy maintenance program, each 15 minutes ⑧

* **G0161** Services performed by a qualified speech-language pathologist, in the home health setting, in the establishment or delivery of a safe and effective speech-language pathology maintenance program, each 15 minutes ⑧

▶ **New** ⤶ **Revised** ✔ **Reinstated** ~~deleted~~ **Deleted** ⊘ **Not covered or valid by Medicare**

☉ **Special coverage instructions** ✳ **Carrier discretion** ⑧ **Bill Part B MAC** ⑧ **Bill DME MAC**

✳ **G0162** Skilled services by a registered nurse (RN) for management and evaluation of the plan of care; each 15 minutes (the patient's underlying condition or complication requires an RN to ensure that essential non-skilled care achieves its purpose in the home health or hospice setting) ⑧

Transmittal No. 824 (CR7182)

✿ **G0166** External counterpulsation, per treatment session ⑧

IOM: 100-03, 1, 20.20

✳ **G0168** Wound closure utilizing tissue adhesive(s) only ⑨

Report for wound closure with only tissue adhesive. If a practitioner utilizes tissue adhesive in addition to staples or sutures to close a wound, HCPCS code G0168 is not separately reportable, but is included in the tissue repair.

The only closure material used for a simple repair, coverage based on payer.

✳ **G0175** Scheduled interdisciplinary team conference (minimum of three exclusive of patient care nursing staff) with patient present ⑧

✿ **G0176** Activity therapy, such as music, dance, art or play therapies not for recreation, related to the care and treatment of patient's disabling mental health problems, per session (45 minutes or more) ⑧

Paid in partial hospitalization

✿ **G0177** Training and educational services related to the care and treatment of patient's disabling mental health problems per session (45 minutes or more) ⑧

Paid in partial hospitalization

✳ **G0179** Physician re-certification for Medicare-covered home health services under a home health plan of care (patient not present), including contacts with home health agency and review of reports of patient status required by physicians to affirm the initial implementation of the plan of care that meets patient's needs, per re-certification period ⑧

The recertification code is used after a patient has received services for at least 60days (or one certification period) when the physician signs the certification after the initial certification period.

✳ **G0180** Physician certification for Medicare-covered home health services under a home health plan of care (patient not present), including contacts with home health agency and review of reports of patient status required by physicians to affirm the initial implementation of the plan of care that meets patient's needs, per certification period ⑧

This code can be billed only when the patient has not received Medicare covered home health services for at least 60days.

✳ **G0181** Physician supervision of a patient receiving Medicare-covered services provided by a participating home health agency (patient not present) requiring complex and multidisciplinary care modalities involving regular physician development and/or revision of care plans, review of subsequent reports of patient status, review of laboratory and other studies, communication (including telephone calls) with other health care professionals involved in the patient's care, integration of new information into the medical treatment plan and/or adjustment of medical therapy, within a calendar month, 30 minutes or more ⑧

✳ **G0182** Physician supervision of a patient under a Medicare-approved hospice (patient not present) requiring complex and multidisciplinary care modalities involving regular physician development and/or revision of care plans, review of subsequent reports of patient status, review of laboratory and other studies, communication (including telephone calls) with other health care professionals involved in the patient's care, integration of new information into the medical treatment plan and/or adjustment of medical therapy, within a calendar month, 30 minutes or more ⑧

✳ **G0186** Destruction of localized lesion of choroid (for example, choroidal neovascularization); photocoagulation, feeder vessel technique (one or more sessions) ⑧

▶ New   ↻ Revised   ✔ Reinstated   ~~deleted~~ Deleted   ⊘ Not covered or valid by Medicare
✿ Special coverage instructions   ✳ Carrier discretion   ⑧ Bill Part B MAC   ⑧ Bill DME MAC

⊘ ~~G0202~~ ~~Screening mammography, bilateral~~ ✖
~~(2-view study of each breast), including~~
~~computer-aided detection (CAD) when~~
~~performed~~

Cross Reference 77067

~~G0204~~ ~~Diagnostic mammography, including~~ ✖
~~computer-aided detection (CAD) when~~
~~performed; bilateral~~

Cross Reference 77066

~~G0206~~ ~~Diagnostic mammography, including~~ ✖
~~computer-aided detection (CAD) when~~
~~performed; unilateral~~

Cross Reference 77065

⊘ **G0219** PET imaging whole body; melanoma
for non-covered indications Ⓑ

Example: Assessing regional lymph
nodes in melanoma.

IOM: 100-03, 4, 220.6

⊘ **G0235** PET imaging, any site, not otherwise
specified Ⓑ

Example: Prostate cancer diagnosis and
initial staging.

IOM: 100-03, 4, 220.6

✳ **G0237** Therapeutic procedures to increase
strength or endurance of respiratory
muscles, face to face, one on one, each
15 minutes (includes monitoring) Ⓑ

✳ **G0238** Therapeutic procedures to improve
respiratory function, other than
described by G0237, one on one, face to
face, per 15 minutes (includes
monitoring) Ⓑ

✳ **G0239** Therapeutic procedures to improve
respiratory function or increase
strength or endurance of respiratory
muscles, two or more individuals
(includes monitoring) Ⓑ

❂ **G0245** Initial physician evaluation and
management of a diabetic patient with
diabetic sensory neuropathy resulting
in a loss of protective sensation (LOPS)
which must include (1) the diagnosis of
LOPS, (2) a patient history, (3) a
physical examination that consist of at
least the following elements: (A) visual
inspection of the forefoot, hindfoot and
toe web spaces, (B) evaluation of a
protective sensation, (C) evaluation of
foot structure and biomechanics,
(D) evaluation of vascular status and
skin integrity, and (E) evaluation and
recommendation of footwear, and
(4) patient education Ⓑ

IOM: 100-03, 1, 70.2.1

❂ **G0246** Follow-up physician evaluation and
management of a diabetic patient with
diabetic sensory neuropathy resulting
in a loss of protective sensation (LOPS)
to include at least the following:
(1) a patient history, (2) a physical
examination that includes: (A) visual
inspection of the forefoot, hindfoot and
toe web spaces, (B) evaluation of
protective sensation, (C) evaluation of
foot structure and biomechanics,
(D) evaluation of vascular status and
skin integrity, and (E) evaluation and
recommendation of footwear, and
(3) patient education Ⓑ

IOM: 100-03, 1, 70.2.1; 100-02, 15, 290

❂ **G0247** Routine foot care by a physician of a
diabetic patient with diabetic sensory
neuropathy resulting in a loss of
protective sensation (LOPS) to include,
the local care of superficial wounds
(i.e., superficial to muscle and fascia)
and at least the following if present:
(1) local care of superficial wounds,
(2) debridement of corns and calluses,
and (3) trimming and debridement of
nails Ⓑ

IOM: 100-03, 1, 70.2.1

❂ **G0248** Demonstration, prior to initiation, of
home INR monitoring for patient with
either mechanical heart valve(s),
chronic atrial fibrillation, or venous
thromboembolism who meets Medicare
coverage criteria, under the direction of
a physician; includes: face-to-face
demonstration of use and care of the
INR monitor, obtaining at least one
blood sample, provision of instructions
for reporting home INR test results,
and documentation of patient's ability
to perform testing and report results Ⓑ

❂ **G0249** Provision of test materials and
equipment for home INR monitoring of
patient with either mechanical heart
valve(s), chronic atrial fibrillation, or
venous thromboembolism who meets
Medicare coverage criteria; includes
provision of materials for use in the
home and reporting of test results to
physician; testing not occurring more
frequently than once a week; testing
materials, billing units of service
include 4 tests Ⓑ

⊗ **G0250** Physician review, interpretation, and patient management of home INR testing for patient with either mechanical heart valve(s), chronic atrial fibrillation, or venous thromboembolism who meets Medicare coverage criteria; testing not occurring more frequently than once a week; billing units of service include 4 tests Ⓑ

⊘ **G0252** PET imaging, full and partial-ring PET scanners only, for initial diagnosis of breast cancer and/or surgical planning for breast cancer (e.g., initial staging of axillary lymph nodes) Ⓑ

IOM: 100-03, 4, 220.6

⊘ **G0255** Current perception threshold/sensory nerve conduction test (SNCT), per limb, any nerve Ⓑ

IOM: 100-03, 2, 160.23

⊗ **G0257** Unscheduled or emergency dialysis treatment for an ESRD patient in a hospital outpatient department that is not certified as an ESRD facility Ⓑ

⊗ **G0259** Injection procedure for sacroiliac joint; arthrography Ⓑ

Replaces 27096 for reporting injections for Medicare beneficiaries

Used by Part A only (facility), not priced by Part B Medicare.

⊗ **G0260** Injection procedure for sacroiliac joint; provision of anesthetic, steroid and/or other therapeutic agent, with or without arthrography Ⓑ

ASCs report when a therapeutic sacroiliac joint injection is administered in ASC

✳ **G0268** Removal of impacted cerumen (one or both ears) by physician on same date of service as audiologic function testing Ⓑ

Report only when a physician, not an audiologist, performs the procedure.

Use with DX 380.4 when performed by physician.

⊗ **G0269** Placement of occlusive device into either a venous or arterial access site, post surgical or interventional procedure (e.g., angioseal plug, vascular plug) Ⓑ

Report for replacement of vasoseal. Hospitals may report the closure device as a supply with C1760. Bundled status on Physician Fee Schedule.

✳ **G0270** Medical nutrition therapy; reassessment and subsequent intervention(s) following second referral in same year for change in diagnosis, medical condition or treatment regimen (including additional hours needed for renal disease), individual, face to face with the patient, each 15 minutes Ⓑ

Requires physician referral for beneficiaries with diabetes or renal disease. Services must be provided by dietitian/nutritionist. Co-insurance and deductible waived.

✳ **G0271** Medical nutrition therapy, reassessment and subsequent intervention(s) following second referral in same year for change in diagnosis, medical condition, or treatment regimen (including additional hours needed for renal disease), group (2 or more individuals), each 30 minutes Ⓑ

Requires physician referral for beneficiaries with diabetes or renal disease. Services must be provided by dietitian/nutritionist. Co-insurance and deductible waived.

⊗ **G0276** Blinded procedure for lumbar stenosis, percutaneous image-guided lumbar decompression (PILD) or placebo-control, performed in an approved coverage with evidence development (CED) clinical trial Ⓑ

⊗ **G0277** Hyperbaric oxygen under pressure, full body chamber, per 30 minute interval Ⓑ

IOM: 100-03, 1, 20.29

✳ **G0278** Iliac and/or femoral artery angiography, non-selective, bilateral or ipsilateral to catheter insertion, performed at the same time as cardiac catheterization and/or coronary angiography, includes positioning or placement of the catheter in the distal aorta or ipsilateral femoral or iliac artery, injection of dye, production of permanent images, and radiologic supervision and interpretation (list separately in addition to primary procedure) Ⓑ

Medicare specific code not reported for iliac injection used as a guiding shot for a closure device

✳ **G0279** Diagnostic digital breast tomosynthesis, unilateral or bilateral (list separately in addition to G0204 or G0206) Ⓑ

▶ **New**   ↻ **Revised**   ✔ **Reinstated**   ~~deleted~~ **Deleted**   ⊘ **Not covered or valid by Medicare**

⊗ **Special coverage instructions**   ✳ **Carrier discretion**   Ⓑ **Bill Part B MAC**   Ⓓ **Bill DME MAC**

* **G0281** Electrical stimulation, (unattended), to one or more areas, for chronic stage III and stage IV pressure ulcers, arterial ulcers, diabetic ulcers, and venous stasis ulcers not demonstrating measurable signs of healing after 30 days of conventional care, as part of a therapy plan of care ⓑ

Reported by encounter/areas and not by site. Therapists report G0281 and G0283 rather than 97014.

⊘ **G0282** Electrical stimulation, (unattended), to one or more areas, for wound care other than described in G0281 ⓑ

IOM: 100-03, 4, 270.1

* **G0283** Electrical stimulation (unattended), to one or more areas for indication(s) other than wound care, as part of a therapy plan of care ⓑ

Reported by encounter/areas and not by site. Therapists report G0281 and G0283 rather than 97014.

* **G0288** Reconstruction, computed tomographic angiography of aorta for surgical planning for vascular surgery ⓑ

* **G0289** Arthroscopy, knee, surgical, for removal of loose body, foreign body, debridement/shaving of articular cartilage (chondroplasty) at the time of other surgical knee arthroscopy in a different compartment of the same knee ⓑ

Add-on code reported with knee arthroscopy code for major procedure performed-reported once per extra compartment

"The code may be reported twice (or with a unit of two) if the physician performs these procedures in two compartments, in addition to the compartment where the main procedure was performed." (http://www.ama-assn.org/resources/doc/cpt/orthopaedics.pdf)

⊙ **G0293** Noncovered surgical procedure(s) using conscious sedation, regional, general or spinal anesthesia in a Medicare qualifying clinical trial, per day ⓑ

⊙ **G0294** Noncovered procedure(s) using either no anesthesia or local anesthesia only, in a Medicare qualifying clinical trial, per day ⓑ

⊘ **G0295** Electromagnetic therapy, to one or more areas, for wound care other than described in G0329 or for other uses ⓑ

IOM: 100-03, 4, 270.1

* **G0296** Counseling visit to discuss need for lung cancer screening (LDCT) using low dose CT scan (service is for eligibility determination and shared decision making) ⓑ

* **G0297** Low dose CT scan (LDCT) for lung cancer screening ⓑ

* **G0299** Direct skilled nursing services of a registered nurse (RN) in the home health or hospice setting, each 15 minutes ⓑ

* **G0300** Direct skilled nursing services of a licensed practical nurse (LPN) in the home health or hospice setting, each 15 minutes ⓑ

* **G0302** Pre-operative pulmonary surgery services for preparation for LVRS, complete course of services, to include a minimum of 16 days of services ⓑ

* **G0303** Pre-operative pulmonary surgery services for preparation for LVRS, 10 to 15 days of services ⓑ

* **G0304** Pre-operative pulmonary surgery services for preparation for LVRS, 1 to 9 days of services ⓑ

* **G0305** Post-discharge pulmonary surgery services after LVRS, minimum of 6 days of services ⓑ

* **G0306** Complete CBC, automated (HgB, HCT, RBC, WBC, without platelet count) and automated WBC differential count ⓑ

* **G0307** Complete CBC, automated (HgB, HCT, RBC, WBC; without platelet count) ⓑ

⊙ **G0328** Colorectal cancer screening; fecal occult blood test, immunoassay, 1-3 simultaneous ⓑ

Co-insurance and deductible waived

Reported for Medicare patients 501; one FOBT per year, with either G0107 (guaiac-based) or G0328 (immunoassay-based)

* **G0329** Electromagnetic therapy, to one or more areas for chronic stage III and stage IV pressure ulcers, arterial ulcers, and diabetic ulcers and venous stasis ulcers not demonstrating measurable signs of healing after 30 days of conventional care as part of a therapy plan of care ⓑ

⊙ **G0333** Pharmacy dispensing fee for inhalation drug(s); initial 30-day supply as a beneficiary ⓑ

Medicare will reimburse an initial dispensing fee to a pharmacy for initial 30-day period of inhalation drugs furnished through DME.

▶ New   ↻ Revised   ✔ Reinstated   ~~deleted~~ Deleted   ⊘ Not covered or valid by Medicare

⊙ Special coverage instructions   * Carrier discretion   ⓑ Bill Part B MAC   ⓑ Bill DME MAC

✳ **G0337** Hospice evaluation and counseling services, pre-election Ⓑ

✳ **G0339** Image-guided robotic linear accelerator-based stereotactic radiosurgery, complete course of therapy in one session or first session of fractionated treatment Ⓑ

✳ **G0340** Image-guided robotic linear accelerator-based stereotactic radiosurgery, delivery including collimator changes and custom plugging, fractionated treatment, all lesions, per session, second through fifth sessions, maximum five sessions per course of treatment Ⓑ

✿ **G0341** Percutaneous islet cell transplant, includes portal vein catheterization and infusion Ⓑ

IOM: 100-03, 4, 260.3; 100-04, 32, 70

✿ **G0342** Laparoscopy for islet cell transplant, includes portal vein catheterization and infusion Ⓑ

IOM: 100-03, 4, 260.3

✿ **G0343** Laparotomy for islet cell transplant, includes portal vein catheterization and infusion Ⓑ

IOM: 100-03, 4, 260.3

~~G0364~~ ~~Bone marrow aspiration performed with bone marrow biopsy through the same incision on the same date of service~~ ✖

✳ **G0365** Vessel mapping of vessels for hemodialysis access (services for preoperative vessel mapping prior to creation of hemodialysis access using an autogenous hemodialysis conduit, including arterial inflow and venous outflow) Ⓑ

Includes evaluation of the relevant arterial and venous vessels. Use modifier 26 for professional component only.

✿ **G0372** Physician service required to establish and document the need for a power mobility device Ⓑ

Providers should bill the E/M code and G0372 on the same claim.

Hospital Services: Observation and Emergency Department

✿ **G0378** Hospital observation service, per hour Ⓑ

Report all related services in addition to G0378. Report units of hours spent in observation (rounded to the nearest hour). Hospitals report the ED or clinic visit with a CPT code or, if applicable, G0379 (direct admit to observation) and G0378 (hospital observation services, per hour).

✿ **G0379** Direct admission of patient for hospital observation care Ⓑ

Report all related services in addition to G0379. Report units of hours spent in observation (rounded to the nearest hour). Hospitals report the ED or clinic visit with a CPT code or, if applicable, G0379 (direct admit to observation) and G0378 (hospital observation services, per hour).

✳ **G0380** Level 1 hospital emergency department visit provided in a type B emergency department; (the ED must meet at least one of the following requirements: (1) it is licensed by the state in which it is located under applicable state law as an emergency room or emergency department; (2) it is held out to the public (by name, posted signs, advertising, or other means) as a place that provides care for emergency medical conditions on an urgent basis without requiring a previously scheduled appointment; or (3) during the calendar year immediately preceding the calendar year in which a determination under 42 CFR 489.24 is being made, based on a representative sample of patient visits that occurred during that calendar year, it provides at least one-third of all of its outpatient visits for the treatment of emergency medical conditions on an urgent basis without requiring a previously scheduled appointment) Ⓑ

▶ **New**   ↻ **Revised**   ✔ **Reinstated**   ~~deleted~~ **Deleted**   ⊘ **Not covered or valid by Medicare**
✿ **Special coverage instructions**   ✳ **Carrier discretion**   Ⓑ **Bill Part B MAC**   Ⓑ **Bill DME MAC**

✳ **G0381** Level 2 hospital emergency department visit provided in a type B emergency department; (the ED must meet at least one of the following requirements: (1) it is licensed by the state in which it is located under applicable state law as an emergency room or emergency department; (2) it is held out to the public (by name, posted signs, advertising, or other means) as a place that provides care for emergency medical conditions on an urgent basis without requiring a previously scheduled appointment; or (3) during the calendar year immediately preceding the calendar year in which a determination under 42 CFR 489.24 is being made, based on a representative sample of patient visits that occurred during that calendar year, it provides at least one-third of all of its outpatient visits for the treatment of emergency medical conditions on an urgent basis without requiring a previously scheduled appointment) ⑧

✳ **G0382** Level 3 hospital emergency department visit provided in a type B emergency department; (the ED must meet at least one of the following requirements: (1) it is licensed by the state in which it is located under applicable state law as an emergency room or emergency department; (2) it is held out to the public (by name, posted signs, advertising, or other means) as a place that provides care for emergency medical conditions on an urgent basis without requiring a previously scheduled appointment; or (3) during the calendar year immediately preceding the calendar year in which a determination under 42 CFR 489.24 is being made, based on a representative sample of patient visits that occurred during that calendar year, it provides at least one-third of all of its outpatient visits for the treatment of emergency medical conditions on an urgent basis without requiring a previously scheduled appointment) ⑧

✳ **G0383** Level 4 hospital emergency department visit provided in a type B emergency department; (the ED must meet at least one of the following requirements: (1) it is licensed by the state in which it is located under applicable state law as an emergency room or emergency department; (2) it is held out to the public (by name, posted signs, advertising, or other means) as a place that provides care for emergency medical conditions on an urgent basis without requiring a previously scheduled appointment; or (3) during the calendar year immediately preceding the calendar year in which a determination under 42 CFR 489.24 is being made, based on a representative sample of patient visits that occurred during that calendar year, it provides at least one-third of all of its outpatient visits for the treatment of emergency medical conditions on an urgent basis without requiring a previously scheduled appointment) ⑧

✳ **G0384** Level 5 hospital emergency department visit provided in a type B emergency department; (the ED must meet at least one of the following requirements: (1) it is licensed by the state in which it is located under applicable state law as an emergency room or emergency department; (2) it is held out to the public (by name, posted signs, advertising, or other means) as a place that provides care for emergency medical conditions on an urgent basis without requiring a previously scheduled appointment; or (3) during the calendar year immediately preceding the calendar year in which a determination under 42 CFR 489.24 is being made, based on a representative sample of patient visits that occurred during that calendar year, it provides at least one-third of all of its outpatient visits for the treatment of emergency medical conditions on an urgent basis without requiring a previously scheduled appointment) ⑧

Trauma Response Team

✪ **G0390** Trauma response team associated with hospital critical care service ⑧

Alcohol Substance Abuse Assessment and Intervention

✳ **G0396**   Alcohol and/or substance (other than tobacco) abuse structured assessment (e.g., audit, DAST), and brief intervention 15 to 30 minutes ⑬

Bill instead of 99408 and 99409

✳ **G0397**   Alcohol and/or substance (other than tobacco) abuse structured assessment (e.g., audit, DAST), and intervention, greater than 30 minutes ⑬

Bill instead of 99408 and 99409

Home Sleep Study Test

✳ **G0398**   Home sleep study test (HST) with type II portable monitor, unattended; minimum of 7 channels: EEG, EOG, EMG, ECG/heart rate, airflow, respiratory effort and oxygen saturation ⑬

✳ **G0399**   Home sleep test (HST) with type III portable monitor, unattended; minimum of 4 channels: 2 respiratory movement/airflow, 1 ECG/heart rate and 1 oxygen saturation ⑬

✳ **G0400**   Home sleep test (HST) with type IV portable monitor, unattended; minimum of 3 channels ⑬

Initial Examination for Medicare Enrollment

✳ **G0402**   Initial preventive physical examination; face-to-face visit, services limited to new beneficiary during the first 12 months of Medicare enrollment ⑬

Depending on circumstances, 99201-99215 may be assigned with modifier 25 to report an E/M service as a significant, separately identifiable service in addition to the Initial Preventive Physical Examination (IPPE), G0402.

Copayment and coinsurance waived, deductible waived.

Electrocardiogram

✳ **G0403**   Electrocardiogram, routine ECG with 12 leads; performed as a screening for the initial preventive physical examination with interpretation and report ⑬

Optional service may be ordered or performed at discretion of physician. Once in a life-time screening, stemming from a referral from Initial Preventive Physical Examination (IPPE). Both deductible and co-payment apply.

✳ **G0404**   Electrocardiogram, routine ECG with 12 leads; tracing only, without interpretation and report, performed as a screening for the initial preventive physical examination ⑬

✳ **G0405**   Electrocardiogram, routine ECG with 12 leads; interpretation and report only, performed as a screening for the initial preventive physical examination ⑬

Follow-up Telehealth Consultation

✳ **G0406**   Follow-up inpatient consultation, limited, physicians typically spend 15 minutes communicating with the patient via telehealth ⑬

These telehealth modifers are required when billing for telehealth services with codes G0406-G0408 and G0425-G0427:

- GT, via interactive audio and video telecommunications system
- GQ, via asynchronous telecommunications system

✳ **G0407**   Follow-up inpatient consultation, intermediate, physicians typically spend 25 minutes communicating with the patient via telehealth ⑬

✳ **G0408**   Follow-up inpatient consultation, complex, physicians typically spend 35 minutes communicating with the patient via telehealth ⑬

Psychological Services

✳ **G0409**   Social work and psychological services, directly relating to and/or furthering the patient's rehabilitation goals, each 15 minutes, face-to-face; individual (services provided by a CORF-qualified social worker or psychologist in a CORF) ⑬

▶ **New**   ↻ **Revised**   ✔ **Reinstated**   ~~deleted~~ **Deleted**   ⊘ **Not covered or valid by Medicare**

✪ **Special coverage instructions**   ✳ **Carrier discretion**   ⑬ **Bill Part B MAC**   ⑬ **Bill DME MAC**

* **G0410** Group psychotherapy other than of a multiple-family group, in a partial hospitalization setting, approximately 45 to 50 minutes Ⓑ

* **G0411** Interactive group psychotherapy, in a partial hospitalization setting, approximately 45 to 50 minutes Ⓑ

Fracture Treatment

* **G0412** Open treatment of iliac spine(s), tuberosity avulsion, or iliac wing fracture(s), unilateral or bilateral for pelvic bone fracture patterns which do not disrupt the pelvic ring includes internal fixation, when performed Ⓑ

* **G0413** Percutaneous skeletal fixation of posterior pelvic bone fracture and/or dislocation, for fracture patterns which disrupt the pelvic ring, unilateral or bilateral, (includes ilium, sacroiliac joint and/or sacrum) Ⓑ

* **G0414** Open treatment of anterior pelvic bone fracture and/or dislocation for fracture patterns which disrupt the pelvic ring, unilateral or bilateral, includes internal fixation when performed (includes pubic symphysis and/or superior/inferior rami) Ⓑ

* **G0415** Open treatment of posterior pelvic bone fracture and/or dislocation, for fracture patterns which disrupt the pelvic ring, unilateral or bilateral, includes internal fixation, when performed (includes ilium, sacroiliac joint and/or sacrum) Ⓑ

Surgical Pathology: Prostate Biopsy

* **G0416** Surgical pathology, gross and microscopic examinations for prostate needle biopsy, any method Ⓑ

This testing requires a facility to have either a CLIA certificate of registration (certificate type code 9), a CLIA certificate of compliance (certificate type code 1), or a CLIA certificate of accreditation (certificate type code 3). A facility without a valid, current, CLIA certificate, with a current CLIA certificate of waiver (certificate type code 2) or with a current CLIA certificate for provider-performed microscopy procedures (certificate type code 4), must not be permitted to be paid for these tests. This code has a TC, 26 (physician), or gobal component.

Educational Services

* **G0420** Face-to-face educational services related to the care of chronic kidney disease; individual, per session, per one hour Ⓑ

CKD is kidney damage of 3months or longer, regardless of the cause of kidney damage. Sessions billed in increments of one hour (if session is less than 1hour, it must last at least 31minutes to be billable. Sessions less than one hour and longer than 31minutes is billable as one session. No more than 6 sessions of KDE services in a beneficiary's lifetime.

* **G0421** Face-to-face educational services related to the care of chronic kidney disease; group, per session, per one hour Ⓑ

Group setting: 2 to 20, report codes G0420 and G0421 with diagnosis code 585.4.

Cardiac and Pulmonary Rehabilitation

* **G0422** Intensive cardiac rehabilitation; with or without continuous ECG monitoring with exercise, per session Ⓑ

Includes the same service as 93798 but at a greater frequency; may be reported with as many as six hourly sessions on a single date of service. Includes medical nutrition services to reduce cardiac disease risk factors.

* **G0423** Intensive cardiac rehabilitation; with or without continuous ECG monitoring; without exercise, per session Ⓑ

Includes the same service as 93797 but at a greater frequency; may be reported with as many as six hourly sessions on a single date of service. Includes medical nutrition services to reduce cardiac disease risk factors.

* **G0424** Pulmonary rehabilitation, including exercise (includes monitoring), one hour, per session, up to two sessions per day Ⓑ

Includes therapeutic services and all related monitoring services to inprove respiratory function. Do not report with G0237, G0238, or G0239.

▶ **New**   ↻ **Revised**   ✔ **Reinstated**   ~~deleted~~ **Deleted**   ⊘ **Not covered or valid by Medicare**

⊛ **Special coverage instructions**   * **Carrier discretion**   Ⓑ **Bill Part B MAC**   Ⓑ **Bill DME MAC**

Initial Telehealth Consultation

✳ **G0425** Telehealth consultation, emergency department or initial inpatient, typically 30 minutes communicating with the patient via telehealth Ⓑ

Problem Focused: Problem focused history and examination, with straightforward medical decision making complexity. Typically 30 minutes communicating with patient via telehealth.

✳ **G0426** Initial inpatient telehealth consultation, emergency department or initial inpatient, typically 50 minutes communicating with the patient via telehealth Ⓑ

Detailed: Detailed history and examination, with moderate medical decision making complexity. Typically 50 minutes communicating with patient via telehealth.

✳ **G0427** Initial inpatient telehealth consultation, emergency department or initial inpatient, typically 70 minutes or more communicating with the patient via telehealth Ⓑ

Comprehensive: Comprehensive history and examination, with high medical decision making complexity. Typically 70 minutes or more communicating with patient via telehealth.

Fillers

⊘ **G0428** Collagen meniscus implant procedure for filling meniscal defects (e.g., cmi, collagen scaffold, menaflex) Ⓑ

✳ **G0429** Dermal filler injection(s) for the treatment of facial lipodystrophy syndrome (LDS) (e.g., as a result of highly active antiretroviral therapy) Ⓑ

Designated for dermal fillers Sculptra® and Radiesse (Medicare). (https://www.cms.gov/ContractorLearningResources/downloads/JA6953.pdf)

Laboratory Screening

✳ **G0432** Infectious agent antibody detection by enzyme immunoassay (EIA) technique, HIV-1 and/or HIV-2, screening Ⓑ

✳ **G0433** Infectious agent antibody detection by enzyme-linked immunosorbent assay (ELISA) technique, HIV-1 and/or HIV-2, screening Ⓑ

Counseling, Wellness, and Screening Services

✳ **G0435** Infectious agent antibody detection by rapid antibody test, HIV-1 and/or HIV-2, screening Ⓑ

✳ **G0438** Annual wellness visit; includes a personalized prevention plan of service (pps), initial visit

✳ **G0439** Annual wellness visit, includes a personalized prevention plan of service (pps), subsequent visit Ⓑ

✳ **G0442** Annual alcohol misuse screening, 15 minutes Ⓑ

✳ **G0443** Brief face-to-face behavioral counseling for alcohol misuse, 15 minutes Ⓑ

✳ **G0444** Annual depression screening, 15 minutes Ⓑ

✳ **G0445** High intensity behavioral counseling to prevent sexually transmitted infection; face-to-face, individual, includes: education, skills training and guidance on how to change sexual behavior; performed semi-annually, 30 minutes Ⓑ

✳ **G0446** Annual, face-to-face intensive behavioral therapy for cardiovascular disease, individual, 15 minutes Ⓑ

✳ **G0447** Face-to-face behavioral counseling for obesity, 15 minutes Ⓑ

✳ **G0448** Insertion or replacement of a permanent pacing cardioverter-defibrillator system with transvenous lead(s), single or dual chamber with insertion of pacing electrode, cardiac venous system, for left ventricular pacing Ⓑ

✳ **G0451** Development testing, with interpretation and report, per standardized instrument form Ⓑ

Miscellaneous Services

✳ **G0452** Molecular pathology procedure; physician interpretation and report Ⓑ

✳ **G0453** Continuous intraoperative neurophysiology monitoring, from outside the operating room (remote or nearby), per patient, (attention directed exclusively to one patient) each 15 minutes (list in addition to primary procedure) Ⓑ

✳ **G0454** Physician documentation of face-to-face visit for durable medical equipment determination performed by nurse practitioner, physician assistant or clinical nurse specialist Ⓑ

▶ **New** ↻ **Revised** ✔ **Reinstated** ~~deleted~~ **Deleted** ⊘ **Not covered or valid by Medicare**
✪ **Special coverage instructions** ✳ **Carrier discretion** Ⓑ **Bill Part B MAC** Ⓓ **Bill DME MAC**

* **G0455** Preparation with instillation of fecal microbiota by any method, including assessment of donor specimen Ⓑ

↻ * **G0458** Low dose rate (LDR) prostate brachytherapy services, composite rate Ⓑ

* **G0459** Inpatient telehealth pharmacologic management, including prescription, use, and review of medication with no more than minimal medical psychotherapy Ⓑ

* **G0460** Autologous platelet rich plasma for chronic wounds/ulcers, including phlebotomy, centrifugation, and all other preparatory procedures, administration and dressings, per treatment Ⓑ

* **G0463** Hospital outpatient clinic visit for assessment and management of a patient Ⓑ

* **G0464** Colorectal cancer screening; stool-based DNA and fecal occult hemoglobin (e.g., KRAS, NDRG4 and BMP3) Ⓠ

Cross Reference 81528

Federally Qualified Health Center Visits

* **G0466** Federally qualified health center (FQHC) visit, new patient; a medically-necessary, face-to-face encounter (one-on-one) between a new patient and a FQHC practitioner during which time one or more FQHC services are rendered and includes a typical bundle of Medicare-covered services that would be furnished per diem to a patient receiving a FQHC visit Ⓑ

* **G0467** Federally qualified health center (FQHC) visit, established patient; a medically-necessary, face-to-face encounter (one-on-one) between an established patient and a FQHC practitioner during which time one or more FQHC services are rendered and includes a typical bundle of Medicare-covered services that would be furnished per diem to a patient receiving a FQHC visit Ⓑ

* **G0468** Federally qualified health center (FQHC) visit, IPPE or AWV; a FQHC visit that includes an initial preventive physical examination (IPPE) or annual wellness visit (AWV) and includes a typical bundle of Medicare-covered services that would be furnished per diem to a patient receiving an IPPE or AWV Ⓠ

* **G0469** Federally qualified health center (FQHC) visit, mental health, new patient; a medically-necessary, face-to-face mental health encounter (one-on-one) between a new patient and a FQHC practitioner during which time one or more FQHC services are rendered and includes a typical bundle of Medicare-covered services that would be furnished per diem to a patient receiving a mental health visit Ⓑ

* **G0470** Federally qualified health center (FQHC) visit, mental health, established patient; a medically-necessary, face-to-face mental health encounter (one-on-one) between an established patient and a FQHC practitioner during which time one or more FQHC services are rendered and includes a typical bundle of Medicare-covered services that would be furnished per diem to a patient receiving a mental health visit Ⓑ

Other Miscellaneous Services

* **G0471** Collection of venous blood by venipuncture or urine sample by catheterization from an individual in a skilled nursing facility (SNF) or by a laboratory on behalf of a home health agency (HHA) Ⓠ

⊚ **G0472** Hepatitis C antibody screening, for individual at high risk and other covered indication(s) Ⓑ

* **G0473** Face-to-face behavioral counseling for obesity, group (2-10), 30 minutes Ⓑ

* **G0475** HIV antigen/antibody, combination assay, screening Ⓑ

* **G0476** Infectious agent detection by nucleic acid (DNA or RNA); human papillomavirus (HPV), high-risk types (e.g., 16, 18, 31, 33, 35, 39, 45, 51, 52, 56, 58, 59, 68) for cervical cancer screening, must be performed in addition to pap test Ⓠ

▶ **New**   ↻ **Revised**   ✔ **Reinstated**   ~~deleted~~ **Deleted**   ⊘ **Not covered or valid by Medicare**
⊛ **Special coverage instructions**   * **Carrier discretion**   Ⓠ **Bill Part B MAC**   Ⓑ **Bill DME MAC**

Drug Tests

✳ **G0480** Drug test(s), definitive, utilizing drug identification methods able to identify individual drugs and distinguish between structural isomers (but not necessarily stereoisomers), including, but not limited to GC/MS (any type, single or tandem) and LC/MS (any type, single or tandem and excluding immunoassays (e.g., IA, EIA, ELISA, EMIT, FPIA) and enzymatic methods (e.g., alcohol dehydrogenase)); qualitative or quantitative, all sources(s), includes specimen validity testing, per day, 1-7 drug class(es), including metabolite(s) if performed Ⓑ

✳ **G0481** Drug test(s), definitive, utilizing drug identification methods able to identify individual drugs and distinguish between structural isomers (but not necessarily stereoisomers), including, but not limited to GC/MS (any type, single or tandem) and LC/MS (any type, single or tandem and excluding immunoassays (e.g., IA, EIA, ELISA, EMIT, FPIA) and enzymatic methods (e.g., alcohol dehydrogenase); qualitative or quantitative, all sources(s), includes specimen validity testing, per day, 8-14 drug class(es), including metabolite(s) if performed Ⓑ

✳ **G0482** Drug test(s), definitive, utilizing drug identification methods able to identify individual drugs and distinguish between structural isomers (but not necessarily stereoisomers), including, but not limited to GC/MS (any type, single or tandem) and LC/MS (any type, single or tandem and excluding immunoassays (e.g., IA, EIA, ELISA, EMIT, FPIA) and enzymatic methods (e.g., alcohol dehydrogenase); qualitative or quantitative, all sources(s), includes specimen validity testing, per day, 15-21 drug class(es), including metabolite(s) if performed Ⓑ

✳ **G0483** Drug test(s), definitive, utilizing drug identification methods able to identify individual drugs and distinguish between structural isomers (but not necessarily stereoisomers), including, but not limited to GC/MS (any type, single or tandem) and LC/MS (any type, single or tandem and excluding immunoassays (e.g., IA, EIA, ELISA, EMIT, FPIA) and enzymatic methods (e.g., alcohol dehydrogenase); qualitative or quantitative, all sources(s), includes specimen validity testing, per day, 22 or more drug class(es), including metabolite(s) if performed Ⓑ

Home Health Nursing Visit: Area of Shortage

✳ **G0490** Face-to-face home health nursing visit by a rural health clinic (RHC) or federally qualified health center (FQHC) in an area with a shortage of home health agencies; (services limited to RN or LPN only) Ⓑ

Dialysis Procedure

✳ **G0491** Dialysis procedure at a Medicare certified esrd facility for acute kidney injury without ESRD Ⓑ

✳ **G0492** Dialysis procedure with single evaluation by a physician or other qualified health care professional for acute kidney injury without ESRD Ⓑ

Home Health or Hospice: Skilled Services

✳ **G0493** Skilled services of a registered nurse (RN) for the observation and assessment of the patient's condition, each 15 minutes (the change in the patient's condition requires skilled nursing personnel to identify and evaluate the patient's need for possible modification of treatment in the home health or hospice setting) Ⓑ

✳ **G0494** Skilled services of a licensed practical nurse (LPN) for the observation and assessment of the patient's condition, each 15 minutes (the change in the patient's condition requires skilled nursing personnel to identify and evaluate the patient's need for possible modification of treatment in the home health or hospice setting) Ⓑ

* **G0495** Skilled services of a registered nurse (RN), in the training and/or education of a patient or family member, in the home health or hospice setting, each 15 minutes Ⓑ

* **G0496** Skilled services of a licensed practical nurse (LPN), in the training and/or education of a patient or family member, in the home health or hospice setting, each 15 minutes Ⓑ

Chemotherapy Administration

* **G0498** Chemotherapy administration, intravenous infusion technique; initiation of infusion in the office/clinic setting using office/clinic pump/ supplies, with continuation of the infusion in the community setting (e.g., home, domiciliary, rest home or assisted living) using a portable pump provided by the office/clinic, includes follow up office/clinic visit at the conclusion of the infusion Ⓑ

Hepatitis B Screening

* **G0499** Hepatitis B screening in non-pregnant, high risk individual includes hepatitis B surface antigen (HBsAG) followed by a neutralizing confirmatory test for initially reactive results, and antibodies to HBsAG (anti-HBs) and hepatitis b core antigen (anti-hbc) Ⓑ

Moderate Sedation Services

* **G0500** Moderate sedation services provided by the same physician or other qualified health care professional performing a gastrointestinal endoscopic service that sedation supports, requiring the presence of an independent trained observer to assist in the monitoring of the patient's level of consciousness and physiological status; initial 15 minutes of intra-service time; patient age 5 years or older (additional time may be reported with 99153, as appropriate) Ⓑ

Resource-Intensive Service

* **G0501** Resource-intensive services for patients for whom the use of specialized mobility-assistive technology (such as adjustable height chairs or tables, patient lift, and adjustable padded leg supports) is medically necessary and used during the provision of an office/ outpatient, evaluation and management visit (list separately in addition to primary service) Ⓑ

Psychiatric Care Management

~~G0502~~ ~~Initial psychiatric collaborative care management, first 70 minutes in the first calendar month of behavioral health care manager activities, in consultation with a psychiatric consultant, and directed by the treating physician or other qualified health care professional, with the following required elements: outreach to and engagement in treatment of a patient directed by the treating physician or other qualified health care professional; initial assessment of the patient, including administration of validated rating scales, with the development of an individualized treatment plan; review by the psychiatric consultant with modifications of the plan if recommended; entering patient in a registry and tracking patient follow-up and progress using the registry, with appropriate documentation, and participation in weekly caseload consultation with the psychiatric consultant; and provision of brief interventions using evidence-based techniques such as behavioral activation, motivational interviewing, and other focused treatment strategies~~ ✖

Cross Reference 99492

▶ **New**   ↻ **Revised**   ✔ **Reinstated**   ~~deleted~~ **Deleted**   ⊘ **Not covered or valid by Medicare**
⊛ **Special coverage instructions**   * **Carrier discretion**   Ⓑ **Bill Part B MAC**   Ⓑ **Bill DME MAC**

G0503 ~~Subsequent psychiatric collaborative care management, first 60 minutes in a subsequent month of behavioral health care manager activities, in consultation with a psychiatric consultant, and directed by the treating physician or other qualified health care professional, with the following required elements: tracking patient follow-up and progress using the registry, with appropriate documentation; participation in weekly caseload consultation with the psychiatric consultant; ongoing collaboration with and coordination of the patient's mental health care with the treating physician or other qualified health care professional and any other treating mental health providers; additional review of progress and recommendations for changes in treatment, as indicated, including medications, based on recommendations provided by the psychiatric consultant; provision of brief interventions using evidence-based techniques such as behavioral activation, motivational interviewing, and other focused treatment strategies; monitoring of patient outcomes using validated rating scales; and relapse prevention planning with patients as they achieve remission of symptoms and/or other treatment goals and are prepared for discharge from active treatment~~ ✖

Cross Reference 99493

G0504 ~~Initial or subsequent psychiatric collaborative care management, each additional 30 minutes in a calendar month of behavioral health care manager activities, in consultation with a psychiatric consultant, and directed by the treating physician or other qualified health care professional (list separately in addition to code for primary procedure); (use G0504 in conjunction with G0502, G0503)~~ ✖

Cross Reference 99494

G0505 ~~Cognition and functional assessment using standardized instruments with development of recorded care plan for the patient with cognitive impairment, history obtained from patient and/or caregiver, in office or other outpatient setting or home or domiciliary or rest home~~ ✖

Cross Reference 99483

✳ **G0506** Comprehensive assessment of and care planning for patients requiring chronic care management services (list separately in addition to primary monthly care management service) Ⓑ

G0507 ~~Care services for behavioral health conditions, at least 20 minutes of clinical staff time, directed by a physician or other qualified health care professional, per calendar month, with the following required elements: initial assessment or follow-up monitoring, including the use of applicable validated rating scales; behavioral health care planning in relation to behavioral/psychiatric health problems, including revision for patients who are not progressing or whose status changes; facilitating and coordinating treatment such as psychotherapy, pharmacotherapy, counseling and/or psychiatric consultation; and continuity of care with a designated member of the care team~~ ✖

Cross Reference 99484

Critical Care Telehealth Consultation

✳ **G0508** Telehealth consultation, critical care, initial , physicians typically spend 60 minutes communicating with the patient and providers via telehealth Ⓑ

✳ **G0509** Telehealth consultation, critical care, subsequent, physicians typically spend 50 minutes communicating with the patient and providers via telehealth Ⓑ

Rural Health Clinic: Management and Care

▶ ✪ **G0511** Rural health clinic or federally qualified health center (RHC or FQHC) only, general care management, 20 minutes or more of clinical staff time for chronic care management services or behavioral health integration services directed by an RHC or FQHC practitioner (physician, NP, PA, or CNM), per calendar month

---

▶ ⊙ **G0512** Rural health clinic or federally qualified health center (RHC/FQHC) only, psychiatric collaborative care model (psychiatric CoCM), 60 minutes or more of clinical staff time for psychiatric CoCM services directed by an RHC or FQHC practitioner (physician, NP, PA, or CNM) and including services furnished by a behavioral health care manager and consultation with a psychiatric consultant, per calendar month

Prolonged Preventive Services

▶ ✳ **G0513** Prolonged preventive service(s) (beyond the typical service time of the primary procedure), in the office or other outpatient setting requiring direct patient contact beyond the usual service; first 30 minutes (list separately in addition to code for preventive service)

▶ ✳ **G0514** Prolonged preventive service(s) (beyond the typical service time of the primary procedure), in the office or other outpatient setting requiring direct patient contact beyond the usual service; each additional 30 minutes (list separately in addition to code G0513 for additional 30 minutes of preventive service)

Cognitive Development

▶ ✳ **G0515** Development of cognitive skills to improve attention, memory, problem solving (includes compensatory training), direct (one-on-one) patient contact, each 15 minutes

Non-biodegradable Drug Delivery Implants: Removal and Insertion

▶ ✳ **G0516** Insertion of non-biodegradable drug delivery implants, 4 or more (services for subdermal rod implant)

▶ ✳ **G0517** Removal of non-biodegradable drug delivery implants, 4 or more (services for subdermal implants)

▶ ✳ **G0518** Removal with reinsertion, non-biodegradable drug delivery implants, 4 or more (services for subdermal implants)

Drug Test

✳ **G0659** Drug test(s), definitive, utilizing drug identification methods able to identify individual drugs and distinguish between structural isomers (but not necessarily stereoisomers), including but not limited to GC/MS (any type, single or tandem) and LC/MS (any type, single or tandem), excluding immunoassays (e.g., IA, EIA, ELISA, EMIT, FPIA) and enzymatic methods (e.g., alcohol dehydrogenase), performed without method or drug-specific calibration, without matrix-matched quality control material, or without use of stable isotope or other universally recognized internal standard(s) for each drug, drug metabolite or drug class per specimen; qualitative or quantitative, all sources, includes specimen validity testing, per day, any number of drug classes

Quality Care Measures: Cataract Surgery

✳ **G0913** Improvement in visual function achieved within 90 days following cataract surgery ⑧

✳ **G0914** Patient care survey was not completed by patient ⑧

✳ **G0915** Improvement in visual function not achieved within 90 days following cataract surgery ⑧

✳ **G0916** Satisfaction with care achieved within 90 days following cataract surgery ⑧

✳ **G0917** Patient satisfaction survey was not completed by patient ⑧

✳ **G0918** Satisfaction with care not achieved within 90 days following cataract surgery ⑧

Guidance

⊙ **G6001** Ultrasonic guidance for placement of radiation therapy fields ⑧

✳ **G6002** Stereoscopic x-ray guidance for localization of target volume for the delivery of radiation therapy ⑧

▶ **New** ⟳ **Revised** ✔ **Reinstated** ~~deleted~~ **Deleted** ⊘ **Not covered or valid by Medicare**
⊙ **Special coverage instructions** ✳ **Carrier discretion** ⑨ **Bill Part B MAC** ⑧ **Bill DME MAC**

Radiation Treatment

* **G6003** Radiation treatment delivery, single treatment area, single port or parallel opposed ports, simple blocks or no blocks: up to 5 mev Ⓑ

* **G6004** Radiation treatment delivery, single treatment area, single port or parallel opposed ports, simple blocks or no blocks: 6-10 mev Ⓑ

* **G6005** Radiation treatment delivery, single treatment area, single port or parallel opposed ports, simple blocks or no blocks: 11-19 mev Ⓑ

* **G6006** Radiation treatment delivery, single treatment area, single port or parallel opposed ports, simple blocks or no blocks: 20 mev or greater Ⓑ

* **G6007** Radiation treatment delivery, 2 separate treatment areas, 3 or more ports on a single treatment area, use of multiple blocks: up to 5 mev Ⓑ

* **G6008** Radiation treatment delivery, 2 separate treatment areas, 3 or more ports on a single treatment area, use of multiple blocks: 6-10 mev Ⓑ

* **G6009** Radiation treatment delivery, 2 separate treatment areas, 3 or more ports on a single treatment area, use of multiple blocks: 11-19 mev Ⓑ

* **G6010** Radiation treatment delivery, 2 separate treatment areas, 3 or more ports on a single treatment area, use of multiple blocks: 20 mev or greater Ⓑ

* **G6011** Radiation treatment delivery, 3 or more separate treatment areas, custom blocking, tangential ports, wedges, rotational beam, compensators, electron beam; up to 5 mev Ⓑ

* **G6012** Radiation treatment delivery, 3 or more separate treatment areas, custom blocking, tangential ports, wedges, rotational beam, compensators, electron beam; 6-10 mev Ⓑ

* **G6013** Radiation treatment delivery, 3 or more separate treatment areas, custom blocking, tangential ports, wedges, rotational beam, compensators, electron beam; 11-19 mev Ⓑ

* **G6014** Radiation treatment delivery, 3 or more separate treatment areas, custom blocking, tangential ports, wedges, rotational beam, compensators, electron beam; 20 mev or greater Ⓑ

* **G6015** Intensity modulated treatment delivery, single or multiple fields/arcs, via narrow spatially and temporally modulated beams, binary, dynamic MLC, per treatment session Ⓑ

* **G6016** Compensator-based beam modulation treatment delivery of inverse planned treatment using 3 or more high resolution (milled or cast) compensator, convergent beam modulated fields, per treatment session Ⓑ

* **G6017** Intra-fraction localization and tracking of target or patient motion during delivery of radiation therapy (e.g., 3D positional tracking, gating, 3D surface tracking), each fraction of treatment Ⓑ

Quality Measures

* **G8395** Left ventricular ejection fraction (LVEF)> = 40% or documentation as normal or mildly depressed left ventricular systolic function Ⓑ

* **G8396** Left ventricular ejection fraction (LVEF) not performed or documented Ⓑ

* **G8397** Dilated macular or fundus exam performed, including documentation of the presence or absence of macular edema and level of severity of retinopathy Ⓑ

* **G8398** Dilated macular or fundus exam not performed Ⓑ

* **G8399** Patient with documented results of a central dual-energy x-ray absorptiometry (DXA) ever being performed Ⓑ

* **G8400** Patient with central dual-energy x-ray absorptiometry (DXA) results not documented Ⓑ

* **G8404** Lower extremity neurological exam performed and documented Ⓑ

* **G8405** Lower extremity neurological exam not performed Ⓑ

* **G8410** Footwear evaluation performed and documented Ⓑ

* **G8415** Footwear evaluation was not performed Ⓑ

* **G8416** Clinician documented that patient was not an eligible candidate for footwear evaluation measure Ⓑ

* **G8417** BMI is documented above normal parameters and a follow-up plan is documented Ⓑ

▶ New   ↻ Revised   ✔ Reinstated   ~~deleted~~ Deleted   ⊘ Not covered or valid by Medicare

☺ Special coverage instructions   ✳ Carrier discretion   Ⓑ Bill Part B MAC   Ⓓ Bill DME MAC

* **G8418** BMI is documented below normal parameters and a follow-up plan is documented ⑧

* **G8419** BMI is documented outside normal parameters, no follow-up plan documented, no reason given ⑧

* **G8420** BMI is documented within normal parameters and no follow-up plan is required ⑧

* **G8421** BMI not documented and no reason is given ⑧

* **G8422** BMI not documented, documentation the patient is not eligible for BMI calculation ⑧

* **G8427** Eligible clinician attests to documenting in the medical record they obtained, updated, or reviewed the patient's current medications ⑧

* **G8428** Current list of medications not documented as obtained, updated, or reviewed by the eligible clinician, reason not given ⑧

↻ * **G8430** Eligible clinician attests to documenting in the medical record the patient is not eligible for a current list of medications being obtained, updated, or reviewed by the eligible clinician ⑧

* **G8431** Screening for depression is documented as being positive and a follow-up plan is documented ⑧

* **G8432** Depression screening not documented, reason not given ⑧

↻ * **G8433** Screening for depression not completed, documented reason ⑧

↻ * **G8442** Pain assessment not documented as being performed, documentation the patient is not eligible for a pain assessment using a standardized tool at the time of the encounter ⑧

* **G8450** Beta-blocker therapy prescribed ⑧

* **G8451** beta therapy for LVEF < 40% not prescribed for reasons documented by the clinician (e.g., low blood pressure, fluid overload, asthma, patients recently treated with an intravenous positive inotropic agent, allergy, intolerance, other medical reasons, patient declined, other patient reasons or other reasons attributable to the healthcare system) ⑧

* **G8452** Beta-blocker therapy not prescribed ⑧

* **G8465** High or very high risk of recurrence of prostate cancer ⑧

* **G8473** Angiotensin converting enzyme (ACE) inhibitor or angiotensin receptor blocker (ARB) therapy prescribed ⑧

* **G8474** Angiotensin converting enzyme (ACE) inhibitor or angiotensin receptor blocker (ARB) therapy not prescribed for reasons documented by the clinician (e.g., allergy, intolerance, pregnancy, renal failure due to ACE inhibitor, diseases of the aortic or mitral valve, other medical reasons) or (e.g., patient declined, other patient reasons) or (e.g., lack of drug availability, other reasons attributable to the health care system) ⑧

* **G8475** Angiotensin converting enzyme (ACE) inhibitor or angiotensin receptor blocker (ARB) therapy not prescribed, reason not given ⑧

* **G8476** Most recent blood pressure has a systolic measurement of < 140 mmHg and a diastolic measurement of < 90 mmHg ⑧

* **G8477** Most recent blood pressure has a systolic measurement of > = 140 mmHg and/or a diastolic measurement of > = 90 mmHg ⑧

* **G8478** Blood pressure measurement not performed or documented, reason not given ⑧

* **G8482** Influenza immunization administered or previously received ⑧

* **G8483** Influenza immunization was not administered for reasons documented by clinician (e.g., patient allergy or other medical reasons, patient declined or other patient reasons, vacine not available or other system reasons) ⑧

* **G8484** Influenza immunization was not administered, reason not given ⑧

* **G8506** Patient receiving angiotensin converting enzyme (ACE) inhibitor or angiotensin receptor blocker (ARB) therapy ⑧

* **G8509** Pain assessment documented as positive using a standardized tool, follow-up plan not documented, reason not given ⑧

* **G8510** Screening for depression is documented as negative, a follow-up plan is not required ⑧

* **G8511** Screening for depression documented as positive, follow up plan not documented, reason not given ⑧

▶ **New**   ↻ **Revised**   ✔ **Reinstated**   ~~deleted~~ **Deleted**   ⊘ **Not covered or valid by Medicare**
⊙ **Special coverage instructions**   ✳ **Carrier discretion**   ⑧ **Bill Part B MAC**   ⑧ **Bill DME MAC**

↻ ✳ **G8535** Elder maltreatment screen not documented; documentation that patient is not eligible for the elder maltreatment screen at the time of the encounter Ⓑ

✳ **G8536** No documentation of an elder maltreatment screen, reason not given Ⓑ

✳ **G8539** Functional outcome assessment documented as positive using a standardized tool and a care plan based on identified deficiencies on the date of functional outcome assessment is documented Ⓑ

↻ ✳ **G8540** Functional outcome assessment not documented as being performed, documentation the patient is not eligible for a functional outcome assessment using a standardized tool at the time of the encounter Ⓑ

✳ **G8541** Functional outcome assessment using a standardized tool not documented, reason not given Ⓑ

✳ **G8542** Functional outcome assessment using a standardized tool is documented; no functional deficiencies identified, care plan not required Ⓑ

✳ **G8543** Documentation of a positive functional outcome assessment using a standardized tool; care plan not documented, reason not given Ⓑ

✳ **G8559** Patient referred to a physician (preferably a physician with training in disorders of the ear) for an otologic evaluation Ⓑ

✳ **G8560** Patient has a history of active drainage from the ear within the previous 90 days Ⓑ

✳ **G8561** Patient is not eligible for the referral for otologic evaluation for patients with a history of active drainage measure Ⓑ

✳ **G8562** Patient does not have a history of active drainage from the ear within the previous 90 days Ⓑ

✳ **G8563** Patient not referred to a physician (preferably a physician with training in disorders of the ear) for an otologic evaluation, reason not given Ⓑ

✳ **G8564** Patient was referred to a physician (preferably a physician with training in disorders of the ear) for an otologic evaluation, reason not specified) Ⓑ

✳ **G8565** Verification and documentation of sudden or rapidly progressive hearing loss Ⓑ

✳ **G8566** Patient is not eligible for the "referral for otologic evaluation for sudden or rapidly progressive hearing loss" measure Ⓑ

✳ **G8567** Patient does not have verification and documentation of sudden or rapidly progressive hearing loss Ⓑ

✳ **G8568** Patient was not referred to a physician (preferably a physician with training in disorders of the ear) for an otologic evaluation, reason not given Ⓑ

✳ **G8569** Prolonged postoperative intubation (>24 hrs) required Ⓑ

✳ **G8570** Prolonged postoperative intubation (>24 hrs) not required Ⓑ

✳ **G8571** Development of deep sternal wound infection/mediastinitis within 30 days postoperatively Ⓑ

✳ **G8572** No deep sternal wound infection/mediastinitis Ⓑ

✳ **G8573** Stroke following isolated CABG surgery Ⓑ

✳ **G8574** No stroke following isolated CABG surgery Ⓑ

✳ **G8575** Developed postoperative renal failure or required dialysis Ⓑ

✳ **G8576** No postoperative renal failure/dialysis not required Ⓑ

✳ **G8577** Re-exploration required due to mediastinal bleeding with or without tamponade, graft occlusion, valve disfunction, or other cardiac reason Ⓑ

✳ **G8578** Re-exploration not required due to mediastinal bleeding with or without tamponade, graft occlusion, valve dysfunction, or other cardiac reason Ⓑ

✳ **G8598** Aspirin or another antiplatelet therapy used Ⓑ

✳ **G8599** Aspirin or another antiplatelet therapy not used, reason not given Ⓑ

✳ **G8600** IV T-PA initiated within three hours (<= 180 minutes) of time last known well Ⓑ

✳ **G8601** IV T-PA not initiated within three hours (<= 180 minutes) of time last known well for reasons documented by clinician Ⓑ

✳ **G8602** IV T-PA not initiated within three hours (<= 180 minutes) of time last known well, reason not given Ⓑ

▶ New	↻ Revised	✔ Reinstated	~~deleted~~ Deleted	⊘ Not covered or valid by Medicare
✪ Special coverage instructions		✳ Carrier discretion	Ⓑ Bill Part B MAC	Ⓓ Bill DME MAC

∗ **G8627** Surgical procedure performed within 30 days following cataract surgery for major complications (e.g., retained nuclear fragments, endophthalmitis, dislocated or wrong power IOL, retinal detachment, or wound dehiscence) ⓖ

∗ **G8628** Surgical procedure not performed within 30 days following cataract surgery for major complications (e.g., retained nuclear fragments, endophthalmitis, dislocated or wrong power IOL, retinal detachment, or wound dehiscence) ⓑ

∗ **G8633** Pharmacologic therapy (other than minierals/vitamins) for osteoporosis prescribed ⓖ

∗ **G8635** Pharmacologic therapy for osteoporosis was not prescribed, reason not given ⓑ

∗ **G8647** Risk-adjusted functional status change residual score for the knee successfully calculated and the score was equal to zero (0) or greater than zero (>0) ⓑ

∗ **G8648** Risk-adjusted functional status change residual score for the knee successfully calculated and the score was less than zero (< 0) ⓑ

∗ **G8649** Risk-adjusted functional status change residual scores for the knee not measured because the patient did not complete FOTO'S status survey near discharge, not appropriate ⓑ

∗ **G8650** Risk-adjusted functional status change residual scores for the knee not measured because the patient did not complete FOTO'S functional intake on admission and/or follow up status survey near discharge, reason not given ⓑ

∗ **G8651** Risk-adjusted functional status change residual score for the hip successfully calculated and the score was equal to zero (0) or greater than zero (>0) ⓑ

∗ **G8652** Risk-adjusted functional status change residual score for the hip successfully calculated and the score was less than zero (< 0) ⓑ

∗ **G8653** Risk-adjusted functional status change residual scores for the hip not measured because the patient did not complete follow up status survey near discharge, patient not appropriate ⓑ

∗ **G8654** Risk-adjusted functional status change residual scores for the hip not measured because the patient did not complete FOTO'S functional intake on admission and/or follow up status survey near discharge, reason not given ⓑ

∗ **G8655** Risk-adjusted functional status change residual score for the foot or ankle successfully calculated and the score was equal to zero (0) or greater than zero (>0) ⓑ

∗ **G8656** Risk-adjusted functional status change residual score for the foot or ankle successfully calculated and the score was less than zero (< 0) ⓑ

∗ **G8657** Risk-adjusted functional status change residual scores for the foot or ankle not measured because the patient did not complete FOTO'S status survey near discharge, patient not appropriate ⓑ

∗ **G8658** Risk-adjusted functional status change residual scores for the foot or ankle not measured because the patient did not complete FOTO'S functional intake on admission and/or follow up status survey near discharge, reason not given ⓑ

∗ **G8659** Risk-adjusted functional status change residual score for the lumbar impairment successfully calculated and the score was equal to zero (0) or greater than zero (> 0) ⓑ

∗ **G8660** Risk-adjusted functional status change residual score for the lumbar impairment successfully calculated and the score was less than zero (<0) ⓑ

∗ **G8661** Risk-adjusted functional status change residual scores for the lumbar impairment not measured because the patient did not complete FOTO'S status survey near discharge, patient not appropriate ⓑ

∗ **G8662** Risk-adjusted functional status change residual scores for the lumbar impairment not measured because the patient did not complete FOTO'S functional intake on admission and/or follow up status survey near discharge, reason not given ⓑ

∗ **G8663** Risk-adjusted functional status change residual score for the shoulder successfully calculated and the score was equal to zero (0) or greater than zero (>0) ⓑ

∗ **G8664** Risk-adjusted functional status change residual score for the shoulder successfully calculated and the score was less than zero (< 0) ⓑ

⁎ **G8665** Risk-adjusted functional status change residual scores for the shoulder not measured because the patient did not complete FOTO'S functional status survey near discharge, patient not appropriate Ⓑ

⁎ **G8666** Risk-adjusted functional status change residual scores for the shoulder not measured because the patient did not complete FOTO'S functional intake on admission and/or follow up status survey near discharge, reason not given Ⓑ

⁎ **G8667** Risk-adjusted functional status change residual score for the elbow, wrist or hand successfully calculated and the score was equal to zero (0) or greater than zero (>0) Ⓑ

⁎ **G8668** Risk-adjusted functional status change residual score for the elbow, wrist or hand successfully calculated and the score was less than zero (< 0) Ⓑ

⁎ **G8669** Risk-adjusted functional status change residual scores for the elbow, wrist or hand not measured because the patient did not complete FOTO'S functional status survey near discharge, patient not appropriate Ⓑ

⁎ **G8670** Risk-adjusted functional status change residual scores for the elbow, wrist or hand not measured because the patient did not complete FOTO'S functional intake on admission and/or follow up status survey near discharge, reason not given Ⓑ

⁎ **G8671** Risk-adjusted functional status change residual score for the neck, cranium, mandible, thoracic spine, ribs, or other general orthopaedic impairment successfully calculated and the score was equal to zero (0) or greater than zero (> 0) Ⓑ

⁎ **G8672** Risk-adjusted functional status change residual score for the neck, cranium, mandible, thoracic spine, ribs, or other general orthopaedic impairment successfully calculated and the score was less than zero (<0) Ⓑ

⁎ **G8673** Risk-adjusted functional status change residual scores for the neck, cranium, mandible, thoracic spine, ribs, or other general orthopaedic impairment not measured because the patient did not complete FOTO'S functional status survey near discharge, patient not appropriate Ⓑ

⁎ **G8674** Risk-adjusted functional status change residual scores for the neck, cranium, mandible, thoracic spine, ribs, or other general orthopaedic impairment not measured because the patient did not complete FOTO'S functional intake on admission and/or follow up status survey near discharge, reason not given Ⓑ

⁎ **G8694** Left ventriucular ejection fraction (LVEF) < 40% Ⓑ

~~G8696 Antithrombotic therapy prescribed at discharge~~ ✖

~~G8697 Antithrombotic therapy not prescribed for documented reasons (e.g., patient had stroke during hospital stay, patient expired during inpatient stay, other medical reason(s)); (e.g., patient left against medical advice, other patient reason(s))~~ ✖

~~G8698 Antithrombotic therapy was not prescribed at discharge, reason not given~~ ✖

⁎ **G8708** Patient not prescribed or dispensed antibiotic Ⓑ

⁎ **G8709** Patient prescribed or dispensed antibiotic for documented medical reason(s) (e.g., intestinal infection, pertussis, bacterial infection, Lyme disease, otitis media, acute sinusitis, acute pharyngitis, acute tonsillitis, chronic sinusitis, infection of the pharynx/larynx/tonsils/adenoids, prostatitis, cellulitis, mastoiditis, or bone infections, acute lymphadenitis, impetigo, skin staph infections, pneumonia/gonococcal infections, venereal disease (syphilis, chlamydia, inflammatory diseases (female reproductive organs), infections of the kidney, cystitis or UTI, and acne) Ⓑ

⁎ **G8710** Patient prescribed or dispensed antibiotic Ⓑ

⁎ **G8711** Prescribed or dispensed antibiotic Ⓑ

⁎ **G8712** Antibiotic not prescribed or dispensed Ⓑ

⁎ **G8721** PT category (primary tumor), PN category (regional lymph nodes), and histologic grade were documented in pathology report Ⓑ

⁎ **G8722** Documentation of medical reason(s) for not including the PT category, the PN category or the histologic grade in the pathology report (e.g., re-excision without residual tumor; non-carcinomasanal canal) Ⓑ

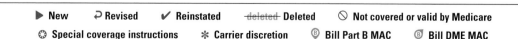

▶ New   ↻ Revised   ✔ Reinstated   ~~deleted~~ Deleted   ⊘ Not covered or valid by Medicare
⊛ Special coverage instructions   ⁎ Carrier discretion   Ⓑ Bill Part B MAC   Ⓓ Bill DME MAC

G8723 — G8841   TEMPORARY PROCEDURES/PROFESSIONAL SERVICES

∗ **G8723**   Specimen site is other than anatomic location of primary tumor Ⓑ

∗ **G8724**   PT category, PN category and histologic grade were not documented in the pathology report, reason not given Ⓑ

∗ **G8730**   Pain assessment documented as positive using a standardized tool and a follow-up plan is documented Ⓑ

∗ **G8731**   Pain assessment using a standardized tool is documented as negative, no follow-up plan required Ⓑ

∗ **G8732**   No documentation of pain assessment, reason not given Ⓑ

∗ **G8733**   Elder maltreatment screen documented as positive and a follow-up plan is documented Ⓑ

∗ **G8734**   Elder maltreatment screen documented as negative, no follow-up required Ⓑ

∗ **G8735**   Elder maltreatment screen documented as positive, follow-up plan not documented, reason not given Ⓑ

∗ **G8749**   Absence of signs of melanoma (cough, dyspnea, tenderness, localized neurologic signs such as weakness, jaundice or any other sign suggesting systemic spread) or absence of symptoms of melanoma (pain, paresthesia, or any other symptom suggesting the possibility of systemic spread of melanoma) Ⓑ

∗ **G8752**   Most recent systolic blood pressure < 140 mmhg Ⓑ

∗ **G8753**   Most recent systolic blood pressure >= 140 mmhg Ⓑ

∗ **G8754**   Most recent diastolic blood pressure < 90 mmhg Ⓑ

∗ **G8755**   Most recent diastolic blood pressure >= 90 mmhg Ⓑ

∗ **G8756**   No documentation of blood pressure measurement, reason not given Ⓑ

∗ **G8783**   Normal blood pressure reading documented, follow-up not required Ⓑ

∗ **G8785**   Blood pressure reading not documented, reason not given Ⓑ

∗ **G8797**   Specimen site other than anatomic location of esophagus Ⓑ

∗ **G8798**   Specimen site other than anatomic location of prostate Ⓑ

∗ **G8806**   Performance of trans-abdominal or trans-vaginal ultrasound Ⓑ

∗ **G8807**   Trans-abdominal or trans-vaginal ultrasound not performed for reasons documented by clinician (e.g., patient has visited the ED multiple times within 72 hours, patient has a documented intrauterine pregnancy [IUP]) Ⓑ

↻ ∗ **G8808**   Trans-abdominal or trans-vaginal ultrasound not performed, reason not given Ⓑ

∗ **G8809**   Rh-immunoglobulin (RhoGAM) ordered Ⓑ

∗ **G8810**   Rh-immunoglobulin (RhoGAM) not ordered for reasons documented by clinician (e.g., patient had prior documented report of RhoGAM within 12 weeks, patient refusal) Ⓑ

∗ **G8811**   Documentation RH-immunoglobulin (RhoGAM) was not ordered, reason not given Ⓑ

∗ **G8815**   Documented reason in the medical records for why the statin therapy was not prescribed (i.e., lower extremity bypass was for a patient with non-artherosclerotic disease) Ⓑ

∗ **G8816**   Statin medication prescribed at discharge Ⓑ

∗ **G8817**   Statin therapy not prescribed at discharge, reason not given Ⓑ

∗ **G8818**   Patient discharge to home no later than post-operative day #7 Ⓑ

∗ **G8825**   Patient not discharged to home by post-operative day #7 Ⓑ

∗ **G8826**   Patient discharge to home no later than post-operative day #2 following EVAR Ⓑ

∗ **G8833**   Patient not discharged to home by post-operative day #2 following EVAR Ⓑ

∗ **G8834**   Patient discharged to home no later than post-operative day #2 following CEA Ⓑ

∗ **G8838**   Patient not discharged to home by post-operative day #2 following CEA Ⓑ

∗ **G8839**   Sleep apnea symptoms assessed, including presence or absence of snoring and daytime sleepiness Ⓑ

∗ **G8840**   Documentation of reason(s) for not documenting an assessment of sleep symptoms (e.g., patient didn't have initial daytime sleepiness, patient visited between initial testing and initiation of therapy) Ⓑ

∗ **G8841**   Sleep apnea symptoms not assessed, reason not given Ⓑ

▶ **New**   ↻ **Revised**   ✔ **Reinstated**   ~~deleted~~ **Deleted**   ⊘ **Not covered or valid by Medicare**
⊕ **Special coverage instructions**   ∗ **Carrier discretion**   Ⓟ **Bill Part B MAC**   Ⓑ **Bill DME MAC**

* **G8842** Apnea Hypopnea Index (AHI) or Respiratory Disturbance Index (RDI) measured at the time of initial diagnosis ⑧

* **G8843** Documentation of reason(s) for not measuring an Apnea Hypopnea Index (AHI) or a Respiratory Disturbance Index (RDI) at the time of initial diagnosis (e.g., psychiatric disease, dementia, patient declined, financial, insurance coverage, test ordered but not yet completed) ⑧

* **G8844** Apnea Hypopnea Index (AHI) or Respiratory Disturbance Index (RDI) not measured at the time of initial diagnosis, reason not given ⑧

* **G8845** Positive airway pressure therapy prescribed ⑧

* **G8846** Moderate or severe obstructive sleep apnea (Apnea Hypopnea Index (AHI) or Respiratory Disturbance Index (RDI) of 15 or greater) ⑧

* **G8849** Documentation of reason(s) for not prescribing positive airway pressure therapy (e.g., patient unable to tolerate, alternative therapies use, patient declined, financial, insurance coverage) ⑧

* **G8850** Positive airway pressure therapy not prescribed, reason not given ⑧

* **G8851** Objective measurement of adherence to positive airway pressure therapy, documented ⑧

* **G8852** Positive airway pressure therapy prescribed ⑧

* **G8854** Documentation of reason(s) for not objectively measuring adherence to positive airway pressure therapy (e.g., patient didn't bring data from continuous positive airway pressure [CPAP], therapy was not yet initiated, not available on machine) ⑧

* **G8855** Objective measurement of adherence to positive airway pressure therapy not performed, reason not given ⑧

* **G8856** Referral to a physician for an otologic evaluation performed ⑧

* **G8857** Patient is not eligible for the referral for otologic evaluation measure (e.g., patients who are already under the care of a physician for acute or chronic dizziness) ⑧

* **G8858** Referral to a physician for an otologic evaluation not performed, reason not given ⑧

* **G8861** Within the past 2 years, central dual-energy x-ray absorptiometry (DXA) ordered and documented, review of systems and medication history or pharmacologic therapy (other than minerals/vitamins) for osteoporosis prescribed ⑧

* **G8863** Patients not assessed for risk of bone loss, reason not given ⑧

* **G8864** Pneumococcal vaccine administered or previously received ⑧

* **G8865** Documentation of medical reason(s) for not administering or previously receiving pneumococcal vaccine (e.g., patient allergic reaction, potential adverse drug reaction) ⑧

* **G8866** Documentation of patient reason(s) for not administering or previously receiving pneumococcal vaccine (e.g., patient refusal) ⑧

* **G8867** Pneumococcal vaccine not administered or previously received, reason not given ⑧

↻ * **G8869** Patient has documented immunity to hepatitis B and initiating anti-TNF therapy ⑧

* **G8872** Excised tissue evaluated by imaging intraoperatively to confirm successful inclusion of targeted lesion ⑧

* **G8873** Patients with needle localization specimens which are not amenable to intraoperative imaging such as MRI needle wire localization, or targets which are tentatively identified on mammogram or ultrasound which do not contain a biopsy marker but which can be verified on intraoperative inspection or pathology (e.g., needle biopsy site where the biopsy marker is remote from the actual biopsy site) ⑧

* **G8874** Excised tissue not evaluated by imaging intraoperatively to confirm successful inclusion of targeted lesion ⑧

* **G8875** Clinician diagnosed breast cancer preoperatively by a minimally invasive biopsy method ⑧

▶ **New**   ↻ **Revised**   ✔ **Reinstated**   ~~deleted~~ **Deleted**   ⊘ **Not covered or valid by Medicare**
✪ **Special coverage instructions**   * **Carrier discretion**   ⑨ **Bill Part B MAC**   ⑧ **Bill DME MAC**

* **G8876** Documentation of reason(s) for not performing minimally invasive biopsy to diagnose breast cancer preoperatively (e.g., lesion too close to skin, implant, chest wall, etc., lesion could not be adequately visualized for needle biopsy, patient condition prevents needle biopsy [weight, breast thickness, etc.], duct excision without imaging abnormality, prophylactic mastectomy, reduction mammoplasty, excisional biopsy performed by another physician) ⑧

* **G8877** Clinician did not attempt to achieve the diagnosis of breast cancer preoperatively by a minimally invasive biopsy method, reason not given ⑧

* **G8878** Sentinel lymph node biopsy procedure performed ⑧

~~G8879   Clinically node negative (T1N0M0 or T2N0M0) invasive breast cancer~~ ✖

↻ * **G8880** Documentation of reason(s) sentinel lymph node biopsy not performed (e.g., reasons could include but not limited to; non-invasive cancer, incidental discovery of breast cancer on prophylactic mastectomy, incidental discovery of breast cancer on reduction mammoplasty, pre-operative biopsy proven lymph node (LN) metastases, inflammatory carcinoma, stage 3 locally advanced cancer, recurrent invasive breast cancer, clinically node positive after neoadjuvant systemic therapy, patient refusal after informed consent) ⑧

* **G8881** Stage of breast cancer is greater than T1N0M0 or T2N0M0 ⑧

* **G8882** Sentinel lymph node biopsy procedure not performed, reason not given ⑧

* **G8883** Biopsy results reviewed, communicated, tracked and documented ⑧

* **G8884** Clinician documented reason that patient's biopsy results were not reviewed ⑧

* **G8885** Biopsy results not reviewed, communicated, tracked or documented ⑧

* **G8907** Patient documented not to have experienced any of the following events: a burn prior to discharge; a fall within the facility; wrong site/side/patient/procedure/implant event; or a hospital transfer or hospital admission upon discharge from the facility ⑧

* **G8908** Patient documented to have received a burn prior to discharge ⑧

* **G8909** Patient documented not to have received a burn prior to discharge ⑧

* **G8910** Patient documented to have experienced a fall within ASC ⑧

* **G8911** Patient documented not to have experienced a fall within ambulatory surgical center ⑧

* **G8912** Patient documented to have experienced a wrong site, wrong side, wrong patient, wrong procedure or wrong implant event ⑧

* **G8913** Patient documented not to have experienced a wrong site, wrong side, wrong patient, wrong procedure or wrong implant event ⑧

* **G8914** Patient documented to have experienced a hospital transfer or hospital admission upon discharge from ASC ⑧

* **G8915** Patient documented not to have experienced a hospital transfer or hospital admission upon discharge from ASC ⑧

* **G8916** Patient with preoperative order for IV antibiotic surgical site infection (SSI) prophylaxis, antibiotic initiated on time ⑧

* **G8917** Patient with preoperative order for IV antibiotic surgical site infection (SSI) prophylaxis, antibiotic not initiated on time ⑧

* **G8918** Patient without preoperative order for IV antibiotic surgical site infection(SSI) prophylaxis ⑧

* **G8923** Left ventricular ejection fraction (LVEF) < 40% or documentation of moderately or severely depressed left ventricular systolic function ⑧

* **G8924** Spirometry test results demonstrate FEV1/FVC <70%, FEV <60% predicted and patient has COPD symptoms (e.g., dyspnea, cough/sputum, wheezing) ⑧

* **G8925** Spirometry test results demonstrate FEV1> = 60% FEV1/FVC> = 70%, predicted or patient does not have COPD symptoms ⑧

* **G8926** Spirometry test not performed or documented, reason not given ⑧

* **G8934** Left ventricular ejection fraction (LVEF) < 40% or documentation of moderately or severely depressed left ventricular systolic function ⑧

▶ New   ↻ Revised   ✔ Reinstated   ~~deleted~~ Deleted   ⊘ Not covered or valid by Medicare

⊙ Special coverage instructions   * Carrier discretion   Ⓑ Bill Part B MAC   Ⓓ Bill DME MAC

✳ **G8935** Clinician prescribed angiotensin converting enzyme (ACE) inhibitor or angiotensin receptor blocker (ARB) therapy Ⓑ

✳ **G8936** Clinician documented that patient was not an eligible candidate for angiotensin converting enzyme (ACE) inhibitor or angiotensin receptor blocker (ARB) therapy (e.g., allergy, intolerance, pregnancy, renal failure due to ace inhibitor, diseases of the aortic or mitral valve, other medical reasons) or (e.g., patient declined, other patient reasons) or (e.g., lack of drug availability, other reasons attributable to the health care system) Ⓑ

✳ **G8937** Clinician did not prescribe angiotensin converting enzyme (ACE) inhibitor or angiotensin receptor blocker (ARB) therapy, reason not given Ⓑ

↺ ✳ **G8938** BMI is documented as being outside of normal limits, follow-up plan is not documented, documentation the patient is not eligible Ⓑ

↺ ✳ **G8939** Pain assessment documented as positive, follow-up plan not documented, documentation the patient is not eligible at the time of the encounter at the time of the encounter Ⓑ

↺ ✳ **G8941** Elder maltreatment screen documented as positive, follow-up plan not documented, documentation the patient is not eligible for follow-up plan at the time of the encounter Ⓑ

✳ **G8942** Functional outcomes assessment using a standardized tool is documented within the previous 30 days and care plan, based on identified deficiencies on the date of the functional outcome assessment, is documented Ⓑ

✳ **G8944** AJCC melanoma cancer stage 0 through IIC melanoma Ⓑ

✳ **G8946** Minimally invasive biopsy method attempted but not diagnostic of breast cancer (e.g., high risk lesion of breast such as atypical ductal hyperplasia, lobular neoplasia, atypical lobular hyperplasia, lobular carcinoma in situ, atypical columnar hyperplasia, flat epithelial atypia, radial scar, complex sclerosing lesion, papillary lesion, or any lesion with spindle cells) Ⓑ

~~G8947~~ ~~One or more neuropsychiatric symptoms~~ ✖

✳ **G8950** Pre-hypertensive or hypertensive blood pressure reading documented, and the indicated follow-up documented Ⓑ

✳ **G8952** Pre-hypertensive or hypertensive blood pressure reading documented, indicated follow-up not documented, reason not given Ⓑ

✳ **G8955** Most recent assessment of adequacy of volume management documented Ⓑ

✳ **G8956** Patient receiving maintenance hemodialysis in an outpatient dialysis facility Ⓑ

✳ **G8958** Assessment of adequacy of volume management not documented, reason not given Ⓑ

✳ **G8959** Clinician treating major depressive disorder communicates to clinician treating comorbid condition Ⓑ

✳ **G8960** Clinician treating major depressive disorder did not communicate to clinician treating comorbid condition, reason not given Ⓑ

✳ **G8961** Cardiac stress imaging test primarily performed on low-risk surgery patient for preoperative evaluation within 30 days preceding this surgery Ⓑ

✳ **G8962** Cardiac stress imaging test performed on patient for any reason including those who did not have low risk surgery or test that was performed more than 30 days preceding low risk surgery Ⓑ

✳ **G8963** Cardiac stress imaging performed primarily for monitoring of asymptomatic patient who had PCI within 2 years Ⓑ

✳ **G8964** Cardiac stress imaging test performed primarily for any other reason than monitoring of asymptomatic patient who had PCI within 2 years (e.g., symptomatic patient, patient greater than 2 years since PCI, initial evaluation, etc.) Ⓑ

✳ **G8965** Cardiac stress imaging test primarily performed on low CHD risk patient for initial detection and risk assessment Ⓑ

✳ **G8966** Cardiac stress imaging test performed on symptomatic or higher than low CHD risk patient or for any reason other than initial detection and risk assessment Ⓑ

↺ ✳ **G8967** Warfarin or another FDA-approved oral anticoagulant is prescribed Ⓑ

↺ ✳ **G8968** Documentation of medical reason(s) for not prescribing warfarin or another FDA-approved anticoagulant (e.g., atrial appendage device in place) Ⓑ

↻ ✳ **G8969** Documentation of patient reason(s) for not prescribing warfarin or another FDA-approved oral anticoagulant that is FDA approved for the prevention of thromboembolism (e.g., patient choice of having atrial appendage device placed) Ⓑ

✳ **G8970** No risk factors or one moderate risk factor for thromboembolism Ⓑ

~~G8971~~ ~~Warfarin or another oral anticoagulant that is FDA approved not prescribed, reason not given~~ ✖

~~G8972~~ ~~One or more high risk factors for thromboembolism or more than one moderate risk factor for thromboembolism~~ ✖

✳ **G8973** Most recent hemoglobin (Hgb) level < 10 g/dl Ⓑ

✳ **G8974** Hemoglobin level measurement not documented, reason not given Ⓑ

✳ **G8975** Documentation of medical reason(s) for patient having a hemoglobin level < 10 g/dl (e.g., patients who have non-renal etiologies of anemia [e.g., sickle cell anemia or other hemoglobinopathies, hypersplenism, primary bone marrow disease, anemia related to chemotherapy for diagnosis of malignancy, postoperative bleeding, active bloodstream or peritoneal infection], other medical reasons) Ⓖ

✳ **G8976** Most recent hemoglobin (Hgb) level>= 10 g/dl Ⓑ

Functional Limitation

✳ **G8978** Mobility: walking & moving around functional limitation, current status, at therapy episode outset and at reporting intervals Ⓑ

✳ **G8979** Mobility: walking & moving around functional limitation, projected goal status, at therapy episode outset, at reporting intervals, and at discharge or to end reporting Ⓑ

✳ **G8980** Mobility: walking & moving around functional limitation, discharge status, at discharge from therapy or to end reporting Ⓑ

✳ **G8981** Changing & maintaining body position functional limitation, current status, at therapy episode outset and at reporting intervals Ⓑ

✳ **G8982** Changing & maintaining body position functional limitation, projected goal status, at therapy episode outset, at reporting intervals, and at discharge or to end reporting Ⓖ

✳ **G8983** Changing & maintaining body position functional limitation, discharge status, at discharge from therapy or to end reporting Ⓑ

✳ **G8984** Carrying, moving & handling objects functional limitation, current status, at therapy episode outset and at reporting intervals Ⓑ

✳ **G8985** Carrying, moving and handling objects, projected goal status, at therapy episode outset, at reporting intervals, and at discharge or to end reporting Ⓑ

✳ **G8986** Carrying, moving & handling objects functional limitation, discharge status, at discharge from therapy or to end reporting Ⓑ

✳ **G8987** Self-care functional limitation, current status, at therapy episode outset and at reporting intervals Ⓑ

✳ **G8988** Self-care functional limitation, projected goal status, at therapy episode outset, at reporting intervals, and at discharge or to end reporting Ⓑ

✳ **G8989** Self-care functional limitation, discharge status, at discharge from therapy or to end reporting Ⓑ

✳ **G8990** Other physical or occupational therapy primary functional limitation, current status, at therapy episode outset and at reporting intervals Ⓑ

✳ **G8991** Other physical or occupational therapy primary functional limitation, projected goal status, at therapy episode outset, at reporting intervals, and at discharge or to end reporting Ⓑ

✳ **G8992** Other physical or occupational therapy primary functional limitation, discharge status, at discharge from therapy or to end reporting Ⓑ

✳ **G8993** Other physical or occupational therapy subsequent functional limitation, current status, at therapy episode outset and at reporting intervals Ⓑ

✳ **G8994** Other physical or occupational therapy subsequent functional limitation, projected goal status, at therapy episode outset, at reporting intervals, and at discharge or to end reporting Ⓑ

✳ **G8995** Other physical or occupational therapy subsequent functional limitation, discharge status, at discharge from therapy or to end reporting Ⓑ

▶ **New**   ↻ **Revised**   ✔ **Reinstated**   ~~deleted~~ **Deleted**   ⊘ **Not covered or valid by Medicare**
⊙ **Special coverage instructions**   ✳ **Carrier discretion**   Ⓑ **Bill Part B MAC**   Ⓓ **Bill DME MAC**

∗ **G8996** Swallowing functional limitation, current status at therapy episode outset and at reporting intervals ⑧

∗ **G8997** Swallowing functional limitation, projected goal status, at therapy episode outset, at reporting intervals, and at discharge or to end reporting ⑧

∗ **G8998** Swallowing functional limitation, discharge status, at discharge from therapy or to end reporting ⑧

∗ **G8999** Motor speech functional limitation, current status at therapy episode outset and at reporting intervals ⑧

Coordinated Care

✪ **G9001** Coordinated care fee, initial rate ⑧

✪ **G9002** Coordinated care fee, maintenance rate ⑧

✪ **G9003** Coordinated care fee, risk adjusted high, initial ⑧

✪ **G9004** Coordinated care fee, risk adjusted low, initial ⑧

✪ **G9005** Coordinated care fee, risk adjusted maintenance ⑧

✪ **G9006** Coordinated care fee, home monitoring ⑧

✪ **G9007** Coordinated care fee, scheduled team conference ⑧

✪ **G9008** Coordinated care fee, physician coordinated care oversight services ⑧

✪ **G9009** Coordinated care fee, risk adjusted maintenance, level 3 ⑧

✪ **G9010** Coordinated care fee, risk adjusted maintenance, level 4 ⑧

✪ **G9011** Coordinated care fee, risk adjusted maintenance, level 5 ⑧

✪ **G9012** Other specified case management services not elsewhere classified ⑧

Demonstration Project

⊘ **G9013** ESRD demo basic bundle Level I ⑧

⊘ **G9014** ESRD demo expanded bundle including venous access and related services ⑧

⊘ **G9016** Smoking cessation counseling, individual, in the absence of or in addition to any other evaluation and management service, per session (6-10 minutes) [demo project code only] ⑧

∗ **G9017** Amantadine hydrochloride, oral, per 100 mg (for use in a Medicare-approved demonstration project) ⑧

∗ **G9018** Zanamivir, inhalation powder, administered through inhaler, per 10 mg (for use in a Medicare-approved demonstration project) ⑧

∗ **G9019** Oseltamivir phosphate, oral, per 75 mg (for use in a Medicare-approved demonstration project) ⑧

∗ **G9020** Rimantadine hydrochloride, oral, per 100 mg (for use in a Medicare-approved demonstration project) ⑧

∗ **G9033** Amantadine hydrochloride, oral brand, per 100 mg (for use in a Medicare-approved demonstration project) ⑧

∗ **G9034** Zanamivir, inhalation powder, administered through inhaler, brand, per 10 mg (for use in a Medicare-approved demonstration project) ⑧

∗ **G9035** Oseltamivir phosphate, oral, brand, per 75 mg (for use in a Medicare-approved demonstration project) ⑧

∗ **G9036** Rimantadine hydrochloride, oral, brand, per 100 mg (for use in a Medicare-approved demonstration project) ⑧

⊘ **G9050** Oncology; primary focus of visit; work-up, evaluation, or staging at the time of cancer diagnosis or recurrence (for use in a Medicare-approved demonstration project) ⑧

⊘ **G9051** Oncology; primary focus of visit; treatment decision-making after disease is staged or restaged, discussion of treatment options, supervising/coordinating active cancer directed therapy or managing consequences of cancer directed therapy (for use in a Medicare-approved demonstration project) ⑧

⊘ **G9052** Oncology; primary focus of visit; surveillance for disease recurrence for patient who has completed definitive cancer-directed therapy and currently lacks evidence of recurrent disease; cancer directed therapy might be considered in the future (for use in a Medicare-approved demonstration project) ⑧

⊘ **G9053** Oncology; primary focus of visit; expectant management of patient with evidence of cancer for whom no cancer directed therapy is being administered or arranged at present; cancer directed therapy might be considered in the future (for use in a Medicare-approved demonstration project) ⑧

▶ **New**　↻ **Revised**　✔ **Reinstated**　~~deleted~~ **Deleted**　⊘ **Not covered or valid by Medicare**

✪ **Special coverage instructions**　∗ **Carrier discretion**　⑧ **Bill Part B MAC**　⑧ **Bill DME MAC**

⊘ **G9054** Oncology; primary focus of visit; supervising, coordinating or managing care of patient with terminal cancer or for whom other medical illness prevents further cancer treatment; includes symptom management, end-of-life care planning, management of palliative therapies (for use in a Medicare-approved demonstration project) Ⓑ

⊘ **G9055** Oncology; primary focus of visit; other, unspecified service not otherwise listed (for use in a Medicare-approved demonstration project) Ⓑ

⊘ **G9056** Oncology; practice guidelines; management adheres to guidelines (for use in a Medicare-approved demonstration project) Ⓑ

⊘ **G9057** Oncology; practice guidelines; management differs from guidelines as a result of patient enrollment in an institutional review board approved clinical trial (for use in a Medicare-approved demonstration project) Ⓑ

⊘ **G9058** Oncology; practice guidelines; management differs from guidelines because the treating physician disagrees with guideline recommendations (for use in a Medicare-approved demonstration project) Ⓑ

⊘ **G9059** Oncology; practice guidelines; management differs from guidelines because the patient, after being offered treatment consistent with guidelines, has opted for alternative treatment or management, including no treatment (for use in a Medicare-approved demonstration project) Ⓑ

⊘ **G9060** Oncology; practice guidelines; management differs from guidelines for reason(s) associated with patient comorbid illness or performance status not factored into guidelines (for use in a Medicare-approved demonstration project) Ⓑ

⊘ **G9061** Oncology; practice guidelines; patient's condition not addressed by available guidelines (for use in a Medicare-approved demonstration project) Ⓑ

⊘ **G9062** Oncology; practice guidelines; management differs from guidelines for other reason(s) not listed (for use in a Medicare-approved demonstration project) Ⓑ

✳ **G9063** Oncology; disease status; limited to non-small cell lung cancer; extent of disease initially established as stage I (prior to neo-adjuvant therapy, if any) with no evidence of disease progression, recurrence, or metastases (for use in a Medicare-approved demonstration project) Ⓑ

✳ **G9064** Oncology; disease status; limited to non-small cell lung cancer; extent of disease initially established as stage II (prior to neo-adjuvant therapy, if any) with no evidence of disease progression, recurrence, or metastases (for use in a Medicare-approved demonstration project) Ⓑ

✳ **G9065** Oncology; disease status; limited to non-small cell lung cancer; extent of disease initially established as stage IIIA (prior to neo-adjuvant therapy, if any) with no evidence of disease progression, recurrence, or metastases (for use in a Medicare-approved demonstration project) Ⓑ

✳ **G9066** Oncology; disease status; limited to non-small cell lung cancer; stage IIIB-IV at diagnosis, metastatic, locally recurrent, or progressive (for use in a Medicare-approved demonstration project) Ⓑ

✳ **G9067** Oncology; disease status; limited to non-small cell lung cancer; extent of disease unknown, staging in progress, or not listed (for use in a Medicare-approved demonstration project) Ⓑ

✳ **G9068** Oncology; disease status; limited to small cell and combined small cell/non-small cell; extent of disease initially established as limited with no evidence of disease progression, recurrence, or metastases (for use in a Medicare-approved demonstration project) Ⓑ

✳ **G9069** Oncology; disease status; small cell lung cancer, limited to small cell and combined small cell/non-small cell; extensive stage at diagnosis, metastatic, locally recurrent, or progressive (for use in a Medicare-approved demonstration project) Ⓑ

✳ **G9070** Oncology; disease status; small cell lung cancer, limited to small cell and combined small cell/non-small cell; extent of disease unknown, staging in progress, or not listed (for use in a Medicare-approved demonstration project) Ⓑ

▶ New	⤺ Revised	✔ Reinstated	~~deleted~~ Deleted	⊘ Not covered or valid by Medicare
⊗ Special coverage instructions		✳ Carrier discretion	Ⓑ Bill Part B MAC	Ⓑ Bill DME MAC

✳ **G9071** Oncology; disease status; invasive female breast cancer (does not include ductal carcinoma in situ); adenocarcinoma as predominant cell type; stage I or stage IIA-IIB; or T3, N1, M0; and ER and/or PR positive; with no evidence of disease progression, recurrence, or metastases (for use in a Medicare-approved demonstration project) Ⓑ

✳ **G9072** Oncology; disease status; invasive female breast cancer (does not include ductal carcinoma in situ); adenocarcinoma as predominant cell type; stage I, or stage IIA-IIB; or T3, N1, M0; and ER and PR negative; with no evidence of disease progression, recurrence, or metastases (for use in a Medicare-approved demonstration project) Ⓑ

✳ **G9073** Oncology; disease status; invasive female breast cancer (does not include ductal carcinoma in situ); adenocarcinoma as predominant cell type; stage IIIA-IIIB; and not T3, N1, M0; and ER and/or PR positive; with no evidence of disease progression, recurrence, or metastases (for use in a Medicare-approved demonstration project) Ⓑ

✳ **G9074** Oncology; disease status; invasive female breast cancer (does not include ductal carcinoma in situ); adenocarcinoma as predominant cell type; stage IIIA-IIIB; and not T3, N1, M0; and ER and PR negative; with no evidence of disease progression, recurrence, or metastases (for use in a Medicare-approved demonstration project) Ⓑ

✳ **G9075** Oncology; disease status; invasive female breast cancer (does not include ductal carcinoma in situ); adenocarcinoma as predominant cell type; M1 at diagnosis, metastatic, locally recurrent, or progressive (for use in a Medicare-approved demonstration project) Ⓖ

✳ **G9077** Oncology; disease status; prostate cancer, limited to adenocarcinoma as predominant cell type; T1-T2c and Gleason 2-7 and PSA <or equal to 20 at diagnosis with no evidence of disease progression, recurrence, or metastases (for use in a Medicare-approved demonstration project) Ⓖ

✳ **G9078** Oncology; disease status; prostate cancer, limited to adenocarcinoma as predominant cell type; T2 or T3a Gleason 8-10 or PSA > 20 at diagnosis with no evidence of disease progression, recurrence, or metastases (for use in a Medicare-approved demonstration project) Ⓖ

✳ **G9079** Oncology; disease status; prostate cancer, limited to adenocarcinoma as predominant cell type; T3b-T4, any N; any T, N1 at diagnosis with no evidence of disease progression, recurrence, or metastases (for use in a Medicare-approved demonstration project) Ⓑ

✳ **G9080** Oncology; disease status; prostate cancer, limited to adenocarcinoma; after initial treatment with rising PSA or failure of PSA decline (for use in a Medicare-approved demonstration project) Ⓖ

✳ **G9083** Oncology; disease status; prostate cancer, limited to adenocarcinoma; extent of disease unknown, staging in progress, or not listed (for use in a Medicare-approved demonstration project) Ⓖ

✳ **G9084** Oncology; disease status; colon cancer, limited to invasive cancer, adenocarcinoma as predominant cell type; extent of disease initially established as T1-3, N0, M0 with no evidence of disease progression, recurrence, or metastases (for use in a Medicare-approved demonstration project) Ⓖ

✳ **G9085** Oncology; disease status; colon cancer, limited to invasive cancer, adenocarcinoma as predominant cell type; extent of disease initially established as T4, N0, M0 with no evidence of disease progression, recurrence, or metastases (for use in a Medicare-approved demonstration project) Ⓑ

✳ **G9086** Oncology; disease status; colon cancer, limited to invasive cancer, adenocarcinoma as predominant cell type; extent of disease initially established as T1-4, N1-2, M0 with no evidence of disease progression, recurrence, or metastases (for use in a Medicare-approved demonstration project) Ⓑ

▶ **New** ⟳ **Revised** ✔ **Reinstated** ~~deleted~~ **Deleted** ⊘ **Not covered or valid by Medicare**
✿ **Special coverage instructions** ✳ **Carrier discretion** Ⓖ **Bill Part B MAC** Ⓑ **Bill DME MAC**

* **G9087** Oncology; disease status; colon cancer, limited to invasive cancer, adenocarcinoma as predominant cell type; M1 at diagnosis, metastatic, locally recurrent, or progressive with current clinical, radiologic, or biochemical evidence of disease (for use in a Medicare-approved demonstration project) Ⓑ

* **G9088** Oncology; disease status; colon cancer, limited to invasive cancer, adenocarcinoma as predominant cell type; M1 at diagnosis, metastatic, locally recurrent, or progressive without current clinical, radiologic, or biochemical evidence of disease (for use in a Medicare-approved demonstration project) Ⓑ

* **G9089** Oncology; disease status; colon cancer, limited to invasive cancer, adenocarcinoma as predominant cell type; extent of disease unknown, staging in progress, or not listed (for use in a Medicare-approved demonstration project) Ⓑ

* **G9090** Oncology; disease status; rectal cancer, limited to invasive cancer, adenocarcinoma as predominant cell type; extent of disease initially established as T1-2, N0, M0 (prior to neo-adjuvant therapy, if any) with no evidence of disease progression, recurrence, or metastases (for use in a Medicare-approved demonstration project) Ⓑ

* **G9091** Oncology; disease status; rectal cancer, limited to invasive cancer, adenocarcinoma as predominant cell type; extent of disease initially established as T3, N0, M0 (prior to neo-adjuvant therapy, if any) with no evidence of disease progression, recurrence, or metastases (for use in a Medicare-approved demonstration project) Ⓑ

* **G9092** Oncology; disease status; rectal cancer, limited to invasive cancer, adenocarcinoma as predominant cell type; extent of disease initially established as T1-3, N1-2, M0 (prior to neo-adjuvant therapy, if any) with no evidence of disease progression, recurrence or metastases (for use in a Medicare-approved demonstration project) Ⓑ

* **G9093** Oncology; disease status; rectal cancer, limited to invasive cancer, adenocarcinoma as predominant cell type; extent of disease initially established as T4, any N, M0 (prior to neo-adjuvant therapy, if any) with no evidence of disease progression, recurrence, or metastases (for use in a Medicare-approved demonstration project) Ⓑ

* **G9094** Oncology; disease status; rectal cancer, limited to invasive cancer, adenocarcinoma as predominant cell type; M1 at diagnosis, metastatic, locally recurrent, or progressive (for use in a Medicare-approved demonstration project) Ⓑ

* **G9095** Oncology; disease status; rectal cancer, limited to invasive cancer, adenocarcinoma as predominant cell type; extent of disease unknown, staging in progress, or not listed (for use in a Medicare-approved demonstration project) Ⓑ

* **G9096** Oncology; disease status; esophageal cancer, limited to adenocarcinoma or squamous cell carcinoma as predominant cell type; extent of disease initially established as T1-T3, N0-N1 or NX (prior to neo-adjuvant therapy, if any) with no evidence of disease progression, recurrence, or metastases (for use in a Medicare-approved demonstration project) Ⓑ

* **G9097** Oncology; disease status; esophageal cancer, limited to adenocarcinoma or squamous cell carcinoma as predominant cell type; extent of disease initially established as T4, any N, M0 (prior to neo-adjuvant therapy, if any) with no evidence of disease progression, recurrence, or metastases (for use in a Medicare-approved demonstration project) Ⓑ

* **G9098** Oncology; disease status; esophageal cancer, limited to adenocarcinoma or squamous cell carcinoma as predominant cell type; M1 at diagnosis, meta-static, locally recurrent, or progressive (for use in a Medicare-approved demonstration project) Ⓑ

* **G9099** Oncology; disease status; esophageal cancer, limited to adenocarcinoma or squamous cell carcinoma as predominant cell type; extent of disease unknown, staging in progress, or not listed (for use in a Medicare-approved demonstration project) Ⓑ

▶ **New**   ↩ **Revised**   ✔ **Reinstated**   ~~deleted~~ **Deleted**   ⊘ **Not covered or valid by Medicare**
✪ **Special coverage instructions**   * **Carrier discretion**   Ⓟ **Bill Part B MAC**   Ⓑ **Bill DME MAC**

✳ **G9100** Oncology; disease status; gastric cancer, limited to adenocarcinoma as predominant cell type; post R0 resection (with or without neoadjuvant therapy) with no evidence of disease recurrence, progression, or metastases (for use in a Medicare-approved demonstration project) Ⓑ

✳ **G9101** Oncology; disease status; gastric cancer, limited to adenocarcinoma as predominant cell type; post R1 or R2 resection (with or without neoadjuvant therapy) with no evidence of disease progression, or metastases (for use in a Medicare-approved demonstration project) Ⓑ

✳ **G9102** Oncology; disease status; gastric cancer, limited to adenocarcinoma as predominant cell type; clinical or pathologic M0, unresectable with no evidence of disease progression, or metastases (for use in a Medicare-approved demonstration project Ⓑ

✳ **G9103** Oncology; disease status; gastric cancer, limited to adenocarcinoma as predominant cell type; clinical or pathologic M1 at diagnosis, metastatic, locally recurrent, or progressive (for use in a Medicare-approved demonstration project) Ⓑ

✳ **G9104** Oncology; disease status; gastric cancer, limited to adenocarcinoma as predominant cell type; extent of disease unknown, staging in progress, or not listed (for use in a Medicare-approved demonstration project Ⓑ

✳ **G9105** Oncology; disease status; pancreatic cancer, limited to adenocarcinoma as predominant cell type; post R0 resection without evidence of disease progression, recurrence, or metastases (for use in a Medicare-approved demonstration project) Ⓑ

✳ **G9106** Oncology; disease status; pancreatic cancer, limited to adenocarcinoma; post R1 or R2 resection with no evidence of disease progression or metastases (for use in a Medicare-approved demonstration project) Ⓑ

✳ **G9107** Oncology; disease status; pancreatic cancer, limited to adenocarcinoma; unresectable at diagnosis, M1 at diagnosis, metastatic, locally recurrent, or progressive (for use in a Medicare-approved demonstration project) Ⓑ

✳ **G9108** Oncology; disease status; pancreatic cancer, limited to adenocarcinoma; extent of disease unknown, staging in progress, or not listed (for use in a Medicare-approved demonstration project) Ⓑ

✳ **G9109** Oncology; disease status; head and neck cancer, limited to cancers of oral cavity, pharynx and larynx with squamous cell as predominant cell type; extent of disease initially established as T1-T2 and N0, M0 (prior to neo-adjuvant therapy, if any) with no evidence of disease progression, recurrence, or metastases (for use in a Medicare-approved demonstration project) Ⓑ

✳ **G9110** Oncology; disease status; head and neck cancer, limited to cancers of oral cavity, pharynx, and larynx with squamous cell as predominant cell type; extent of disease initially established as T3-4 and/ or N1-3, M0 (prior to neo-adjuvant therapy, if any) with no evidence of disease progression, recurrence, or metastases (for use in a Medicare-approved demonstration project) Ⓑ

✳ **G9111** Oncology; disease status; head and neck cancer, limited to cancers of oral cavity, pharynx and larynx with squamous cell as predominant cell type; M1 at diagnosis, metastatic, locally recurrent, or progressive (for use in a Medicare-approved demonstration project) Ⓑ

✳ **G9112** Oncology; disease status; head and neck cancer, limited to cancers of oral cavity, pharynx and larynx with squamous cell as predominant cell type; extent of disease unknown, staging in progress, or not listed (for use in a Medicare-approved demonstration project) Ⓑ

✳ **G9113** Oncology; disease status; ovarian cancer, limited to epithelial cancer; pathologic stage IA-B (grade 1) without evidence of disease progression, recurrence, or metastases (for use in a Medicare-approved demonstration project) Ⓑ

✳ **G9114** Oncology; disease status; ovarian cancer, limited to epithelial cancer; pathologic stage IA-B (grade 2-3); or stage IC (all grades); or stage II; without evidence of disease progression, recurrence, or metastases (for use in a Medicare-approved demonstration project) Ⓑ

▶ New	↻ Revised	✔ Reinstated	deleted Deleted	⊘ Not covered or valid by Medicare
✪ Special coverage instructions		✳ Carrier discretion	Ⓑ Bill Part B MAC	Ⓓ Bill DME MAC

✳ **G9115** Oncology; disease status; ovarian cancer, limited to epithelial cancer; pathologic stage III-IV; without evidence of progression, recurrence, or metastases (for use in a Medicare-approved demonstration project) Ⓑ

✳ **G9116** Oncology; disease status; ovarian cancer, limited to epithelial cancer; evidence of disease progression, or recurrence and/or platinum resistance (for use in a Medicare-approved demonstration project) Ⓑ

✳ **G9117** Oncology; disease status; ovarian cancer, limited to epithelial cancer; extent of disease unknown, staging in progress, or not listed (for use in a Medicare-approved demonstration project) Ⓑ

✳ **G9123** Oncology; disease status; chronic myelogenous leukemia, limited to Philadelphia chromosome positive and/or BCR-ABL positive; chronic phase not in hematologic, cytogenetic, or molecular remission (for use in a Medicare-approved demonstration project) Ⓑ

✳ **G9124** Oncology; disease status; chronic myelogenous leukemia, limited to Philadelphia chromosome positive and/or BCR-ABL positive; accelerated phase not in hematologic cytogenetic, or molecular remission (for use in a Medicare-approved demonstration project) Ⓑ

✳ **G9125** Oncology; disease status; chronic myelogenous leukemia, limited to Philadelphia chromosome positive and/or BCR-ABL positive; blast phase not in hematologic, cytogenetic, or molecular remission (for use in a Medicare-approved demonstration project) Ⓑ

✳ **G9126** Oncology; disease status; chronic myelogenous leukemia, limited to Philadelphia chromosome positive and/or BCR-ABL positive; in hematologic, cytogenetic, or molecular remission (for use in a Medicare-approved demonstration project) Ⓑ

✳ **G9128** Oncology: disease status; limited to multiple myeloma, systemic disease; smouldering, stage I (for use in a Medicare-approved demonstration project) Ⓑ

✳ **G9129** Oncology; disease status; limited to multiple myeloma, systemic disease; stage II or higher (for use in a Medicare-approved demonstration project) Ⓑ

✳ **G9130** Oncology; disease status; limited to multiple myeloma, systemic disease; extent of disease unknown, staging in progress, or not listed (for use in a Medicare-approved demonstration project) Ⓑ

✳ **G9131** Oncology; disease status; invasive female breast cancer (does not include ductal carcinoma in situ); adenocarcinoma as predominant cell type; extent of disease unknown, staging in progress, or not listed (for use in a Medicare-approved demonstration project) Ⓑ

✳ **G9132** Oncology; disease status; prostate cancer, limited to adenocarcinoma; hormone-refractory/androgen-independent (e.g., rising PSA on anti-androgen therapy or post-orchiectomy); clinical metastases (for use in a Medicare-approved demonstration project) Ⓑ

✳ **G9133** Oncology; disease status; prostate cancer, limited to adenocarcinoma; hormone-responsive; clinical metastases or M1 at diagnosis (for use in a Medicare-approved demonstration project) Ⓑ

✳ **G9134** Oncology; disease status; non-Hodgkin's lymphoma, any cellular classification; stage I, II at diagnosis, not relapsed, not refractory (for use in a Medicare-approved demonstration project) Ⓑ

✳ **G9135** Oncology; disease status; non-Hodgkin's lymphoma, any cellular classification; stage III, IV, not relapsed, not refractory (for use in a Medicare-approved demonstration project) Ⓑ

✳ **G9136** Oncology; disease status; non-Hodgkin's lymphoma, transformed from original cellular diagnosis to a second cellular classification (for use in a Medicare-approved demonstration project) Ⓑ

✳ **G9137** Oncology; disease status; non-Hodgkin's lymphoma, any cellular classification; relapsed/refractory (for use in a Medicare-approved demonstration project) Ⓑ

✳ **G9138** Oncology; disease status; non-Hodgkin's lymphoma, any cellular classification; diagnostic evaluation, stage not determined, evaluation of possible relapse or non-response to therapy, or not listed (for use in a Medicare-approved demonstration project) Ⓑ

▶ **New**   ↩ **Revised**   ✔ **Reinstated**   deleted **Deleted**   ⊘ **Not covered or valid by Medicare**
⊕ **Special coverage instructions**   ✳ **Carrier discretion**   Ⓑ **Bill Part B MAC**   Ⓖ **Bill DME MAC**

✳ **G9139** Oncology; disease status; chronic myelogenous leukemia, limited to Philadelphia chromosome positive and/or BCR-ABL positive; extent of disease unknown, staging in progress, not listed (for use in a Medicare-approved demonstration project) ⑧

✳ **G9140** Frontier extended stay clinic demonstration; for a patient stay in a clinic approved for the CMS demonstration project; the following measures should be present: the stay must be equal to or greater than 4 hours; weather or other conditions must prevent transfer or the case falls into a category of monitoring and observation cases that are permitted by the rules of the demonstration; there is a maximum frontier extended stay clinic (FESC) visit of 48 hours, except in the case when weather or other conditions prevent transfer; payment is made on each period up to 4 hours, after the first 4 hours ⑧

Warfarin Responsiveness Testing

✳ **G9143** Warfarin responsiveness testing by genetic technique using any method, any number of specimen(s) ⑧

This would be a once-in-a-lifetime test unless there is a reason to believe that the patient's personal genetic characteristics would change over time. (https://www.cms.gov/ContractorLearningResources/downloads/JA6715.pdf)

Outpatient IV Insulin Treatment

⊘ **G9147** Outpatient intravenous insulin treatment (OIVIT) either pulsatile or continuous, by any means, guided by the results of measurements for: respiratory quotient; and/or, urine urea nitrogen (UUN); and/or, arterial, venous or capillary glucose; and/or potassium concentration ⑧

On December 23, 2009, CMS issued a national non-coverage decision on the use of OIVIT. CR 6775.

Not covered on Physician Fee Schedule

Quality Assurance

✳ **G9148** National committee for quality assurance - level 1 medical home ⑧

✳ **G9149** National committee for quality assurance - level 2 medical home ⑧

✳ **G9150** National committee for quality assurance - level 3 medical home ⑧

✳ **G9151** MAPCP demonstration - state provided services ⑧

✳ **G9152** MAPCP demonstration - community health teams ⑨

✳ **G9153** MAPCP demonstration - physician incentive pool ⑨

Wheelchair Evaluation

✳ **G9156** Evaluation for wheelchair requiring face to face visit with physician ⑧

Cardiac Monitoring

✳ **G9157** Transesophageal doppler measurement of cardiac output (including probe placement, image acquisition, and interpretation per course of treatment) for monitoring purposes ⑧

Functional Limitation

✳ **G9158** Motor speech functional limitation, discharge status, at discharge from therapy or to end reporting ⑧

✳ **G9159** Spoken language comprehension functional limitation, current status at therapy episode outset and at reporting intervals ⑧

✳ **G9160** Spoken language comprehension functional limitation, projected goal status at therapy episode outset, at reporting intervals, and at discharge or to end reporting ⑧

✳ **G9161** Spoken language comprehension functional limitation, discharge status at discharge from therapy or to end reporting ⑧

✳ **G9162** Spoken language expression functional limitation, current status at therapy episode outset and at reporting intervals ⑧

* **G9163** Spoken language expression functional limitation, projected goal status at therapy episode outset, at reporting intervals, and at discharge or to end reporting ⑧

* **G9164** Spoken language expression functional limitation, discharge status at discharge from therapy or to end reporting ⑧

* **G9165** Attention functional limitation, current status at therapy episode outset and at reporting intervals ⑧

* **G9166** Attention functional limitation, projected goal status at therapy episode outset, at reporting intervals, and at discharge or to end reporting ⑧

* **G9167** Attention functional limitation, discharge status at discharge from therapy or to end reporting ⑧

* **G9168** Memory functional limitation, current status at therapy episode outset and at reporting intervals ⑧

* **G9169** Memory functional limitation, projected goal status at therapy episode outset, at reporting intervals, and at discharge or to end reporting ⑧

* **G9170** Memory functional limitation, discharge status at discharge from therapy or to end reporting ⑧

* **G9171** Voice functional limitation, current status at therapy episode outset and at reporting intervals ⑧

* **G9172** Voice functional limitation, projected goal status at therapy episode outset, at reporting intervals, and at discharge or to end reporting ⑧

* **G9173** Voice functional limitation, discharge status at discharge from therapy or to end reporting ⑧

* **G9174** Other speech language pathology functional limitation, current status at therapy episode outset and at reporting intervals ⑧

* **G9175** Other speech language pathology functional limitation, projected goal status at therapy episode outset, at reporting intervals, and at discharge or to end reporting ⑧

* **G9176** Other speech language pathology functional limitation, discharge status at discharge from therapy or to end reporting ⑧

* **G9186** Motor speech functional limitation, projected goal status at therapy episode outset, at reporting intervals, and at discharge or to end reporting ⑧

Bundled Payment Care Improvement

* **G9187** Bundled payments for care improvement initiative home visit for patient assessment performed by a qualified health care professional for individuals not considered homebound including, but not limited to, assessment of safety, falls, clinical status, fluid status, medication reconciliation/management, patient compliance with orders/plan of care, performance of activities of daily living, appropriateness of care setting; (for use only in the Medicare-approved bundled payments for care improvement initiative); may not be billed for a 30-day period covered by a transitional care management code ⑨

Quality Measures: Miscellaneous

* **G9188** Beta-blocker therapy not prescribed, reason not given ⑧

* **G9189** Beta-blocker therapy prescribed or currently being taken ⑧

* **G9190** Documentation of medical reason(s) for not prescribing beta-blocker therapy (e.g., allergy, intolerance, other medical reasons) ⑧

* **G9191** Documentation of patient reason(s) for not prescribing beta-blocker therapy (e.g., patient declined, other patient reasons) ⑧

* **G9192** Documentation of system reason(s) for not prescribing beta-blocker therapy (e.g., other reasons attributable to the health care system) ⑧

* **G9196** Documentation of medical reason(s) for not ordering a first or second generation cephalosporin for antimicrobial prophylaxis (e.g., patients enrolled in clinical trials, patients with documented infection prior to surgical procedure of interest, patients who were receiving antibiotics more than 24 hours prior to surgery [except colon surgery patients taking oral prophylactic antibiotics], patients who were receiving antibiotics within 24 hours prior to arrival [except colon surgery patients taking oral prophylactic antibiotics], other medical reason(s)) ⑧

✳ **G9197** Documentation of order for first or second generation cephalosporin for antimicrobial prophylaxis Ⓑ

✳ **G9198** Order for first or second generation cephalosporin for antimicrobial prophylaxis was not documented, reason not given Ⓑ

✳ **G9212** DSM-IVTM criteria for major depressive disorder documented at the initial evaluation Ⓑ

✳ **G9213** DSM-IV-TR criteria for major depressive disorder not documented at the initial evaluation, reason not otherwise specified Ⓑ

✳ **G9223** Pneumocystis jiroveci pneumonia prophylaxis prescribed within 3 months of low CD4+ cell count below 500 cells/mm3 or a CD4 percentage below 15% Ⓑ

✳ **G9225** Foot exam was not performed, reason not given Ⓑ

✳ **G9226** Foot examination performed (includes examination through visual inspection, sensory exam with 10-g monofilament plus testing any one of the following: vibration using 128-hz tuning fork, pinprick sensation, ankle reflexes, or vibration perception threshold, and pulse exam; report when all of the 3 components are completed) Ⓑ

↻ ✳ **G9227** Functional outcome assessment documented, care plan not documented, documentation the patient is not eligible for a care plan at the time of the encounter Ⓑ

✳ **G9228** Chlamydia, gonorrhea and syphilis screening results documented (report when results are present for all of the 3 screenings) Ⓑ

✳ **G9229** Chlamydia, gonorrhea, and syphilis screening results not documented (patient refusal is the only allowed exception) Ⓑ

✳ **G9230** Chlamydia, gonorrhea, and syphilis not screened, reason not given Ⓑ

✳ **G9231** Documentation of end stage renal disease (ESRD), dialysis, renal transplant before or during the measurement period or pregnancy during the measurement period Ⓑ

✳ **G9232** Clinician treating major depressive disorder did not communicate to clinician treating comorbid condition for specified patient reason (e.g., patient is unable to communicate the diagnosis of a comorbid condition; the patient is unwilling to communicate the diagnosis of a comorbid condition; or the patient is unaware of the comorbid condition, or any other specified patient reason) Ⓑ

✳ **G9239** Documentation of reasons for patient initiating maintenance hemodialysis with a catheter as the mode of vascular access (e.g., patient has a maturing AVF/AVG, time-limited trial of hemodialysis, other medical reasons, patient declined AVF/AVG, other patient reasons, patient followed by reporting nephrologist for fewer than 90 days, other system reasons) Ⓑ

✳ **G9240** Patient whose mode of vascular access is a catheter at the time maintenance hemodialysis is initiated Ⓑ

✳ **G9241** Patient whose mode of vascular access is not a catheter at the time maintenance hemodialysis is initiated Ⓑ

✳ **G9242** Documentation of viral load equal to or greater than 200 copies/ml or viral load not performed Ⓑ

✳ **G9243** Documentation of viral load less than 200 copies/ml Ⓑ

✳ **G9246** Patient did not have at least one medical visit in each 6 month period of the 24 month measurement period, with a minimum of 60 days between medical visits Ⓑ

✳ **G9247** Patient had at least one medical visit in each 6 month period of the 24 month measurement period, with a minimum of 60 days between medical visits Ⓑ

✳ **G9250** Documentation of patient pain brought to a comfortable level within 48 hours from initial assessment Ⓑ

✳ **G9251** Documentation of patient with pain not brought to a comfortable level within 48 hours from initial assessment Ⓑ

✳ **G9254** Documentation of patient discharged to home later than post-operative day 2 following CAS Ⓑ

✳ **G9255** Documentation of patient discharged to home no later than post operative day 2 following CAS Ⓑ

↻ ✳ **G9256** Documentation of patient death following CAS Ⓑ

↻ ✳ **G9257** Documentation of patient stroke following CAS Ⓑ

↻ ✳ **G9258** Documentation of patient stroke following CEA Ⓑ

↻ ✳ **G9259** Documentation of patient survival and absence of stroke following CAS Ⓑ

↻ ✳ **G9260** Documentation of patient death following CEA Ⓑ

↻ ✳ **G9261** Documentation of patient survival and absence of stroke following CEA Ⓑ

↻ ✳ **G9262** Documentation of patient death in the hospital following endovascular AAA repair Ⓑ

↻ ✳ **G9263** Documentation of patient discharged alive following endovascular AAA repair Ⓑ

✳ **G9264** Documentation of patient receiving maintenance hemodialysis for greater than or equal to 90 days with a catheter for documented reasons (e.g., other medical reasons, patient declined AVF/AVG, other patient reasons) Ⓑ

✳ **G9265** Patient receiving maintenance hemodialysis for greater than or equal to 90 days with a catheter as the mode of vascular access Ⓑ

✳ **G9266** Patient receiving maintenance hemodialysis for greater than or equal to 90 days without a catheter as the mode of vascular access Ⓑ

✳ **G9267** Documentation of patient with one or more complications or mortality within 30 days Ⓑ

✳ **G9268** Documentation of patient with one or more complications within 90 days Ⓑ

✳ **G9269** Documentation of patient without one or more complications and without mortality within 30 days Ⓑ

✳ **G9270** Documentation of patient without one or more complications within 90 days Ⓑ

✳ **G9273** Blood pressure has a systolic value of <140 and a diastolic value of <90 Ⓑ

✳ **G9274** Blood pressure has a systolic value of =140 and a diastolic value of = 90 or systolic value <140 and diastolic value = 90 or systolic value = 140 and diastolic value <90 Ⓑ

✳ **G9275** Documentation that patient is a current non-tobacco user Ⓑ

✳ **G9276** Documentation that patient is a current tobacco user Ⓑ

✳ **G9277** Documentation that the patient is on daily aspirin or anti-platelet or has documentation of a valid contraindication or exception to aspirin/anti-platelet; contraindications/exceptions include anti-coagulant use, allergy to aspirin or anti-platelets, history of gastrointestinal bleed and bleeding disorder; additionally, the following exceptions documented by the physician as a reason for not taking daily aspirin or anti-platelet are acceptable (use of non-steroidal anti-inflammatory agents, documented risk for drug interaction, uncontrolled hypertension defined as > 180 systolic or > 110 diastolic or gastroesophageal reflux) Ⓑ

✳ **G9278** Documentation that the patient is not on daily aspirin or anti-platelet regimen Ⓑ

✳ **G9279** Pneumococcal screening performed and documentation of vaccination received prior to discharge Ⓑ

✳ **G9280** Pneumococcal vaccination not administered prior to discharge, reason not specified Ⓑ

✳ **G9281** Screening performed and documentation that vaccination not indicated/patient refusal Ⓑ

✳ **G9282** Documentation of medical reason(s) for not reporting the histological type or NSCLC-NOS classification with an explanation (e.g., biopsy taken for other purposes in a patient with a history of non-small cell lung cancer or other documented medical reasons) Ⓑ

✳ **G9283** Non small cell lung cancer biopsy and cytology specimen report documents classification into specific histologic type or classified as NSCLC-NOS with an explanation Ⓑ

✳ **G9284** Non small cell lung cancer biopsy and cytology specimen report does not document classification into specific histologic type or classified as NSCLC-NOS with an explanation Ⓑ

✳ **G9285** Specimen site other than anatomic location of lung or is not classified as non small cell lung cancer Ⓑ

✳ **G9286** Antibiotic regimen prescribed within 10 days after onset of symptoms Ⓑ

✳ **G9287** Antibiotic regimen not prescribed within 10 days after onset of symptoms Ⓑ

TEMPORARY PROCEDURES/PROFESSIONAL SERVICES

G9256 – G9287

▶ **New**   ↻ **Revised**   ✔ **Reinstated**   ~~deleted~~ **Deleted**   ⊘ **Not covered or valid by Medicare**
⊛ **Special coverage instructions**   ✳ **Carrier discretion**   Ⓑ **Bill Part B MAC**   Ⓑ **Bill DME MAC**

❋ **G9288** Documentation of medical reason(s) for not reporting the histological type or NSCLC-NOS classification with an explanation (e.g., a solitary fibrous tumor in a person with a history of non-small cell carcinoma or other documented medical reasons) Ⓑ

❋ **G9289** Non-small cell lung cancer biopsy and cytology specimen report documents classification into specific histologic type or classified as NSCLC-NOS with an explanation Ⓑ

❋ **G9290** Non-small cell lung cancer biopsy and cytology specimen report does not document classification into specific histologic type or classified as NSCLC-NOS with an explanation Ⓑ

❋ **G9291** Specimen site other than anatomic location of lung, is not classified as non small cell lung cancer or classified as NSCLC-NOS Ⓑ

❋ **G9292** Documentation of medical reason(s) for not reporting PT category and a statement on thickness and ulceration and for PT1, mitotic rate (e.g., negative skin biopsies in a patient with a history of melanoma or other documented medical reasons) Ⓑ

❋ **G9293** Pathology report does not include the PT category and a statement on thickness and ulceration and for PT1, mitotic rate Ⓑ

❋ **G9294** Pathology report includes the PT category and a statement on thickness and ulceration and for PT1, mitotic rate Ⓑ

❋ **G9295** Specimen site other than anatomic cutaneous location Ⓑ

❋ **G9296** Patients with documented shared decision-making including discussion of conservative (non-surgical) therapy (e.g., NSAIDs, analgesics, weight loss, exercise, injections) prior to the procedure Ⓑ

❋ **G9297** Shared decision-making including discussion of conservative (non-surgical) therapy (e.g., NSAIDs, analgesics, weight loss, exercise, injections) prior to the procedure not documented, reason not given Ⓑ

❋ **G9298** Patients who are evaluated for venous thromboembolic and cardiovascular risk factors within 30 days prior to the procedure (e.g., history of DVT, PE, MI, arrhythmia and stroke) Ⓑ

❋ **G9299** Patients who are not evaluated for venous thromboembolic and cardiovascular risk factors within 30 days prior to the procedure (e.g., history of DVT, PE, MI, arrhythmia and stroke, reason not given) Ⓑ

❋ **G9300** Documentation of medical reason(s) for not completely infusing the prophylactic antibiotic prior to the inflation of the proximal tourniquet (e.g., a tourniquet was not used) Ⓑ

❋ **G9301** Patients who had the prophylactic antibiotic completely infused prior to the inflation of the proximal tourniquet Ⓑ

❋ **G9302** Prophylactic antibiotic not completely infused prior to the inflation of the proximal tourniquet, reason not given Ⓑ

❋ **G9303** Operative report does not identify the prosthetic implant specifications including the prosthetic implant manufacturer, the brand name of the prosthetic implant and the size of each prosthetic implant, reason not given Ⓑ

❋ **G9304** Operative report identifies the prosthetic implant specifications including the prosthetic implant manufacturer, the brand name of the prosthetic implant and the size of each prosthetic implant Ⓑ

❋ **G9305** Intervention for presence of leak of endoluminal contents through an anastomosis not required Ⓑ

❋ **G9306** Intervention for presence of leak of endoluminal contents through an anastomosis required Ⓑ

❋ **G9307** No return to the operating room for a surgical procedure, for complications of the principal operative procedure, within 30 days of the principal operative procedure Ⓑ

❋ **G9308** Unplanned return to the operating room for a surgical procedure, for complications of the principal operative procedure, within 30 days of the principal operative procedure Ⓑ

❋ **G9309** No unplanned hospital readmission within 30 days of principal procedure Ⓑ

❋ **G9310** Unplanned hospital readmission within 30 days of principal procedure Ⓑ

❋ **G9311** No surgical site infection Ⓑ

❋ **G9312** Surgical site infection Ⓑ

↻ ✳ **G9313** Amoxicillin, with or without clavulanate, not prescribed as first line antibiotic at the time of diagnosis for documented reason ⑬

✳ **G9314** Amoxicillin, with or without clavulanate, not prescribed as first line antibiotic at the time of diagnosis, reason not given ⑬

✳ **G9315** Documentation amoxicillin, with or without clavulanate, prescribed as a first line antibiotic at the time of diagnosis ⑬

✳ **G9316** Documentation of patient-specific risk assessment with a risk calculator based on multi-institutional clinical data, the specific risk calculator used, and communication of risk assessment from risk calculator with the patient or family ⑬

✳ **G9317** Documentation of patient-specific risk assessment with a risk calculator based on multi-institutional clinical data, the specific risk calculator used, and communication of risk assessment from risk calculator with the patient or family not completed ⑬

✳ **G9318** Imaging study named according to standardized nomenclature ⑬

✳ **G9319** Imaging study not named according to standardized nomenclature, reason not given ⑬

✳ **G9321** Count of previous CT (any type of CT) and cardiac nuclear medicine (myocardial perfusion) studies documented in the 12-month period prior to the current study ⑬

✳ **G9322** Count of previous CT and cardiac nuclear medicine (myocardial perfusion) studies not documented in the 12-month period prior to the current study, reason not given ⑬

✳ **G9326** CT studies performed not reported to a radiation dose index registry that is capable of collecting at a minimum all necessary data elements, reason not given ⑬

✳ **G9327** CT studies performed reported to a radiation dose index registry that is capable of collecting at a minimum all necessary data elements ⑬

✳ **G9329** DICOM format image data available to non-affiliated external healthcare facilities or entities on a secure, media free, reciprocally searchable basis with patient authorization for at least a 12-month period after the study not documented in final report, reason not given ⑬

✳ **G9340** Final report documented that DICOM format image data available to non-affiliated external healthcare facilities or entities on a secure, media free, reciprocally searchable basis with patient authorization for at least a 12-month period after the study ⑬

✳ **G9341** Search conducted for prior patient CT studies completed at non-affiliated external healthcare facilities or entities within the past 12-months and are available through a secure, authorized, media-free, shared archive prior to an imaging study being performed ⑬

✳ **G9342** Search not conducted prior to an imaging study being performed for prior patient CT studies completed at non-affiliated external healthcare facilities or entities within the past 12-months and are available through a secure, authorized, media-free, shared archive, reason not given ⑬

✳ **G9344** Due to system reasons search not conducted for DICOM format images for prior patient CT imaging studies completed at non-affiliated external healthcare facilities or entities within the past 12 months that are available through a secure, authorized, media-free, shared archive (e.g., non-affiliated external healthcare facilities or entities does not have archival abilities through a shared archival system) ⑬

✳ **G9345** Follow-up recommendations documented according to recommended guidelines for incidentally detected pulmonary nodules (e.g., follow-up CT imaging studies needed or that no follow-up is needed) based at a minimum on nodule size and patient risk factors ⑬

✳ **G9347** Follow-up recommendations not documented according to recommended guidelines for incidentally detected pulmonary nodules, reason not given ⑬

↻ ✳ **G9348** CT scan of the paranasal sinuses ordered at the time of diagnosis for documented reasons ⑬

✳ **G9349** Documentation of a CT scan of the paranasal sinuses ordered at the time of diagnosis or received within 28 days after date of diagnosis ⑬

✳ **G9350** CT scan of the paranasal sinuses not ordered at the time of diagnosis or received within 28 days after date of diagnosis ⑬

▶ **New**   ↻ **Revised**   ✔ **Reinstated**   deleted **Deleted**   ⊘ **Not covered or valid by Medicare**
✪ **Special coverage instructions**   ✳ **Carrier discretion**   ⑨ **Bill Part B MAC**   ⑬ **Bill DME MAC**

❋ **G9351** More than one CT scan of the paranasal sinuses ordered or received within 90 days after diagnosis Ⓑ

❋ **G9352** More than one CT scan of the paranasal sinuses ordered or received within 90 days after the date of diagnosis, reason not given Ⓑ

❋ **G9353** More than one CT scan of the paranasal sinuses ordered or received within 90 days after the date of diagnosis for documented reasons (e.g., patients with complications, second CT obtained prior to surgery, other medical reasons) Ⓑ

❋ **G9354** One CT scan or no CT scan of the paranasal sinuses ordered within 90 days after the date of diagnosis Ⓑ

❋ **G9355** Elective delivery or early induction not performed Ⓑ

❋ **G9356** Elective delivery or early induction performed Ⓑ

❋ **G9357** Post-partum screenings, evaluations and education performed Ⓑ

❋ **G9358** Post-partum screenings, evaluations and education not performed Ⓑ

❋ **G9359** Documentation of negative or managed positive TB screen with further evidence that TB is not active within one year of patient visit Ⓑ

❋ **G9360** No documentation of negative or managed positive TB screen Ⓑ

❋ **G9361** Medical indication for induction [documentation of reason(s) for elective delivery (c-section) or early induction (e.g., hemorrhage and placental complications, hypertension, preeclampsia and eclampsia, rupture of membranes-premature or prolonged, maternal conditions complicating pregnancy/delivery, fetal conditions complicating pregnancy/delivery, late pregnancy, prior uterine surgery, or participation in clinical trial)] Ⓑ

❋ **G9364** Sinusitis caused by, or presumed to be caused by, bacterial infection Ⓑ

❋ **G9365** One high-risk medication ordered Ⓑ

❋ **G9366** One high-risk medication not ordered Ⓑ

❋ **G9367** At least two different high-risk medications ordered Ⓑ

❋ **G9368** At least two different high-risk medications not ordered Ⓑ

❋ **G9380** Patient offered assistance with end of life issues during the measurement period Ⓑ

~~G9381~~ ~~Documentation of medical reason(s)~~ ✖ ~~for not offering assistance with end of life issues (e.g., patient in hospice care, patient in terminal phase) during the measurement period~~

❋ **G9382** Patient not offered assistance with end of life issues during the measurement period Ⓑ

❋ **G9383** Patient received screening for HCV infection within the 12 month reporting period Ⓑ

↻ ❋ **G9384** Documentation of medical reason(s) for not receiving annual screening for HCV infection (e.g., decompensated cirrhosis indicating advanced disease [i.e., ascites, esophageal variceal bleeding, hepatic encephalopathy], hepatocellular carcinoma, waitlist for organ transplant, limited life expectancy, other medical reasons) Ⓑ

❋ **G9385** Documentation of patient reason(s) for not receiving annual screening for HCV infection (e.g., patient declined, other patient reasons) Ⓑ

❋ **G9386** Screening for HCV infection not received within the 12 month reporting period, reason not given Ⓑ

❋ **G9389** Unplanned rupture of the posterior capsule requiring vitrectomy during cataract surgery Ⓑ

❋ **G9390** No unplanned rupture of the posterior capsule requiring vitrectomy during cataract surgery Ⓑ

❋ **G9393** Patient with an initial PHQ-9 score greater than nine who achieves remission at twelve months as demonstrated by a twelve month (+/- 30 days) phq-9 score of less than five Ⓑ

❋ **G9394** Patient who had a diagnosis of bipolar disorder or personality disorder, death, permanent nursing home resident or receiving hospice or palliative care any time during the measurement or assessment period Ⓑ

❋ **G9395** Patient with an initial PHQ-9 score greater than nine who did not achieve remission at twelve months as demonstrated by a twelve month (+/- 30 days) phq-9 score greater than or equal to five Ⓑ

❋ **G9396** Patient with an initial PHQ-9 score greater than nine who was not assessed for remission at twelve months (+/- 30 days) Ⓑ

▶ New   ↻ Revised   ✔ Reinstated   ~~deleted~~ Deleted   ⊘ Not covered or valid by Medicare

⊗ Special coverage instructions   ❋ Carrier discretion   Ⓑ Bill Part B MAC   Ⓓ Bill DME MAC

* **G9399** Documentation in the patient record of a discussion between the physician/clinician and the patient that includes all of the following: treatment choices appropriate to genotype, risks and benefits, evidence of effectiveness, and patient preferences toward the outcome of the treatment Ⓑ

* **G9400** Documentation of medical or patient reason(s) for not discussing treatment options; medical reasons: patient is not a candidate for treatment due to advanced physical or mental health comorbidity (including active substance use); currently receiving antiviral treatment; successful antiviral treatment (with sustained virologic response) prior to reporting period; other documented medical reasons; patient reasons: patient unable or unwilling to participate in the discussion or other patient reasons Ⓑ

* **G9401** No documentation of a discussion in the patient record of a discussion between the physician or other qualified healthcare professional and the patient that includes all of the following: treatment choices appropriate to genotype, risks and benefits, evidence of effectiveness, and patient preferences toward treatment Ⓑ

* **G9402** Patient received follow-up on the date of discharge or within 30 days after discharge Ⓑ

* **G9403** Clinician documented reason patient was not able to complete 30 day follow-up from acute inpatient setting discharge (e.g., patient death prior to follow-up visit, patient non-compliant for visit follow-up) Ⓑ

* **G9404** Patient did not receive follow-up on the date of discharge or within 30 days after discharge Ⓑ

* **G9405** Patient received follow-up within 7 days from discharge Ⓑ

* **G9406** Clinician documented reason patient was not able to complete 7 day follow-up from acute inpatient setting discharge (i.e patient death prior to follow-up visit, patient non-compliance for visit follow-up) Ⓑ

* **G9407** Patient did not receive follow-up on or within 7 days after discharge Ⓑ

* **G9408** Patients with cardiac tamponade and/or pericardiocentesis occurring within 30 days Ⓑ

* **G9409** Patients without cardiac tamponade and/or pericardiocentesis occurring within 30 days Ⓑ

* **G9410** Patient admitted within 180 days, status post CIED implantation, replacement, or revision with an infection requiring device removal or surgical revision Ⓑ

* **G9411** Patient not admitted within 180 days, status post CIED implantation, replacement, or revision with an infection requiring device removal or surgical revision Ⓑ

* **G9412** Patient admitted within 180 days, status post CIED implantation, replacement, or revision with an infection requiring device removal or surgical revision Ⓑ

* **G9413** Patient not admitted within 180 days, status post CIED implantation, replacement, or revision with an infection requiring device removal or surgical revision Ⓑ

* **G9414** Patient had one dose of meningococcal vaccine on or between the patient's 11th and 13th birthdays Ⓑ

* **G9415** Patient did not have one dose of meningococcal vaccine on or between the patient's 11th and 13th birthdays Ⓑ

* **G9416** Patient had one tetanus, diphtheria toxoids and acellular pertussis vaccine (Tdap) or one tetanus, diphtheria toxoids vaccine (Td) on or between the patient's 10th and 13th birthdays Ⓑ

* **G9417** Patient did not have one tetanus, diphtheria toxoids and acellular pertussis vaccine (Tdap) on or between the patient's 10th and 13th birthdays Ⓑ

* **G9418** Primary non-small cell lung cancer biopsy and cytology specimen report documents classification into specific histologic type or classified as NSCLC-NOS with an explanation Ⓑ

* **G9419** Documentation of medical reason(s) for not including the histological type or NSCLC-NOS classification with an explanation (e.g., biopsy taken for other purposes in a patient with a history of primary non-small cell lung cancer or other documented medical reasons) Ⓑ

* **G9420** Specimen site other than anatomic location of lung or is not classified as primary non-small cell lung cancer Ⓑ

▶ New   ↻ Revised   ✔ Reinstated   deleted Deleted   ⊘ Not covered or valid by Medicare

⊙ Special coverage instructions   * Carrier discretion   Ⓑ Bill Part B MAC   Ⓖ Bill DME MAC

* **G9421** Primary non-small cell lung cancer biopsy and cytology specimen report does not document classification into specific histologic type or classified as NSCLC-NOS with an explanation ⓑ

* **G9422** Primary lung carcinoma resection report documents pT category, pN category and for non-small cell lung cancer, histologic type (squamous cell carcinoma, adenocarcinoma and not nsclc-nos) ⓑ

* **G9423** Documentation of medical reason for not including pT category, pN category and histologic type [for patient with appropriate exclusion criteria (e.g., metastatic disease, benign tumors, malignant tumors other than carcinomas, inadequate surgical specimens)] ⓑ

* **G9424** Specimen site other than anatomic location of lung, or classified as NSCLC-NOS ⓑ

* **G9425** Primary lung carcinoma resection report does not document pT category, pN category and for non-small cell lung cancer, histologic type (squamous cell carcinoma,adenocarcinoma) ⓑ

* **G9426** Improvement in median time from ED arrival to initial ED oral or parenteral pain medication administration performed for ED admitted patients ⓑ

* **G9427** Improvement in median time from ED arrival to initial ED oral or parenteral pain medication administration not performed for ED admitted patients ⓑ

* **G9428** Pathology report includes the pT category and a statement on thickness and ulceration and for pT1, mitotic rate ⓑ

* **G9429** Documentation of medical reason(s) for not including pT category and a statement on thickness and ulceration and for pT1, mitotic rate (e.g., negative skin biopsies in a patient with a history of melanoma or other documented medical reasons) ⓑ

* **G9430** Specimen site other than anatomic cutaneous location ⓑ

* **G9431** Pathology report does not include the pT category and a statement on thickness and ulceration and for pT1, mitotic rate ⓑ

* **G9432** Asthma well-controlled based on the ACT, C-ACT, ACQ, or ATAQ score and results documented ⓑ

* **G9434** Asthma not well-controlled based on the ACT, C-ACT, ACQ, or ATAQ score, or specified asthma control tool not used, reason not given ⓑ

* **G9448** Patients who were born in the years 1945-1965 ⓑ

* **G9449** History of receiving blood transfusions prior to 1992 ⓑ

* **G9450** History of injection drug use ⓑ

* **G9451** Patient received one-time screening for HCV infection ⓑ

* **G9452** Documentation of medical reason(s) for not receiving one-time screening for HCV infection (e.g., decompensated cirrhosis indicating advanced disease [i.e., ascites, esophageal variceal bleeding, hepatic encephalopathy], hepatocellular carcinoma, waitlist for organ transplant, limited life expectancy, other medical reasons) ⓑ

* **G9453** Documentation of patient reason(s) for not receiving one-time screening for HCV infection (e.g., patient declined, other patient reasons) ⓑ

* **G9454** One-time screening for HCV infection not received within 12 month reporting period and no documentation of prior screening for HCV infection, reason not given ⓑ

* **G9455** Patient underwent abdominal imaging with ultrasound, contrast enhanced CT or contrast MRI for HCC ⓑ

* **G9456** Documentation of medical or patient reason(s) for not ordering or performing screening for HCC. medical reason: comorbid medical conditions with expected survival <5 years, hepatic decompensation and not a candidate for liver transplantation, or other medical reasons; patient reasons: patient declined or other patient reasons (e.g., cost of tests, time related to accessing testing equipment) ⓑ

* **G9457** Patient did not undergo abdominal imaging and did not have a documented reason for not undergoing abdominal imaging in the reporting period ⓑ

▶ New   ↻ Revised   ✔ Reinstated   ~~deleted~~ Deleted   ⊘ Not covered or valid by Medicare
✪ Special coverage instructions   * Carrier discretion   ⓑ Bill Part B MAC   ⑧ Bill DME MAC

✱ **G9458** Patient documented as tobacco user and received tobacco cessation intervention (must include at least one of the following: advice given to quit smoking or tobacco use, counseling on the benefits of quitting smoking or tobacco use, assistance with or referral to external smoking or tobacco cessation support programs, or current enrollment in smoking or tobacco use cessation program) if identified as a tobacco user ⑧

✱ **G9459** Currently a tobacco non-user ⑧

✱ **G9460** Tobacco assessment or tobacco cessation intervention not performed, reason not given ⑧

✱ **G9468** Patient not receiving corticosteroids greater than or equal to 10 mg/day of prednisone equivalents for 60 or greater consecutive days or a single prescription equating to 600 mg prednisone or greater for all fills ⑧

✱ **G9469** Patients who have received or are receiving corticosteroids greater than or equal to 10 mg/day of prednisone equivalents for 60 or greater consecutive days or a single prescription equating to 600 mg prednisone or greater for all fills ⑧

✱ **G9470** Patients not receiving corticosteroids greater than or equal to 10 mg/day of prednisone equivalents for 60 or greater consecutive days or a single prescription equating to 600 mg prednisone or greater for all fills ⑧

✱ **G9471** Within the past 2 years, central dual-energy x-ray absorptiometry (DXA) not ordered or documented ⑧

✱ **G9472** Within the past 2 years, central dual-energy x-ray absorptiometry (DXA) not ordered and documented, no review of systems and no medication history or pharmacologic therapy (other than minerals/vitamins) for osteoporosis prescribed ⑧

✱ **G9473** Services performed by chaplain in the hospice setting, each 15 minutes ⑧

✱ **G9474** Services performed by dietary counselor in the hospice setting, each 15 minutes ⑧

✱ **G9475** Services performed by other counselor in the hospice setting, each 15 minutes ⑧

✱ **G9476** Services performed by volunteer in the hospice setting, each 15 minutes ⑧

✱ **G9477** Services performed by care coordinator in the hospice setting, each 15 minutes ⑧

✱ **G9478** Services performed by other qualified therapist in the hospice setting, each 15 minutes ⑧

✱ **G9479** Services performed by qualified pharmacist in the hospice setting, each 15 minutes ⑧

✱ **G9480** Admission to Medicare Care Choice Model program (MCCM) ⑧

✱ **G9481** Remote in-home visit for the evaluation and management of a new patient for use only in the Medicare-approved comprehensive care for joint replacement model, which requires these 3 key components: a problem focused history; a problem focused examination; and straightforward medical decision making, furnished in real time using interactive audio and video technology. Counseling and coordination of care with other physicians, other qualified health care professionals or agencies are provided consistent with the nature of the problem(s) and the needs of the patient or the family or both. Usually, the presenting problem(s) are self limited or minor. Typically, 10 minutes are spent with the patient or family or both via real time, audio and video intercommunications technology ⑧

✱ **G9482** Remote in-home visit for the evaluation and management of a new patient for use only in the Medicare-approved comprehensive care for joint replacement model, which requires these 3 key components: an expanded problem focused history; an expanded problem focused examination; straightforward medical decision making, furnished in real time using interactive audio and video technology. Counseling and coordination of care with other physicians, other qualified health care professionals or agencies are provided consistent with the nature of the problem(s) and the needs of the patient or the family or both. Usually, the presenting problem(s) are of low to moderate severity. Typically, 20 minutes are spent with the patient or family or both via real time, audio and video intercommunications technology ⑧

▶ **New**   ↻ **Revised**   ✔ **Reinstated**   ~~deleted~~ **Deleted**   ⊘ **Not covered or valid by Medicare**
⊙ **Special coverage instructions**   ✱ **Carrier discretion**   ⑧ **Bill Part B MAC**   ⑧ **Bill DME MAC**

✳ **G9483** Remote in-home visit for the evaluation and management of a new patient for use only in the Medicare-approved comprehensive care for joint replacement model, which requires these 3 key components: a detailed history; a detailed examination; medical decision making of low complexity, furnished in real time using interactive audio and video technology. Counseling and coordination of care with other physicians, other qualified health care professionals or agencies are provided consistent with the nature of the problem(s) and the needs of the patient or the family or both. Usually, the presenting problem(s) are of moderate severity. Typically, 30 minutes are spent with the patient or family or both via real time, audio and video intercommunications technology Ⓑ

✳ **G9484** Remote in-home visit for the evaluation and management of a new patient for use only in the Medicare-approved comprehensive care for joint replacement model, which requires these 3 key components: a comprehensive history; a comprehensive examination; medical decision making of moderate complexity, furnished in real time using interactive audio and video technology. Counseling and coordination of care with other physicians, other qualified health care professionals or agencies are provided consistent with the nature of the problem(s) and the needs of the patient or the family or both. Usually, the presenting problem(s) are of moderate to high severity. Typically, 45 minutes are spent with the patient or family or both via real time, audio and video intercommunications technology Ⓑ

✳ **G9485** Remote in-home visit for the evaluation and management of a new patient for use only in the Medicare-approved comprehensive care for joint replacement model, which requires these 3 key components: a comprehensive history; a comprehensive examination; medical decision making of high complexity, furnished in real time using interactive audio and video technology. Counseling and coordination of care with other physicians, other qualified health care professionals or agencies are provided consistent with the nature of the problem(s) and the needs of the patient or the family or both. Usually, the presenting problem(s) are of moderate to high severity. Typically, 60 minutes are spent with the patient or family or both via real time, audio and video intercommunications technology Ⓑ

✳ **G9486** Remote in-home visit for the evaluation and management of an established patient for use only in the Medicare-approved comprehensive care for joint replacement model, which requires at least 2 of the following 3 key components: a problem focused history; a problem focused examination; straightforward medical decision making, furnished in real time using interactive audio and video technology. Counseling and coordination of care with other physicians, other qualified health care professionals or agencies are provided consistent with the nature of the problem(s) and the needs of the patient or the family or both. Usually, the presenting problem(s) are self limited or minor. Typically, 10 minutes are spent with the patient or family or both via real time, audio and video intercommunications technology Ⓑ

▶ **New**   ↻ **Revised**   ✔ **Reinstated**   ~~deleted~~ **Deleted**   ⊘ **Not covered or valid by Medicare**

✪ **Special coverage instructions**   ✳ **Carrier discretion**   Ⓑ **Bill Part B MAC**   Ⓑ **Bill DME MAC**

* **G9487** Remote in-home visit for the evaluation and management of an established patient for use only in the Medicare-approved comprehensive care for joint replacement model, which requires at least 2 of the following 3 key components: an expanded problem focused history; an expanded problem focused examination; medical decision making of low complexity, furnished in real time using interactive audio and video technology. Counseling and coordination of care with other physicians, other qualified health care professionals or agencies are provided consistent with the nature of the problem(s) and the needs of the patient or the family or both. Usually, the presenting problem(s) are of low to moderate severity. Typically, 15 minutes are spent with the patient or family or both via real time, audio and video intercommunications technology ⑧

* **G9488** Remote in-home visit for the evaluation and management of an established patient for use only in the Medicare-approved comprehensive care for joint replacement model, which requires at least 2 of the following 3 key components: a detailed history; a detailed examination; medical decision making of moderate complexity, furnished in real time using interactive audio and video technology. Counseling and coordination of care with other physicians, other qualified health care professionals or agencies are provided consistent with the nature of the problem(s) and the needs of the patient or the family or both. Usually, the presenting problem(s) are of moderate to high severity. Typically, 25 minutes are spent with the patient or family or both via real time, audio and video intercommunications technology ⑧

* **G9489** Remote in-home visit for the evaluation and management of an established patient for use only in the Medicare-approved comprehensive care for joint replacement model, which requires at least 2 of the following 3 key components: a comprehensive history; a comprehensive examination; medical decision making of high complexity, furnished in real time using interactive audio and video technology. Counseling and coordination of care with other physicians, other qualified health care professionals or agencies are provided consistent with the nature of the problem(s) and the needs of the patient or the family or both. Usually, the presenting problem(s) are of moderate to high severity. Typically, 40 minutes are spent with the patient or family or both via real time, audio and video intercommunications technology ⑧

* **G9490** Comprehensive care for joint replacement model, home visit for patient assessment performed by clinical staff for an individual not considered homebound, including, but not necessarily limited to patient assessment of clinical status, safety/fall prevention, functional status/ambulation, medication reconciliation/management, compliance with orders/plan of care, performance of activities of daily living, and ensuring beneficiary connections to community and other services. (for use only in the Medicare-approved CJR model); may not be billed for a 30 day period covered by a transitional care management code ⑧

~~G9496~~ ~~Documentation of reason for not detecting adenoma(s) or other neoplasm. (e.g., neoplasm detected is only diagnosed as traditional serrated adenoma, sessile serrated polyp, or sessile serrated adenoma~~ ✖

* **G9497** Received instruction from the anesthesiologist or proxy prior to the day of surgery to abstain from smoking on the day of surgery ⑧

* **G9498** Antibiotic regimen prescribed ⑧

* **G9500** Radiation exposure indices, or exposure time and number of fluorographic images in final report for procedures using fluoroscopy, documented ⑧

* **G9501** Radiation exposure indices, or exposure time and number of fluorographic images not documented in final report for procedure using fluoroscopy, reason not given ⑧

▶ **New**   ↺ **Revised**   ✔ **Reinstated**   ~~deleted~~ **Deleted**   ⊘ **Not covered or valid by Medicare**
⊙ **Special coverage instructions**   ✳ **Carrier discretion**   ⑨ **Bill Part B MAC**   ⑧ **Bill DME MAC**

✳ **G9502** Documentation of medical reason for not performing foot exam (i.e., patients who have had either a bilateral amputation above or below the knee, or both a left and right amputation above or below the knee before or during the measurement period) ⓑ

✳ **G9503** Patient taking tamsulosin hydrochloride ⓑ

↻ ✳ **G9504** Documented reason for not assessing Hepatitis B virus (HBV) status (e.g. patient not initiating anti-TNF therapy, patient declined) prior to initiating anti-TNF therapy ⓑ

✳ **G9505** Antibiotic regimen prescribed within 10 days after onset of symptoms for documented medical reason ⓑ

✳ **G9506** Biologic immune response modifier prescribed ⓑ

✳ **G9507** Documentation that the patient is on a statin medication or has documentation of a valid contraindication or exception to statin medications; contraindications/exceptions that can be defined by diagnosis codes include pregnancy during the measurement period, active liver disease, rhabdomyolysis, end stage renal disease on dialysis and heart failure; provider documented contraindications/ exceptions include breastfeeding during the measurement period, woman of child-bearing age not actively taking birth control, allergy to statin, drug interaction (HIV protease inhibitors, nefazodone, cyclosporine, gemfibrozil, and danazol) and intolerance (with supporting documentation of trying a statin at least once within the last 5 years or diagnosis codes for myositis or toxic myopathy related to drugs) ⓑ

✳ **G9508** Documentation that the patient is not on a statin medication ⓑ

✳ **G9509** Remission at twelve months as demonstrated by a twelve month (+/-30 days) PHQ-9 score of less than 5 ⓑ

✳ **G9510** Remission at twelve months not demonstrated by a twelve month (+/-30 days) PHQ-9 score of less than five; either PHQ-9 score was not assessed or is greater than or equal to 5 ⓑ

✳ **G9511** Index date PHQ-9 score greater than 9 documented during the twelve month denominator identification period ⓑ

✳ **G9512** Individual had a PDC of 0.8 or greater ⓑ

✳ **G9513** Individual did not have a PDC of 0.8 or greater ⓑ

✳ **G9514** Patient required a return to the operating room within 90 days of surgery ⓑ

✳ **G9515** Patient did not require a return to the operating room within 90 days of surgery ⓑ

✳ **G9516** Patient achieved an improvement in visual acuity, from their preoperative level, within 90 days of surgery ⓖ

✳ **G9517** Patient did not achieve an improvement in visual acuity, from their preoperative level, within 90 days of surgery, reason not given ⓑ

✳ **G9518** Documentation of active injection drug use ⓑ

✳ **G9519** Patient achieves final refraction (spherical equivalent) +/- 0.5 diopters of their planned refraction within 90 days of surgery ⓑ

✳ **G9520** Patient does not achieve final refraction (spherical equivalent) +/- 0.5 diopters of their planned refraction within 90 days of surgery ⓑ

✳ **G9521** Total number of emergency department visits and inpatient hospitalizations less than two in the past 12 months ⓑ

✳ **G9522** Total number of emergency department visits and inpatient hospitalizations equal to or greater than two in the past 12 months or patient not screened, reason not given ⓑ

✳ **G9523** Patient discontinued from hemodialysis or peritoneal dialysis ⓖ

✳ **G9524** Patient was referred to hospice care ⓑ

✳ **G9525** Documentation of patient reason(s) for not referring to hospice care (e.g., patient declined, other patient reasons) ⓑ

✳ **G9526** Patient was not referred to hospice care, reason not given ⓑ

✳ **G9529** Patient with minor blunt head trauma had an appropriate indication(s) for a head CT ⓑ

✳ **G9530** Patient presented within 24 hours of a minor blunt head trauma with a GCS score of 15 and had a head CT ordered for trauma by an emergency care provider ⓑ

▶ **New**   ↻ **Revised**   ✔ **Reinstated**   ~~deleted~~ **Deleted**   ⊘ **Not covered or valid by Medicare**
✪ **Special coverage instructions**   ✳ **Carrier discretion**   ⓑ **Bill Part B MAC**   ⓖ **Bill DME MAC**

* **G9531** Patient has documentation of ventricular shunt, brain tumor, multisystem trauma, pregnancy, or is currently taking an antiplatelet medication including: asa/dipyridamole, clopidogrel, prasugrel, ticlopidine, ticagrelor or cilstazol) Ⓑ

* **G9532** Patient's head injury occurred greater than 24 hours before presentation to the emergency department, or has a GCS score less than 15 or does not have a GCSs score documented, or had a head CT for trauma ordered by someone other than an emergency care provider, or was ordered for a reason other than trauma Ⓑ

* **G9533** Patient with minor blunt head trauma did not have an appropriate indication(s) for a head CT Ⓑ

* **G9534** Advanced brain imaging (CTA, CT, MRA or MRI) was not ordered Ⓑ

* **G9535** Patients with a normal neurological examination Ⓑ

* **G9536** Documentation of medical reason(s) for ordering an advanced brain imaging study (i.e., patient has an abnormal neurological examination; patient has the coexistence of seizures, or both; recent onset of severe headache; change in the type of headache; signs of increased intracranial pressure (e.g., papilledema, absent venous pulsations on funduscopic examination, altered mental status, focal neurologic deficits, signs of meningeal irritation); HIV-positive patients with a new type of headache; immunocompromised patient with unexplained headache symptoms; patient on coagulopathy/anti-coagulation or anti-platelet therapy; very young patients with unexplained headache symptoms) Ⓑ

* **G9537** Documentation of system reason(s) for ordering an advanced brain imaging study (i.e., needed as part of a clinical trial; other clinician ordered the study) Ⓑ

* **G9538** Advanced brain imaging (cta, ct, mra or mri) was ordered Ⓑ

* **G9539** Intent for potential removal at time of placement Ⓑ

* **G9540** Patient alive 3 months post procedure Ⓑ

↻ * **G9541** Filter removed within 3 months of placement Ⓑ

* **G9542** Documented re-assessment for the appropriateness of filter removal within 3 months of placement Ⓑ

* **G9543** Documentation of at least two attempts to reach the patient to arrange a clinical re-assessment for the appropriateness of filter removal within 3 months of placement Ⓑ

* **G9544** Patients that do not have the filter removed, documented re-assessment for the appropriateness of filter removal, or documentation of at least two attempts to reach the patient to arrange a clinical re-assessment for the appropriateness of filter removal within 3 months of placement Ⓑ

* **G9547** Incidental finding: liver lesion <= 0.5 cm, cystic kidney lesion <1.0 cm or adrenal lesion <= 1.0 cm Ⓑ

* **G9548** Final reports for abdominal imaging studies with follow-up imaging recommended Ⓑ

* **G9549** Documentation of medical reason(s) that follow-up imaging is indicated (e.g., patient has a known malignancy that can metastasize, other medical reason(s) such as fever in an immunocompromised patient) Ⓑ

* **G9550** Final reports for abdominal imaging studies with follow-up imaging not recommended Ⓑ

* **G9551** Final reports for abdominal imaging studies without an incidentally found lesion noted: liver lesion <= 0.5 cm, cystic kidney lesion <1.0 cm or adrenal lesion <= 1.0 cm noted or no lesion found Ⓑ

* **G9552** Incidental thyroid nodule <1.0 cm noted in report Ⓑ

* **G9553** Prior thyroid disease diagnosis Ⓑ

* **G9554** Final reports for CT, CTA, MRI or MRA of the chest or neck or ultrasound of the neck with follow-up imaging recommended Ⓑ

* **G9555** Documentation of medical reason(s) for recommending follow up imaging (e.g., patient has multiple endocrine neoplasia, patient has cervical lymphadenopathy, other medical reason(s)) Ⓑ

* **G9556** Final reports for CT, CTA, MRI or MRA of the chest or neck or ultrasound of the neck with follow-up imaging not recommended Ⓑ

* **G9557** Final reports for CT, CTA, MRI or MRA studies of the chest or neck or ultrasound of the neck without an incidentally found thyroid nodule <1.0 cm noted or no nodule found Ⓑ

▶ New   ↻ Revised   ✔ Reinstated   ~~deleted~~ Deleted   ⊘ Not covered or valid by Medicare
⚙ Special coverage instructions   * Carrier discretion   Ⓑ Bill Part B MAC   Ⓓ Bill DME MAC

* **G9558** Patient treated with a beta-lactam antibiotic as definitive therapy ⑧

* **G9559** Documentation of medical reason(s) for not prescribing a beta-lactam antibiotic (e.g., allergy, intolerance to beta-lactam antibiotics) ⑧

* **G9560** Patient not treated with a beta-lactam antibiotic as definitive therapy, reason not given ⑧

* **G9561** Patients prescribed opiates for longer than six weeks ⑧

* **G9562** Patients who had a follow-up evaluation conducted at least every three months during opioid therapy ⑧

* **G9563** Patients who did not have a follow-up evaluation conducted at least every three months during opioid therapy ⑧

* **G9573** Remission at six months as demonstrated by a six month (+/-30 days) PHQ-9 score of less than five ⑧

* **G9574** Remission at six months not demonstrated by a six month (+/-30 days) PHQ-9 score of less than five; either PHQ-9 score was not assessed or is greater than or equal to five ⑧

* **G9577** Patients prescribed opiates for longer than six weeks ⑧

* **G9578** Documentation of signed opioid treatment agreement at least once during opioid therapy ⑧

* **G9579** No documentation of signed an opioid treatment agreement at least once during opioid therapy ⑧

* **G9580** Door to puncture time of less than 2 hours ⑧

* **G9582** Door to puncture time of greater than 2 hours, no reason given ⑧

* **G9583** Patients prescribed opiates for longer than six weeks ⑧

* **G9584** Patient evaluated for risk of misuse of opiates by using a brief validated instrument (e.g., opioid risk tool, SOAPP-R) or patient interviewed at least once during opioid therapy ⑧

* **G9585** Patient not evaluated for risk of misuse of opiates by using a brief validated instrument (e.g., opioid risk tool, SOAPP-R) or patient not interviewed at least once during opioid therapy ⑧

* **G9593** Pediatric patient with minor blunt head trauma classified as low risk according to the pecarn Prediction Rules ⑧

* **G9594** Patient presented within 24 hours of a minor blunt head trauma with a GCS score of 15 and had a head CT ordered for trauma by an emergency care provider ⑧

* **G9595** Patient has documentation of ventricular shunt, brain tumor, coagulopathy, including thrombocytopenia ⑧

* **G9596** Pediatric patient's head injury occurred greater than 24 hours before presentation to the emergency department, or has a GCS score less than 15 or does not have a GCS score documented, or had a head CT for trauma ordered by someone other than an emergency care provider, or was ordered for a reason other than trauma ⑧

* **G9597** Pediatric patient with minor blunt head trauma not classified as low risk according to the pecarn Prediction Rules ⑧

* **G9598** Aortic aneurysm 5.5 - 5.9 cm maximum diameter on centerline formatted CT or minor diameter on axial formatted CT ⑧

* **G9599** Aortic aneurysm 6.0 cm or greater maximum diameter on centerline formatted CT or minor diameter on axial formatted CT ⑧

* **G9600** Symptomatic AAAS that required urgent/emergent (non-elective) repair ⑧

* **G9601** Patient discharge to home no later than post-operative day #7 ⑧

* **G9602** Patient not discharged to home by post-operative day #7 ⑧

* **G9603** Patient survey score improved from baseline following treatment ⑧

* **G9604** Patient survey results not available ⑧

* **G9605** Patient survey score did not improve from baseline following treatment ⑧

* **G9606** Intraoperative cystoscopy performed to evaluate for lower tract injury ⑧

⤺ * **G9607** Documented medical reasons for not performing intraoperative cystoscopy (e.g., urethral pathology precluding cystoscopy, any patient who has a congenital or acquired absence of the urethra) or in the case of patient death ⑧

* **G9608** Intraoperative cystoscopy not performed to evaluate for lower tract injury ⑧

* **G9609** Documentation of an order for anti-platelet agents ⑧

▶ New   ⤺ Revised   ✔ Reinstated   deleted Deleted   ⊘ Not covered or valid by Medicare
☼ Special coverage instructions   ✳ Carrier discretion   ⑨ Bill Part B MAC   ⑧ Bill DME MAC

* **G9610** Documentation of medical reason(s) in the patient's record for not ordering anti-platelet agents Ⓑ

* **G9611** Order for anti-platelet agents was not documented in the patient's record, reason not given Ⓑ

* **G9612** Photodocumentation of one or more cecal landmarks to establish a complete examination Ⓑ

* **G9613** Documentation of post-surgical anatomy (e.g., right hemicolectomy, ileocecal resection, etc.) Ⓑ

* **G9614** No photodocumentation of cecal landmarks to establish a complete examination Ⓑ

* **G9615** Preoperative assessment documented Ⓑ

* **G9616** Documentation of reason(s) for not documenting a preoperative assessment (e.g., patient with a gynecologic or other pelvic malignancy noted at the time of surgery) Ⓑ

* **G9617** Preoperative assessment not documented, reason not given Ⓑ

* **G9618** Documentation of screening for uterine malignancy or those that had an ultrasound and/or endometrial sampling of any kind Ⓑ

* **G9620** Patient not screened for uterine malignancy, or those that have not had an ultrasound and/or endometrial sampling of any kind, reason not given Ⓑ

* **G9621** Patient identified as an unhealthy alcohol user when screened for unhealthy alcohol use using a systematic screening method and received brief counseling Ⓑ

* **G9622** Patient not identified as an unhealthy alcohol user when screened for unhealthy alcohol use using a systematic screening method Ⓑ

* **G9623** Documentation of medical reason(s) for not screening for unhealthy alcohol use (e.g., limited life expectancy, other medical reasons) Ⓑ

↻ * **G9624** Patient not screened for unhealthy alcohol use using a systematic screening method or patient did not receive brief counseling if identified as an unhealthy alcohol user, reason not given Ⓑ

* **G9625** Patient sustained bladder injury at the time of surgery or discovered subsequently up to 1 month post-surgery Ⓑ

* **G9626** Documented medical reason for reporting bladder injury (e.g., gynecologic or other pelvic malignancy documented, concurrent surgery involving bladder pathology, injury that occurs during urinary incontinence procedure, patient death from non-medical causes not related to surgery, patient died during procedure without evidence of bladder injury) Ⓑ

* **G9627** Patient did not sustain bladder injury at the time of surgery nor discovered subsequently up to 1 month post-surgery Ⓑ

* **G9628** Patient sustained bowel injury at the time of surgery or discovered subsequently up to 1 month post-surgery Ⓑ

* **G9629** Documented medical reasons for not reporting bowel injury (e.g., gynecologic or other pelvic malignancy documented, planned (e.g., not due to an unexpected bowel injury) resection and/or re-anastomosis of bowel, or patient death from non-medical causes not related to surgery, patient died during procedure without evidence of bowel injury) Ⓑ

* **G9630** Patient did not sustain a bowel injury at the time of surgery nor discovered subsequently up to 1 month post-surgery Ⓑ

* **G9631** Patient sustained ureter injury at the time of surgery or discovered subsequently up to 1 month post-surgery Ⓑ

* **G9632** Documented medical reasons for not reporting ureter injury (e.g., gynecologic or other pelvic malignancy documented, concurrent surgery involving bladder pathology, injury that occurs during a urinary incontinence procedure, patient death from non-medical causes not related to surgery, patient died during procedure without evidence of ureter injury) Ⓑ

* **G9633** Patient did not sustain ureter injury at the time of surgery nor discovered subsequently up to 1 month post-surgery Ⓑ

* **G9634** Health-related quality of life assessed with tool during at least two visits and quality of life score remained the same or improved Ⓑ

▶ New   ↻ Revised   ✔ Reinstated   ~~deleted~~ Deleted   ⊘ Not covered or valid by Medicare

✺ Special coverage instructions   ✳ Carrier discretion   Ⓑ Bill Part B MAC   Ⓑ Bill DME MAC

✳ **G9635** Health-related quality of life not assessed with tool for documented reason(s) (e.g., patient has a cognitive or neuropsychiatric impairment that impairs his/her ability to complete the HRQOL survey, patient has the inability to read and/or write in order to complete the HRQOL questionnaire) Ⓑ

✳ **G9636** Health-related quality of life not assessed with tool during at least two visits or quality of life score declined Ⓑ

↻ ✳ **G9637** At least two orders for the same high-risk medications Ⓑ

↻ ✳ **G9638** At least two orders for the same high-risk medications not ordered Ⓑ

✳ **G9639** Major amputation or open surgical bypass not required within 48 hours of the index endovascular lower extremity revascularization procedure Ⓑ

✳ **G9640** Documentation of planned hybrid or staged procedure Ⓑ

✳ **G9641** Major amputation or open surgical bypass required within 48 hours of the index endovascular lower extremity revascularization procedure Ⓑ

✳ **G9642** Current smokers (e.g., cigarette, cigar, pipe, e-cigarette or marijuana) Ⓑ

✳ **G9643** Elective surgery Ⓑ

✳ **G9644** Patients who abstained from smoking prior to anesthesia on the day of surgery or procedure Ⓑ

✳ **G9645** Patients who did not abstain from smoking prior to anesthesia on the day of surgery or procedure Ⓑ

✳ **G9646** Patients with 90 day MRS score of 0 to 2 Ⓑ

✳ **G9647** Patients in whom MRS score could not be obtained at 90 day follow-up Ⓑ

✳ **G9648** Patients with 90 day MRS score greater than 2 Ⓑ

✳ **G9649** Psoriasis assessment tool documented meeting any one of the specified benchmarks (e.g., PGA; 6-point scale), body surface area (BSA), psoriasis area and severity index (PASI) and/or dermatology life quality index (DLQI) Ⓑ

✳ **G9651** Psoriasis assessment tool documented not meeting any one of the specified benchmarks (e.g., (pga; 6-point scale), body surface area (bsa), psoriasis area and severity index (pasi) and/or dermatology life quality index) (dlqi)) or psoriasis assessment tool not documented Ⓑ

✳ **G9654** Monitored anesthesia care (mac) Ⓑ

✳ **G9655** A transfer of care protocol or handoff tool/checklist that includes the required key handoff elements is used Ⓑ

↻ ✳ **G9656** Patient transferred directly from anesthetizing location to PACU or other non-ICU location Ⓑ

✳ **G9658** A transfer of care protocol or handoff tool/checklist that includes the required key handoff elements is not used Ⓑ

✳ **G9659** Patients greater than 85 years of age who did not have a history of colorectal cancer or valid medical reason for the colonoscopy, including: iron deficiency anemia, lower gastrointestinal bleeding, Crohn's Disease (i.e., regional enteritis), familial adenomatous polyposis, lynch syndrome (i.e., hereditary non-polyposis colorectal cancer), inflammatory bowel disease, ulcerative colitis, abnormal finding of gastrointestinal tract, or changes in bowel habits Ⓑ

✳ **G9660** Documentation of medical reason(s) for a colonoscopy performed on a patient greater than 85 years of age (e.g., last colonoscopy incomplete, last colonoscopy had inadequate prep, iron deficiency anemia, lower gastrointestinal bleeding, Crohn's Disease (i.e., regional enteritis), familial history of adenomatous polyposis, lynch syndrome (i.e., hereditary non-polyposis colorectal cancer), inflammatory bowel disease, ulcerative colitis, abnormal finding of gastrointestinal tract, or changes in bowel habits) Ⓑ

✳ **G9661** Patients greater than 85 years of age who received a routine colonoscopy for a reason other than the following: an assessment of signs/symptoms of GI tract illness, and/or the patient is considered high risk, and/or to follow-up on previously diagnosed advance lesions Ⓑ

✳ **G9662** Previously diagnosed or have an active diagnosis of clinical ascvd Ⓑ

✳ **G9663** Any fasting or direct ldl-c laboratory test result = 190 mg/dL Ⓑ

✳ **G9664** Patients who are currently statin therapy users or received an order (prescription) for statin therapy Ⓑ

✳ **G9665** Patients who are not currently statin therapy users or did not receive an order (prescription) for statin therapy Ⓑ

▶ New ↻ Revised ✔ Reinstated ~~deleted~~ Deleted ⃠ Not covered or valid by Medicare
✪ Special coverage instructions ✳ Carrier discretion Ⓑ Bill Part B MAC Ⓖ Bill DME MAC

* **G9666** The highest fasting or direct ldl-c laboratory test result of 70-189 mg/dL in the measurement period or two years prior to the beginning of the measurement period Ⓑ

* **G9674** Patients with clinical ascvd diagnosis Ⓑ

* **G9675** Patients who have ever had a fasting or direct laboratory result of ldl-c = 190 mg/dl Ⓑ

* **G9676** Patients aged 40 to 75 years at the beginning of the measurement period with type 1 or type 2 diabetes and with an ldl-c result of 70-189 mg/dl recorded as the highest fasting or direct laboratory test result in the measurement year or during the two years prior to the beginning of the measurement period Ⓑ

* **G9678** Oncology care model (OCM) monthly enhanced oncology services (MEOS) payment for OCM enhanced services. G9678 payments may only be made to OCM practitioners for ocm beneficiaries for the furnishment of enhanced services as defined in the OCM participation agreement Ⓑ

* **G9679** This code is for onsite acute care treatment of a nursing facility resident with pneumonia; may only be billed once per day per beneficiary Ⓑ

* **G9680** This code is for onsite acute care treatment of a nursing facility resident with CHF; may only be billed once per day per beneficiary Ⓑ

* **G9681** This code is for onsite acute care treatment of a resident with COPD or asthma; may only be billed once per day per beneficiary Ⓑ

* **G9682** This code is for the onsite acute care treatment a nursing facility resident with a skin infection; may only be billed once per day per beneficiary Ⓑ

* **G9683** This code is for the onsite acute care treatment of a nursing facility resident with fluid or electrolyte disorder or dehydration (similar pattern); may only be billed once per day per beneficiary Ⓑ

* **G9684** This code is for the onsite acute care treatment of a nursing facility resident for a UTI; may only be billed once per day per beneficiary Ⓑ

* **G9685** This code is for the evaluation and management of a beneficiary's acute change in condition in a nursing facility Ⓑ

* **G9686** Onsite nursing facility conference, that is separate and distinct from an evaluation and management visit, including qualified practitioner and at least one member of the nursing facility interdisciplinary care team Ⓑ

* **G9687** Hospice services provided to patient any time during the measurement period Ⓑ

* **G9688** Patients using hospice services any time during the measurement period Ⓑ

* **G9689** Patient admitted for performance of elective carotid intervention Ⓑ

* **G9690** Patient receiving hospice services any time during the measurement period Ⓑ

* **G9691** Patient had hospice services any time during the measurement period Ⓑ

* **G9692** Hospice services received by patient any time during the measurement period Ⓑ

* **G9693** Patient use of hospice services any time during the measurement period Ⓑ

* **G9694** Hospice services utilized by patient any time during the measurement period Ⓑ

* **G9695** Long-acting inhaled bronchodilator prescribed Ⓑ

* **G9696** Documentation of medical reason(s) for not prescribing a long-acting inhaled bronchodilator Ⓑ

* **G9697** Documentation of patient reason(s) for not prescribing a long-acting inhaled bronchodilator Ⓑ

* **G9698** Documentation of system reason(s) for not prescribing a long-acting inhaled bronchodilator Ⓑ

* **G9699** Long-acting inhaled bronchodilator not prescribed, reason not otherwise specified Ⓑ

* **G9700** Patients who use hospice services any time during the measurement period Ⓑ

* **G9701** Children who are taking antibiotics in the 30 days prior to the date of the encounter during which the diagnosis was established Ⓑ

* **G9702** Patients who use hospice services any time during the measurement period Ⓑ

* **G9703** Children who are taking antibiotics in the 30 days prior to the diagnosis of pharyngitis Ⓑ

* **G9704** AJCC breast cancer stage I: T1 mic or T1a documented Ⓑ

* **G9705** AJCC breast cancer stage I: T1b (tumor> 0.5 cm but <= 1 cm in greatest dimension) documented Ⓑ

▶ New   ↻ Revised   ✔ Reinstated   ~~deleted~~ Deleted   ⊘ Not covered or valid by Medicare

✪ Special coverage instructions   * Carrier discretion   Ⓟ Bill Part B MAC   Ⓑ Bill DME MAC

214

* **G9706** Low (or very low) risk of recurrence, prostate cancer Ⓑ

* **G9707** Patient received hospice services any time during the measurement period Ⓑ

* **G9708** Women who had a bilateral mastectomy or who have a history of a bilateral mastectomy or for whom there is evidence of a right and a left unilateral mastectomy Ⓑ

* **G9709** Hospice services used by patient any time during the measurement period Ⓑ

* **G9710** Patient was provided hospice services any time during the measurement period Ⓑ

* **G9711** Patients with a diagnosis or past history of total colectomy or colorectal cancer Ⓑ

* **G9712** Documentation of medical reason(s) for prescribing or dispensing antibiotic (e.g., intestinal infection, pertussis, bacterial infection, Lyme disease, otitis media, acute sinusitis, acute pharyngitis, acute tonsillitis, chronic sinusitis, infection of the pharynx/larynx/tonsils/adenoids, prostatitis, cellulitis/ mastoiditis/bone infections, acute lymphadenitis, impetigo, skin staph infections, pneumonia, gonococcal infections/venereal disease (syphilis, chlamydia, inflammatory diseases [female reproductive organs]), infections of the kidney, cystitis/UTI, acne, HIV disease/asymptomatic HIV, cystic fibrosis, disorders of the immune system, malignancy neoplasms, chronic bronchitis, emphysema, bronchiectasis, extrinsic allergic alveolitis, chronic airway obstruction, chronic obstructive asthma, pneumoconiosis and other lung disease due to external agents, other diseases of the respiratory system, and tuberculosis Ⓑ

* **G9713** Patients who use hospice services any time during the measurement period Ⓑ

* **G9714** Patient is using hospice services any time during the measurement period Ⓑ

* **G9715** Patients who use hospice services any time during the measurement period Ⓑ

↻ * **G9716** BMI is documented as being outside of normal limits, follow-up plan is not completed for documented reason Ⓑ

↻ * **G9717** Documentation stating the patient has an active diagnosis of depression or has a diagnosed bipolar disorder, therefore screening or follow-up not required Ⓑ

* **G9718** Hospice services for patient provided any time during the measurement period Ⓑ

* **G9719** Patient is not ambulatory, bed ridden, immobile, confined to chair, wheelchair bound, dependent on helper pushing wheelchair, independent in wheelchair or minimal help in wheelchair Ⓑ

* **G9720** Hospice services for patient occurred any time during the measurement period Ⓑ

* **G9721** Patient not ambulatory, bed ridden, immobile, confined to chair, wheelchair bound, dependent on helper pushing wheelchair, independent in wheelchair or minimal help in wheelchair Ⓑ

* **G9722** Documented history of renal failure or baseline serum creatinine = 4.0 mg/dl; renal transplant recipients are not considered to have preoperative renal failure, unless, since transplantation the CR has been or is 4.0 or higher Ⓑ

* **G9723** Hospice services for patient received any time during the measurement period Ⓑ

* **G9724** Patients who had documentation of use of anticoagulant medications overlapping the measurement year Ⓑ

* **G9725** Patients who use hospice services any time during the measurement period Ⓑ

* **G9726** Patient refused to participate Ⓑ

* **G9727** Patient unable to complete the FOTO knee intake prom at admission and discharge due to blindness, illiteracy, severe mental incapacity or language incompatibility and an adequate proxy is not available Ⓑ

* **G9728** Patient refused to participate Ⓑ

* **G9729** Patient unable to complete the FOTO hip intake prom at admission and discharge due to blindness, illiteracy, severe mental incapacity or language incompatibility and an adequate proxy is not available Ⓑ

* **G9730** Patient refused to participate Ⓑ

* **G9731** Patient unable to complete the FOTO foot or ankle intake prom at admission and discharge due to blindness, illiteracy, severe mental incapacity or language incompatibility and an adequate proxy is not available Ⓑ

* **G9732** Patient refused to participate Ⓑ

▶ New ↻ Revised ✔ Reinstated deleted Deleted ⊘ Not covered or valid by Medicare

✹ Special coverage instructions ✱ Carrier discretion Ⓟ Bill Part B MAC Ⓑ Bill DME MAC

* **G9733** Patient unable to complete the FOTO lumbar intake prom at admission and discharge due to blindness, illiteracy, severe mental incapacity or language incompatibility and an adequate proxy is not available ⑧

* **G9734** Patient refused to participate ⑧

* **G9735** Patient unable to complete the FOTO shoulder intake prom at admission and discharge due to blindness, illiteracy, severe mental incapacity or language incompatibility and an adequate proxy is not available ⑧

* **G9736** Patient refused to participate ⑧

* **G9737** Patient unable to complete the FOTO elbow, wrist or hand intake prom at admission and discharge due to blindness, illiteracy, severe mental incapacity or language incompatibility and an adequate proxy is not available ⑧

* **G9738** Patient refused to participate ⑧

* **G9739** Patient unable to complete the foto general orthopedic intake prom at admission and discharge due to blindness, illiteracy, severe mental incapacity or language incompatibility and an adequate proxy is not available ⑧

* **G9740** Hospice services given to patient any time during the measurement period ⑧

* **G9741** Patients who use hospice services any time during the measurement period ⑧

* **G9742** Psychiatric symptoms assessed ⑧

* **G9743** Psychiatric symptoms not assessed, reason not otherwise specified ⑧

↺ * **G9744** Patient not eligible due to active diagnosis of hypertension ⑧

↺ * **G9745** Documented reason for not screening or recommending a follow-up for high blood pressure ⑧

* **G9746** Patient has mitral stenosis or prosthetic heart valves or patient has transient or reversible cause of AF (e.g., pneumonia, hyperthyroidism, pregnancy, cardiac surgery) ⑧

* **G9747** Patient is undergoing palliative dialysis with a catheter ⑧

* **G9748** Patient approved by a qualified transplant program and scheduled to receive a living donor kidney transplant ⑧

* **G9749** Patient is undergoing palliative dialysis with a catheter ⑧

* **G9750** Patient approved by a qualified transplant program and scheduled to receive a living donor kidney transplant ⑧

* **G9751** Patient died at any time during the 24-month measurement period ⑧

* **G9752** Emergency surgery ⑧

* **G9753** Documentation of medical reason for not conducting a search for DICOM format images for prior patient CT imaging studies completed at non-affiliated external healthcare facilities or entities within the past 12 months that are available through a secure, authorized, media-free, shared archive (e.g., trauma, acute myocardial infarction, stroke, aortic aneurysm where time is of the essence) ⑧

* **G9754** A finding of an incidental pulmonary nodule ⑧

* **G9755** Documentation of medical reason(s) that follow-up imaging is indicated (e.g., patient has a known malignancy that can metastasize, other medical reason(s) ⑧

* **G9756** Surgical procedures that included the use of silicone oil ⑧

* **G9757** Surgical procedures that included the use of silicone oil ⑧

↺ * **G9758** Patient in hospice at any time during the measurement period ⑧

* **G9759** History of preoperative posterior capsule rupture ⑧

* **G9760** Patients who use hospice services any time during the measurement period ⑧

* **G9761** Patients who use hospice services any time during the measurement period ⑧

↺ * **G9762** Patient had at least two HPV vaccines (with at least 146 days between the two) or three HPV vaccines on or between the patient's 9th and 13th birthdays ⑧

↺ * **G9763** Patient did not have at least two HPV vaccines (with at least 146 days between the two) or three HPV vaccines on or between the patient's 9th and 13th birthdays ⑧

↺ * **G9764** Patient has been treated with an oral systemic or biologic medication for psoriasis vulgaris ⑧

▶ New   ↺ Revised   ✔ Reinstated   ~~deleted~~ Deleted   ⊘ Not covered or valid by Medicare
✪ Special coverage instructions   ✳ Carrier discretion   ⑧ Bill Part B MAC   ⑧ Bill DME MAC

↻ ✳ **G9765** Documentation that the patient declined therapy change or alternative therapies were unavailable, has documented contraindications, or has not been treated with an oral systemic or biologic for at least six consecutive months (e.g., experienced adverse effects or lack of efficacy with all other therapy options) in order to achieve better disease control as measured by PGA, BSA, PASI, or DLQI ⑧

✳ **G9766** Patients who are transferred from one institution to another with a known diagnosis of CVA for endovascular stroke treatment ⑧

✳ **G9767** Hospitalized patients with newly diagnosed CVA considered for endovascular stroke treatment ⑧

✳ **G9768** Patients who utilize hospice services any time during the measurement period ⑧

✳ **G9769** Patient had a bone mineral density test in the past two years or received osteoporosis medication or therapy in the past 12 months ⑧

✳ **G9770** Peripheral nerve block (PNB) ⑧

✳ **G9771** At least 1 body temperature measurement equal to or greater than 35.5 degrees Celsius (or 95.9 degrees Fahrenheit) achieved within the 30 minutes immediately before or the 15 minutes immediately after anesthesia end time ⑧

✳ **G9772** Documentation of one of the following medical reason(s) for not achieving at least 1 body temperature measurement equal to or greater than 35.5 degrees Celsius (or 95.9 degrees Fahrenheit) achieved within the 30 minutes immediately before or the 15 minutes immediately after anesthesia end time (e.g., emergency cases, intentional hypothermia, etc.) ⑧

✳ **G9773** At least 1 body temperature measurement equal to or greater than 35.5 degrees Celsius (or 95.9 degrees Fahrenheit) not achieved within the 30 minutes immediately before or the 15 minutes immediately after anesthesia end time ⑧

✳ **G9774** Patients who have had a hysterectomy ⑧

✳ **G9775** Patient received at least 2 prophylactic pharmacologic anti-emetic agents of different classes preoperatively and/or intraoperatively ⑧

✳ **G9776** Documentation of medical reason for not receiving at least 2 prophylactic pharmacologic anti-emetic agents of different classes preoperatively and/or intraoperatively (e.g., intolerance or other medical reason) ⑧

✳ **G9777** Patient did not receive at least 2 prophylactic pharmacologic anti-emetic agents of different classes preoperatively and/or intraoperatively ⑧

✳ **G9778** Patients who have a diagnosis of pregnancy ⑧

✳ **G9779** Patients who are breastfeeding ⑧

✳ **G9780** Patients who have a diagnosis of rhabdomyolysis ⑧

✳ **G9781** Documentation of medical reason(s) for not currently being a statin therapy user or receive an order (prescription) for statin therapy (e.g., patient with adverse effect, allergy or intolerance to statin medication therapy, patients who are receiving palliative care, patients with active liver disease or hepatic disease or insufficiency, and patients with end stage renal disease [ESRD]) ⑧

✳ **G9782** History of or active diagnosis of familial or pure hypercholesterolemia ⑧

✳ **G9783** Documentation of patients with diabetes who have a most recent fasting or direct LDL-C laboratory test result <70 mg/dl and are not taking statin therapy ⑧

↻ ✳ **G9784** Pathologists/dermatopathologists providing a second opinion on a biopsy ⑧

↻ ✳ **G9785** Pathology report diagnosing cutaneous basal cell carcinoma or squamous cell carcinoma (to include in situ disease) sent from the pathologist/dermatopathologist to the biopsying clinician for review within 7 days from the time when the tissue specimen was received by the pathologist ⑧

↻ ✳ **G9786** Pathology report diagnosing cutaneous basal cell carcinoma or squamous cell carcinoma (to include in situ disease) was not sent from the pathologist/dermatopathologist to the biopsying clinician for review within 7 days from the time when the tissue specimen was received by the pathologist ⑧

✳ **G9787** Patient alive as of the last day of the measurement year ⑧

✳ **G9788** Most recent bp is less than or equal to 140/90 mm hg ⑧

▶ New	↻ Revised	✔ Reinstated	~~deleted~~ Deleted	⊘ Not covered or valid by Medicare
⊛ Special coverage instructions	✳ Carrier discretion	⑨ Bill Part B MAC	⑧ Bill DME MAC	

* **G9789** Blood pressure recorded during inpatient stays, emergency room visits, urgent care visits, and patient self-reported BP's (home and health fair BP results) Ⓑ

* **G9790** Most recent BP is greater than 140/90 mm hg, or blood pressure not documented Ⓑ

* **G9791** Most recent tobacco status is tobacco free Ⓑ

* **G9792** Most recent tobacco status is not tobacco free Ⓑ

* **G9793** Patient is currently on a daily aspirin or other antiplatelet Ⓑ

↻ * **G9794** Documentation of medical reason(s) for not on a daily aspirin or other antiplatelet (e.g., history of gastrointestinal bleed, intra-cranial bleed, idiopathic thrombocytopenic purpura (ITP), gastric bypass or documentation of active anticoagulant use during the measurement period) Ⓑ

* **G9795** Patient is not currently on a daily aspirin or other antiplatelet Ⓑ

* **G9796** Patient is currently on a statin therapy Ⓑ

* **G9797** Patient is not on a statin therapy Ⓑ

* **G9798** Discharge(s) for AMI between July 1 of the year prior measurement year to June 30 of the measurement period Ⓑ

* **G9799** Patients with a medication dispensing event indicator of a history of asthma any time during the patient's history through the end of the measure period Ⓑ

* **G9800** Patients who are identified as having an intolerance or allergy to beta-blocker therapy Ⓑ

* **G9801** Hospitalizations in which the patient was transferred directly to a non-acute care facility for any diagnosis' Ⓑ

* **G9802** Patients who use hospice services any time during the measurement period Ⓑ

* **G9803** Patient prescribed a 180-day course of treatment with beta-blockers post discharge for AMI Ⓑ

* **G9804** Patient was not prescribed a 180-day course of treatment with beta-blockers post discharge for AMI Ⓑ

* **G9805** Patients who use hospice services any time during the measurement period Ⓑ

* **G9806** Patients who received cervical cytology or an HPV test Ⓑ

* **G9807** Patients who did not receive cervical cytology or an HPV test Ⓑ

* **G9808** Any patients who had no asthma controller medications dispensed during the measurement year Ⓑ

* **G9809** Patients who use hospice services any time during the measurement period Ⓑ

* **G9810** Patient achieved a pDC of at least 75% for their asthma controller medication Ⓑ

* **G9811** Patient did not achieve a pDC of at least 75% for their asthma controller medication Ⓑ

* **G9812** Patient died including all deaths occurring during the hospitalization in which the operation was performed, even if after 30 days, and those deaths occurring after discharge from the hospital, but within 30 days of the procedure Ⓑ

* **G9813** Patient did not die within 30 days of the procedure or during the index hospitalization Ⓑ

↻ * **G9814** Death occurring during the index acute care hospitalization Ⓑ

↻ * **G9815** Death did not occur during the index acute care hospitalization Ⓑ

↻ * **G9816** Death occurring after discharge from the hospital but within 30 days post procedure Ⓑ

↻ * **G9817** Death did not occur after discharge from the hospital within 30 days post procedure Ⓑ

* **G9818** Documentation of sexual activity Ⓑ

* **G9819** Patients who use hospice services any time during the measurement period Ⓑ

* **G9820** Documentation of a chlamydia screening test with proper follow-up Ⓑ

* **G9821** No documentation of a chlamydia screening test with proper follow-up Ⓑ

* **G9822** Women who had an endometrial ablation procedure during the year prior to the index date (exclusive of the index date) Ⓑ

* **G9823** Endometrial sampling or hysteroscopy with biopsy and results documented Ⓑ

* **G9824** Endometrial sampling or hysteroscopy with biopsy and results not documented Ⓑ

* **G9825** HER-2/neu negative or undocumented/ unknown Ⓑ

* **G9826** Patient transferred to practice after initiation of chemotherapy Ⓑ

* **G9827** HER2-targeted therapies not administered during the initial course of treatment Ⓑ

✳ **G9828** HER2-targeted therapies administered during the initial course of treatment ⑧

✳ **G9829** Breast adjuvant chemotherapy administered ⑧

✳ **G9830** HER-2/neu positive ⑧

✳ **G9831** AJCC stage at breast cancer diagnosis = II or III ⑧

✳ **G9832** AJCC stage at breast cancer diagnosis = I (Ia or Ib) and T-stage at breast cancer diagnosis does not equal = T1, T1a, T1b ⑧

✳ **G9833** Patient transfer to practice after initiation of chemotherapy ⑧

✳ **G9834** Patient has metastatic disease at diagnosis ⑧

✳ **G9835** Trastuzumab administered within 12 months of diagnosis ⑧

✳ **G9836** Reason for not administering trastuzumab documented (e.g., patient declined, patient died, patient transferred, contraindication or other clinical exclusion, neoadjuvant chemotherapy or radiation not complete) ⑧

✳ **G9837** Trastuzumab not administered within 12 months of diagnosis ⑧

✳ **G9838** Patient has metastatic disease at diagnosis ⑧

✳ **G9839** Anti-EGFR monoclonal antibody therapy ⑧

↺ ✳ **G9840** Ras (KRas and NRas) gene mutation testing performed before initiation of anti-EGFR MoAb ⑧

↺ ✳ **G9841** Ras (KRas and NRas) gene mutation testing not performed before initiation of anti-EGFR MoAb ⑧

✳ **G9842** Patient has metastatic disease at diagnosis ⑧

↺ ✳ **G9843** Ras (KRas and NRas) gene mutation ⑧

✳ **G9844** Patient did not receive anti-EGFR monoclonal antibody therapy ⑧

✳ **G9845** Patient received anti-EGFR monoclonal antibody therapy ⑧

✳ **G9846** Patients who died from cancer ⑧

✳ **G9847** Patient received chemotherapy in the last 14 days of life ⑧

✳ **G9848** Patient did not receive chemotherapy in the last 14 days of life ⑧

✳ **G9849** Patients who died from cancer ⑧

✳ **G9850** Patient had more than one emergency department visit in the last 30 days of life ⑧

✳ **G9851** Patient had one or less emergency department visits in the last 30 days of life ⑧

✳ **G9852** Patients who died from cancer ⑧

✳ **G9853** Patient admitted to the ICU in the last 30 days of life ⑧

✳ **G9854** Patient was not admitted to the ICU in the last 30 days of life ⑧

✳ **G9855** Patients who died from cancer ⑧

✳ **G9856** Patient was not admitted to hospice ⑧

✳ **G9857** Patient admitted to hospice ⑧

✳ **G9858** Patient enrolled in hospice ⑧

✳ **G9859** Patients who died from cancer ⑧

✳ **G9860** Patient spent less than three days in hospice care ⑧

✳ **G9861** Patient spent greater than or equal to three days in hospice care ⑧

✳ **G9862** Documentation of medical reason(s) for not recommending at least a 10 year follow-up interval (e.g., inadequate prep, familial or personal history of colonic polyps, patient had no adenoma and age is = 66 years old, or life expectancy <10 years old, other medical reasons) ⑧

▶ ✳ **G9890** Dilated macular exam performed, including documentation of the presence or absence of macular thickening or geographic atrophy or hemorrhage and the level of macular degeneration severity

▶ ✳ **G9891** Documentation of medical reason(s) for not performing a dilated macular examination

▶ ✳ **G9892** Documentation of patient reason(s) for not performing a dilated macular examination

▶ ✳ **G9893** Dilated macular exam was not performed, reason not otherwise specified

▶ ✳ **G9894** Androgen deprivation therapy prescribed/administered in combination with external beam radiotherapy to the prostate

▶ ✳ **G9895** Documentation of medical reason(s) for not prescribing/administering androgen deprivation therapy in combination with external beam radiotherapy to the prostate (e.g., salvage therapy)

▶ ✳ **G9896** Documentation of patient reason(s) for not prescribing/administering androgen deprivation therapy in combination with external beam radiotherapy to the prostate

---

▶ New   ↺ Revised   ✔ Reinstated   deleted Deleted   ⊘ Not covered or valid by Medicare
✪ Special coverage instructions   ✳ Carrier discretion   ⑧ Bill Part B MAC   ⑧ Bill DME MAC

▶ ✳ **G9897** Patients who were not prescribed/administered androgen deprivation therapy in combination with external beam radiotherapy to the prostate, reason not given

▶ ✳ **G9898** Patient age 65 or older in institutional special needs plans (SNP) or residing in long-term care with POS code 32, 33, 34, 54, or 56 any time during the measurement period

▶ ✳ **G9899** Screening, diagnostic, film, digital or digital breast tomosynthesis (3D) mammography results documented and reviewed

▶ ✳ **G9900** Screening, diagnostic, film, digital or digital breast tomosynthesis (3D) mammography results were not documented and reviewed, reason not otherwise specified

▶ ✳ **G9901** Patient age 65 or older in institutional special needs plans (SNP) or residing in long-term care with pos code 32, 33, 34, 54, or 56 any time during the measurement period

▶ ✳ **G9902** Patient screened for tobacco use and identified as a tobacco user

▶ ✳ **G9903** Patient screened for tobacco use and identified as a tobacco non-user

▶ ✳ **G9904** Documentation of medical reason(s) for not screening for tobacco use (e.g., limited life expectancy, other medical reason)

▶ ✳ **G9905** Patient not screened for tobacco use, reason not given

▶ ✳ **G9906** Patient identified as a tobacco user received tobacco cessation intervention (counseling and/or pharmacotherapy)

▶ ✳ **G9907** Documentation of medical reason(s) for not providing tobacco cessation intervention (e.g., limited life expectancy, other medical reason)

▶ ✳ **G9908** Patient identified as tobacco user did not receive tobacco cessation intervention (counseling and/or pharmacotherapy), reason not given

▶ ✳ **G9909** Documentation of medical reason(s) for not providing tobacco cessation intervention if identified as a tobacco user (e.g., limited life expectancy, other medical reason)

▶ ✳ **G9910** Patients age 65 or older in institutional special needs plans (SNP) or residing in long-term care with pos code 32, 33, 34, 54, or 56 anytime during the measurement period

▶ ✳ **G9911** Clinically node negative (t1n0m0 or t2n0m0) invasive breast cancer before or after neoadjuvant systemic therapy

▶ ✳ **G9912** Hepatitis B virus (HBV) status assessed and results interpreted prior to initiating anti-TNF (tumor necrosis factor) therapy

▶ ✳ **G9913** Hepatitis B virus (HBV) status not assessed and results interpreted prior to initiating anti-TNF (tumor necrosis factor) therapy, reason not given

▶ ✳ **G9914** Patient receiving an anti-TNF agent

▶ ✳ **G9915** No record of HBV results documented

▶ ✳ **G9916** Functional status performed once in the last 12 months

▶ ✳ **G9917** Documentation of medical reason(s) for not performing functional status (e.g., patient is severely impaired and caregiver knowledge is limited, other medical reason)

▶ ✳ **G9918** Functional status not performed, reason not otherwise specified

▶ ✳ **G9919** Screening performed and positive and provision of recommendations

▶ ✳ **G9920** Screening performed and negative

▶ ✳ **G9921** No screening performed, partial screening performed or positive screen without recommendations and reason is not given or otherwise specified

▶ ✳ **G9922** Safety concerns screen provided and if positive then documented mitigation recommendations

▶ ✳ **G9923** Safety concerns screen provided and negative

▶ ✳ **G9924** Documentation of medical reason(s) for not providing safety concerns screen or for not providing recommendations, orders or referrals for positive screen (e.g., patient in palliative care, other medical reason)

▶ ✳ **G9925** Safety concerns screening not provided, reason not otherwise specified

▶ ✳ **G9926** Safety concerns screening positive screen is without provision of mitigation recommendations, including but not limited to referral to other resources

▶ ✳ **G9927** Documentation of system reason(s) for not prescribing warfarin or another FDA-approved anticoagulation due to patient being currently enrolled in a clinical trial related to af/atrial flutter treatment

---

▶ New   ↻ Revised   ✔ Reinstated   ~~deleted~~ Deleted   ⊘ Not covered or valid by Medicare

⊕ Special coverage instructions   ✳ Carrier discretion   Ⓑ Bill Part B MAC   Ⓑ Bill DME MAC

▶ ✳ **G9928** Warfarin or another FDA-approved anticoagulant not prescribed, reason not given

▶ ✳ **G9929** Patient with transient or reversible cause of AF (e.g., pneumonia, hyperthyroidism, pregnancy, cardiac surgery)

▶ ✳ **G9930** Patients who are receiving comfort care only

▶ ✳ **G9931** Documentation of CHA2DS2-VASc risk score of 0 or 1

▶ ✳ **G9932** Documentation of patient reason(s) for not having records of negative or managed positive TB screen (e.g., patient does not return for mantoux (ppd) skin test evaluation)

▶ ✳ **G9933** Adenoma(s) or colorectal cancer detected during screening colonoscopy

▶ ✳ **G9934** Documentation that neoplasm detected is only diagnosed as traditional serrated adenoma, sessile serrated polyp, or sessile serrated adenoma

▶ ✳ **G9935** Adenoma(s) or colorectal cancer not detected during screening colonoscopy

▶ ✳ **G9936** Surveillance colonoscopy - personal history of colonic polyps, colon cancer, or other malignant neoplasm of rectum, rectosigmoid junction, and anus

▶ ✳ **G9937** Diagnostic colonoscopy

▶ ✳ **G9938** Patients age 65 or older in institutional special needs plans (SNP) or residing in long-term care with POS code 32, 33, 34, 54, or 56 any time during the measurement period

▶ ✳ **G9939** Pathologists/dermatopathologists is the same clinician who performed the biopsy

▶ ✳ **G9940** Documentation of medical reason(s) for not on a statin (e.g., pregnancy, in vitro fertilization, clomiphene rx, esrd, cirrhosis, muscular pain and disease during the measurement period or prior year)

▶ ✳ **G9941** Back pain was measured by the visual analog scale (VAS) within three months preoperatively and at three months (6 - 20 weeks) postoperatively

▶ ✳ **G9942** Patient had any additional spine procedures performed on the same date as the lumbar discectomy/laminotomy

▶ ✳ **G9943** Back pain was not measured by the visual analog scale (VAS) within three months preoperatively and at three months (6 - 20 weeks) postoperatively

▶ ✳ **G9944** Back pain was measured by the visual analog scale (VAS) within three months preoperatively and at one year (9 to 15 months) postoperatively

▶ ✳ **G9945** Patient had cancer, fracture or infection related to the lumbar spine or patient had idiopathic or congenital scoliosis

▶ ✳ **G9946** Back pain was not measured by the visual analog scale (VAS) within three months preoperatively and at one year (9 to 15 months) postoperatively

▶ ✳ **G9947** Leg pain was measured by the visual analog scale (VAS) within three months preoperatively and at three months (6 to 20 weeks) postoperatively

▶ ✳ **G9948** Patient had any additional spine procedures performed on the same date as the lumbar discectomy/laminotomy

▶ ✳ **G9949** Leg pain was not measured by the visual analog scale (VAS) within three months preoperatively and at three months (6 to 20 weeks) postoperatively

▶ ✳ **G9954** Patient exhibits 2 or more risk factors for post-operative vomiting

▶ ✳ **G9955** Cases in which an inhalational anesthetic is used only for induction

▶ ✳ **G9956** Patient received combination therapy consisting of at least two prophylactic pharmacologic anti-emetic agents of different classes preoperatively and/or intraoperatively

▶ ✳ **G9957** Documentation of medical reason for not receiving combination therapy consisting of at least two prophylactic pharmacologic anti-emetic agents of different classes preoperatively and/or intraoperatively (e.g., intolerance or other medical reason)

▶ ✳ **G9958** Patient did not receive combination therapy consisting of at least two prophylactic pharmacologic anti-emetic agents of different classes preoperatively and/or intraoperatively

▶ ✳ **G9959** Systemic antimicrobials not prescribed

▶ ✳ **G9960** Documentation of medical reason(s) for prescribing systemic antimicrobials

▶ ✳ **G9961** Systemic antimicrobials prescribed

▶ New	↻ Revised	✔ Reinstated	deleted Deleted	⊘ Not covered or valid by Medicare
✪ Special coverage instructions		✳ Carrier discretion	⑨ Bill Part B MAC	⑧ Bill DME MAC

▶ ✳ **G9962** Embolization endpoints are documented separately for each embolized vessel and ovarian artery angiography or embolization performed in the presence of variant uterine artery anatomy

▶ ✳ **G9963** Embolization endpoints are not documented separately for each embolized vessel or ovarian artery angiography or embolization not performed in the presence of variant uterine artery anatomy

▶ ✳ **G9964** Patient received at least one well-child visit with a PCP during the performance period

▶ ✳ **G9965** Patient did not receive at least one well-child visit with a PCP during the performance period

▶ ✳ **G9966** Children who were screened for risk of developmental, behavioral and social delays using a standardized tool with interpretation and report

▶ ✳ **G9967** Children who were not screened for risk of developmental, behavioral and social delays using a standardized tool with interpretation and report

▶ ✳ **G9968** Patient was referred to another provider or specialist during the performance period

▶ ✳ **G9969** Provider who referred the patient to another provider received a report from the provider to whom the patient was referred

▶ ✳ **G9970** Provider who referred the patient to another provider did not receive a report from the provider to whom the patient was referred

▶ ✳ **G9974** Dilated macular exam performed, including documentation of the presence or absence of macular thickening or geographic atrophy or hemorrhage and the level of macular degeneration severity

▶ ✳ **G9975** Documentation of medical reason(s) for not performing a dilated macular examination

▶ ✳ **G9976** Documentation of patient reason(s) for not performing a dilated macular examination

▶ ✳ **G9977** Dilated macular exam was not performed, reason not otherwise specified

▶ New   ↻ Revised   ✔ Reinstated   ~~deleted~~ Deleted   ⊘ Not covered or valid by Medicare

✪ Special coverage instructions   ✳ Carrier discretion   Ⓑ Bill Part B MAC   Ⓓ Bill DME MAC

BEHAVIORAL HEALTH AND/OR SUBSTANCE ABUSE TREATMENT SERVICES (H0001-H9999)

NOTE: Used by Medicaid state agencies because no national code exists to meet the reporting needs of these agencies.

⊘ **H0001** Alcohol and/or drug assessment

⊘ **H0002** Behavioral health screening to determine eligibility for admission to treatment program

⊘ **H0003** Alcohol and/or drug screening; laboratory analysis of specimens for presence of alcohol and/or drugs

⊘ **H0004** Behavioral health counseling and therapy, per 15 minutes

⊘ **H0005** Alcohol and/or drug services; group counseling by a clinician

⊘ **H0006** Alcohol and/or drug services; case management

⊘ **H0007** Alcohol and/or drug services; crisis intervention (outpatient)

⊘ **H0008** Alcohol and/or drug services; sub-acute detoxification (hospital inpatient)

⊘ **H0009** Alcohol and/or drug services; acute detoxification (hospital inpatient)

⊘ **H0010** Alcohol and/or drug services; sub-acute detoxification (residential addiction program inpatient)

⊘ **H0011** Alcohol and/or drug services; acute detoxification (residential addiction program inpatient)

⊘ **H0012** Alcohol and/or drug services; sub-acute detoxification (residential addiction program outpatient)

⊘ **H0013** Alcohol and/or drug services; acute detoxification (residential addiction program outpatient)

⊘ **H0014** Alcohol and/or drug services; ambulatory detoxification

⊘ **H0015** Alcohol and/or drug services; intensive outpatient (treatment program that operates at least 3 hours/day and at least 3 days/week and is based on an individualized treatment plan), including assessment, counseling; crisis intervention, and activity therapies or education

⊘ **H0016** Alcohol and/or drug services; medical/somatic (medical intervention in ambulatory setting)

⊘ **H0017** Behavioral health; residential (hospital residential treatment program), without room and board, per diem

⊘ **H0018** Behavioral health; short-term residential (non-hospital residential treatment program), without room and board, per diem

⊘ **H0019** Behavioral health; long-term residential (non-medical, non-acute care in a residential treatment program where stay is typically longer than 30 days), without room and board, per diem

⊘ **H0020** Alcohol and/or drug services; methadone administration and/or service (provision of the drug by a licensed program)

⊘ **H0021** Alcohol and/or drug training service (for staff and personnel not employed by providers)

⊘ **H0022** Alcohol and/or drug intervention service (planned facilitation)

⊘ **H0023** Behavioral health outreach service (planned approach to reach a targeted population)

⊘ **H0024** Behavioral health prevention information dissemination service (one-way direct or non-direct contact with service audiences to affect knowledge and attitude)

⊘ **H0025** Behavioral health prevention education service (delivery of services with target population to affect knowledge, attitude and/or behavior)

⊘ **H0026** Alcohol and/or drug prevention process service, community-based (delivery of services to develop skills of impactors)

⊘ **H0027** Alcohol and/or drug prevention environmental service (broad range of external activities geared toward modifying systems in order to mainstream prevention through policy and law)

⊘ **H0028** Alcohol and/or drug prevention problem identification and referral service (e.g., student assistance and employee assistance programs), does not include assessment

⊘ **H0029** Alcohol and/or drug prevention alternatives service (services for populations that exclude alcohol and other drug use e.g., alcohol-free social events)

⊘ **H0030** Behavioral health hotline service

⊘ **H0031** Mental health assessment, by non-physician

⊘ **H0032** Mental health service plan development by non-physician

⊘ **H0033** Oral medication administration, direct observation

---

▶ **New** ↻ **Revised** ✔ **Reinstated** ~~deleted~~ **Deleted** ⊘ **Not covered or valid by Medicare**
✪ **Special coverage instructions** ✳ **Carrier discretion** Ⓟ **Bill Part B MAC** Ⓑ **Bill DME MAC**

⊘ **H0034** Medication training and support, per 15 minutes

⊘ **H0035** Mental health partial hospitalization, treatment, less than 24 hours

⊘ **H0036** Community psychiatric supportive treatment, face-to-face, per 15 minutes

⊘ **H0037** Community psychiatric supportive treatment program, per diem

⊘ **H0038** Self-help/peer services, per 15 minutes

⊘ **H0039** Assertive community treatment, face-to-face, per 15 minutes

⊘ **H0040** Assertive community treatment program, per diem

⊘ **H0041** Foster care, child, non-therapeutic, per diem

⊘ **H0042** Foster care, child, non-therapeutic, per month

⊘ **H0043** Supported housing, per diem

⊘ **H0044** Supported housing, per month

⊘ **H0045** Respite care services, not in the home, per diem

⊘ **H0046** Mental health services, not otherwise specified

⊘ **H0047** Alcohol and/or other drug abuse services, not otherwise specified

⊘ **H0048** Alcohol and/or other drug testing: collection and handling only, specimens other than blood

⊘ **H0049** Alcohol and/or drug screening

⊘ **H0050** Alcohol and/or drug services, brief intervention, per 15 minutes

⊘ **H1000** Prenatal care, at-risk assessment

⊘ **H1001** Prenatal care, at-risk enhanced service; antepartum management

⊘ **H1002** Prenatal care, at-risk enhanced service; care coordination

⊘ **H1003** Prenatal care, at-risk enhanced service; education

⊘ **H1004** Prenatal care, at-risk enhanced service; follow-up home visit

⊘ **H1005** Prenatal care, at-risk enhanced service package (includes H1001-H1004)

⊘ **H1010** Non-medical family planning education, per session

⊘ **H1011** Family assessment by licensed behavioral health professional for state defined purposes

⊘ **H2000** Comprehensive multidisciplinary evaluation

⊘ **H2001** Rehabilitation program, per 1/2 day

⊘ **H2010** Comprehensive medication services, per 15 minutes

⊘ **H2011** Crisis intervention service, per 15 minutes

⊘ **H2012** Behavioral health day treatment, per hour

⊘ **H2013** Psychiatric health facility service, per diem

⊘ **H2014** Skills training and development, per 15 minutes

⊘ **H2015** Comprehensive community support services, per 15 minutes

⊘ **H2016** Comprehensive community support services, per diem

⊘ **H2017** Psychosocial rehabilitation services, per 15 minutes

⊘ **H2018** Psychosocial rehabilitation services, per diem

⊘ **H2019** Therapeutic behavioral services, per 15 minutes

⊘ **H2020** Therapeutic behavioral services, per diem

⊘ **H2021** Community-based wrap-around services, per 15 minutes

⊘ **H2022** Community-based wrap-around services, per diem

⊘ **H2023** Supported employment, per 15 minutes

⊘ **H2024** Supported employment, per diem

⊘ **H2025** Ongoing support to maintain employment, per 15 minutes

⊘ **H2026** Ongoing support to maintain employment, per diem

⊘ **H2027** Psychoeducational service, per 15 minutes

⊘ **H2028** Sexual offender treatment service, per 15 minutes

⊘ **H2029** Sexual offender treatment service, per diem

⊘ **H2030** Mental health clubhouse services, per 15 minutes

⊘ **H2031** Mental health clubhouse services, per diem

⊘ **H2032** Activity therapy, per 15 minutes

⊘ **H2033** Multisystemic therapy for juveniles, per 15 minutes

⊘ **H2034** Alcohol and/or drug abuse halfway house services, per diem

⊘ **H2035** Alcohol and/or other drug treatment program, per hour

⊘ **H2036** Alcohol and/or other drug treatment program, per diem

⊘ **H2037** Developmental delay prevention activities, dependent child of client, per 15 minutes

▶ New	↻ Revised	✔ Reinstated	~~deleted~~ Deleted	⊘ Not covered or valid by Medicare
⊕ Special coverage instructions		✳ Carrier discretion	⑨ Bill Part B MAC	⑩ Bill DME MAC

DRUGS OTHER THAN CHEMOTHERAPY DRUGS (J0100-J8999)

Injection

↻✹ **J0120** Injection, tetracycline, up to 250 mg ⑧ ⑧

IOM: 100-02, 15, 50

✳ **J0129** Injection, abatacept, 10 mg (code may be used for medicare when drug administered under the direct supervision of a physician, not for use when drug is self administered) ⑧ ⑧

↻✹ **J0130** Injection, abciximab, 10 mg ⑧ ⑧

IOM: 100-02, 15, 50

✳ **J0131** Injection, acetaminophen, 10 mg ⑧ ⑧

↻✳ **J0132** Injection, acetylcysteine, 100 mg ⑧ ⑧

✳ **J0133** Injection, acyclovir, 5 mg ⑧ ⑧

✳ **J0135** Injection, adalimumab, 20 mg ⑧ ⑧

IOM: 100-02, 15, 50

✹ **J0153** Injection, adenosine, 1 mg (not to be used to report any adenosine phosphate compounds) ⑧ ⑧

✹ **J0171** Injection, adrenalin, epinephrine, 0.1 mg ⑧ ⑧

IOM: 100-02, 15, 50

✳ **J0178** Injection, aflibercept, 1 mg ⑧ ⑧

✳ **J0180** Injection, agalsidase beta, 1 mg ⑧ ⑧

IOM: 100-02, 15, 50

✹ **J0190** Injection, biperiden lactate, per 5 mg ⑧ ⑧

IOM: 100-02, 15, 50

✹ **J0200** Injection, alatrofloxacin mesylate, 100 mg ⑧ ⑧

IOM: 100-02, 15, 50

✳ **J0202** Injection, alemtuzumab, 1 mg ⑧ ⑧

✹ **J0205** Injection, alglucerase, per 10 units ⑧ ⑧

IOM: 100-02, 15, 50

✹ **J0207** Injection, amifostine, 500 mg ⑧ ⑧

IOM: 100-02, 15, 50

✹ **J0210** Injection, methyldopate HCL, up to 250 mg ⑧ ⑧

IOM: 100-02, 15, 50

↻✳ **J0215** Injection, alefacept, 0.5 mg ⑧ ⑧

✳ **J0220** Injection, alglucosidase alfa, not otherwise specified, 10 mg ⑧ ⑧

✳ **J0221** Injection, alglucosidase alfa, (lumizyme), 10 mg ⑧ ⑧

✹ **J0256** Injection, alpha 1-proteinase inhibitor (human), not otherwise specified, 10 mg ⑧ ⑧

IOM: 100-02, 15, 50

✹ **J0257** Injection, alpha 1 proteinase inhibitor (human), (glassia), 10 mg ⑧ ⑧

IOM: 100-02, 15, 50

✹ **J0270** Injection, alprostadil, per 1.25 mcg (Code may be used for Medicare when drug administered under the direct supervision of a physician, not for use when drug is self administered) ⑧ ⑧

IOM: 100-02, 15, 50

✹ **J0275** Alprostadil urethral suppository (Code may be used for Medicare when drug administered under the direct supervision of a physician, not for use when drug is self administered) ⑧ ⑧

IOM: 100-02, 15, 50

✳ **J0278** Injection, amikacin sulfate, 100 mg ⑧ ⑧

✹ **J0280** Injection, aminophylline, up to 250 mg ⑧ ⑧

IOM: 100-02, 15, 50

✹ **J0282** Injection, amiodarone hydrochloride, 30 mg ⑧ ⑧

IOM: 100-02, 15, 50

✹ **J0285** Injection, amphotericin B, 50 mg ⑧ ⑧

IOM: 100-02, 15, 50

✹ **J0287** Injection, amphotericin B lipid complex, 10 mg ⑧ ⑧

IOM: 100-02, 15, 50

✹ **J0288** Injection, amphotericin B cholesteryl sulfate complex, 10 mg ⑧ ⑧

IOM: 100-02, 15, 50

✹ **J0289** Injection, amphotericin B liposome, 10 mg ⑧ ⑧

IOM: 100-02, 15, 50

✹ **J0290** Injection, ampicillin sodium, 500 mg ⑧ ⑧

IOM: 100-02, 15, 50

✹ **J0295** Injection, ampicillin sodium/sulbactam sodium, per 1.5 gm ⑧ ⑧

IOM: 100-02, 15, 50

✹ **J0300** Injection, amobarbital, up to 125 mg ⑧ ⑧

IOM: 100-02, 15, 50

✹ **J0330** Injection, succinylcholine chloride, up to 20 mg ⑧ ⑧

IOM: 100-02, 15, 50

✳ **J0348** Injection, anidulafungin, 1 mg ⑧ ⑧

▶ New   ↻ Revised   ✔ Reinstated   ~~deleted~~ Deleted   ⊘ Not covered or valid by Medicare
✹ Special coverage instructions   ✳ Carrier discretion   ⑧ Bill Part B MAC   ⑧ Bill DME MAC

⊛ **J0350** Injection, anistreplase, per 30 units Ⓑ Ⓖ

IOM: 100-02, 15, 50

⊛ **J0360** Injection, hydralazine hydrochloride, up to 20 mg Ⓑ Ⓖ

IOM: 100-02, 15, 50

✳ **J0364** Injection, apomorphine hydrochloride, 1 mg Ⓑ Ⓖ

↻ ⊛ **J0365** Injection, aprotinin, 10,000 KIU Ⓑ Ⓖ

IOM: 100-02, 15, 50

⊛ **J0380** Injection, metaraminol bitartrate, per 10 mg Ⓑ Ⓖ

IOM: 100-02, 15, 50

⊛ **J0390** Injection, chloroquine hydrochloride, up to 250 mg Ⓑ Ⓖ

Benefit only for diagnosed malaria or amebiasis

IOM: 100-02, 15, 50

⊛ **J0395** Injection, arbutamine HCL, 1 mg Ⓑ Ⓖ

IOM: 100-02, 15, 50

↻ ✳ **J0400** Injection, aripiprazole, intramuscular, 0.25 mg Ⓑ Ⓖ

✳ **J0401** Injection, aripiprazole, extended release, 1 mg Ⓑ Ⓖ

⊛ **J0456** Injection, azithromycin, 500 mg Ⓑ Ⓖ

IOM: 100-02, 15, 50

⊛ **J0461** Injection, atropine sulfate, 0.01 mg Ⓑ Ⓖ

IOM: 100-02, 15, 50

↻ ⊛ **J0470** Injection, dimercaprol, per 100 mg Ⓑ Ⓖ

IOM: 100-02, 15, 50

⊛ **J0475** Injection, baclofen, 10 mg Ⓑ Ⓖ

IOM: 100-02, 15, 50

⊛ **J0476** Injection, baclofen 50 mcg for intrathecal trial Ⓑ Ⓖ

IOM: 100-02, 15, 50

⊛ **J0480** Injection, basiliximab, 20 mg Ⓑ Ⓖ

IOM: 100-02, 15, 50

✳ **J0485** Injection, belatacept, 1 mg Ⓑ Ⓖ

✳ **J0490** Injection, belimumab, 10 mg Ⓑ Ⓖ

⊛ **J0500** Injection, dicyclomine HCL, up to 20 mg Ⓑ Ⓖ

IOM: 100-02, 15, 50

⊛ **J0515** Injection, benztropine mesylate, per 1 mg Ⓑ Ⓖ

IOM: 100-02, 15, 50

⊛ **J0520** Injection, bethanechol chloride, myotonachol or urecholine, up to 5 mg Ⓑ Ⓖ

IOM: 100-02, 15, 50

✳ **J0558** Injection, penicillin G benzathine and penicillin G procaine, 100,000 units Ⓑ Ⓖ

⊛ **J0561** Injection, penicillin G benzathine, 100,000 units Ⓑ Ⓖ

IOM: 100-02, 15, 50

▶ ✳ **J0565** Injection, bezlotoxumab, 10 mg

✳ **J0570** Buprenorphine implant, 74.2 mg

⊛ **J0571** Buprenorphine, oral, 1 mg Ⓑ Ⓖ

⊛ **J0572** Buprenorphine/naloxone, oral, less than or equal to 3 mgbuprenorphine Ⓑ Ⓖ

⊛ **J0573** Buprenorphine/naloxone, oral, greater than 3 mg, but less than or equal to 6 mg buprenorphine Ⓑ Ⓖ

⊛ **J0574** Buprenorphine/naloxone, oral, greater than 6 mg, but less than or equal to 10 mg buprenorphine Ⓑ Ⓖ

⊛ **J0575** Buprenorphine/naloxone, oral, greater than 10 mg buprenorphine Ⓑ Ⓖ

↻ ✳ **J0583** Injection, bivalirudin, 1 mg Ⓑ Ⓖ

⊛ **J0585** Injection, onabotulinumtoxinaA, 1 unit Ⓑ Ⓖ

IOM: 100-02, 15, 50

✳ **J0586** Injection, abobotulinumtoxinaA, 5 units Ⓑ Ⓖ

⊛ **J0587** Injection, rimabotulinumtoxinB, 100 units Ⓑ Ⓖ

IOM: 100-02, 15, 50

✳ **J0588** Injection, incobotulinumtoxin A, 1 unit Ⓑ Ⓖ

⊛ **J0592** Injection, buprenorphine hydrochloride, 0.1 mg Ⓑ Ⓖ

IOM: 100-02, 15, 50

✳ **J0594** Injection, busulfan, 1 mg Ⓑ Ⓖ

✳ **J0595** Injection, butorphanol tartrate, 1 m eg Ⓑ Ⓖ

✳ **J0596** Injection, C1 esterase inhibitor (recombinant), ruconest, 10 units Ⓑ Ⓖ

✳ **J0597** Injection, C-1 esterase inhibitor (human), Berinert,10 units Ⓑ Ⓖ

✳ **J0598** Injection, C1 esterase inhibitor (human), cinryze, 10 units Ⓑ Ⓖ

⊛ **J0600** Injection, edetate calcium disodium, up to 1000 mg Ⓑ Ⓖ

IOM: 100-02, 15, 50

▶ **New**   ↻ **Revised**   ✔ **Reinstated**   ~~deleted~~ **Deleted**   ⊘ **Not covered or valid by Medicare**

⊛ **Special coverage instructions**   ✳ **Carrier discretion**   Ⓑ **Bill Part B MAC**   Ⓖ **Bill DME MAC**

▶ ✿ **J0604** Cinacalcet, oral, 1 mg, (for ESRD on dialysis)

▶ ✿ **J0606** Injection, etelcalcetide, 0.1 mg

✿ **J0610** Injection, calcium gluconate, per 10 ml Ⓑ Ⓓ

IOM: 100-02, 15, 50

✿ **J0620** Injection, calcium glycerophosphate and calcium lactate, per 10 ml Ⓑ Ⓓ

IOM: 100-02, 15, 50

✿ **J0630** Injection, calcitonin (salmon), up to 400 units Ⓑ Ⓓ

IOM: 100-02, 15, 50

✿ **J0636** Injection, calcitriol, 0.1 mcg Ⓑ Ⓓ

Non-dialysis use

IOM: 100-02, 15, 50

✳ **J0637** Injection, caspofungin acetate, 5 mg Ⓑ Ⓓ

✳ **J0638** Injection, canakinumab, 1 mg Ⓑ Ⓓ

✿ **J0640** Injection, leucovorin calcium, per 50 mg Ⓑ Ⓓ

IOM: 100-02, 15, 50

✿ **J0641** Injection, levoleucovorin calcium, 0.5 mg Ⓑ Ⓓ

Part of treatment regimen for osteosarcoma

✿ **J0670** Injection, mepivacaine HCL, per 10 ml Ⓑ Ⓓ

IOM: 100-02, 15, 50

✿ **J0690** Injection, cefezolin sodium, 500 mg Ⓑ Ⓓ

IOM: 100-02, 15, 50

✳ **J0692** Injection, cefepime HCL, 500 mg Ⓑ Ⓓ

✿ **J0694** Injection, cefoxitin sodium, 1 gm Ⓑ Ⓓ

IOM: 100-02, 15, 50,

Cross Reference Q0090

✳ **J0695** Injection, ceftolozane 50 mg and tazobactam25 mg Ⓑ Ⓓ

✿ **J0696** Injection, ceftriaxone sodium, per 250 mg Ⓑ Ⓓ

IOM: 100-02, 15, 50

✿ **J0697** Injection, sterile cefuroxime sodium, per 750 mg Ⓑ Ⓓ

IOM: 100-02, 15, 50

✿ **J0698** Injection, cefotaxime sodium, per gm Ⓑ Ⓓ

IOM: 100-02, 15, 50

✿ **J0702** Injection, betamethasone acetate 3 mg and betamethasone sodium phosphate 3 mg Ⓑ Ⓓ

IOM: 100-02, 15, 50

✳ **J0706** Injection, caffeine citrate, 5 mg Ⓑ Ⓓ

✿ **J0710** Injection, cephapirin sodium, up to 1 gm Ⓑ Ⓓ

IOM: 100-02, 15, 50

✳ **J0712** Injection, ceftaroline fosamil, 10 mg Ⓑ Ⓓ

✿ **J0713** Injection, ceftazidime, per 500 mg Ⓑ Ⓓ

IOM: 100-02, 15, 50

✳ **J0714** Injection, ceftazidime and avibactam, 0.5 g/0.125 g Ⓑ Ⓓ

✿ **J0715** Injection, ceftizoxime sodium, per 500 mg Ⓑ Ⓓ

IOM: 100-02, 15, 50

✳ **J0716** Injection, centruroides immune F(ab)2, up to 120 milligrams Ⓑ Ⓓ

✳ **J0717** Injection, certolizumab pegol, 1 mg (code may be used for Medicare when drug administered under the direct supervision of a physician, not for use when drug is self administered) Ⓑ Ⓓ

↻ ✿ **J0720** Injection, chloramphenicol sodium succinate, up to 1 gm Ⓑ Ⓓ

IOM: 100-02, 15, 50

↻ ✿ **J0725** Injection, chorionic gonadotropin, per 1,000 USP units Ⓑ Ⓓ

IOM: 100-02, 15, 50

✿ **J0735** Injection, clonidine hydrochloride (HCL), 1 mg Ⓑ Ⓓ

IOM: 100-02, 15, 50

✿ **J0740** Injection, cidofovir, 375 mg Ⓑ Ⓓ

IOM: 100-02, 15, 50

✿ **J0743** Injection, cilastatin sodium; imipenem, per 250 mg Ⓑ Ⓓ

IOM: 100-02, 15, 50

✳ **J0744** Injection, ciprofloxacin for intravenous infusion, 200 mg Ⓑ Ⓓ

✿ **J0745** Injection, codeine phosphate, per 30 mg Ⓑ Ⓓ

IOM: 100-02, 15, 50

✿ **J0770** Injection, colistimethate sodium, up to 150 mg Ⓑ Ⓓ

IOM: 100-02, 15, 50

✳ **J0775** Injection, collagenase, clostridium histolyticum, 0.01 mg Ⓑ Ⓓ

✿ **J0780** Injection, prochlorperazine, up to 10 mg Ⓑ Ⓓ

IOM: 100-02, 15, 50

✿ **J0795** Injection, corticorelin ovine triflutate, 1 microgram Ⓑ Ⓓ

IOM: 100-02, 15, 50

▶ **New**   ↻ **Revised**   ✔ **Reinstated**   ~~deleted~~ **Deleted**   ⊘ **Not covered or valid by Medicare**

✿ **Special coverage instructions**   ✳ **Carrier discretion**   Ⓑ **Bill Part B MAC**   Ⓓ **Bill DME MAC**

⊛ **J0800** Injection, corticotropin, up to 40 units Ⓑ Ⓑ

IOM: 100-02, 15, 50

↻⁎ **J0833** Injection, cosyntropin, not otherwise specified, 0.25 mg Ⓑ Ⓑ

⁎ **J0834** Injection, cosyntropin (Cortrosyn), 0.25 mg Ⓟ Ⓑ

⁎ **J0840** Injection, crotalidae polyvalent immune fab (ovine), up to 1 gram Ⓑ Ⓑ

⊛ **J0850** Injection, cytomegalovirus immune globulin intravenous (human), per vial Ⓟ Ⓑ

Prophylaxis to prevent cytomegalovirus disease associated with transplantation of kidney, lung, liver, pancreas, and heart.

IOM: 100-02, 15, 50

⁎ **J0875** Injection, dalbavancin, 5 mg Ⓑ Ⓑ

⁎ **J0878** Injection, daptomycin, 1 mg Ⓑ Ⓑ

⊛ **J0881** Injection, darbepoetin alfa, 1 microgram (non-ESRD use) Ⓟ Ⓑ

⊛ **J0882** Injection, darbepoetin alfa, 1 microgram (for ESRD on dialysis) Ⓟ Ⓑ

IOM: 100-02, 6, 10; 100-04, 4, 240

⊛ **J0883** Injection, argatroban, 1 mg (for non-ESRD use)

IOM: 100-02, 15, 50

↻⊛ **J0884** Injection, argatroban, 1 mg (for ESRD on dialysis)

IOM: 100-02, 15, 50

⊛ **J0885** Injection, epoetin alfa, (for non-ESRD use), 1000 units Ⓟ Ⓑ

IOM: 100-02, 15, 50

⊛ **J0887** Injection, epoetin beta, 1 microgram, (for ESRD on dialysis) Ⓟ Ⓑ

↻⊛ **J0888** Injection, epoetin beta, 1 microgram, (for non ESRD use) Ⓟ Ⓑ

⁎ **J0890** Injection, peginesatide, 0.1 mg (for ESRD on dialysis) Ⓑ Ⓑ

⁎ **J0894** Injection, decitabine, 1 mg Ⓑ Ⓑ

Indicated for treatment of myelodysplastic syndromes (MDS)

⊛ **J0895** Injection, deferoxamine mesylate, 500 mg Ⓟ ⒷIOM: 100-02, 15, 50,

IOM: 100-02, 15, 50,

Cross Reference Q0087

⁎ **J0897** Injection, denosumab, 1 mg Ⓑ Ⓑ

⊛ **J0945** Injection, brompheniramine maleate, per 10 mg Ⓑ Ⓑ

IOM: 100-02, 15, 50

⊛ **J1000** Injection, depo-estradiol cypionate, up to 5 mg Ⓟ Ⓑ

IOM: 100-02, 15, 50

⊛ **J1020** Injection, methylprednisolone acetate, 20 mg Ⓑ Ⓑ

IOM: 100-02, 15, 50

⊛ **J1030** Injection, methylprednisolone acetate, 40 mg Ⓑ Ⓑ

IOM: 100-02, 15, 50

⊛ **J1040** Injection, methylprednisolone acetate, 80 mg Ⓑ Ⓑ

IOM: 100-02, 15, 50

⁎ **J1050** Injection, medroxyprogesterone acetate, 1 mg Ⓑ Ⓑ

⊛ **J1071** Injection, testosterone cypionate, 1 mg

⊛ **J1094** Injection, dexamethasone acetate, 1 mg Ⓑ Ⓑ

IOM: 100-02, 15, 50

⊛ **J1100** Injection, dexamethasone sodium phosphate, 1 mg Ⓑ Ⓑ

IOM: 100-02, 15, 50

↻⊛ **J1110** Injection, dihydroergotamine mesylate, per 1 mg Ⓑ Ⓑ

IOM: 100-02, 15, 50

⊛ **J1120** Injection, acetazolamide sodium, up to 500 mg Ⓟ Ⓑ

IOM: 100-02, 15, 50

↻⁎ **J1130** Injection, diclofenac sodium, 0.5 mg

⊛ **J1160** Injection, digoxin, up to 0.5 mg Ⓑ Ⓑ

IOM: 100-02, 15, 50

⊛ **J1162** Injection, digoxin immune Fab (ovine), per vial Ⓑ Ⓑ

IOM: 100-02, 15, 50

⊛ **J1165** Injection, phenytoin sodium, per 50 mg Ⓑ Ⓑ

IOM: 100-02, 15, 50

⊛ **J1170** Injection, hydromorphone, up to 4 mg Ⓑ Ⓑ

IOM: 100-02, 15, 50

⊛ **J1180** Injection, dyphylline, up to 500 mg Ⓑ Ⓑ

IOM: 100-02, 15, 50

⊛ **J1190** Injection, dexrazoxane hydrochloride, per 250 mg Ⓑ Ⓑ

IOM: 100-02, 15, 50

⊛ **J1200** Injection, diphenhydramine HCL, up to 50 mg Ⓑ Ⓑ

IOM: 100-02, 15, 50

↻ ✿ **J1205** Injection, chlorothiazide sodium, per 500 mg Ⓑ Ⓑ

IOM: 100-02, 15, 50

✿ **J1212** Injection, DMSO, dimethyl sulfoxide, 50%, 50 ml Ⓑ Ⓑ

IOM: 100-02, 15, 50; 100-03, 4, 230.12

✿ **J1230** Injection, methadone HCL, up to 10 mg Ⓑ Ⓑ

IOM: 100-02, 15, 50

✿ **J1240** Injection, dimenhydrinate, up to 50 mg Ⓑ Ⓑ

IOM: 100-02, 15, 50

✿ **J1245** Injection, dipyridamole, per 10 mg Ⓑ Ⓑ

IOM: 100-04, 15, 50; 100-04, 12, 30.6

✿ **J1250** Injection, dobutamine HCL, per 250 mg Ⓑ Ⓑ

IOM: 100-02, 15, 50

✿ **J1260** Injection, dolasetron mesylate, 10 mg Ⓑ Ⓑ

IOM: 100-02, 15, 50

✳ **J1265** Injection, dopamine HCL, 40 mg Ⓑ Ⓑ

✳ **J1267** Injection, doripenem, 10 mg Ⓑ Ⓑ

✳ **J1270** Injection, doxercalciferol, 1 mcg Ⓑ Ⓑ

✳ **J1290** Injection, ecallantide, 1 mg Ⓑ Ⓑ

✳ **J1300** Injection, eculizumab, 10 mg Ⓑ Ⓑ

✿ **J1320** Injection, amitriptyline HCL, up to 20 mg Ⓑ Ⓑ

IOM: 100-02, 15, 50

✳ **J1322** Injection, elosulfase alfa, 1 mg Ⓑ Ⓑ

↻ ✳ **J1324** Injection, enfuvirtide, 1 mg Ⓑ Ⓑ

✿ **J1325** Injection, epoprostenol, 0.5 mg Ⓑ Ⓑ

IOM: 100-02, 15, 50

✿ **J1327** Injection, eptifibatide, 5 mg Ⓑ Ⓑ

IOM: 100-02, 15, 50

✿ **J1330** Injection, ergonovine maleate, up to 0.2 mg Ⓑ Ⓑ

IOM: 100-02, 15, 50

Benefit limited to obstetrical diagnosis

✳ **J1335** Injection, ertapenem sodium, 500 mg Ⓑ Ⓑ

✿ **J1364** Injection, erythromycin lactobionate, per 500 mg Ⓑ Ⓑ

IOM: 100-02, 15, 50

✿ **J1380** Injection, estradiol valerate, up to 10 mg Ⓑ Ⓑ

IOM: 100-02, 15, 50

✿ **J1410** Injection, estrogen conjugated, per 25 mg Ⓑ Ⓑ

IOM: 100-02, 15, 50

▶ ✳ **J1428** Injection, eteplirsen, 10 mg

✿ **J1430** Injection, ethanolamine oleate, 100 mg Ⓑ Ⓑ

IOM: 100-02, 15, 50

✿ **J1435** Injection, estrone, per 1 mg Ⓑ Ⓑ

IOM: 100-02, 15, 50

✿ **J1436** Injection, etidronate disodium, per 300 mg Ⓑ Ⓑ

IOM: 100-02, 15, 50

✿ **J1438** Injection, etanercept, 25 mg (Code may be used for Medicare when drug administered under the direct supervision of a physician, not for use when drug is self-administered.) Ⓑ Ⓑ

IOM: 100-02, 15, 50

✳ **J1439** Injection, ferric carboxymaltose, 1 mg Ⓑ Ⓑ

✿ **J1442** Injection, filgrastim (G-CSF), excludes biosimilars, 1 microgram Ⓑ Ⓑ

✳ **J1443** Injection, ferric pyrophosphate citrate solution, 0.1 mg of iron Ⓑ Ⓑ

✿ **J1447** Injection, TBO-filgrastim, 1 microgram Ⓑ Ⓑ

IOM: 100-02, 15, 50

✿ **J1450** Injection, fluconazole, 200 mg Ⓑ Ⓑ

IOM: 100-02, 15, 50

✿ **J1451** Injection, fomepizole, 15 mg Ⓑ Ⓑ

IOM: 100-02, 15, 50

✿ **J1452** Injection, fomivirsen sodium, intraocular, 1.65 mg Ⓑ Ⓑ

IOM: 100-02, 15, 50

✳ **J1453** Injection, fosaprepitant, 1 mg Ⓑ Ⓑ

Prevents chemotherapy-induced nausea and vomiting

✿ **J1455** Injection, foscarnet sodium, per 1000 mg Ⓑ Ⓑ

IOM: 100-02, 15, 50

✳ **J1457** Injection, gallium nitrate, 1 mg Ⓑ Ⓑ

✳ **J1458** Injection, galsulfase, 1 mg Ⓑ Ⓑ

✳ **J1459** Injection, immune globulin (Privigen), intravenous, non-lyophilized (e.g., liquid), 500 mg Ⓑ Ⓑ

✿ **J1460** Injection, gamma globulin, intramuscular, 1 cc Ⓑ Ⓑ

IOM: 100-02, 15, 50

▶ ✳ **J1555** Injection, immune globulin (cuvitru), 100 mg

▶ **New** ↻ **Revised** ✔ **Reinstated** ~~deleted~~ **Deleted** ⊘ **Not covered or valid by Medicare**

✿ **Special coverage instructions** ✳ **Carrier discretion** Ⓑ **Bill Part B MAC** Ⓑ **Bill DME MAC**

✳ **J1556** Injection, immune globulin (Bivigam), 500 mg Ⓑ Ⓑ

✳ **J1557** Injection, immune globulin, (gammaplex), intravenous, non-lyophilized (e.g., liquid), 500 mg Ⓑ Ⓑ

✳ **J1559** Injection, immune globulin, (hizentra), 100 mg Ⓑ Ⓑ

✿ **J1560** Injection, gamma globulin, intramuscular, over 10 cc Ⓑ Ⓑ

IOM: 100-02, 15, 50

✿ **J1561** Injection, immune globulin, (Gamunex-C/Gammaked), non-lyophilized (e.g., liquid), 500 mg Ⓑ Ⓑ

IOM: 100-02, 15, 50

✳ **J1562** Injection, immune globulin (Vivaglobin), 100 mg Ⓑ Ⓑ

✿ **J1566** Injection, immune globulin, intravenous, lyophilized (e.g., powder), not otherwise specified, 500 mg Ⓑ Ⓑ

IOM: 100-02, 15, 50

✳ **J1568** Injection, immune globulin, (Octagam), intravenous, non-lyophilized (e.g., liquid), 500 mg Ⓑ Ⓑ

✿ **J1569** Injection, immune globulin, (Gammagard Liquid), non-lyophilized, (e.g., liquid), 500 mg Ⓑ Ⓑ

IOM: 100-02, 15, 50

✿ **J1570** Injection, ganciclovir sodium, 500 mg Ⓑ Ⓑ

IOM: 100-02, 15, 50

✿ **J1571** Injection, hepatitis B immune globulin (HepaGam B), intramuscular, 0.5 ml Ⓑ Ⓑ

IOM: 100-02, 15, 50

✿ **J1572** Injection, immune globulin, (flebogamma/flebogamma DIF) intravenous, non-lyophilized (e.g., liquid), 500 mg Ⓑ Ⓑ

IOM: 100-02, 15, 50

✳ **J1573** Injection, hepatitis B immune globulin (HepaGam B), intravenous, 0.5 ml Ⓑ Ⓑ

✳ **J1575** Injection, immune globulin/hyaluronidase, (HYQVIA), 100 mg immunoglobulin Ⓑ Ⓑ

✿ **J1580** Injection, Garamycin, gentamicin, up to 80 mg Ⓑ Ⓑ

IOM: 100-02, 15, 50

✿ **J1595** Injection, glatiramer acetate, 20 mg Ⓑ Ⓑ

IOM: 100-02, 15, 50

✳ **J1599** Injection, immune globulin, intravenous, non-lyophilized (e.g., liquid), not otherwise specified, 500 mg Ⓑ Ⓑ

✿ **J1600** Injection, gold sodium thiomalate, up to 50 mg Ⓑ Ⓑ

IOM: 100-02, 15, 50

✳ **J1602** Injection, golimumab, 1 mg, for intravenous use Ⓑ Ⓑ

✿ **J1610** Injection, glucagon hydrochloride, per 1 mg Ⓑ Ⓑ

IOM: 100-02, 15, 50

✿ **J1620** Injection, gonadorelin hydrochloride, per 100 mcg Ⓑ Ⓑ

IOM: 100-02, 15, 50

✿ **J1626** Injection, granisetron hydrochloride, 100 mcg Ⓑ Ⓑ

IOM: 100-02, 15, 50

▶ ✳ **J1627** Injection, granisetron, extended-release, 0.1 mg Ⓑ Ⓑ

✿ **J1630** Injection, haloperidol, up to 5 mg Ⓑ Ⓑ

IOM: 100-02, 15, 50

✿ **J1631** Injection, haloperidol decanoate, per 50 mg Ⓑ Ⓑ

IOM: 100-02, 15, 50

✿ **J1640** Injection, hemin, 1 mg Ⓑ Ⓑ

IOM: 100-02, 15, 50

✿ **J1642** Injection, heparin sodium, (heparin lock flush), per 10 units Ⓑ Ⓑ

IOM: 100-02, 15, 50

✿ **J1644** Injection, heparin sodium, per 1000 units Ⓑ Ⓑ

IOM: 100-02, 15, 50

✿ **J1645** Injection, dalteparin sodium, per 2500 IU Ⓑ Ⓑ

IOM: 100-02, 15, 50

✳ **J1650** Injection, enoxaparin sodium, 10 mg Ⓑ Ⓑ

✿ **J1652** Injection, fondaparinux sodium, 0.5 mg Ⓑ Ⓑ

IOM: 100-02, 15, 50

✳ **J1655** Injection, tinzaparin sodium, 1000 IU Ⓑ Ⓑ

✿ **J1670** Injection, tetanus immune globulin, human, up to 250 units Ⓑ Ⓑ

Indicated for transient protection against tetanus post-exposure to tetanus (V03.7).

IOM: 100-02, 15, 50

✿ **J1675** Injection, histrelin acetate, 10 micrograms Ⓑ Ⓑ

IOM: 100-02, 15, 50

✿ **J1700** Injection, hydrocortisone acetate, up to 25 mg Ⓑ Ⓑ

IOM: 100-02, 15, 50

▶ New	↻ Revised	✔ Reinstated	~~deleted~~ Deleted	⊘ Not covered or valid by Medicare
✿ Special coverage instructions		✳ Carrier discretion	Ⓑ Bill Part B MAC	Ⓑ Bill DME MAC

⚙ **J1710** Injection, hydrocortisone sodium phosphate, up to 50 mg Ⓑ Ⓓ

IOM: 100-02, 15, 50

⚙ **J1720** Injection, hydrocortisone sodium succinate, up to 100 mg Ⓑ Ⓓ

IOM: 100-02, 15, 50

~~J1725 Injection, hydroxyprogesterone caproate, 1 mg~~ ✖

▶ ✱ **J1726** Injection, hydroxyprogesterone caproate, (makena), 10 mg

▶ ✱ **J1729** Injection, hydroxyprogesterone caproate, not otherwise specified, 10 mg

↻⚙ **J1730** Injection, diazoxide, up to 300 mg Ⓑ Ⓓ

IOM: 100-02, 15, 50

✱ **J1740** Injection, ibandronate sodium, 1 mg Ⓑ Ⓓ

✱ **J1741** Injection, ibuprofen, 100 mg Ⓑ Ⓓ

⚙ **J1742** Injection, ibutilide fumarate, 1 mg Ⓑ Ⓓ

IOM: 100-02, 15, 50

✱ **J1743** Injection, idursulfase, 1 mg Ⓑ Ⓓ

✱ **J1744** Injection, icatibant, 1 mg Ⓑ Ⓓ

⚙ **J1745** Injection, infliximab, excludes biosimilar, 10 mg Ⓑ Ⓓ

Report total number of 10 mg increments administered

For biosimilar, Inflectra, report Q5102

IOM: 100-02, 15, 50

⚙ **J1750** Injection, iron dextran, 50 mg Ⓑ Ⓓ

IOM: 100-02, 15, 50

✱ **J1756** Injection, iron sucrose, 1 mg Ⓑ Ⓓ

⚙ **J1786** Injection, imiglucerase, 10 units Ⓑ Ⓓ

IOM: 100-02, 15, 50

⚙ **J1790** Injection, droperidol, up to 5 mg Ⓑ Ⓓ

IOM: 100-02, 15, 50

⚙ **J1800** Injection, propranolol HCL, up to 1 mg Ⓑ Ⓓ

IOM: 100-02, 15, 50

⚙ **J1810** Injection, droperidol and fentanyl citrate, up to 2 ml ampule Ⓑ Ⓓ

IOM: 100-02, 15, 50

⚙ **J1815** Injection, insulin, per 5 units Ⓑ Ⓓ

IOM: 100-02, 15, 50; 100-03, 4, 280.14

✱ **J1817** Insulin for administration through DME (i.e., insulin pump) per 50 units Ⓑ Ⓓ

✱ **J1826** Injection, interferon beta-1a, 30 mcg Ⓑ Ⓓ

⚙ **J1830** Injection, interferon beta-1b, 0.25 mg (Code may be used for Medicare when drug administered under the direct supervision of a physician, not for use when drug is self administered) Ⓑ Ⓓ

IOM: 100-02, 15, 50

✱ **J1833** Injection, isavuconazonium, 1 mg Ⓑ Ⓓ

✱ **J1835** Injection, itraconazole, 50 mg Ⓑ Ⓓ

⚙ **J1840** Injection, kanamycin sulfate, up to 500 mg Ⓑ Ⓓ

IOM: 100-02, 15, 50

⚙ **J1850** Injection, kanamycin sulfate, up to 75 mg Ⓑ Ⓓ

IOM: 100-02, 15, 50

⚙ **J1885** Injection, ketorolac tromethamine, per 15 mg Ⓑ Ⓓ

IOM: 100-02, 15, 50

⚙ **J1890** Injection, cephalothin sodium, up to 1 gram Ⓑ Ⓓ

IOM: 100-02, 15, 50

✱ **J1930** Injection, lanreotide, 1 mg Ⓑ Ⓓ

Treats acromegaly and symptoms caused by neuroendocrine tumors

✱ **J1931** Injection, laronidase, 0.1 mg Ⓑ Ⓓ

⚙ **J1940** Injection, furosemide, up to 20 mg Ⓑ Ⓓ

IOM: 100-02, 15, 50

✱ **J1942** Injection, aripiprazole lauroxil, 1 mg

↻⚙ **J1945** Injection, lepirudin, 50 mg Ⓑ Ⓓ

IOM: 100-02, 15, 50

⚙ **J1950** Injection, leuprolide acetate (for depot suspension), per 3.75 mg Ⓑ Ⓓ

IOM: 100-02, 15, 50

✱ **J1953** Injection, levetiracetam, 10 mg Ⓑ Ⓓ

⚙ **J1955** Injection, levocarnitine, per 1 gm Ⓑ Ⓓ

IOM: 100-02, 15, 50

⚙ **J1956** Injection, levofloxacin, 250 mg Ⓑ Ⓓ

IOM: 100-02, 15, 50

⚙ **J1960** Injection, levorphanol tartrate, up to 2 mg Ⓑ Ⓓ

IOM: 100-02, 15, 50

⚙ **J1980** Injection, hyoscyamine sulfate, up to 0.25 mg Ⓑ Ⓓ

IOM: 100-02, 15, 50

⚙ **J1990** Injection, chlordiazepoxide HCL, up to 100 mg Ⓑ Ⓓ

IOM: 100-02, 15, 50

⚙ **J2001** Injection, lidocaine HCL for intravenous infusion, 10 mg Ⓑ Ⓓ

IOM: 100-02, 15, 50

▶ New	↻ Revised	✔ Reinstated	~~deleted~~ Deleted	⊘ Not covered or valid by Medicare
⚙ Special coverage instructions		✱ Carrier discretion	Ⓑ Bill Part B MAC	Ⓓ Bill DME MAC

⊛ **J2010** Injection, lincomycin HCL, up to 300 mg Ⓑ Ⓑ

IOM: 100-02, 15, 50

↻ ✳ **J2020** Injection, linezolid, 200 mg Ⓑ Ⓑ

⊛ **J2060** Injection, lorazepam, 2 mg Ⓑ Ⓑ

IOM: 100-02, 15, 50

⊛ **J2150** Injection, mannitol, 25% in 50 ml Ⓑ Ⓑ

IOM: 100-02, 15, 50

✳ **J2170** Injection, mecasermin, 1 mg Ⓑ Ⓑ

⊛ **J2175** Injection, meperidine hydrochloride, per 100 mg Ⓑ Ⓑ

IOM: 100-02, 15, 50

⊛ **J2180** Injection, meperidine and promethazine HCL, up to 50 mg Ⓑ Ⓑ

IOM: 100-02, 15, 50

✳ **J2182** Injection, mepolizumab, 1 mg

✳ **J2185** Injection, meropenem, 100 mg Ⓑ Ⓑ

⊛ **J2210** Injection, methylergonovine maleate, up to 0.2 mg Ⓑ Ⓑ

Benefit limited to obstetrical diagnoses for prevention and control of post-partum hemorrhage

IOM: 100-02, 15, 50

✳ **J2212** Injection, methylnaltrexone, 0.1 mg Ⓑ Ⓑ

✳ **J2248** Injection, micafungin sodium, 1 mg Ⓑ Ⓑ

⊛ **J2250** Injection, midazolam hydrochloride, per 1 mg Ⓑ Ⓑ

IOM: 100-02, 15, 50

↻ ⊛ **J2260** Injection, milrinone lactate, 5 mg Ⓑ Ⓑ

IOM: 100-02, 15, 50

✳ **J2265** Injection, minocycline hydrochloride, 1 mg Ⓑ Ⓑ

⊛ **J2270** Injection, morphine sulfate, up to 10 mg Ⓑ Ⓑ

IOM: 100-02, 15, 50

↻ ⊛ **J2274** Injection, morphine sulfate, preservative-free for epidural or intrathecal use, 10 mg Ⓑ Ⓑ

IOM: 100-03, 4, 280.1; 100-02, 15, 50

⊛ **J2278** Injection, ziconotide, 1 microgram Ⓑ Ⓑ

✳ **J2280** Injection, moxifloxacin, 100 mg Ⓑ Ⓑ

⊛ **J2300** Injection, nalbuphine hydrochloride, per 10 mg Ⓑ Ⓑ

IOM: 100-02, 15, 50

⊛ **J2310** Injection, naloxone hydrochloride, per 1 mg Ⓑ Ⓑ

IOM: 100-02, 15, 50

✳ **J2315** Injection, naltrexone, depot form, 1 mg Ⓑ Ⓑ

⊛ **J2320** Injection, nandrolone decanoate, up to 50 mg Ⓑ Ⓑ

IOM: 100-02, 15, 50

✳ **J2323** Injection, natalizumab, 1 mg Ⓑ Ⓑ

⊛ **J2325** Injection, nesiritide, 0.1 mg Ⓑ Ⓑ

IOM: 100-02, 15, 50

▶ ✳ **J2326** Injection, nusinersen, 0.1 mg

▶ ✳ **J2350** Injection, ocrelizumab, 1 mg

✳ **J2353** Injection, octreotide, depot form for intramuscular injection, 1 mg Ⓑ Ⓑ

✳ **J2354** Injection, octreotide, non-depot form for subcutaneous or intravenous injection, 25 mcg Ⓑ Ⓑ

⊛ **J2355** Injection, oprelvekin, 5 mg Ⓑ Ⓑ

IOM: 100-02, 15, 50

✳ **J2357** Injection, omalizumab, 5 mg Ⓑ Ⓑ

↻ ✳ **J2358** Injection, olanzapine, long-acting, 1 mg Ⓑ Ⓑ

⊛ **J2360** Injection, orphenadrine citrate, up to 60 mg Ⓑ Ⓑ

IOM: 100-02, 15, 50

⊛ **J2370** Injection, phenylephrine HCL, up to 1 ml Ⓑ Ⓑ

IOM: 100-02, 15, 50

⊛ **J2400** Injection, chloroprocaine hydrochloride, per 30 ml Ⓑ Ⓑ

IOM: 100-02, 15, 50

⊛ **J2405** Injection, ondansetron hydrochloride, per 1 mg Ⓑ Ⓑ

IOM: 100-02, 15, 50

⊛ **J2407** Injection, oritavancin, 10 mg Ⓑ Ⓑ

IOM: 100-02, 15, 50

⊛ **J2410** Injection, oxymorphone HCL, up to 1 mg Ⓑ Ⓑ

IOM: 100-02, 15, 50

✳ **J2425** Injection, palifermin, 50 micrograms Ⓑ Ⓑ

✳ **J2426** Injection, paliperidone palmitate extended release, 1 mg Ⓑ Ⓑ

⊛ **J2430** Injection, pamidronate disodium, per 30 mg Ⓑ Ⓑ

IOM: 100-02, 15, 50

⊛ **J2440** Injection, papaverine HCL, up to 60 mg Ⓑ Ⓑ

IOM: 100-02, 15, 50

⊛ **J2460** Injection, oxytetracycline HCL, up to 50 mg Ⓑ Ⓑ

IOM: 100-02, 15, 50

▶ New   ↻ Revised   ✔ Reinstated   ~~deleted~~ Deleted   ⊘ Not covered or valid by Medicare

⊛ Special coverage instructions   ✳ Carrier discretion   Ⓑ Bill Part B MAC   Ⓑ Bill DME MAC

✳ **J2469** Injection, palonosetron HCL, 25 mcg ⑧ ⑥

Example: 0.25 mgm dose = 10 units. Example of use is acute, delayed, nausea and vomiting due to chemotherapy

✪ **J2501** Injection, paricalcitol, 1 mcg ⑧ ⑥

IOM: 100-02, 15, 50

✳ **J2502** Injection, pasireotide long acting, 1 mg ⑨ ⑥

✳ **J2503** Injection, pegaptanib sodium, 0.3 mg ⑧ ⑥

✪ **J2504** Injection, pegademase bovine, 25 IU ⑨ ⑥

IOM: 100-02, 15, 50

✳ **J2505** Injection, pegfilgrastim, 6 mg ⑧ ⑥

Report 1 unit per 6 mg.

✳ **J2507** Injection, pegloticase, 1 mg ⑧ ⑥

↻✪ **J2510** Injection, penicillin G procaine, aqueous, up to 600,000 units ⑧ ⑥

IOM: 100-02, 15, 50

✪ **J2513** Injection, pentastarch, 10% solution, 100 ml ⑨ ⑥

IOM: 100-02, 15, 50

✪ **J2515** Injection, pentobarbital sodium, per 50 mg ⑨ ⑥

IOM: 100-02, 15, 50

✪ **J2540** Injection, penicillin G potassium, up to 600,000 units ⑨ ⑥

IOM: 100-02, 15, 50

✪ **J2543** Injection, piperacillin sodium/ tazobactam sodium, 1 gram/ 0.125 grams (1.125 grams) ⑧ ⑥

IOM: 100-02, 15, 50

✪ **J2545** Pentamidine isethionate, inhalation solution, FDA-approved final product, non-compounded, administered through DME, unit dose form, per 300 mg ⑨ ⑥

✳ **J2547** Injection, peramivir, 1 mg ⑧ ⑥

✪ **J2550** Injection, promethazine HCL, up to 50 mg ⑨ ⑥

Administration of phenergan suppository considered part of E/M encounter

IOM: 100-02, 15, 50

✪ **J2560** Injection, phenobarbital sodium, up to 120 mg ⑨ ⑥

IOM: 100-02, 15, 50

✳ **J2562** Injection, plerixafor, 1 mg ⑧ ⑥

FDA approved for non-Hodgkin lymphoma and multiple myeloma in 2008.

✪ **J2590** Injection, oxytocin, up to 10 units ⑨ ⑥

IOM: 100-02, 15, 50

✪ **J2597** Injection, desmopressin acetate, per 1 mcg ⑨ ⑥

IOM: 100-02, 15, 50

✪ **J2650** Injection, prednisolone acetate, up to 1 ml ⑨ ⑥

IOM: 100-02, 15, 50

↻✪ **J2670** Injection, tolazoline HCL, up to 25 mg ⑨ ⑥

IOM: 100-02, 15, 50

✪ **J2675** Injection, progesterone, per 50 mg ⑨ ⑥

IOM: 100-02, 15, 50

✪ **J2680** Injection, fluphenazine decanoate, up to 25 mg ⑨ ⑥

IOM: 100-02, 15, 50

✪ **J2690** Injection, procainamide HCL, up to 1 gm ⑨ ⑥

Benefit limited to obstetrical diagnoses

IOM: 100-02, 15, 50

✪ **J2700** Injection, oxacillin sodium, up to 250 mg ⑨ ⑥

IOM: 100-02, 15, 50

✳ **J2704** Injection, propofol, 10 mg ⑧ ⑥

✪ **J2710** Injection, neostigmine methylsulfate, up to 0.5 mg ⑨ ⑥

IOM: 100-02, 15, 50

✪ **J2720** Injection, protamine sulfate, per 10 mg ⑨ ⑥

IOM: 100-02, 15, 50

✳ **J2724** Injection, protein C concentrate, intravenous, human, 10 IU ⑧ ⑥

✪ **J2725** Injection, protirelin, per 250 mcg ⑧ ⑥

IOM: 100-02, 15, 50

↻✪ **J2730** Injection, pralidoxime chloride, up to 1 gm ⑨ ⑥

IOM: 100-02, 15, 50

✪ **J2760** Injection, phentolamine mesylate, up to 5 mg ⑨ ⑥

IOM: 100-02, 15, 50

✪ **J2765** Injection, metoclopramide HCL, up to 10 mg ⑨ ⑥

IOM: 100-02, 15, 50

✪ **J2770** Injection, quinupristin/dalfopristin, 500 mg (150/350) ⑨ ⑥

IOM: 100-02, 15, 50

▶ **New**   ↻ **Revised**   ✔ **Reinstated**   ~~deleted~~ **Deleted**   ⊘ **Not covered or valid by Medicare**
✪ **Special coverage instructions**   ✳ **Carrier discretion**   ⑨ **Bill Part B MAC**   ⑥ **Bill DME MAC**

* **J2778** Injection, ranibizumab, 0.1 mg Ⓑ Ⓑ

  May be reported for exudative senile macular degeneration (wet AMD) with 67028 (RT or LT)

☺ **J2780** Injection, ranitidine hydrochloride, 25 mg Ⓑ Ⓑ

  IOM: 100-02, 15, 50

* **J2783** Injection, rasburicase, 0.5 mg Ⓑ Ⓑ

* **J2785** Injection, regadenoson, 0.1 mg Ⓑ Ⓑ

  One billing unit equal to 0.1 mg of regadenoson

* **J2786** Injection, reslizumab, 1 mg

☺ **J2788** Injection, Rho D immune globulin, human, minidose, 50 mcg (250 IU) Ⓠ Ⓑ

  IOM: 100-02, 15, 50

☺ **J2790** Injection, Rho D immune globulin, human, full dose, 300 mcg (1500 IU) Ⓠ Ⓑ

  Administered to pregnant female to prevent hemolistic disease of newborn. Report 90384 to private payer

  IOM: 100-02, 15, 50

☺ **J2791** Injection, Rho(D) immune globulin (human), (Rhophylac), intramuscular or intravenous, 100 IU Ⓑ Ⓑ

  Agent must be billed per 100 IU in both physician office and hospital outpatient settings

  IOM: 100-02, 15, 50

☺ **J2792** Injection, Rho D immune globulin intravenous, human, solvent detergent, 100 IU Ⓑ Ⓑ

  IOM: 100-02, 15, 50

☺ **J2793** Injection, rilonacept, 1 mg Ⓑ Ⓑ

  IOM: 100-02, 15, 50

* **J2794** Injection, risperidone, long acting, 0.5 mg Ⓠ Ⓑ

* **J2795** Injection, ropivacaine hydrochloride, 1 mg Ⓠ Ⓑ

* **J2796** Injection, romiplostim, 10 micrograms Ⓑ Ⓑ

  Stimulates bone marrow megakarocytes to produce platelets (i.e., ITP).

☺ **J2800** Injection, methocarbamol, up to 10 ml Ⓑ Ⓑ

  IOM: 100-02, 15, 50

* **J2805** Injection, sincalide, 5 micrograms Ⓑ Ⓑ

☺ **J2810** Injection, theophylline, per 40 mg Ⓠ Ⓑ

  IOM: 100-02, 15, 50

☺ **J2820** Injection, sargramostim (GM-CSF), 50 mcg Ⓠ Ⓑ

  IOM: 100-02, 15, 50

* **J2840** Injection, sebelipase alfa, 1 mg

☺ **J2850** Injection, secretin, synthetic, human, 1 microgram Ⓠ Ⓑ

  IOM: 100-02, 15, 50

* **J2860** Injection, siltuximab, 10 mg Ⓠ Ⓑ

☺ **J2910** Injection, aurothioglucose, up to 50 mg Ⓠ Ⓑ

  IOM: 100-02, 15, 50

☺ **J2916** Injection, sodium ferric gluconate complex in sucrose injection, 12.5 mg Ⓠ Ⓑ

  IOM: 100-02, 15, 50

☺ **J2920** Injection, methylprednisolone sodium succinate, up to 40 mg Ⓠ Ⓠ

  IOM: 100-02, 15, 50

☺ **J2930** Injection, methylprednisolone sodium succinate, up to 125 mg Ⓠ Ⓠ

  IOM: 100-02, 15, 50

☺ **J2940** Injection, somatrem, 1 mg Ⓑ Ⓑ

  IOM: 100-02, 15, 50

☺ **J2941** Injection, somatropin, 1 mg Ⓠ Ⓑ

  IOM: 100-02, 15, 50

☺ **J2950** Injection, promazine HCL, up to 25 mg Ⓑ Ⓑ

  IOM: 100-02, 15, 50

☺ **J2993** Injection, reteplase, 18.1 mg Ⓑ Ⓑ

☺ **J2995** Injection, streptokinase, per 250,000 IU Ⓑ Ⓑ

  Bill 1 unit for each 250,000 IU

  IOM: 100-02, 15, 50

☺ **J2997** Injection, alteplase recombinant, 1 mg Ⓑ Ⓑ

  Thrombolytic agent, treatment of occluded catheters. Bill units of 1 mg administered.

  IOM: 100-02, 15, 50

☺ **J3000** Injection, streptomycin, up to 1 gm Ⓠ Ⓑ

  IOM: 100-02, 15, 50

☺ **J3010** Injection, fentanyl citrate, 0.1 mg Ⓠ Ⓑ

  IOM: 100-02, 15, 50

☺ **J3030** Injection, sumatriptan succinate, 6 mg (Code may be used for Medicare when drug administered under the direct supervision of a physician, not for use when drug is self administered) Ⓑ Ⓑ

  IOM: 100-02, 15, 50

* **J3060** Injection, taliglucerase alfa, 10 units Ⓠ Ⓑ

☺ **J3070** Injection, pentazocine, 30 mg Ⓠ Ⓑ

  IOM: 100-02, 15, 50

▶ **New**   ↻ **Revised**   ✔ **Reinstated**   ~~deleted~~ **Deleted**   ⊘ **Not covered or valid by Medicare**

☺ **Special coverage instructions**   * **Carrier discretion**   Ⓠ **Bill Part B MAC**   Ⓑ **Bill DME MAC**

✳ **J3090** Injection, tedizolid phosphate, 1 mg Ⓑ Ⓖ

✳ **J3095** Injection, televancin, 10 mg Ⓑ Ⓖ

Prescribed for the treatment of adults with complicated skin and skin structure infections (cSSSI) of the following Gram-positive microorganisms: Staphylococcus aureus; Streptococcus pyogenes, Streptococcus agalactiae, Streptococcus anginosusgroup. Separately payable under the ASC payment system.

✳ **J3101** Injection, tenecteplase, 1 mg Ⓑ Ⓖ

✪ **J3105** Injection, terbutaline sulfate, up to 1 mg Ⓑ Ⓖ

IOM: 100-02, 15, 50

✪ **J3110** Injection, teriparatide, 10 mcg Ⓑ Ⓖ

✪ **J3121** Injection, testosterone enanthate, 1 mg Ⓑ Ⓖ

✪ **J3145** Injection, testosterone undecanoate, 1 mg Ⓑ Ⓖ

✪ **J3230** Injection, chlorpromazine HCL, up to 50 mg Ⓑ Ⓖ

IOM: 100-02, 15, 50

✪ **J3240** Injection, thyrotropin alfa, 0.9 mg provided in 1.1 mg vial Ⓑ Ⓖ

IOM: 100-02, 15, 50

✳ **J3243** Injection, tigecycline, 1 mg Ⓑ Ⓖ

✳ **J3246** Injection, tirofiban HCL, 0.25 mg Ⓑ Ⓖ

✪ **J3250** Injection, trimethobenzamide HCL, up to 200 mg Ⓑ Ⓖ

IOM: 100-02, 15, 50

✪ **J3260** Injection, tobramycin sulfate, up to 80 mg Ⓑ Ⓖ

IOM: 100-02, 15, 50

✳ **J3262** Injection, tocilizumab, 1 mg Ⓑ Ⓖ

Indicated for the treatment of adult patients with moderately to severely active rheumatoid arthritis (RA) who have had an inadequate response to one or more tumor necrosis factor (TNF) antagonist therapies.

✪ **J3265** Injection, torsemide, 10 mg/ml Ⓑ Ⓖ

IOM: 100-02, 15, 50

✪ **J3280** Injection, thiethylperazine maleate, up to 10 mg Ⓑ Ⓖ

IOM: 100-02, 15, 50

✳ **J3285** Injection, treprostinil, 1 mg Ⓑ Ⓖ

✪ **J3300** Injection, triamcinolone acetonide, preservative free, 1 mg Ⓑ Ⓖ

✪ **J3301** Injection, triamcinolone acetonide, not otherwise specified, 10 mg Ⓑ Ⓖ

IOM: 100-02, 15, 50

✪ **J3302** Injection, triamcinolone diacetate, per 5 mg Ⓑ Ⓖ

IOM: 100-02, 15, 50

✪ **J3303** Injection, triamcinolone hexacetonide, per 5 mg Ⓑ Ⓖ

IOM: 100-02, 15, 50

✪ **J3305** Injection, trimetrexate glucuronate, per 25 mg Ⓑ Ⓖ

IOM: 100-02, 15, 50

✪ **J3310** Injection, perphenazine, up to 5 mg Ⓑ Ⓖ

IOM: 100-02, 15, 50

✪ **J3315** Injection, triptorelin pamoate, 3.75 mg Ⓑ Ⓖ

IOM: 100-02, 15, 50

✪ **J3320** Injection, spectinomycin dihydrochloride, up to 2 gm Ⓑ Ⓖ

IOM: 100-02, 15, 50

✪ **J3350** Injection, urea, up to 40 gm Ⓑ Ⓖ

IOM: 100-02, 15, 50

↻✪ **J3355** Injection, urofollitropin, 75 IU Ⓑ Ⓖ

IOM: 100-02, 15, 50

✳ **J3357** Ustekinumab, for subcutaneous injection, 1 mg Ⓑ Ⓖ

▶✳ **J3358** Ustekinumab, for intravenous injection, 1 mg

Cross Reference Q9989

✪ **J3360** Injection, diazepam, up to 5 mg Ⓑ Ⓖ

IOM: 100-02, 15, 50

✪ **J3364** Injection, urokinase, 5000 IU vial Ⓑ Ⓖ

IOM: 100-02, 15, 50

↻✪ **J3365** Injection, IV, urokinase, 250,000 IU vial Ⓑ Ⓖ

IOM: 100-02, 15, 50

Cross Reference Q0089

✪ **J3370** Injection, vancomycin HCL, 500 mg Ⓑ Ⓖ

IOM: 100-02, 15, 50

✪ **J3380** Injection, vedolizumab, 1 mg Ⓑ Ⓖ

✳ **J3385** Injection, velaglucerase alfa, 100 units Ⓑ Ⓖ

Enzyme replacement therapy in Gaucher Disease that results from a specific enzyme deficiency in the body, caused by a genetic mutation received from both parents. Type 1 is the most prevalent Ashkenazi Jewish genetic disease, occurring in one in every 1,000.

✪ **J3396** Injection, verteporfin, 0.1 mg Ⓑ Ⓖ

IOM: 100-03, 1, 80.2; 100-03, 1, 80.3

▶ New ↻ Revised ✔ Reinstated deleted Deleted ⊘ Not covered or valid by Medicare
✪ Special coverage instructions ✳ Carrier discretion Ⓑ Bill Part B MAC Ⓖ Bill DME MAC

235

⊗ **J3400** Injection, triflupromazine HCL, up to 20 mg Ⓑ Ⓑ

IOM: 100-02, 15, 50

⊗ **J3410** Injection, hydroxyzine HCL, up to 25 mg Ⓑ Ⓑ

IOM: 100-02, 15, 50

✳ **J3411** Injection, thiamine HCL, 100 mg Ⓑ Ⓑ

✳ **J3415** Injection, pyridoxine HCL, 100 mg Ⓑ Ⓑ

⊗ **J3420** Injection, vitamin B-12 cyanocobalamin, up to 1000 mcg Ⓑ Ⓑ

Medicare carriers may have local coverage decisions regarding vitamin B12 injections that provide reimbursement only for patients with certain types of anemia and other conditions.

IOM: 100-02, 15, 50; 100-03, 2, 150.6

⊗ **J3430** Injection, phytonadione (vitamin K), per 1 mg Ⓑ Ⓑ

IOM: 100-02, 15, 50

⊗ **J3465** Injection, voriconazole, 10 mg Ⓑ Ⓑ

IOM: 100-02, 15, 50

⊗ **J3470** Injection, hyaluronidase, up to 150 units Ⓑ Ⓑ

IOM: 100-02, 15, 50

⊗ **J3471** Injection, hyaluronidase, ovine, preservative free, per 1 USP unit (up to 999 USP units) Ⓑ Ⓑ

⊗ **J3472** Injection, hyaluronidase, ovine, preservative free, per 1000 USP units Ⓑ Ⓑ

⊗ **J3473** Injection, hyaluronidase, recombinant, 1 USP unit Ⓑ Ⓑ

IOM: 100-02, 15, 50

⊗ **J3475** Injection, magnesium sulfate, per 500 mg Ⓑ Ⓑ

IOM: 100-02, 15, 50

⊗ **J3480** Injection, potassium chloride, per 2 meq Ⓑ Ⓑ

IOM: 100-02, 15, 50

⊗ **J3485** Injection, zidovudine, 10 mg Ⓑ Ⓑ

IOM: 100-02, 15, 50

✳ **J3486** Injection, ziprasidone mesylate, 10 mg Ⓑ Ⓑ

↻ ✳ **J3489** Injection, zoledronic acid, 1 mg Ⓑ Ⓑ

⊗ **J3490** Unclassified drugs Ⓑ Ⓑ

Bill on paper. Bill one unit. Identify drug and total dosage in "Remarks" field.

IOM: 100-02, 15, 50

⊘ **J3520** Edetate disodium, per 150 mg Ⓑ Ⓑ

IOM: 100-03, 1, 20.21; 100-03, 1, 20.22

⊗ **J3530** Nasal vaccine inhalation Ⓑ Ⓑ

IOM: 100-02, 15, 50

⊘ **J3535** Drug administered through a metered dose inhaler Ⓑ Ⓑ

IOM: 100-02, 15, 50

⊘ **J3570** Laetrile, amygdalin, vitamin B-17 Ⓑ Ⓑ

IOM: 100-03, 1, 30.7

✳ **J3590** Unclassified biologics Ⓑ

Bill on paper. Bill one unit. Identify drug and total dosage in "Remarks" field.

⊗ **J7030** Infusion, normal saline solution, 1000 cc Ⓑ Ⓑ

IOM: 100-02, 15, 50

⊗ **J7040** Infusion, normal saline solution, sterile (500 ml= 1 unit) Ⓑ Ⓑ

IOM: 100-02, 15, 50

⊗ **J7042** 5% dextrose/normal saline (500 ml = 1 unit) Ⓑ Ⓑ

IOM: 100-02, 15, 50

⊗ **J7050** Infusion, normal saline solution, 250 cc Ⓑ Ⓑ

IOM: 100-02, 15, 50

⊗ **J7060** 5% dextrose/water (500 ml = 1 unit) Ⓑ Ⓑ

IOM: 100-02, 15, 50

⊗ **J7070** Infusion, D 5 W, 1000 cc Ⓑ Ⓑ

IOM: 100-02, 15, 50

⊗ **J7100** Infusion, dextran 40, 500 ml Ⓑ Ⓑ

IOM: 100-02, 15, 50

⊗ **J7110** Infusion, dextran 75, 500 ml Ⓑ Ⓑ

IOM: 100-02, 15, 50

⊗ **J7120** Ringer's lactate infusion, up to 1000 cc Ⓑ Ⓑ

Replacement fluid or electrolytes.

IOM: 100-02, 15, 50

⊗ **J7121** 5% dextrose in lactated ringers infusion, up to 1000 cc Ⓑ Ⓑ

IOM: 100-02, 15, 50

⊗ **J7131** Hypertonic saline solution, 1 ml Ⓑ Ⓑ

IOM: 100-02, 15, 50

Clotting Factors

✳ **J7175** Injection, Factor X, (human), 1 IU Ⓑ

✳ **J7178** Injection, human fibrinogen concentrate, 1 mg Ⓑ

▶ New	↻ Revised	✔ Reinstated	~~deleted~~ Deleted	⊘ Not covered or valid by Medicare
⊗ Special coverage instructions		✳ Carrier discretion	Ⓑ Bill Part B MAC	Ⓑ Bill DME MAC

✪ **J7179** Injection, von Willebrand factor (recombinant), (vonvendi), 1 IU VWF:RCo Ⓑ

✳ **J7180** Injection, factor XIII (antihemophilic factor, human), 1 IU Ⓑ

✳ **J7181** Injection, factor XIII a-subunit, (recombinant), per IU Ⓑ

✳ **J7182** Injection, factor VIII, (antihemophilic factor, recombinant), (novoeight), per IU Ⓑ

✪ **J7183** Injection, von Willebrand factor complex (human), wilate, 1 IU VWF:RCo Ⓑ

IOM: 100-02, 15, 50

✳ **J7185** Injection, Factor VIII (antihemophilic factor, recombinant) (Xyntha), per IU Ⓑ

✪ **J7186** Injection, anti-hemophilic factor VIII/von Willebrand factor complex (human), per factor VIII IU Ⓑ

IOM: 100-02, 15, 50

✪ **J7187** Injection, von Willebrand factor complex (HUMATE-P), per IU VWF:RCo Ⓑ

IOM: 100-02, 15, 50

✪ **J7188** Injection, factor VIII (antihemophilic factor, recombinant), (obizur), per IU Ⓑ

IOM: 100-02, 15, 50

✪ **J7189** Factor VIIa (anti-hemophilic factor, recombinant), per 1 microgram Ⓑ

IOM: 100-02, 15, 50

✪ **J7190** Factor VIII anti-hemophilic factor, human, per IU Ⓑ

IOM: 100-02, 15, 50

⮌ ✪ **J7191** Factor VIII, anti-hemophilic factor (porcine), per IU Ⓑ

IOM: 100-02, 15, 50

✪ **J7192** Factor VIII (anti-hemophilic factor, recombinant) per IU, not otherwise specified Ⓑ

IOM: 100-02, 15, 50

✪ **J7193** Factor IX (anti-hemophilic factor, purified, non-recombinant) per IU Ⓑ

IOM: 100-02, 15, 50

✪ **J7194** Factor IX, complex, per IU Ⓑ

IOM: 100-02, 15, 50

✪ **J7195** Injection, Factor IX (anti-hemophilic factor, recombinant) per IU, not otherwise specified Ⓑ

IOM: 100-02, 15, 50

⮌ ✳ **J7196** Injection, antithrombin recombinant, 50 IU Ⓑ

✪ **J7197** Anti-thrombin III (human), per IU Ⓑ

IOM: 100-02, 15, 50

✪ **J7198** Anti-inhibitor, per IU Ⓑ

Diagnosis examples: 286.0 Congenital Factor VIII disorder; 286.1 Congenital Factor IX disorder; 286.4 VonWillebrand's disease

IOM: 100-02, 15, 50; 100-03, 2, 110.3

✪ **J7199** Hemophilia clotting factor, not otherwise classified Ⓑ

IOM: 100-02, 15, 50; 100-03, 2, 110.3

✪ **J7200** Injection, factor IX, (antihemophilic factor, recombinant), rixubis, per IU Ⓑ

IOM: 100-02, 15, 50

✪ **J7201** Injection, factor IX, fc fusion protein (recombinant), alprolix, 1 IU Ⓑ

IOM: 100-02, 15, 50

✪ **J7202** Injection, Factor IX, albumin fusion protein, (recombinant), idelvion, 1 IU

✪ **J7205** Injection, factor VIII Fc fusion protein (recombinant), per IU Ⓑ

✪ **J7207** Injection, Factor VIII, (antihemophilic factor, recombinant), PEGylated, 1 IU

✳ **J7209** Injection, Factor VIII, (antihemophilic factor, recombinant), (Nuwiq), 1 IU

▶ ✳ **J7210** Injection, Factor VIII, (antihemophilic factor, recombinant), (afstyla), 1 i.u.

▶ ✳ **J7211** Injection, Factor VIII, (antihemophilic factor, recombinant), (kovaltry), 1 i.u.

Contraceptives

▶ ⊘ **J7296** Levonorgestrel-releasing intrauterine contraceptive system, (kyleena), 19.5 mg

Cross Reference Q9984

⊘ **J7297** Levonorgestrel-releasing intrauterine contraceptive system (liletta), 52 mg Ⓑ

⊘ **J7298** Levonorgestrel-releasing intrauterine contraceptive system (mirena), 52 mg Ⓑ

⊘ **J7300** Intrauterine copper contraceptive Ⓑ

Report IUD insertion with 58300. Bill usual and customary charge.

⊘ **J7301** Levonorgestrel-releasing intrauterine contraceptive system (skyla), 13.5 mg Ⓑ

⊘ **J7303** Contraceptive supply, hormone containing vaginal ring, each Ⓑ

⊘ **J7304** Contraceptive supply, hormone containing patch, each Ⓑ

Only billed by Family Planning Clinics

⊘ **J7306** Levonorgestrel (contraceptive) implant system, including implants and supplies Ⓑ

⊘ **J7307** Etonogestrel (contraceptive) implant system, including implant and supplies Ⓑ

Aminolevulinic Acid HCL

✳ **J7308** Aminolevulinic acid HCL for topical administration, 20%, single unit dosage form (354 mg) Ⓑ

↻⊗ **J7309** Methyl aminolevulinate (MAL) for topical administration, 16.8%, 1 gram Ⓑ

Ganciclovir

↻⊗ **J7310** Ganciclovir, 4.5 mg, long-acting implant Ⓑ

IOM: 100-02, 15, 50

Ophthalmic Drugs

✳ **J7311** Fluocinolone acetonide, intravitreal implant Ⓑ

Treatment of chronic noninfectious posterior segment uveitis

✳ **J7312** Injection, dexamethasone, intravitreal implant, 0.1 mg Ⓑ

To bill for Ozurdex services submit the following codes: J7312 and 67028 with the modifier -22 (for the increased work difficulty and increased risk). Indicated for the treatment of macular edema occurring after branch retinal vein occlusion (BRVO) or central retinal vein occlusion (CRVO) and non-infectious uveitis affecting the posterior segment of the eye.

✳ **J7313** Injection, fluocinolone acetonide, intravitreal implant, 0.01 mg Ⓑ

✳ **J7315** Mitomycin, ophthalmic, 0.2 mg Ⓑ

✳ **J7316** Injection, ocriplasmin, 0.125 mg Ⓑ

Hyaluronan

↻✳ **J7320** Hyaluronan or derivitive, genvisc 850, for intra-articular injection, 1 mg Ⓑ

↻✳ **J7321** Hyaluronan or derivative, Hyalgan, Supartz or Visco-3, for intra-articular injection, per dose Ⓑ

Therapeutic goal is to restore visco-elasticity of synovial hyaluronan, thereby decreasing pain, improving mobility and restoring natural protective functions of hyaluronan in joint

✳ **J7322** Hyaluronan or derivative, hymovis, for intra-articular injection, 1 mg Ⓑ

✳ **J7323** Hyaluronan or derivative, Euflexxa, for intra-articular injection, per dose Ⓑ

✳ **J7324** Hyaluronan or derivative, Orthovisc, for intra-articular injection, per dose Ⓑ

✳ **J7325** Hyaluronan or derivative, Synvisc or Synvisc-One, for intra-articular injection, 1 mg Ⓑ

✳ **J7326** Hyaluronan or derivative, Gel-One, for intra-articular injection, per dose Ⓑ

✳ **J7327** Hyaluronan or derivative, monovisc, for intra-articular injection, per dose Ⓑ

↻✳ **J7328** Hyaluronan or derivative, gelsyn-3, for intra-articular injection, 0.1 mg Ⓑ

Miscellaneous Drugs

✳ **J7330** Autologous cultured chondrocytes, implant Ⓑ

✳ **J7336** Capsaicin 8% patch, per square centimeter Ⓑ

✳ **J7340** Carbidopa 5 mg/levodopa 20 mg enteral suspension, 100 ml Ⓑ

✳ **J7342** Instillation, ciprofloxacin otic suspension, 6 mg Ⓑ

▶⊗ **J7345** Aminolevulinic acid hcl for topical administration, 10% gel, 10 mg

Immunosuppressive Drugs (Includes Non-injectibles)

⊗ **J7500** Azathioprine, oral, 50 mg Ⓑ Ⓓ

IOM: 100-02, 15, 50

⊗ **J7501** Azathioprine, parenteral, 100 mg Ⓑ Ⓓ

IOM: 100-02, 15, 50

⊗ **J7502** Cyclosporine, oral, 100 mg Ⓑ Ⓓ

IOM: 100-02, 15, 50

▶ New   ↻ Revised   ✔ Reinstated   ~~deleted~~ Deleted   ⊘ Not covered or valid by Medicare

⊗ Special coverage instructions   ✳ Carrier discretion   Ⓑ Bill Part B MAC   Ⓓ Bill DME MAC

⊛ **J7503** Tacrolimus, extended release, (Envarsus XR), oral, 0.25 mg ⑨ ⑥

IOM: 100-02, 15, 50

⊛ **J7504** Lymphocyte immune globulin, antithymocyte globulin, equine, parenteral, 250 mg ⑧ ⑧

IOM: 100-02, 15, 50; 100-03, 2, 110.3

⊛ **J7505** Muromonab-CD3, parenteral, 5 mg ⑨ ⑧

IOM: 100-02, 15, 50

⊛ **J7507** Tacrolimus, immediate release, oral, 1 mg ⑨ ⑧

IOM: 100-02, 15, 50

↺ ⊛ **J7508** Tacrolimus, extended release, (Astagraf XL), oral, 0.1 mg ⑧ ⑧

IOM: 100-02, 15, 50

⊛ **J7509** Methylprednisolone oral, per 4 mg ⑨ ⑧

IOM: 100-02, 15, 50

⊛ **J7510** Prednisolone oral, per 5 mg ⑧ ⑧

IOM: 100-02, 15, 50

✱ **J7511** Lymphocyte immune globulin, antithymocyte globulin, rabbit, parenteral, 25 mg ⑧ ⑧

⊛ **J7512** Prednisone, immediate release or delayed release, oral, 1 mg ⑧ ⑧

IOM: 100-02, 15, 50

↺ ⊛ **J7513** Daclizumab, parenteral, 25 mg ⑧ ⑧

IOM: 100-02, 15, 50

✱ **J7515** Cyclosporine, oral, 25 mg ⑧ ⑧

✱ **J7516** Cyclosporin, parenteral, 250 mg ⑧ ⑧

✱ **J7517** Mycophenolate mofetil, oral, 250 mg ⑧ ⑧

⊛ **J7518** Mycophenolic acid, oral, 180 mg ⑧ ⑧

IOM: 100-04, 4, 240; 100-4, 17, 80.3.1

⊛ **J7520** Sirolimus, oral, 1 mg ⑨ ⑧

IOM: 100-02, 15, 50

⊛ **J7525** Tacrolimus, parenteral, 5 mg ⑧ ⑧

IOM: 100-02, 15, 50

⊛ **J7527** Everolimus, oral, 0.25 mg ⑧ ⑧

IOM: 100-02, 15, 50

⊛ **J7599** Immunosuppressive drug, not otherwise classified ⑧ ⑧

Bill on paper. Bill one unit. Identify drug and total dosage in "Remarks" field.

IOM: 100-02, 15, 50

Inhalation Solutions

✱ **J7604** Acetylcysteine, inhalation solution, compounded product, administered through DME, unit dose form, per gram ⑨ ⑧

✱ **J7605** Arformoterol, inhalation solution, FDA approved final product, non-compounded, administered through DME, unit dose form, 15 micrograms ⑨ ⑧

Maintenance treatment of bronchoconstriction in patients with chronic obstructive pulmonary disease (COPD).

✱ **J7606** Formoterol fumarate, inhalation solution, FDA approved final product, non-compounded, administered through DME, unit dose form, 20 micrograms ⑨ ⑧

✱ **J7607** Levalbuterol, inhalation solution, compounded product, administered through DME, concentrated form, 0.5 mg ⑨ ⑧

⊛ **J7608** Acetylcysteine, inhalation solution, FDA-approved final product, non-compounded, administered through DME, unit dose form, per gram ⑧ ⑧

✱ **J7609** Albuterol, inhalation solution, compounded product, administered through DME, unit dose, 1 mg ⑨ ⑧

Patient's home, medications—such as a albuterol when administered through a nebulizer—are considered DME and are payable under Part B.

✱ **J7610** Albuterol, inhalation solution, compounded product, administered through DME, concentrated form, 1 mg ⑨ ⑧

⊛ **J7611** Albuterol, inhalation solution, FDA-approved final product, non-compounded, administered through DME, concentrated form, 1 mg ⑨ ⑧

Report once for each milligram administered. For example, 2 mg of concentrated albuterol (usually diluted with saline), reported with J7611×2.

⊛ **J7612** Levalbuterol, inhalation solution, FDA-approved final product, non-compounded, administered through DME, concentrated form, 0.5 mg ⑨ ⑧

⊛ **J7613** Albuterol, inhalation solution, FDA-approved final product, non-compounded, administered through DME, unit dose, 1 mg ⑨ ⑧

⊕ **J7614** Levalbuterol, inhalation solution, FDA-approved final product, non-compounded, administered through DME, unit dose, 0.5 mg ⑨ ⑧

✳ **J7615** Levalbuterol, inhalation solution, compounded product, administered through DME, unit dose, 0.5 mg ⑨ ⑧

⊕ **J7620** Albuterol, up to 2.5 mg and ipratropium bromide, up to 0.5 mg,FDA-approved final product, non-compounded, administered through DME ⑨ ⑧

✳ **J7622** Beclomethasone, inhalation solution, compounded product, administered through DME, unit dose form, per mg ⑧ ⑧

✳ **J7624** Betamethasone, inhalation solution, compounded product, administered through DME, unit dose form, per mg ⑧ ⑧

✳ **J7626** Budesonide inhalation solution, FDA-approved final product, non-compounded, administered through DME, unit dose form, up to 0.5 mg ⑨ ⑧

✳ **J7627** Budesonide, inhalation solution, compounded product, administered through DME, unit dose form, up to 0.5 mg ⑧ ⑧

⊕ **J7628** Bitolterol mesylate, inhalation solution, compounded product, administered through DME, concentrated form, per milligram ⑧ ⑧

⊕ **J7629** Bitolterol mesylate, inhalation solution, compounded product, administered through DME, unit dose form, per milligram ⑧ ⑧

⊕ **J7631** Cromolyn sodium, inhalation solution, FDA-approved final product, non-compounded, administered through DME, unit dose form, per 10 milligrams ⑧ ⑧

✳ **J7632** Cromolyn sodium, inhalation solution, compounded product, administered through DME, unit dose form, per 10 milligrams ⑧ ⑧

✳ **J7633** Budesonide, inhalation solution, FDA-approved final product, non-compounded, administered through DME, concentrated form, per 0.25 milligram ⑨ ⑧

✳ **J7634** Budesonide, inhalation solution, compounded product, administered through DME, concentrated form, per 0.25 milligram ⑧ ⑧

⊕ **J7635** Atropine, inhalation solution, compounded product, administered through DME, concentrated form, per milligram ⑨ ⑧

⊕ **J7636** Atropine, inhalation solution, compounded product, administered through DME, unit dose form, per milligram ⑨ ⑧

⊕ **J7637** Dexamethasone, inhalation solution, compounded product, administered through DME, concentrated form, per milligram ⑨ ⑧

⊕ **J7638** Dexamethasone, inhalation solution, compounded product, administered through DME, unit dose form, per milligram ⑨ ⑧

⊕ **J7639** Dornase alfa, inhalation solution, FDA-approved final product, non-compounded, administered through DME, unit dose form, per milligram ⑧ ⑧

✳ **J7640** Formoterol, inhalation solution, compounded product, administered through DME, unit dose form, 12 micrograms ⑨ ⑧

✳ **J7641** Flunisolide, inhalation solution, compounded product, administered through DME, unit dose, per milligram ⑧ ⑧

⊕ **J7642** Glycopyrrolate, inhalation solution, compounded product, administered through DME, concentrated form, per milligram ⑨ ⑧

⊕ **J7643** Glycopyrrolate, inhalation solution, compounded product, administered through DME, unit dose form, per milligram ⑨ ⑧

⊕ **J7644** Ipratropium bromide, inhalation solution, FDA-approved final product, non-compounded, administered through DME, unit dose form, per milligram ⑨ ⑧

✳ **J7645** Ipratropium bromide, inhalation solution, compounded product, administered through DME, unit dose form, per milligram ⑨ ⑧

✳ **J7647** Isoetharine HCL, inhalation solution, compounded product, administered through DME, concentrated form, per milligram ⑨ ⑧

⊕ **J7648** Isoetharine HCL, inhalation solution, FDA-approved final product, non-compounded, administered through DME, concentrated form, per milligram ⑨ ⑧

▶ New	⟳ Revised	✔ Reinstated	~~deleted~~ Deleted	⊘ Not covered or valid by Medicare
⊕ Special coverage instructions		✳ Carrier discretion	⑨ Bill Part B MAC	⑧ Bill DME MAC

✿ **J7649** Isoetharine HCL, inhalation solution, FDA-approved final product, non-compounded, administered through DME, unit dose form, per milligram ⑨ ⑧

✳ **J7650** Isoetharine HCL, inhalation solution, compounded product, administered through DME, unit dose form, per milligram ⑧ ⑧

✳ **J7657** Isoproterenol HCL, inhalation solution, compounded product, administered through DME, concentrated form, per milligram ⑨ ⑧

✿ **J7658** Isoproterenol HCL inhalation solution, FDA-approved final product, non-compounded, administered through DME, concentrated form, per milligram ⑨ ⑧

✿ **J7659** Isoproterenol HCL, inhalation solution, FDA-approved final product, non-compounded, administered through DME, unit dose form, per milligram ⑨ ⑧

✳ **J7660** Isoproterenol HCL, inhalation solution, compounded product, administered through DME, unit dose form, per milligram ⑨ ⑧

✳ **J7665** Mannitol, administered through an inhaler, 5 mg ⑧ ⑧

✳ **J7667** Metaproterenol sulfate, inhalation solution, compounded product, concentrated form, per 10 milligrams ⑨ ⑧

✿ **J7668** Metaproterenol sulfate, inhalation solution, FDA-approved final product, non-compounded, administered through DME, concentrated form, per 10 milligrams ⑧ ⑧

✿ **J7669** Metaproterenol sulfate, inhalation solution, FDA-approved final product, non-compounded, administered through DME, unit dose form, per 10 milligrams ⑧ ⑧

✳ **J7670** Metaproterenol sulfate, inhalation solution, compounded product, administered through DME, unit dose form, per 10 milligrams ⑧ ⑧

✳ **J7674** Methacholine chloride administered as inhalation solution through a nebulizer, per 1 mg ⑧ ⑧

✳ **J7676** Pentamidine isethionate, inhalation solution, compounded product, administered through DME, unit dose form, per 300 mg ⑧ ⑧

✿ **J7680** Terbutaline sulfate, inhalation solution, compounded product, administered through DME, concentrated form, per milligram ⑧ ⑧

✿ **J7681** Terbutaline sulfate, inhalation solution, compounded product, administered through DME, unit dose form, per milligram ⑧ ⑧

✿ **J7682** Tobramycin, inhalation solution, FDA-approved final product, non-compounded unit dose form, administered through DME, per 300 milligrams ⑧ ⑧

✿ **J7683** Triamcinolone, inhalation solution, compounded product, administered through DME, concentrated form, per milligram ⑧ ⑧

✿ **J7684** Triamcinolone, inhalation solution, compounded product, administered through DME, unit dose form, per milligram ⑧ ⑧

✳ **J7685** Tobramycin, inhalation solution, compounded product, administered through DME, unit dose form, per 300 milligrams ⑨ ⑧

✳ **J7686** Treprostinil, inhalation solution, FDA-approved final product, non-compounded, administered through DME, unit dose form, 1.74 mg ⑧ ⑧

Not Otherwise Classified/Specified

✿ **J7699** NOC drugs, inhalation solution administered through DME ⑧ ⑧

✿ **J7799** NOC drugs, other than inhalation drugs, administered through DME ⑨ ⑧

Bill on paper. Bill one unit and identify drug and total dosage in the "Remark" field.

IOM: 100-02, 15, 110.3

✿ **J7999** Compounded drug, not otherwise classified ⑧ ⑧

✿ **J8498** Antiemetic drug, rectal/suppository, not otherwise specified ⑧

⊘ **J8499** Prescription drug, oral, non chemotherapeutic, NOS ⑨ ⑧

IOM: 100-02, 15, 50

Oral Anti-Cancer Drugs

✿ **J8501** Aprepitant, oral, 5 mg ⑧

↺ ✿ **J8510** Busulfan; oral, 2 mg ⑧

IOM: 100-02, 15, 50; 100-04, 4, 240; 100-04, 17, 80.1.1

▶ **New** ↺ **Revised** ✔ **Reinstated** deleted **Deleted** ⊘ **Not covered or valid by Medicare** ✿ **Special coverage instructions** ✳ **Carrier discretion** ⑨ **Bill Part B MAC** ⑧ **Bill DME MAC**

⊘ **J8515** Cabergoline, oral, 0.25 mg Ⓑ
IOM: 100-02, 15, 50; 100-04, 4, 240

✪ **J8520** Capecitabine, oral, 150 mg Ⓑ
IOM: 100-02, 15, 50; 100-04, 4, 240; 100-04, 17, 80.1.1

✪ **J8521** Capecitabine, oral, 500 mg Ⓑ
IOM: 100-02, 15, 50; 100-04, 4, 240; 100-04, 17, 80.1.1

✪ **J8530** Cyclophosphamide; oral, 25 mg Ⓑ
IOM: 100-02, 15, 50; 100-04, 4, 240; 100-04, 17, 80.1.1

✪ **J8540** Dexamethasone, oral, 0.25 mg Ⓑ

✪ **J8560** Etoposide; oral, 50 mg Ⓑ
IOM: 100-02, 15, 50; 100-04, 4, 230.1; 100-04, 4, 240; 100-04, 17, 80.1.1

✻ **J8562** Fludarabine phosphate, oral, 10 mg Ⓑ

✪ **J8565** Gefitinib, oral, 250 mg Ⓑ

✪ **J8597** Antiemetic drug, oral, not otherwise specified Ⓑ

✪ **J8600** Melphalan; oral, 2 mg Ⓑ
IOM: 100-02, 15, 50; 100-04, 4, 240; 100-04, 17, 80.1.1

✪ **J8610** Methotrexate; oral, 2.5 mg Ⓑ
IOM: 100-02, 15, 50; 100-04, 4, 240; 100-04, 17, 80.1.1

↺✻ **J8650** Nabilone, oral, 1 mg Ⓑ

✪ **J8655** Netupitant 300 mg and palonosetron 0.5 mg Ⓑ

✪ **J8670** Rolapitant, oral, 1 mg

↺✪ **J8700** Temozolomide, oral, 5 mg Ⓑ
IOM: 100-02, 15, 50; 100-04, 4, 240

✻ **J8705** Topotecan, oral, 0.25 mg Ⓑ
Treatment for ovarian and lung cancers, etc. Report J9350 (Topotecan, 4 mg) for intravenous version

✪ **J8999** Prescription drug, oral, chemotherapeutic, NOS Ⓑ
IOM: 100-02, 15, 50; 100-04, 4, 250; 100-04, 17, 80.1.1; 100-04, 17, 80.1.2

CHEMOTHERAPY DRUGS (J9000-J9999)

NOTE: These codes cover the cost of the chemotherapy drug only, not to include the administration

✪ **J9000** Injection, doxorubicin hydrochloride, 10 mg Ⓟ Ⓑ
IOM: 100-02, 15, 50

✪ **J9015** Injection, aldesleukin, per single use vial Ⓟ Ⓑ
IOM: 100-02, 15, 50

✻ **J9017** Injection, arsenic trioxide, 1 mg Ⓟ Ⓑ

✪ **J9019** Injection, asparaginase (Erwinaze), 1,000 IU Ⓟ Ⓑ
IOM: 100-02, 15, 50

✪ **J9020** Injection, asparaginase, not otherwise specified 10,000 units Ⓟ Ⓑ
IOM: 100-02, 15, 50

▶✻ **J9022** Injection, atezolizumab, 10 mg

▶✻ **J9023** Injection, avelumab, 10 mg

✻ **J9025** Injection, azacitidine, 1 mg Ⓟ Ⓑ

✻ **J9027** Injection, clofarabine, 1 mg Ⓑ Ⓑ

✪ **J9031** BCG (intravesical), per instillation Ⓟ Ⓑ
IOM: 100-02, 15, 50

✻ **J9032** Injection, belinostat, 10 mg Ⓑ Ⓑ

✻ **J9033** Injection, bendamustine HCL (treanda), 1 mg Ⓟ Ⓑ
Treatment for form of non-Hodgkin's lymphoma; standard administration time is as an intravenous infusion over 30 minutes

✻ **J9034** Injection, bendamustine hcl (bendeka), 1 mg

✻ **J9035** Injection, bevacizumab, 10 mg Ⓑ Ⓑ
For malignant neoplasm of breast, considered J9207.

✻ **J9039** Injection, blinatumomab, 1 microgram Ⓟ Ⓑ

✪ **J9040** Injection, bleomycin sulfate, 15 units Ⓟ Ⓑ
IOM: 100-02, 15, 50

✻ **J9041** Injection, bortezomib, 0.1 mg Ⓟ Ⓑ

✻ **J9042** Injection, brentuximab vedotin, 1 mg Ⓟ Ⓑ

✻ **J9043** Injection, cabazitaxel, 1 mg Ⓟ Ⓑ

✪ **J9045** Injection, carboplatin, 50 mg Ⓟ Ⓑ
IOM: 100-02, 15, 50

✻ **J9047** Injection, carfilzomib, 1 mg Ⓟ Ⓑ

✪ **J9050** Injection, carmustine, 100 mg Ⓟ Ⓑ
IOM: 100-02, 15, 50

✻ **J9055** Injection, cetuximab, 10 mg Ⓟ Ⓑ

✪ **J9060** Injection, cisplatin, powder or solution, 10 mg Ⓟ Ⓑ
IOM: 100-02, 15, 50

✪ **J9065** Injection, cladribine, per 1 mg Ⓟ Ⓑ
IOM: 100-02, 15, 50

⊛ **J9070** Cyclophosphamide, 100 mg ⑧ ⑥
IOM: 100-02, 15, 50

✳ **J9098** Injection, cytarabine liposome, 10 mg ⑧ ⑥

⊛ **J9100** Injection, cytarabine, 100 mg ⑧ ⑧
IOM: 100-02, 15, 50

⊛ **J9120** Injection, dactinomycin, 0.5 mg ⑧ ⑧
IOM: 100-02, 15, 50

⊛ **J9130** Dacarbazine, 100 mg ⑧ ⑥
IOM: 100-02, 15, 50

⊛ **J9145** Injection, daratumumab, 10 mg
IOM: 100-02, 15, 50

⊛ **J9150** Injection, daunorubicin, 10 mg ⑧ ⑥
IOM: 100-02, 15, 50

↺⊛ **J9151** Injection, daunorubicin citrate, liposomal formulation, 10 mg ⑧ ⑧
IOM: 100-02, 15, 50

✳ **J9155** Injection, degarelix, 1 mg ⑧ ⑧
Report 1 unit for every 1 mg.

✳ **J9160** Injection, denileukin diftitox, 300 micrograms ⑧ ⑥

⊛ **J9165** Injection, diethylstilbestrol diphosphate, 250 mg ⑧ ⑧
IOM: 100-02, 15, 50

⊛ **J9171** Injection, docetaxel, 1 mg ⑧ ⑧
Report 1 unit for every 1 mg.
IOM: 100-02, 15, 50

⊛ **J9175** Injection, Elliott's B solution, 1 ml ⑧ ⑧
IOM: 100-02, 15, 50

✳ **J9176** Injection, elotuzumab, 1 mg

✳ **J9178** Injection, epirubicin HCL, 2 mg ⑧ ⑧

✳ **J9179** Injection, eribulin mesylate, 0.1 mg ⑧ ⑥

⊛ **J9181** Injection, etoposide, 10 mg ⑧ ⑧

↺⊛ **J9185** Injection, fludarabine phosphate, 50 mg ⑧ ⑥
IOM: 100-02, 15, 50

⊛ **J9190** Injection, fluorouracil, 500 mg ⑧ ⑧
IOM: 100-02, 15, 50

↺⊛ **J9200** Injection, floxuridine, 500 mg ⑧ ⑥
IOM: 100-02, 15, 50

⊛ **J9201** Injection, gemcitabine hydrochloride, 200 mg ⑧ ⑥
IOM: 100-02, 15, 50

⊛ **J9202** Goserelin acetate implant, per 3.6 mg ⑧ ⑧
IOM: 100-02, 15, 50

▶✳ **J9203** Injection, gemtuzumab ozogamicin, 0.1 mg

⊛ **J9205** Injection, irinotecan liposome, 1 mg
IOM: 100-02, 15, 50

⊛ **J9206** Injection, irinotecan, 20 mg ⑧ ⑧
IOM: 100-02, 15, 50

✳ **J9207** Injection, ixabepilone, 1 mg ⑧ ⑧

↺⊛ **J9208** Injection, ifosfamide, 1 gm ⑧ ⑧
IOM: 100-02, 15, 50

⊛ **J9209** Injection, mesna, 200 mg ⑧ ⑧
IOM: 100-02, 15, 50

⊛ **J9211** Injection, idarubicin hydrochloride, 5 mg ⑧ ⑧
IOM: 100-02, 15, 50

⊛ **J9212** Injection, interferon alfacon-1, recombinant, 1 mcg ⑧ ⑧
IOM: 100-02, 15, 50

↺⊛ **J9213** Injection, interferon, alfa-2a, recombinant, 3 million units ⑧ ⑧
IOM: 100-02, 15, 50

⊛ **J9214** Injection, interferon, alfa-2b, recombinant, 1 million units ⑧ ⑧
IOM: 100-02, 15, 50

⊛ **J9215** Injection, interferon, alfa-n3 (human leukocyte derived), 250,000 IU ⑧ ⑧
IOM: 100-02, 15, 50

⊛ **J9216** Injection, interferon, gamma-1B, 3 million units ⑧ ⑧
IOM: 100-02, 15, 50

⊛ **J9217** Leuprolide acetate (for depot suspension), 7.5 mg ⑧ ⑧
IOM: 100-02, 15, 50

⊛ **J9218** Leuprolide acetate, per 1 mg ⑧ ⑧
IOM: 100-02, 15, 50

↺⊛ **J9219** Leuprolide acetate implant, 65 mg ⑧ ⑧
IOM: 100-02, 15, 50

⊛ **J9225** Histrelin implant (Vantas), 50 mg ⑧ ⑧
IOM: 100-02, 15, 50

⊛ **J9226** Histrelin implant (Supprelin LA), 50 mg ⑧ ⑧
IOM: 100-02, 15, 50

✳ **J9228** Injection, ipilimumab, 1 mg ⑧ ⑧

⊛ **J9230** Injection, mechlorethamine hydrochloride, (nitrogen mustard), 10 mg ⑧ ⑧
IOM: 100-02, 15, 50

▶ **New**   ↺ **Revised**   ✔ **Reinstated**   ~~deleted~~ **Deleted**   ⊘ **Not covered or valid by Medicare**
⊛ **Special coverage instructions**   ✳ **Carrier discretion**   ⑧ **Bill Part B MAC**   ⑧ **Bill DME MAC**

✺ **J9245** Injection, melphalan hydrochloride, 50 mg Ⓑ Ⓑ

IOM: 100-02, 15, 50

✺ **J9250** Methotrexate sodium, 5 mg Ⓑ Ⓑ

IOM: 100-02, 15, 50

✺ **J9260** Methotrexate sodium, 50 mg Ⓑ Ⓑ

IOM: 100-02, 15, 50

✳ **J9261** Injection, nelarabine, 50 mg Ⓑ Ⓑ

✳ **J9262** Injection, omacetaxine mepesuccinate, 0.01 mg Ⓑ Ⓑ

↻ ✳ **J9263** Injection, oxaliplatin, 0.5 mg Ⓑ Ⓑ

Eloxatin, platinum-based anticancer drug that destroys cancer cells

✳ **J9264** Injection, paclitaxel protein-bound particles, 1 mg Ⓑ Ⓑ

✺ **J9266** Injection, pegaspargase, per single dose vial Ⓑ Ⓑ

IOM: 100-02, 15, 50

✺ **J9267** Injection, paclitaxel, 1 mg Ⓑ Ⓑ

✺ **J9268** Injection, pentostatin, 10 mg Ⓑ Ⓑ

IOM: 100-02, 15, 50

✺ **J9270** Injection, plicamycin, 2.5 mg Ⓑ Ⓑ

IOM: 100-02, 15, 50

✳ **J9271** Injection, pembrolizumab, 1 mg Ⓑ Ⓑ

✺ **J9280** Injection, mitomycin, 5 mg Ⓑ Ⓑ

IOM: 100-02, 15, 50

▶ ✳ **J9285** Injection, olaratumab, 10 mg Ⓑ Ⓑ

✺ **J9293** Injection, mitoxantrone hydrochloride, per 5 mg Ⓑ Ⓑ

IOM: 100-02, 15, 50

✳ **J9295** Injection, necitumumab, 1 mg

✺ **J9299** Injection, nivolumab, 1 mg Ⓑ Ⓑ

✳ **J9300** Injection, gemtuzumab ozogamicin, 5 mg

✳ **J9301** Injection, obinutuzumab, 10 mg Ⓑ Ⓑ

✳ **J9302** Injection, ofatumumab, 10 mg Ⓑ Ⓑ

✳ **J9303** Injection, panitumumab, 10 mg Ⓑ Ⓑ

✳ **J9305** Injection, pemetrexed, 10 mg Ⓑ Ⓑ

✳ **J9306** Injection, pertuzumab, 1 mg Ⓑ Ⓑ

✳ **J9307** Injection, pralatrexate, 1 mg Ⓑ Ⓑ

✳ **J9308** Injection, ramucirumab, 5 mg Ⓑ Ⓑ

✺ **J9310** Injection, rituximab, 100 mg Ⓑ Ⓑ

IOM: 100-02, 15, 50

✳ **J9315** Injection, romidepsin, 1 mg Ⓑ Ⓑ

✺ **J9320** Injection, streptozocin, 1 gram Ⓑ Ⓑ

IOM: 100-02, 15, 50

✳ **J9325** Injection, talimogene laherparepvec, per 1 million plaque forming units

✳ **J9328** Injection, temozolomide, 1 mg Ⓑ Ⓑ

Intravenous formulation, not for oral administration

✳ **J9330** Injection, temsirolimus, 1 mg Ⓑ Ⓑ

Treatment for advanced renal cell carcinoma; standard administration is intravenous infusion greater than 30-60 minutes

✺ **J9340** Injection, thiotepa, 15 mg Ⓑ Ⓑ

IOM: 100-02, 15, 50

↻ ✳ **J9351** Injection, topotecan, 0.1 mg Ⓑ Ⓑ

✳ **J9352** Injection, trabectedin, 0.1 mg

✳ **J9354** Injection, ado-trastuzumab emtansine, 1 mg Ⓑ Ⓑ

✳ **J9355** Injection, trastuzumab, 10 mg Ⓑ Ⓑ

✺ **J9357** Injection, valrubicin, intravesical, 200 mg Ⓑ Ⓑ

IOM: 100-02, 15, 50

✺ **J9360** Injection, vinblastine sulfate, 1 mg Ⓑ Ⓑ

IOM: 100-02, 15, 50

✺ **J9370** Vincristine sulfate, 1 mg Ⓑ Ⓑ

IOM: 100-02, 15, 50

✳ **J9371** Injection, vincristine sulfate liposome, 1 mg Ⓑ Ⓑ

✺ **J9390** Injection, vinorelbine tartrate, 10 mg Ⓑ Ⓑ

IOM: 100-02, 15, 50

✳ **J9395** Injection, fulvestrant, 25 mg Ⓑ Ⓑ

✳ **J9400** Injection, ziv-aflibercept, 1 mg Ⓑ Ⓑ

✺ **J9600** Injection, porfimer sodium, 75 mg Ⓑ Ⓑ

IOM: 100-02, 15, 50

✺ **J9999** Not otherwise classified, antineoplastic drugs Ⓑ Ⓑ

Bill on paper, bill one unit, and identify drug and total dosage in "Remarks" field. Include invoice of cost or NDC number in "Remarks" field.

IOM: 100-02, 15, 50; 100-03, 2, 110.2

▶ New   ↻ Revised   ✔ Reinstated   ~~deleted~~ Deleted   ⊘ Not covered or valid by Medicare

✺ Special coverage instructions   ✳ Carrier discretion   Ⓑ Bill Part B MAC   Ⓑ Bill DME MAC

TEMPORARY CODES ASSIGNED TO DME REGIONAL CARRIERS (K0000-K9999)

NOTE: This section contains national codes assigned by CMS on a temporary basis and for the exclusive use of the durable medical equipment regional carriers (DMERC).

Wheelchairs and Accessories

* K0001   Standard wheelchair ⑧

  Capped rental

* K0002   Standard hemi (low seat) wheelchair ⑧

  Capped rental

* K0003   Lightweight wheelchair ⑧

  Capped rental

* K0004   High strength, lightweight wheelchair ⑧

  Capped rental

* K0005   Ultralightweight wheelchair ⑧

  Capped rental. Inexpensive and routinely purchased DME

* K0006   Heavy duty wheelchair ⑧

  Capped rental

* K0007   Extra heavy duty wheelchair ⑧

  Capped rental

☼ K0008   Custom manual wheelchair/base ⑧

* K0009   Other manual wheelchair/base ⑧

  Not otherwise classified

* K0010   Standard - weight frame motorized/power wheelchair ⑧

  Capped rental. Codes K0010-K0014 are not for manual wheelchairs with add-on power packs. Use the appropriate code for the manual wheelchair base provided (K0001-K0009) and code K0460

* K0011   Standard - weight frame motorized/power wheelchair with programmable control parameters for speed adjustment, tremor dampening, acceleration control and braking ⑧

  Capped rental. A patient who requires a power wheelchair usually is totally nonambulatory and has severe weakness of the upper extremities due to a neurologic or muscular disease/condition.

* K0012   Lightweight portable motorized/power wheelchair ⑧

  Capped rental

☼ K0013   Custom motorized/power wheelchair base ⑧

* K0014   Other motorized/power wheelchair base ⑧

  Capped rental

* K0015   Detachable, non-adjustable height armrest, replacement only, each ⑧

  Inexpensive and routinely purchased DME

* K0017   Detachable, adjustable height armrest, base, replacement only, each ⑥

  Inexpensive and routinely purchased DME

* K0018   Detachable, adjustable height armrest, upper portion, replacement only, each ⑥

  Inexpensive and routinely purchased DME

* K0019   Arm pad, replacement only, each ⑥

  Inexpensive and routinely purchased DME

* K0020   Fixed, adjustable height armrest, pair ⑧

  Inexpensive and routinely purchased DME

* K0037   High mount flip-up footrest, replacement only, each ⑧

  Inexpensive and routinely purchased DME

* K0038   Leg strap, each ⑥

  Inexpensive and routinely purchased DME

* K0039   Leg strap, H style, each ⑥

  Inexpensive and routinely purchased DME

* K0040   Adjustable angle footplate, each ⑧

  Inexpensive and routinely purchased DME

* K0041   Large size footplate, each ⑧

  Inexpensive and routinely purchased DME

* K0042   Standard size footplate, replacement only, each ⑧

  Inexpensive and routinely purchased DME

▶ New	↻ Revised	✔ Reinstated	deleted Deleted	⊘ Not covered or valid by Medicare
☼ Special coverage instructions		✳ Carrier discretion	Ⓑ Bill Part B MAC	Ⓓ Bill DME MAC

245

TEMPORARY CODES ASSIGNED TO DME REGIONAL CARRIERS   K0001 – K0042

* **K0043** Footrest, lower extension tube, replacement only, each Ⓑ

  Inexpensive and routinely purchased DME

* **K0044** Footrest, upper hanger bracket, replacement only, each Ⓑ

  Inexpensive and routinely purchased DME

* **K0045** Footrest, complete assembly, replacement only, each Ⓑ

  Inexpensive and routinely purchased DME

* **K0046** Elevating legrest, lower extension tube, replacement only, each Ⓑ

  Inexpensive and routinely purchased DME

* **K0047** Elevating legrest, upper hanger bracket, replacement only, each Ⓑ

  Inexpensive and routinely purchased DME

* **K0050** Ratchet assembly, replacement only Ⓑ

  Inexpensive and routinely purchased DME

* **K0051** Cam release assembly, footrest or legrests, replacement only, each Ⓑ

  Inexpensive and routinely purchased DME

* **K0052** Swing-away, detachable footrests, replacement only, each Ⓑ

  Inexpensive and routinely purchased DME

* **K0053** Elevating footrests, articulating (telescoping), each Ⓑ

  Inexpensive and routinely purchased DME

* **K0056** Seat height less than 17" or equal to or greater than 21" for a high strength, lightweight, or ultralightweight wheelchair Ⓑ

  Inexpensive and routinely purchased DME

* **K0065** Spoke protectors, each Ⓑ

  Inexpensive and routinely purchased DME

* **K0069** Rear wheel assembly, complete, with solid tire, spokes or molded, replacement only, each Ⓑ

  Inexpensive and routinely purchased DME

* **K0070** Rear wheel assembly, complete, with pneumatic tire, spokes or molded, replacement only, each Ⓑ

  Inexpensive and routinely purchased DME

* **K0071** Front caster assembly, complete, with pneumatic tire, replacement only, each Ⓑ

  Caster assembly includes a caster fork (E2396), wheel rim, and tire. Inexpensive and routinely purchased DME

* **K0072** Front caster assembly, complete, with semi-pneumatic tire, replacement only, each Ⓑ

  Inexpensive and routinely purchased DME

* **K0073** Caster pin lock, each Ⓑ

  Inexpensive and routinely purchased DME

* **K0077** Front caster assembly, complete, with solid tire, replacement only, each Ⓑ

* **K0098** Drive belt for power wheelchair, replacement only Ⓑ

  Inexpensive and routinely purchased DME

* **K0105** IV hanger, each Ⓑ

  Inexpensive and routinely purchased DME

* **K0108** Wheelchair component or accessory, not otherwise specified Ⓑ

⊙ **K0195** Elevating leg rests, pair (for use with capped rental wheelchair base) Ⓑ

  Medically necessary replacement items are covered if rollabout chair or transport chair covered

  IOM: 100-03, 4, 280.1

Infusion Pump, Supplies, and Batteries

⊙ **K0455** Infusion pump used for uninterrupted parenteral administration of medication (e.g., epoprostenol or treprostinol) Ⓑ

  An EIP may also be referred to as an external insulin pump, ambulatory pump, or mini-infuser. CMN/DIF required. Frequent and substantial service DME

  IOM: 100-03, 1, 50.3

▶ New   ↻ Revised   ✔ Reinstated   ~~deleted~~ Deleted   ⊘ Not covered or valid by Medicare
⊙ Special coverage instructions   ✱ Carrier discretion   Ⓟ Bill Part B MAC   Ⓑ Bill DME MAC

✪ **K0462** Temporary replacement for patient owned equipment being repaired, any type Ⓑ

Only report for maintenance and service for an item for which initial claim was paid. The term power mobility device (PMD) includes power operated vehicles (POVs) and power wheelchairs (PWCs). Not Otherwise Classified.

IOM: 100-04, 20, 40.1

✪ **K0552** Supplies for external non-insulin drug infusion pump, syringe type cartridge, sterile, each Ⓑ

Supplies

IOM: 100-03, 1, 50.3

▶ ✪ **K0553** Supply allowance for therapeutic continuous glucose monitor (CGM), includes all supplies and accessories, 1 month supply = 1 unit of service

▶ ✪ **K0554** Receiver (monitor), dedicated, for use with therapeutic glucose continuous monitor system

✳ **K0601** Replacement battery for external infusion pump owned by patient, silver oxide, 1.5 volt, each Ⓑ

Inexpensive and routinely purchased DME

✳ **K0602** Replacement battery for external infusion pump owned by patient, silver oxide, 3 volt, each Ⓑ

Inexpensive and routinely purchased DME

✳ **K0603** Replacement battery for external infusion pump owned by patient, alkaline, 1.5 volt, each Ⓑ

Inexpensive and routinely purchased DME

✳ **K0604** Replacement battery for external infusion pump owned by patient, lithium, 3.6 volt, each Ⓑ

Inexpensive and routinely purchased DME

✳ **K0605** Replacement battery for external infusion pump owned by patient, lithium, 4.5 volt, each Ⓑ

Inexpensive and routinely purchased DME

Defibrillator and Accessories

✳ **K0606** Automatic external defibrillator, with integrated electrocardiogram analysis, garment type Ⓑ

Capped rental

✳ **K0607** Replacement battery for automated external defibrillator, garment type only, each Ⓑ

Inexpensive and routinely purchased DME

✳ **K0608** Replacement garment for use with automated external defibrillator, each Ⓑ

Inexpensive and routinely purchased DME

✳ **K0609** Replacement electrodes for use with automated external defibrillator, garment type only, each Ⓑ

Supplies

Miscellaneous

✳ **K0669** Wheelchair accessory, wheelchair seat or back cushion, does not meet specific code criteria or no written coding verification from DME PDAC Ⓑ

Inexpensive and routinely purchased DME

✳ **K0672** Addition to lower extremity orthosis, removable soft interface, all components, replacement only, each Ⓑ

Prosthetics/Orthotics

✳ **K0730** Controlled dose inhalation drug delivery system Ⓑ

Inexpensive and routinely purchased DME

✳ **K0733** Power wheelchair accessory, 12 to 24 amp hour sealed lead acid battery, each (e.g., gel cell, absorbed glassmat) Ⓑ

Inexpensive and routinely purchased DME

✳ **K0738** Portable gaseous oxygen system, rental; home compressor used to fill portable oxygen cylinders; includes portable containers, regulator, flowmeter, humidifier, cannula or mask, and tubing Ⓑ

Oxygen and oxygen equipment

▶ New	↻ Revised	✔ Reinstated	deleted Deleted	⊘ Not covered or valid by Medicare
✪ Special coverage instructions	✳ Carrier discretion	Ⓟ Bill Part B MAC	Ⓑ Bill DME MAC	

* **K0739** Repair or nonroutine service for durable medical equipment other than oxygen equipment requiring the skill of a technician, labor component, per 15 minutes ⑨ Ⓑ

⊘ **K0740** Repair or nonroutine service for oxygen equipment requiring the skill of a technician, labor component, per 15 minutes Ⓑ

* **K0743** Suction pump, home model, portable, for use on wounds Ⓑ

* **K0744** Absorptive wound dressing for use with suction pump, home model, portable, pad size 16 square inches or less Ⓑ

* **K0745** Absorptive wound dressing for use with suction pump, home model, portable, pad size more than 16 square inches but less than or equal to 48 square inches Ⓑ

* **K0746** Absorptive wound dressing for use with suction pump, home model, portable, pad size greater than 48 square inches Ⓑ

Power Mobility Devices

* **K0800** Power operated vehicle, group 1 standard, patient weight capacity up to and including 300 pounds Ⓑ

  Power mobility device (PMD) includes power operated vehicles (POVs) and power wheelchairs (PWCs). Inexpensive and routinely purchased DME

* **K0801** Power operated vehicle, group 1 heavy duty, patient weight capacity 301 to 450 pounds Ⓑ

  Inexpensive and routinely purchased DME

* **K0802** Power operated vehicle, group 1 very heavy duty, patient weight capacity 451 to 600 pounds Ⓑ

  Inexpensive and routinely purchased DME

* **K0806** Power operated vehicle, group 2 standard, patient weight capacity up to and including 300 pounds Ⓑ

  Inexpensive and routinely purchased DME

* **K0807** Power operated vehicle, group 2 heavy duty, patient weight capacity 301 to 450 pounds Ⓑ

  Inexpensive and routinely purchased DME

* **K0808** Power operated vehicle, group 2 very heavy duty, patient weight capacity 451 to 600 pounds Ⓑ

  Inexpensive and routinely purchased DME

* **K0812** Power operated vehicle, not otherwise classified Ⓑ

  Not Otherwise Classified.

* **K0813** Power wheelchair, group 1 standard, portable, sling/solid seat and back, patient weight capacity up to and including 300 pounds Ⓑ

  Capped rental

* **K0814** Power wheelchair, group 1 standard, portable, captains chair, patient weight capacity up to and including 300 pounds Ⓑ

  Capped rental

* **K0815** Power wheelchair, group 1 standard, sling/solid seat and back, patient weight capacity up to and including 300 pounds Ⓑ

  Capped rental

* **K0816** Power wheelchair, group 1 standard, captains chair, patient weight capacity up to and including 300 pounds Ⓑ

  Capped rental

* **K0820** Power wheelchair, group 2 standard, portable, sling/solid seat/back, patient weight capacity up to and including 300 pounds Ⓑ

  Capped rental

* **K0821** Power wheelchair, group 2 standard, portable, captains chair, patient weight capacity up to and including 300 pounds Ⓑ

  Capped rental

* **K0822** Power wheelchair, group 2 standard, sling/solid seat/back, patient weight capacity up to and including 300 pounds Ⓑ

  Capped rental

* **K0823** Power wheelchair, group 2 standard, captains chair, patient weight capacity up to and including 300 pounds Ⓑ

  Capped rental

* **K0824** Power wheelchair, group 2 heavy duty, sling/solid seat/back, patient weight capacity 301 to 450 pounds Ⓑ

  Capped rental

▶ **New**   ↻ **Revised**   ✔ **Reinstated**   ~~deleted~~ **Deleted**   ⊘ **Not covered or valid by Medicare**
⊕ **Special coverage instructions**   ✳ **Carrier discretion**   ⑨ **Bill Part B MAC**   ⑤ **Bill DME MAC**

* **K0825** Power wheelchair, group 2 heavy duty, captains chair, patient weight capacity 301 to 450 pounds Ⓑ

  Capped rental

* **K0826** Power wheelchair, group 2 very heavy duty, sling/solid seat/back, patient weight capacity 451 to 600 pounds Ⓑ

  Capped rental

* **K0827** Power wheelchair, group 2 very heavy duty, captains chair, patient weight capacity 451 to 600 pounds Ⓑ

  Capped rental

* **K0828** Power wheelchair, group 2 extra heavy duty, sling/solid seat/back, patient weight capacity 601 pounds or more Ⓑ

  Capped rental

* **K0829** Power wheelchair, group 2 extra heavy duty, captains chair, patient weight 601 pounds or more Ⓑ

  Capped rental

* **K0830** Power wheelchair, group 2 standard, seat elevator, sling/solid seat/back, patient weight capacity up to and including 300 pounds Ⓑ

  Capped rental

* **K0831** Power wheelchair, group 2 standard, seat elevator, captains chair, patient weight capacity up to and including 300 pounds Ⓑ

* **K0835** Power wheelchair, group 2 standard, single power option, sling/solid seat/back, patient weight capacity up to and including 300 pounds Ⓑ

  Capped rental

* **K0836** Power wheelchair, group 2 standard, single power option, captains chair, patient weight capacity up to and including 300 pounds Ⓑ

  Capped rental

* **K0837** Power wheelchair, group 2 heavy duty, single power option, sling/solid seat/back, patient weight capacity 301 to 450 pounds Ⓑ

  Capped rental

* **K0838** Power wheelchair, group 2 heavy duty, single power option, captains chair, patient weight capacity 301 to 450 pounds Ⓑ

  Capped rental

* **K0839** Power wheelchair, group 2 very heavy duty, single power option, sling/solid seat/back, patient weight capacity 451 to 600 pounds Ⓑ

  Capped rental

* **K0840** Power wheelchair, group 2 extra heavy duty, single power option, sling/solid seat/back, patient weight capacity 601 pounds or more Ⓑ

  Capped rental

* **K0841** Power wheelchair, group 2 standard, multiple power option, sling/solid seat/back, patient weight capacity up to and including 300 pounds Ⓑ

  Capped rental

* **K0842** Power wheelchair, group 2 standard, multiple power option, captains chair, patient weight capacity up to and including 300 pounds Ⓑ

  Capped rental

* **K0843** Power wheelchair, group 2 heavy duty, multiple power option, sling/solid seat/back, patient weight capacity 301 to 450 pounds Ⓑ

  Capped rental

* **K0848** Power wheelchair, group 3 standard, sling/solid seat/back, patient weight capacity up to and including 300 pounds Ⓑ

  Capped rental

* **K0849** Power wheelchair, group 3 standard, captains chair, patient weight capacity up to and including 300 pounds Ⓑ

  Capped rental

* **K0850** Power wheelchair, group 3 heavy duty, sling/solid seat/back, patient weight capacity 301 to 450 pounds Ⓑ

  Capped rental

* **K0851** Power wheelchair, group 3 heavy duty, captains chair, patient weight capacity 301 to 450 pounds Ⓑ

  Capped rental

* **K0852** Power wheelchair, group 3 very heavy duty, sling/solid seat/back, patient weight capacity 451 to 600 pounds Ⓑ

  Capped rental

* **K0853** Power wheelchair, group 3 very heavy duty, captains chair, patient weight capacity 451 to 600 pounds Ⓑ

  Capped rental

▶ New   ⟳ Revised   ✔ Reinstated   ~~deleted~~ Deleted   ⊘ Not covered or valid by Medicare
✿ Special coverage instructions   ✳ Carrier discretion   Ⓑ Bill Part B MAC   Ⓓ Bill DME MAC

TEMPORARY CODES ASSIGNED TO DME REGIONAL CARRIERS   K0825 — K0853

249

✳ **K0854** Power wheelchair, group 3 extra heavy duty, sling/solid seat/back, patient weight capacity 601 pounds or more Ⓑ

Capped rental

✳ **K0855** Power wheelchair, group 3 extra heavy duty, captains chair, patient weight capacity 601 pounds or more Ⓑ

Capped rental

✳ **K0856** Power wheelchair, group 3 standard, single power option, sling/solid seat/back, patient weight capacity up to and including 300 pounds Ⓑ

Capped rental

✳ **K0857** Power wheelchair, group 3 standard, single power option, captains chair, patient weight capacity up to and including 300 pounds Ⓑ

Capped rental

✳ **K0858** Power wheelchair, group 3 heavy duty, single power option, sling/solid seat/back, patient weight 301 to 450 pounds Ⓑ

Capped rental

✳ **K0859** Power wheelchair, group 3 heavy duty, single power option, captains chair, patient weight capacity 301 to 450 pounds Ⓑ

Capped rental

✳ **K0860** Power wheelchair, group 3 very heavy duty, single power option, sling/solid seat/back, patient weight capacity 451 to 600 pounds Ⓑ

Capped rental

✳ **K0861** Power wheelchair, group 3 standard, multiple power option, sling/solid seat/back, patient weight capacity up to and including 300 pounds Ⓑ

Capped rental

✳ **K0862** Power wheelchair, group 3 heavy duty, multiple power option, sling/solid seat/back, patient weight capacity 301 to 450 pounds Ⓑ

Capped rental

✳ **K0863** Power wheelchair, group 3 very heavy duty, multiple power option, sling/solid seat/back, patient weight capacity 451 to 600 pounds Ⓑ

Capped rental

✳ **K0864** Power wheelchair, group 3 extra heavy duty, multiple power option, sling/solid seat/back, patient weight capacity 601 pounds or more Ⓑ

Capped rental

✳ **K0868** Power wheelchair, group 4 standard, sling/solid seat/back, patient weight capacity up to and including 300 pounds Ⓑ

Capped rental

✳ **K0869** Power wheelchair, group 4 standard, captains chair, patient weight capacity up to and including 300 pounds Ⓑ

Capped rental

✳ **K0870** Power wheelchair, group 4 heavy duty, sling/solid seat/back, patient weight capacity 301 to 450 pounds Ⓑ

Capped rental

✳ **K0871** Power wheelchair, group 4 very heavy duty, sling/solid seat/back, patient weight capacity 451 to 600 pounds Ⓑ

Capped rental

✳ **K0877** Power wheelchair, group 4 standard, single power option, sling/solid seat/back, patient weight capacity up to and including 300 pounds Ⓑ

Capped rental

✳ **K0878** Power wheelchair, group 4 standard, single power option, captains chair, patient weight capacity up to and including 300 pounds Ⓑ

Capped rental

✳ **K0879** Power wheelchair, group 4 heavy duty, single power option, sling/solid seat/back, patient weight capacity 301 to 450 pounds Ⓑ

Capped rental

✳ **K0880** Power wheelchair, group 4 very heavy duty, single power option, sling/solid seat/back, patient weight 451 to 600 pounds Ⓑ

Capped rental

✳ **K0884** Power wheelchair, group 4 standard, multiple power option, sling/solid seat/back, patient weight capacity up to and including 300 pounds Ⓑ

Capped rental

✳ **K0885** Power wheelchair, group 4 standard, multiple power option, captains chair, patient weight capacity up to and including 300 pounds Ⓑ

Capped rental

✳ **K0886** Power wheelchair, group 4 heavy duty, multiple power option, sling/solid seat/back, patient weight capacity 301 to 450 pounds Ⓑ

Capped rental

▶ New   ↻ Revised   ✔ Reinstated   ~~deleted~~ Deleted   ⊘ Not covered or valid by Medicare
Ⓢ Special coverage instructions   ✳ Carrier discretion   Ⓟ Bill Part B MAC   Ⓑ Bill DME MAC

✳ **K0890** Power wheelchair, group 5 pediatric, single power option, sling/solid seat/back, patient weight capacity up to and including 125 pounds Ⓑ

Capped rental

✳ **K0891** Power wheelchair, group 5 pediatric, multiple power option, sling/solid seat/back, patient weight capacity up to and including 125 pounds Ⓑ

Capped rental

✳ **K0898** Power wheelchair, not otherwise classified Ⓑ

✳ **K0899** Power mobility device, not coded by DME PDAC or does not meet criteria Ⓑ

Customized DME: Other than Wheelchair

✪ **K0900** Customized durable medical equipment, other than wheelchair Ⓑ

▶ New   ↩ Revised   ✔ Reinstated   ~~deleted~~ Deleted   ⊘ Not covered or valid by Medicare
✪ Special coverage instructions   ✳ Carrier discretion   Ⓑ Bill Part B MAC   Ⓑ Bill DME MAC

TEMPORARY CODES ASSIGNED TO DME REGIONAL CARRIERS   K0890 – K0900

251

ORTHOTICS (L0100-L4999)

NOTE: DMEPOS fee schedule: https://www.cms.gov/Medicare/Medicare-Fee-for-Service-Payment/DMEPOSFeeSched/DMEPOS-Fee-Schedule.html

Cervical Orthotics

* **L0112** Cranial cervical orthosis, congenital torticollis type, with or without soft interface material, adjustable range of motion joint, custom fabricated ⓑ

* **L0113** Cranial cervical orthosis, torticollis type, with or without joint, with or without soft interface material, prefabricated, includes fitting and adjustment ⓑ

* **L0120** Cervical, flexible, non-adjustable, prefabricated, off-the-shelf (foam collar) ⓑ

> Cervical orthoses, including soft and rigid devices may be used as nonoperative management for cervical trauma

* **L0130** Cervical, flexible, thermoplastic collar, molded to patient ⓑ

* **L0140** Cervical, semi-rigid, adjustable (plastic collar) ⓑ

* **L0150** Cervical, semi-rigid, adjustable molded chin cup (plastic collar with mandibular/occipital piece) ⓑ

* **L0160** Cervical, semi-rigid, wire frame occipital/mandibular support, prefabricated, off-the-shelf ⓑ

* **L0170** Cervical, collar, molded to patient model ⓑ

* **L0172** Cervical, collar, semi-rigid thermoplastic foam, two-piece, prefabricated, off-the-shelf ⓑ

* **L0174** Cervical, collar, semi-rigid, thermoplastic foam, two piece with thoracic extension, prefabricated, off-the-shelf ⓑ

Multiple Post Collar: Cervical

* **L0180** Cervical, multiple post collar, occipital/mandibular supports, adjustable ⓑ

* **L0190** Cervical, multiple post collar, occipital/mandibular supports, adjustable cervical bars (SOMI, Guilford, Taylor types) ⓑ

* **L0200** Cervical, multiple post collar, occipital/mandibular supports, adjustable cervical bars, and thoracic extension ⓑ

Thoracic Rib Belt

* **L0220** Thoracic, rib belt, custom fabricated ⓑ

Thoracic-Lumbar-Sacral Orthotics

* **L0450** TLSO, flexible, provides trunk support, upper thoracic region, produces intracavitary pressure to reduce load on the intervertebral disks with rigid stays or panel(s), includes shoulder straps and closures, prefabricated, off-the-shelf ⓑ

> Used to immobilize specified area of spine, and is generally worn under clothing

* **L0452** TLSO, flexible, provides trunk support, upper thoracic region, produces intracavitary pressure to reduce load on the intervertebral disks with rigid stays or panel(s), includes shoulder straps and closures, custom fabricated ⓑ

* **L0454** TLSO flexible, provides trunk support, extends from sacrococcygeal junction to above T-9 vertebra, restricts gross trunk motion in the sagittal plane, produces intracavitary pressure to reduce load on the intervertebral disks with rigid stays or panel(s), includes shoulder straps and closures, prefabricated item that has been trimmed, bent, molded, assembled, or otherwise customized to fit a specific patient by an individual with expertise ⓑ

> Used to immobilize specified areas of spine; and is generally designed to be worn under clothing; not specifically designed for patients in wheelchairs

* **L0455** TLSO, flexible, provides trunk support, extends from sacrococcygeal junction to above T-9 vertebra, restricts gross trunk motion in the sagittal plane, produces intracavitary pressure to reduce load on the intervertebral disks with rigid stays or panel(s), includes shoulder straps and closures, prefabricated, off-the-shelf ⓑ

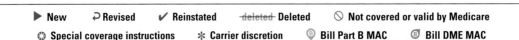

▶ New　↻ Revised　✔ Reinstated　~~deleted~~ Deleted　⊘ Not covered or valid by Medicare
⊙ Special coverage instructions　* Carrier discretion　ⓟ Bill Part B MAC　ⓑ Bill DME MAC

✳ **L0456** TLSO, flexible, provides trunk support, thoracic region, rigid posterior panel and soft anterior apron, extends from the sacrococcygeal junction and terminates just inferior to the scapular spine, restricts gross trunk motion in the sagittal plane, produces intracavitary pressure to reduce load on the intervertebral disks, includes straps and closures, prefabricated item that has been trimmed, bent, molded, assembled, or otherwise customized to fit a specific patient by an individual with expertise Ⓑ

✳ **L0457** TLSO, flexible, provides trunk support, thoracic region, rigid posterior panel and soft anterior apron, extends from the sacrococcygeal junction and terminates just inferior to the scapular spine, restricts gross trunk motion in the sagittal plane, produces intracavitary pressure to reduce load on the intervertebral disks, includes straps and closures, prefabricated, off-the-shelf Ⓑ

✳ **L0458** TLSO, triplanar control, modular segmented spinal system, two rigid plastic shells, posterior extends from the sacrococcygeal junction and terminates just inferior to the scapular spine, anterior extends from the symphysis pubis to the xiphoid, soft liner, restricts gross trunk motion in the sagittal, coronal, and transverse planes, lateral strength is provided by overlapping plastic and stabilizing closures, includes straps and closures, prefabricated, includes fitting and adjustment Ⓑ

To meet Medicare's definition of body jacket, orthosis has to have rigid plastic shell that circles trunk with overlapping edges and stabilizing closures, and entire circumference of shell must be made of same rigid material.

✳ **L0460** TLSO, triplanar control, modular segmented spinal system, two rigid plastic shells, posterior extends from the sacrococcygeal junction and terminates just inferior to the scapular spine, anterior extends from the symphysis pubis to the sternal notch, soft liner, restricts gross trunk motion in the sagittal, coronal, and transverse planes, lateral strength is provided by overlapping plastic and stabilizing closures, includes straps and closures, prefabricated item that has been trimmed, bent, molded, assembled, or otherwise customized to fit a specific patient by an individual with expertise Ⓑ

✳ **L0462** TLSO, triplanar control, modular segmented spinal system, three rigid plastic shells, posterior extends from the sacrococcygeal junction and terminates just inferior to the scapular spine, anterior extends from the symphysis pubis to the sternal notch, soft liner, restricts gross trunk motion in the sagittal, coronal, and transverse planes, lateral strength is provided by overlapping plastic and stabilizing closures, includes straps and closures, prefabricated, includes fitting and adjustment Ⓖ

✳ **L0464** TLSO, triplanar control, modular segmented spinal system, four rigid plastic shells, posterior extends from sacrococcygeal junction and terminates just inferior to scapular spine, anterior extends from symphysis pubis to the sternal notch, soft liner, restricts gross trunk motion in sagittal, coronal, and transverse planes, lateral strength is provided by overlapping plastic and stabilizing closures, includes straps and closures, prefabricated, includes fitting and adjustment Ⓖ

✳ **L0466** TLSO, sagittal control, rigid posterior frame and flexible soft anterior apron with straps, closures and padding, restricts gross trunk motion in sagittal plane, produces intracavitary pressure to reduce load on intervertebral disks, prefabricated item that has been trimmed, bent, molded, assembled, or otherwise customized to fit a specific patient by an individual with expertise Ⓑ

✳ **L0467** TLSO, sagittal control, rigid posterior frame and flexible soft anterior apron with straps, closures and padding, restricts gross trunk motion in sagittal plane, produces intracavitary pressure to reduce load on intervertebral disks, prefabricated, off-the-shelf Ⓑ

✳ **L0468** TLSO, sagittal-coronal control, rigid posterior frame and flexible soft anterior apron with straps, closures and padding, extends from sacrococcygeal junction over scapulae, lateral strength provided by pelvic, thoracic, and lateral frame pieces, restricts gross trunk motion in sagittal, and coronal planes, produces intracavitary pressure to reduce load on intervertebral disks, prefabricated item that has been trimmed, bent, molded, assembled, or otherwise customized to fit a specific patient by an individual with expertise Ⓑ

▶ New   ↻ Revised   ✔ Reinstated   ~~deleted~~ Deleted   ⊘ Not covered or valid by Medicare

✿ Special coverage instructions   ✳ Carrier discretion   Ⓑ Bill Part B MAC   Ⓖ Bill DME MAC

✳ **L0469** TLSO, sagittal-coronal control, rigid posterior frame and flexible soft anterior apron with straps, closures and padding, extends from sacrococcygeal junction over scapulae, lateral strength provided by pelvic, thoracic, and lateral frame pieces, restricts gross trunk motion in sagittal and coronal planes, produces intracavitary pressure to reduce load on intervertebral disks, prefabricated, off-the-shelf Ⓑ

✳ **L0470** TLSO, triplanar control, rigid posterior frame and flexible soft anterior apron with straps, closures and padding, extends from sacrococcygeal junction to scapula, lateral strength provided by pelvic, thoracic, and lateral frame pieces, rotational strength provided by subclavicular extensions, restricts gross trunk motion in sagittal, coronal, and transverse planes, provides intracavitary pressure to reduce load on the intervertebral disks, includes fitting and shaping the frame, prefabricated, includes fitting and adjustment Ⓑ

✳ **L0472** TLSO, triplanar control, hyperextension, rigid anterior and lateral frame extends from symphysis pubis to sternal notch with two anterior components (one pubic and one sternal), posterior and lateral pads with straps and closures, limits spinal flexion, restricts gross trunk motion in sagittal, coronal, and transverse planes, includes fitting and shaping the frame, prefabricated, includes fitting and adjustment Ⓑ

✳ **L0480** TLSO, triplanar control, one piece rigid plastic shell without interface liner, with multiple straps and closures, posterior extends from sacrococcygeal junction and terminates just inferior to scapular spine, anterior extends from symphysis pubis to sternal notch, anterior or posterior opening, restricts gross trunk motion in sagittal, coronal, and transverse planes, includes a carved plaster or CAD-CAM model, custom fabricated Ⓑ

✳ **L0482** TLSO, triplanar control, one piece rigid plastic shell with interface liner, multiple straps and closures, posterior extends from sacrococcygeal junction and terminates just inferior to scapular spine, anterior extends from symphysis pubis to sternal notch, anterior or posterior opening, restricts gross trunk motion in sagittal, coronal, and transverse planes, includes a carved plaster or CAD-CAM model, custom fabricated Ⓑ

✳ **L0484** TLSO, triplanar control, two piece rigid plastic shell without interface liner, with multiple straps and closures, posterior extends from sacrococcygeal junction and terminates just inferior to scapular spine, anterior extends from symphysis pubis to sternal notch, lateral strength is enhanced by overlapping plastic, restricts gross trunk motion in the sagittal, coronal, and transverse planes, includes a carved plaster or CAD-CAM model, custom fabricated Ⓑ

✳ **L0486** TLSO, triplanar control, two piece rigid plastic shell with interface liner, multiple straps and closures, posterior extends from sacrococcygeal junction and terminates just inferior to scapular spine, anterior extends from symphysis pubis to sternal notch, lateral strength is enhanced by overlapping plastic, restricts gross trunk motion in the sagittal, coronal, and transverse planes, includes a carved plaster or CAD-CAM model, custom fabricated Ⓑ

✳ **L0488** TLSO, triplanar control, one piece rigid plastic shell with interface liner, multiple straps and closures, posterior extends from sacrococcygeal junction and terminates just inferior to scapular spine, anterior extends from symphysis pubis to sternal notch, anterior or posterior opening, restricts gross trunk motion in sagittal, coronal, and transverse planes, prefabricated, includes fitting and adjustment Ⓑ

✳ **L0490** TLSO, sagittal-coronal control, one piece rigid plastic shell, with overlapping reinforced anterior, with multiple straps and closures, posterior extends from sacrococcygeal junction and terminates at or before the T-9 vertebra, anterior extends from symphysis pubis to xiphoid, anterior opening, restricts gross trunk motion in sagittal and coronal planes, prefabricated, includes fitting and adjustment Ⓑ

✳ **L0491** TLSO, sagittal-coronal control, modular segmented spinal system, two rigid plastic shells, posterior extends from the sacrococcygeal junction and terminates just inferior to the scapular spine, anterior extends from the symphysis pubis to the xiphoid, soft liner, restricts gross trunk motion in the sagittal and coronal planes, lateral strength is provided by overlapping plastic and stabilizing closures, includes straps and closures, prefabricated, includes fitting and adjustment Ⓑ

▶ New	↻ Revised	✔ Reinstated	̶d̶e̶l̶e̶t̶e̶d̶ Deleted	⊘ Not covered or valid by Medicare
✪ Special coverage instructions		✳ Carrier discretion	Ⓑ Bill Part B MAC	Ⓑ Bill DME MAC

* **L0492** TLSO, sagittal-coronal control, modular segmented spinal system, three rigid plastic shells, posterior extends from the sacrococcygeal junction and terminates just inferior to the scapular spine, anterior extends from the symphysis pubis to the xiphoid, soft liner, restricts gross trunk motion in the sagittal and coronal planes, lateral strength is provided by overlapping plastic and stabilizing closures, includes straps and closures, prefabricated, includes fitting and adjustment Ⓑ

Sacroilliac Orthotics

* **L0621** Sacroiliac orthosis, flexible, provides pelvic-sacral support, reduces motion about the sacroiliac joint, includes straps, closures, may include pendulous abdomen design, prefabricated, off-the-shelf Ⓑ

* **L0622** Sacroiliac orthosis, flexible, provides pelvic-sacral support, reduces motion about the sacroiliac joint, includes straps, closures, may include pendulous abdomen design, custom fabricated Ⓑ

    Type of custom-fabricated device for which impression of specific body part is made (e.g., by means of plaster cast, or CAD-CAM [computer-aided design] technology); impression then used to make specific patient model

* **L0623** Sacroiliac orthosis, provides pelvic-sacral support, with rigid or semi-rigid panels over the sacrum and abdomen, reduces motion about the sacroiliac joint, includes straps, closures, may include pendulous abdomen design, prefabricated, off-the-shelf Ⓑ

* **L0624** Sacroiliac orthosis, provides pelvic-sacral support, with rigid or semi-rigid panels placed over the sacrum and abdomen, reduces motion about the sacroiliac joint, includes straps, closures, may include pendulous abdomen design, custom fabricated Ⓑ

    Custom fitted

Lumbar Orthotics

* **L0625** Lumbar orthosis, flexible, provides lumbar support, posterior extends from L-1 to below L-5 vertebra, produces intracavitary pressure to reduce load on the intervertebral discs, includes straps, closures, may include pendulous abdomen design, shoulder straps, stays, prefabricated, off-the-shelf Ⓑ

* **L0626** Lumbar orthosis, sagittal control, with rigid posterior panel(s), posterior extends from L-1 to below L-5 vertebra, produces intracavitary pressure to reduce load on the intervertebral discs, includes straps, closures, may include padding, stays, shoulder straps, pendulous abdomen design, prefabricated item that has been trimmed, bent, molded, assembled, or otherwise customized to fit a specific patient by an individual with expertise Ⓑ

* **L0627** Lumbar orthosis, sagittal control, with rigid anterior and posterior panels, posterior extends from L-1 to below L-5 vertebra, produces intracavitary pressure to reduce load on the intervertebral discs, includes straps, closures, may include padding, shoulder straps, pendulous abdomen design, prefabricated item that has been trimmed, bent, molded, assembled, or otherwise customized to fit a specific patient by an individual with expertise Ⓑ

Lumbar-Sacral Orthotics

* **L0628** Lumbar-sacral orthosis, flexible, provides lumbo-sacral support, posterior extends from sacrococcygeal junction to T-9 vertebra, produces intracavitary pressure to reduce load on the intervertebral discs, includes straps, closures, may include stays, shoulder straps, pendulous abdomen design, prefabricated, off-the-shelf Ⓑ

* **L0629** Lumbar-sacral orthosis, flexible, provides lumbo-sacral support, posterior extends from sacrococcygeal junction to T-9 vertebra, produces intracavitary pressure to reduce load on the intervertebral discs, includes straps, closures, may include stays, shoulder straps, pendulous abdomen design, custom fabricated Ⓑ

    Custom fitted

▶ New   ↻ Revised   ✔ Reinstated   ~~deleted~~ Deleted   ⊘ Not covered or valid by Medicare

✿ Special coverage instructions   ✳ Carrier discretion   Ⓟ Bill Part B MAC   Ⓑ Bill DME MAC

✳ **L0630** Lumbar-sacral orthosis, sagittal control, with rigid posterior panel(s), posterior extends from sacrococcygeal junction to T-9 vertebra, produces intracavitary pressure to reduce load on the intervertebral discs, includes straps, closures, may include padding, stays, shoulder straps, pendulous abdomen design, prefabricated item that has been trimmed, bent, molded, assembled, or otherwise customized to fit a specific patient by an individual with expertise ⑧

✳ **L0631** Lumbar-sacral orthosis, sagittal control, with rigid anterior and posterior panels, posterior extends from sacrococcygeal junction to T-9 vertebra, produces intracavitary pressure to reduce load on the intervertebral discs, includes straps, closures, may include padding, shoulder straps, pendulous abdomen design, prefabricated item that has been trimmed, bent, molded, assembled, or otherwise customized to fit a specific patient by an individual with expertise ⑧

✳ **L0632** Lumbar-sacral orthosis, sagittal control, with rigid anterior and posterior panels, posterior extends from sacrococcygeal junction to T-9 vertebra, produces intracavitary pressure to reduce load on the intervertebral discs, includes straps, closures, may include padding, shoulder straps, pendulous abdomen design, custom fabricated ⑧

Custom fitted

✳ **L0633** Lumbar-sacral orthosis, sagittal-coronal control, with rigid posterior frame/panel(s), posterior extends from sacrococcygeal junction to T-9 vertebra, lateral strength provided by rigid lateral frame/panels, produces intracavitary pressure to reduce load on intervertebral discs, includes straps, closures, may include padding, stays, shoulder straps, pendulous abdomen design, prefabricated item that has been trimmed, bent, molded, assembled, or otherwise customized to fit a specific patient by an individual with expertise ⑧

✳ **L0634** Lumbar-sacral orthosis, sagittal-coronal control, with rigid posterior frame/panel(s), posterior extends from sacrococcygeal junction to T-9 vertebra, lateral strength provided by rigid lateral frame/panel(s), produces intracavitary pressure to reduce load on intervertebral discs, includes straps, closures, may include padding, stays, shoulder straps, pendulous abdomen design, custom fabricated ⑧

Custom fitted

✳ **L0635** Lumbar-sacral orthosis, sagittal-coronal control, lumbar flexion, rigid posterior frame/panel(s), lateral articulating design to flex the lumbar spine, posterior extends from sacrococcygeal junction to T-9 vertebra, lateral strength provided by rigid lateral frame/panel(s), produces intracavitary pressure to reduce load on intervertebral discs, includes straps, closures, may include padding, anterior panel, pendulous abdomen design, prefabricated, includes fitting and adjustment ⑧

✳ **L0636** Lumbar sacral orthosis, sagittal-coronal control, lumbar flexion, rigid posterior frame/panels, lateral articulating design to flex the lumbar spine, posterior extends from sacrococcygeal junction to T-9 vertebra, lateral strength provided by rigid lateral frame/panels, produces intracavitary pressure to reduce load on intervertebral discs, includes straps, closures, may include padding, anterior panel, pendulous abdomen design, custom fabricated ⑧

Custom fitted

✳ **L0637** Lumbar-sacral orthosis, sagittal-coronal control, with rigid anterior and posterior frame/panels, posterior extends from sacrococcygeal junction to T-9 vertebra, lateral strength provided by rigid lateral frame/panels, produces intracavitary pressure to reduce load on intervertebral discs, includes straps, closures, may include padding, shoulder straps, pendulous abdomen design, prefabricated item that has been trimmed, bent, molded, assembled, or otherwise customized to fit a specific patient by an individual with expertise ⑧

▶ New   ↻ Revised   ✔ Reinstated   ~~deleted~~ Deleted   ⊘ Not covered or valid by Medicare

✪ Special coverage instructions   ✳ Carrier discretion   ⑨ Bill Part B MAC   ⑧ Bill DME MAC

L0638 Lumbar-sacral orthosis, sagittal-coronal control, with rigid anterior and posterior frame/panels, posterior extends from sacrococcygeal junction to T-9 vertebra, lateral strength provided by rigid lateral frame/panels, produces intracavitary pressure to reduce load on intervertebral discs, includes straps, closures, may include padding, shoulder straps, pendulous abdomen design, custom fabricated Ⓑ

L0639 Lumbar-sacral orthosis, sagittal-coronal control, rigid shell(s)/panel(s), posterior extends from sacrococcygeal junction to T-9 vertebra, anterior extends from symphysis pubis to xyphoid, produces intracavitary pressure to reduce load on the intervertebral discs, overall strength is provided by overlapping rigid material and stabilizing closures, includes straps, closures, may include soft interface, pendulous abdomen design, prefabricated item that has been trimmed, bent, molded, assembled, or otherwise customized to fit a specific patient by an individual with expertise Ⓑ

Characterized by rigid plastic shell that encircles trunk with overlapping edges and stabilizing closures and provides high degree of immobility

L0640 Lumbar-sacral orthosis, sagittal-coronal control, rigid shell(s)/panel(s), posterior extends from sacrococcygeal junction to T-9 vertebra, anterior extends from symphysis pubis to xyphoid, produces intracavitary pressure to reduce load on the intervertebral discs, overall strength is provided by overlapping rigid material and stabilizing closures, includes straps, closures, may include soft interface, pendulous abdomen design, custom fabricated Ⓑ

Custom fitted

Lumbar Orthotics

L0641 Lumbar orthosis, sagittal control, with rigid posterior panel(s), posterior extends from L-1 to below L-5 vertebra, produces intracavitary pressure to reduce load on the intervertebral discs, includes straps, closures, may include padding, stays, shoulder straps, pendulous abdomen design, prefabricated, off-the-shelf Ⓑ

L0642 Lumbar orthosis, sagittal control, with rigid anterior and posterior panels, posterior extends from L-1 to below L-5 vertebra, produces intracavitary pressure to reduce load on the intervertebral discs, includes straps, closures, may include padding, shoulder straps, pendulous abdomen design, prefabricated, off-the-shelf Ⓑ

Lumbar-Sacral Orthotics

L0643 Lumbar-sacral orthosis, sagittal control, with rigid posterior panel(s), posterior extends from sacrococcygeal junction to T-9 vertebra, produces intracavitary pressure to reduce load on the intervertebral discs, includes straps, closures, may include padding, stays, shoulder straps, pendulous abdomen design, prefabricated, off-the-shelf Ⓑ

L0648 Lumbar-sacral orthosis, sagittal control, with rigid anterior and posterior panels, posterior extends from sacrococcygeal junction to T-9 vertebra, produces intracavitary pressure to reduce load on the intervertebral discs, includes straps, closures, may include padding, shoulder straps, pendulous abdomen design, prefabricated, off-the-shelf Ⓑ

L0649 Lumbar-sacral orthosis, sagittal-coronal control, with rigid posterior frame/panel(s), posterior extends from sacrococcygeal junction to T-9 vertebra, lateral strength provided by rigid lateral frame/panels, produces intracavitary pressure to reduce load on intervertebral discs, includes straps, closures, may include padding, stays, shoulder straps, pendulous abdomen design, prefabricated, off-the-shelf Ⓑ

L0650 Lumbar-sacral orthosis, sagittal-coronal control, with rigid anterior and posterior frame/panel(s), posterior extends from sacrococcygeal junction to T-9 vertebra, lateral strength provided by rigid lateral frame/panel(s), produces intracavitary pressure to reduce load on intervertebral discs, includes straps, closures, may include padding, shoulder straps, pendulous abdomen design, prefabricated, off-the-shelf Ⓑ

▶ New   ↻ Revised   ✔ Reinstated   ~~deleted~~ Deleted   ⊘ Not covered or valid by Medicare
✪ Special coverage instructions   ✱ Carrier discretion   Ⓟ Bill Part B MAC   Ⓑ Bill DME MAC

* **L0651**   Lumbar-sacral orthosis, sagittal-coronal control, rigid shell(s)/panel(s), posterior extends from sacrococcygeal junction to T-9 vertebra, anterior extends from symphysis pubis to xyphoid, produces intracavitary pressure to reduce load on the intervertebral discs, overall strength is provided by overlapping rigid material and stabilizing closures, includes straps, closures, may include soft interface, pendulous abdomen design, prefabricated, off-the-shelf ⑧

Cervical-Thoracic-Lumbar-Sacral

* **L0700**   Cervical-thoracic-lumbar-sacral-orthoses (CTLSO), anterior-posterior-lateral control, molded to patient model, (Minerva type) ⑧

* **L0710**   CTLSO, anterior-posterior-lateral-control, molded to patient model, with interface material, (Minerva type) ⑧

HALO Procedure

* **L0810**   HALO procedure, cervical halo incorporated into jacket vest ⑧

* **L0820**   HALO procedure, cervical halo incorporated into plaster body jacket ⑧

* **L0830**   HALO procedure, cervical halo incorporated into Milwaukee type orthosis ⑧

* **L0859**   Addition to HALO procedure, magnetic resonance image compatible systems, rings and pins, any material ⑧

* **L0861**   Addition to HALO procedure, replacement liner/interface material ⑧

Additions to Spinal Orthotics

NOTE: TLSO - Thoraci-lumbar-sacral orthoses/ Spinal orthoses may be prefabricated, prefitted, or custom fabricated. Conservative treatment for back pain may include the use of spinal orthoses.

* **L0970**   TLSO, corset front ⑧
* **L0972**   LSO, corset front ⑧
* **L0974**   TLSO, full corset ⑧
* **L0976**   LSO, full corset ⑧
* **L0978**   Axillary crutch extension ⑧
* **L0980**   Peroneal straps, prefabricated, off-the-shelf, pair ⑧

* **L0982**   Stocking supporter grips, prefabricated, off-the-shelf, set of four (4) ⑧

Convenience item

* **L0984**   Protective body sock, prefabricated, off-the-shelf, each ⑧

Garment made of cloth or similar material that is worn under spinal orthosis and is not primarily medical in nature

* **L0999**   Addition to spinal orthosis, not otherwise specified ⑧

Orthotic Devices: Scoliosis Procedures

NOTE: Orthotic care of scoliosis differs from other orthotic care in that the treatment is more dynamic in nature and uses ongoing continual modification of the orthosis to the patient's changing condition. This coding structure uses the proper names, or eponyms, of the procedures because they have historic and universal acceptance in the profession. It should be recognized that variations to the basic procedures described by the founders/developers are accepted in various medical and orthotic practices throughout the country. All procedures include a model of patient when indicated.

* **L1000**   Cervical-thoracic-lumbar-sacral orthosis (CTLSO) (Milwaukee), inclusive of furnishing initial orthosis, including model ⑧

* **L1001**   Cervical thoracic lumbar sacral orthosis, immobilizer, infant size, prefabricated, includes fitting and adjustment ⑧

* **L1005**   Tension based scoliosis orthosis and accessory pads, includes fitting and adjustment ⑧

* **L1010**   Addition to cervical-thoracic-lumbar-sacral orthosis (CTLSO) or scoliosis orthosis, axilla sling ⑧

* **L1020**   Addition to CTLSO or scoliosis orthosis, kyphosis pad ⑧

* **L1025**   Addition to CTLSO or scoliosis orthosis, kyphosis pad, floating ⑧

* **L1030**   Addition to CTLSO or scoliosis orthosis, lumbar bolster pad ⑧

* **L1040**   Addition to CTLSO or scoliosis orthosis, lumbar or lumbar rib pad ⑧

* **L1050**   Addition to CTLSO or scoliosis orthosis, sternal pad ⑧

* **L1060**   Addition to CTLSO or scoliosis orthosis, thoracic pad ⑧

▶ New   ↪ Revised   ✔ Reinstated   ~~deleted~~ Deleted   ⊘ Not covered or valid by Medicare
✪ Special coverage instructions   * Carrier discretion   ⑨ Bill Part B MAC   ⑤ Bill DME MAC

* **L1070** Addition to CTLSO or scoliosis orthosis, trapezius sling Ⓑ

* **L1080** Addition to CTLSO or scoliosis orthosis, outrigger Ⓑ

* **L1085** Addition to CTLSO or scoliosis orthosis, outrigger, bilateral with vertical extensions Ⓑ

* **L1090** Addition to CTLSO or scoliosis orthosis, lumbar sling Ⓑ

* **L1100** Addition to CTLSO or scoliosis orthosis, ring flange, plastic or leather Ⓑ

* **L1110** Addition to CTLSO or scoliosis orthosis, ring flange, plastic or leather, molded to patient model Ⓑ

* **L1120** Addition to CTLSO, scoliosis orthosis, cover for upright, each Ⓑ

Thoracic-Lumbar-Sacral (Low Profile)

* **L1200** Thoracic-lumbar-sacral-orthosis (TLSO), inclusive of furnishing initial orthosis only Ⓑ

* **L1210** Addition to TLSO, (low profile), lateral thoracic extension Ⓑ

* **L1220** Addition to TLSO, (low profile), anterior thoracic extension Ⓑ

* **L1230** Addition to TLSO, (low profile), Milwaukee type superstructure Ⓑ

* **L1240** Addition to TLSO, (low profile), lumbar derotation pad Ⓑ

* **L1250** Addition to TLSO, (low profile), anterior ASIS pad Ⓑ

* **L1260** Addition to TLSO, (low profile), anterior thoracic derotation pad Ⓑ

* **L1270** Addition to TLSO, (low profile), abdominal pad Ⓑ

* **L1280** Addition to TLSO, (low profile), rib gusset (elastic), each Ⓑ

* **L1290** Addition to TLSO, (low profile), lateral trochanteric pad Ⓑ

Other Scoliosis Procedures

* **L1300** Other scoliosis procedure, body jacket molded to patient model Ⓑ

* **L1310** Other scoliosis procedure, postoperative body jacket Ⓑ

* **L1499** Spinal orthosis, not otherwise specified Ⓑ

Orthotic Devices: Lower Limb (L1600-L3649)

NOTE: the procedures in L1600-L2999 are considered as base or basic procedures and may be modified by listing procedure from the Additions Sections and adding them to the base procedure.

Hip: Flexible

* **L1600** Hip orthosis, abduction control of hip joints, flexible, frejka type with cover, prefabricated item that has been trimmed, bent, molded, assembled, or otherwise customized to fit a specific patient by an individual with expertise Ⓑ

* **L1610** Hip orthosis, abduction control of hip joints, flexible, (frejka cover only), prefabricated item that has been trimmed, bent, molded, assembled, or otherwise customized to fit a specific patient by an individual with expertise Ⓑ

* **L1620** Hip orthosis, abduction control of hip joints, flexible, (Pavlik harness), prefabricated item that has been trimmed, bent, molded, assembled, or otherwise customized to fit a specific patient by an individual with expertise Ⓑ

* **L1630** Hip orthosis, abduction control of hip joints, semi-flexible (Von Rosen type), custom-fabricated Ⓑ

* **L1640** Hip orthosis, abduction control of hip joints, static, pelvic band or spreader bar, thigh cuffs, custom-fabricated Ⓑ

* **L1650** Hip orthosis, abduction control of hip joints, static, adjustable, (Ilfled type), prefabricated, includes fitting and adjustment Ⓑ

* **L1652** Hip orthosis, bilateral thigh cuffs with adjustable abductor spreader bar, adult size, prefabricated, includes fitting and adjustment, any type Ⓑ

* **L1660** Hip orthosis, abduction control of hip joints, static, plastic, prefabricated, includes fitting and adjustment Ⓑ

* **L1680** Hip orthosis, abduction control of hip joints, dynamic, pelvic control, adjustable hip motion control, thigh cuffs (Rancho hip action type), custom fabrication Ⓑ

* **L1685** Hip orthosis, abduction control of hip joint, postoperative hip abduction type, custom fabricated Ⓑ

▶ New   ↻ Revised   ✔ Reinstated   ~~deleted~~ Deleted   ⊘ Not covered or valid by Medicare

☼ Special coverage instructions   * Carrier discretion   Ⓟ Bill Part B MAC   Ⓑ Bill DME MAC

* **L1686** Hip orthosis, abduction control of hip joint, postoperative hip abduction type, prefabricated, includes fitting and adjustment Ⓑ

* **L1690** Combination, bilateral, lumbo-sacral, hip, femur orthosis providing adduction and internal rotation control, prefabricated, includes fitting and adjustment Ⓑ

Legg Perthes

* **L1700** Legg-Perthes orthosis, (Toronto type), custom-fabricated Ⓑ

* **L1710** Legg-Perthes orthosis, (Newington type), custom-fabricated Ⓑ

* **L1720** Legg-Perthes orthosis, trilateral, (Tachdjian type), custom-fabricated Ⓑ

* **L1730** Legg-Perthes orthosis, (Scottish Rite type), custom-fabricated Ⓑ

* **L1755** Legg-Perthes orthosis, (Patten bottom type), custom-fabricated Ⓑ

Knee (KO)

* **L1810** Knee orthosis, elastic with joints, prefabricated item that has been trimmed, bent, molded, assembled, or otherwise customized to fit a specific patient by an individual with expertise Ⓑ

* **L1812** Knee orthosis, elastic with joints, prefabricated, off-the-shelf Ⓑ

* **L1820** Knee orthosis, elastic with condylar pads and joints, with or without patellar control, prefabricated, includes fitting and adjustment Ⓑ

* **L1830** Knee orthosis, immobilizer, canvas longitudinal, prefabricated, off-the-shelf Ⓑ

* **L1831** Knee orthosis, locking knee joint(s), positional orthosis, prefabricated, includes fitting and adjustment Ⓑ

* **L1832** Knee orthosis, adjustable knee joints (unicentric or polycentric), positional orthosis, rigid support, prefabricated item that has been trimmed, bent, molded, assembled, or otherwise customized to fit a specific patient by an individual with expertise Ⓑ

* **L1833** Knee orthosis, adjustable knee joints (unicentric or polycentric), positional orthosis, rigid support, prefabricated, off-the-shelf Ⓑ

* **L1834** Knee orthosis, without knee joint, rigid, custom-fabricated Ⓑ

* **L1836** Knee orthosis, rigid, without joint(s), includes soft interface material, prefabricated, off-the-shelf Ⓑ

* **L1840** Knee orthosis, derotation, medial-lateral, anterior cruciate ligament, custom fabricated Ⓑ

* **L1843** Knee orthosis, single upright, thigh and calf, with adjustable flexion and extension joint (unicentric or polycentric), medial-lateral and rotation control, with or without varus/valgus adjustment, prefabricated item that has been trimmed, bent, molded, assembled, or otherwise customized to fit a specific patient by an individual with expertise Ⓑ

* **L1844** Knee orthosis, single upright, thigh and calf, with adjustable flexion and extension joint (unicentric or polycentric), medial-lateral and rotation control, with or without varus/ valgus adjustment, custom fabricated Ⓑ

* **L1845** Knee orthosis, double upright, thigh and calf, with adjustable flexion and extension joint (unicentric or polycentric), medial-lateral and rotation control, with or without varus/valgus adjustment, prefabricated item that has been trimmed, bent, molded, assembled, or otherwise customized to fit a specific patient by an individual with expertise Ⓑ

* **L1846** Knee orthrosis, double upright, thigh and calf, with adjustable flexion and extension joint (unicentric or polycentric), medial-lateral and rotation control, with or without varus/ valgus adjustment, custom fabricated Ⓑ

* **L1847** Knee orthosis, double upright with adjustable joint, with inflatable air support chamber(s), prefabricated item that has been trimmed, bent, molded, assembled, or otherwise customized to fit a specific patient by an individual with expertise Ⓑ

* **L1848** Knee orthosis, double upright with adjustable joint, with inflatable air support chamber(s), prefabricated, off-the-shelf Ⓑ

* **L1850** Knee orthosis, Swedish type, prefabricated, off-the-shelf Ⓑ

* **L1851** Knee orthosis (KO), single upright, thigh and calf, with adjustable flexion and extension joint (unicentric or polycentric), medial-lateral and rotation control, with or without varus/valgus adjustment, prefabricated, off-the-shelf

---

▶ New   ⟲ Revised   ✔ Reinstated   ~~deleted~~ Deleted   ⊘ Not covered or valid by Medicare

✿ Special coverage instructions   ✱ Carrier discretion   Ⓑ Bill Part B MAC   Ⓑ Bill DME MAC

* **L1852** Knee orthosis (KO), double upright, thigh and calf, with adjustable flexion and extension joint (unicentric or polycentric), medial-lateral and rotation control, with or without varus/valgus adjustment, prefabricated, off-the-shelf

* **L1860** Knee orthosis, modification of supracondylar prosthetic socket, custom fabricated (SK) Ⓑ

Ankle-Foot (AFO)

* **L1900** Ankle foot orthosis (AFO), spring wire, dorsiflexion assist calf band, custom-fabricated Ⓑ

* **L1902** Ankle orthosis, ankle gauntlet or similiar, with or without joints, prefabricated, off-the-shelf Ⓖ

* **L1904** Ankle orthosis, ankle gauntlet or similiar, with or without joints, custom fabricated Ⓑ

* **L1906** Ankle foot orthosis, multiligamentus ankle support, prefabricated, off-the-shelf Ⓖ

* **L1907** Ankle orthosis, supramalleolar with straps, with or without interface/pads, custom fabricated Ⓑ

* **L1910** Ankle foot orthosis, posterior, single bar, clasp attachment to shoe counter, prefabricated, includes fitting and adjustment Ⓖ

* **L1920** Ankle foot orthosis, single upright with static or adjustable stop (Phelps or Perlstein type), custom fabricated Ⓑ

* **L1930** Ankle-foot orthosis, plastic or other material, prefabricated, includes fitting and adjustment Ⓑ

* **L1932** AFO, rigid anterior tibial section, total carbon fiber or equal material, prefabricated, includes fitting and adjustment Ⓑ

* **L1940** Ankle foot orthosis, plastic or other material, custom fabricated Ⓖ

* **L1945** Ankle foot orthosis, plastic, rigid anterior tibial section (floor reaction), custom fabricated Ⓖ

* **L1950** Ankle foot orthosis, spiral, (Institute of Rehabilitation Medicine type), plastic, custom fabricated Ⓑ

* **L1951** Ankle foot orthosis, spiral, (Institute of Rehabilitative Medicine type), plastic or other material, prefabricated, includes fitting and adjustment Ⓑ

* **L1960** Ankle foot orthosis, posterior solid ankle, plastic, custom fabricated Ⓑ

* **L1970** Ankle foot orthosis, plastic, with ankle joint, custom fabricated Ⓑ

* **L1971** Ankle foot orthosis, plastic or other material with ankle joint, prefabricated, includes fitting and adjustment Ⓖ

* **L1980** Ankle foot orthosis, single upright free plantar dorsiflexion, solid stirrup, calf band/cuff (single bar 'BK' orthosis), custom fabricated Ⓖ

* **L1990** Ankle foot orthosis, double upright free plantar dorsiflexion, solid stirrup, calf band/cuff (double bar 'BK' orthosis), custom fabricated Ⓖ

Hip-Knee-Ankle-Foot (or Any Combination)

NOTE: L2000, L2020, and L2036 are base procedures to be used with any knee joint. L2010 and L2030 are to be used only with no knee joint.

* **L2000** Knee ankle foot orthosis, single upright, free knee, free ankle, solid stirrup, thigh and calf bands/cuffs (single bar 'AK' orthosis), custom-fabricated Ⓑ

* **L2005** Knee ankle foot orthosis, any material, single or double upright, stance control, automatic lock and swing phase release, any type activation; includes ankle joint, any type, custom fabricated Ⓑ

* **L2010** Knee ankle foot orthosis, single upright, free ankle, solid stirrup, thigh and calf bands/cuffs (single bar 'AK' orthosis), without knee joint, custom-fabricated Ⓑ

* **L2020** Knee ankle foot orthosis, double upright, free knee, free ankle, solid stirrup, thigh and calf bands/cuffs (double bar 'AK' orthosis), custom fabricated Ⓑ

* **L2030** Knee ankle foot orthosis, double upright, free ankle, solid stirrup, thigh and calf bands/cuffs (double bar 'AK' orthosis), without knee joint, custom fabricated Ⓑ

* **L2034** Knee ankle foot orthosis, full plastic, single upright, with or without free motion knee, medial lateral rotation control, with or without free motion ankle, custom fabricated Ⓑ

* **L2035** Knee ankle foot orthosis, full plastic, static (pediatric size), without free motion ankle, prefabricated, includes fitting and adjustment Ⓖ

▶ **New**   ↻ **Revised**   ✔ **Reinstated**   ~~deleted~~ **Deleted**   ⊘ **Not covered or valid by Medicare**
✪ **Special coverage instructions**   ✳ **Carrier discretion**   Ⓟ **Bill Part B MAC**   Ⓖ **Bill DME MAC**

✳ **L2036**   Knee ankle foot orthosis, full plastic, double upright, with or without free motion knee, with or without free motion ankle, custom fabricated Ⓑ

✳ **L2037**   Knee ankle foot orthosis, full plastic, single upright, with or without free motion knee, with or without free motion ankle, custom fabricated Ⓑ

✳ **L2038**   Knee ankle foot orthosis, full plastic, with or without free motion knee, multi-axis ankle, custom fabricated Ⓑ

Torsion Control: Hip-Knee-Ankle-Foot (TLSO)

✳ **L2040**   Hip knee ankle foot orthosis, torsion control, bilateral rotation straps, pelvic band/belt, custom fabricated Ⓑ

✳ **L2050**   Hip knee ankle foot orthosis, torsion control, bilateral torsion cables, hip joint, pelvic band/belt, custom fabricated Ⓑ

✳ **L2060**   Hip knee ankle foot orthosis, torsion control, bilateral torsion cables, ball bearing hip joint, pelvic band/belt, custom fabricated Ⓑ

✳ **L2070**   Hip knee ankle foot orthosis, torsion control, unilateral rotation straps, pelvic band/belt, custom fabricated Ⓑ

✳ **L2080**   Hip knee ankle foot orthosis, torsion control, unilateral torsion cable, hip joint, pelvic band/belt, custom fabricated Ⓑ

✳ **L2090**   Hip knee ankle foot orthosis, torsion control, unilateral torsion cable, ball bearing hip joint, pelvic band/belt, custom fabricated Ⓑ

Fracture Orthotics: Ankle-Foot and Knee-Ankle-Foot

✳ **L2106**   Ankle foot orthosis, fracture orthosis, tibial fracture cast orthosis, thermoplastic type casting material, custom fabricated Ⓑ

✳ **L2108**   Ankle foot orthosis, fracture orthosis, tibial fracture cast orthosis, custom fabricated Ⓑ

✳ **L2112**   Ankle foot orthosis, fracture orthosis, tibial fracture orthosis, soft, prefabricated, includes fitting and adjustment Ⓑ

✳ **L2114**   Ankle foot orthosis, fracture orthosis, tibial fracture orthosis, semi-rigid, prefabricated, includes fitting and adjustment Ⓑ

✳ **L2116**   Ankle foot orthosis, fracture orthosis, tibial fracture orthosis, rigid, prefabricated, includes fitting and adjustment Ⓑ

✳ **L2126**   Knee ankle foot orthosis, fracture orthosis, femoral fracture cast orthosis, thermoplastic type casting material, custom fabricated Ⓑ

✳ **L2128**   Knee ankle foot orthosis, fracture orthosis, femoral fracture cast orthosis, custom fabricated Ⓑ

✳ **L2132**   KAFO, femoral fracture cast orthosis, soft, prefabricated, includes fitting and adjustment Ⓑ

✳ **L2134**   KAFO, femoral fracture cast orthosis, semi-rigid, prefabricated, includes fitting and adjustment Ⓑ

✳ **L2136**   KAFO, fracture orthosis, femoral fracture cast orthosis, rigid, prefabricated, includes fitting and adjustment Ⓑ

Additions to Fracture Orthotics

✳ **L2180**   Addition to lower extremity fracture orthosis, plastic shoe insert with ankle joints Ⓑ

✳ **L2182**   Addition to lower extremity fracture orthosis, drop lock knee joint Ⓑ

✳ **L2184**   Addition to lower extremity fracture orthosis, limited motion knee joint Ⓑ

✳ **L2186**   Addition to lower extremity fracture orthosis, adjustable motion knee joint, Lerman type Ⓑ

✳ **L2188**   Addition to lower extremity fracture orthosis, quadrilateral brim Ⓑ

✳ **L2190**   Addition to lower extremity fracture orthosis, waist belt Ⓑ

✳ **L2192**   Addition to lower extremity fracture orthosis, hip joint, pelvic band, thigh flange, and pelvic belt Ⓑ

Additions to Lower Extremity Orthotics

✳ **L2200**   Addition to lower extremity, limited ankle motion, each joint Ⓑ

✳ **L2210**   Addition to lower extremity, dorsiflexion assist (plantar flexion resist), each joint Ⓑ

✳ **L2220**   Addition to lower extremity, dorsiflexion and plantar flexion assist/resist, each joint Ⓑ

✳ **L2230**   Addition to lower extremity, split flat caliper stirrups and plate attachment Ⓑ

✳ **L2232**   Addition to lower extremity orthosis, rocker bottom for total contact ankle foot orthosis, for custom fabricated orthosis only Ⓑ

✳ **L2240**   Addition to lower extremity, round caliper and plate attachment Ⓑ

▶ New	↻ Revised	✔ Reinstated	deleted Deleted	⃠ Not covered or valid by Medicare
✿ Special coverage instructions		✳ Carrier discretion	Ⓟ Bill Part B MAC	Ⓓ Bill DME MAC

* **L2250** Addition to lower extremity, foot plate, molded to patient model, stirrup attachment Ⓑ

* **L2260** Addition to lower extremity, reinforced solid stirrup (Scott-Craig type) Ⓑ

* **L2265** Addition to lower extremity, long tongue stirrup Ⓑ

* **L2270** Addition to lower extremity, varus/valgus correction ('T') strap, padded/lined or malleolus pad Ⓑ

* **L2275** Addition to lower extremity, varus/valgus correction, plastic modification, padded/lined Ⓑ

* **L2280** Addition to lower extremity, molded inner boot Ⓑ

* **L2300** Addition to lower extremity, abduction bar (bilateral hip involvement), jointed, adjustable Ⓑ

* **L2310** Addition to lower extremity, abduction bar-straight Ⓑ

* **L2320** Addition to lower extremity, non-molded lacer, for custom fabricated orthosis only Ⓑ

* **L2330** Addition to lower extremity, lacer molded to patient model, for custom fabricated orthosis only Ⓑ

    Used whether closure is lacer or Velcro

* **L2335** Addition to lower extremity, anterior swing band Ⓑ

* **L2340** Addition to lower extremity, pre-tibial shell, molded to patient model Ⓑ

* **L2350** Addition to lower extremity, prosthetic type, (BK) socket, molded to patient model, (used for 'PTB' and 'AFO' orthoses) Ⓑ

* **L2360** Addition to lower extremity, extended steel shank Ⓑ

* **L2370** Addition to lower extremity, Patten bottom Ⓑ

* **L2375** Addition to lower extremity, torsion control, ankle joint and half solid stirrup Ⓑ

* **L2380** Addition to lower extremity, torsion control, straight knee joint, each joint Ⓑ

* **L2385** Addition to lower extremity, straight knee joint, heavy duty, each joint Ⓑ

* **L2387** Addition to lower extremity, polycentric knee joint, for custom fabricated knee ankle foot orthosis, each joint Ⓑ

* **L2390** Addition to lower extremity, offset knee joint, each joint Ⓑ

* **L2395** Addition to lower extremity, offset knee joint, heavy duty, each joint Ⓑ

* **L2397** Addition to lower extremity orthosis, suspension sleeve Ⓑ

Additions to Straight Knee or Offset Knee Joints

* **L2405** Addition to knee joint, drop lock, each Ⓑ

* **L2415** Addition to knee lock with integrated release mechanism (bail, cable, or equal), any material, each joint Ⓑ

* **L2425** Addition to knee joint, disc or dial lock for adjustable knee flexion, each joint Ⓑ

* **L2430** Addition to knee joint, ratchet lock for active and progressive knee extension, each joint Ⓑ

* **L2492** Addition to knee joint, lift loop for drop lock ring Ⓑ

Additions to Thigh/Weight Bearing Gluteal/Ischial Weight Bearing

* **L2500** Addition to lower extremity, thigh/weight bearing, gluteal/ischial weight bearing, ring Ⓑ

* **L2510** Addition to lower extremity, thigh/weight bearing, quadri-lateral brim, molded to patient model Ⓑ

* **L2520** Addition to lower extremity, thigh/weight bearing, quadri-lateral brim, custom fitted Ⓑ

* **L2525** Addition to lower extremity, thigh/weight bearing, ischial containment/narrow M-L brim molded to patient model Ⓑ

* **L2526** Addition to lower extremity, thigh/weight bearing, ischial containment/narrow M-L brim, custom fitted Ⓑ

* **L2530** Addition to lower extremity, thigh-weight bearing, lacer, non-molded Ⓑ

* **L2540** Addition to lower extremity, thigh/weight bearing, lacer, molded to patient model Ⓑ

* **L2550** Addition to lower extremity, thigh/weight bearing, high roll cuff Ⓑ

Additions to Pelvic and Thoracic Control

* **L2570** Addition to lower extremity, pelvic control, hip joint, Clevis type two position joint, each Ⓑ

* **L2580** Addition to lower extremity, pelvic control, pelvic sling Ⓑ

▶ New ↻ Revised ✔ Reinstated deleted Deleted ⊘ Not covered or valid by Medicare ✿ Special coverage instructions ✻ Carrier discretion Ⓟ Bill Part B MAC Ⓑ Bill DME MAC

ORTHOTICS L2250 – L2580

263

* **L2600** Addition to lower extremity, pelvic control, hip joint, Clevis type, or thrust bearing, free, each Ⓑ

* **L2610** Addition to lower extremity, pelvic control, hip joint, Clevis or thrust bearing, lock, each Ⓑ

* **L2620** Addition to lower extremity, pelvic control, hip joint, heavy duty, each Ⓑ

* **L2622** Addition to lower extremity, pelvic control, hip joint, adjustable flexion, each Ⓑ

* **L2624** Addition to lower extremity, pelvic control, hip joint, adjustable flexion, extension, abduction control, each Ⓑ

* **L2627** Addition to lower extremity, pelvic control, plastic, molded to patient model, reciprocating hip joint and cables Ⓖ

* **L2628** Addition to lower extremity, pelvic control, metal frame, reciprocating hip joint and cables Ⓖ

* **L2630** Addition to lower extremity, pelvic control, band and belt, unilateral Ⓖ

* **L2640** Addition to lower extremity, pelvic control, band and belt, bilateral Ⓖ

* **L2650** Addition to lower extremity, pelvic and thoracic control, gluteal pad, each Ⓑ

* **L2660** Addition to lower extremity, thoracic control, thoracic band Ⓑ

* **L2670** Addition to lower extremity, thoracic control, paraspinal uprights Ⓑ

* **L2680** Addition to lower extremity, thoracic control, lateral support uprights Ⓑ

General Additions

* **L2750** Addition to lower extremity orthosis, plating chrome or nickel, per bar Ⓑ

* **L2755** Addition to lower extremity orthosis, high strength, lightweight material, all hybrid lamination/prepreg composite, per segment, for custom fabricated orthosis only Ⓑ

* **L2760** Addition to lower extremity orthosis, extension, per extension, per bar (for lineal adjustment for growth) Ⓑ

* **L2768** Orthotic side bar disconnect device, per bar Ⓖ

* **L2780** Addition to lower extremity orthosis, non-corrosive finish, per bar Ⓑ

* **L2785** Addition to lower extremity orthosis, drop lock retainer, each Ⓑ

* **L2795** Addition to lower extremity orthosis, knee control, full kneecap Ⓖ

* **L2800** Addition to lower extremity orthosis, knee control, knee cap, medial or lateral pull, for use with custom fabricated orthosis only Ⓖ

* **L2810** Addition to lower extremity orthosis, knee control, condylar pad Ⓑ

* **L2820** Addition to lower extremity orthosis, soft interface for molded plastic, below knee section Ⓖ

Only report if soft interface provided, either leather or other material

* **L2830** Addition to lower extremity orthosis, soft interface for molded plastic, above knee section Ⓖ

* **L2840** Addition to lower extremity orthosis, tibial length sock, fracture or equal, each Ⓖ

* **L2850** Addition to lower extremity orthosis, femoral length sock, fracture or equal, each Ⓖ

⊘ **L2861** Addition to lower extremity joint, knee or ankle, concentric adjustable torsion style mechanism for custom fabricated orthotics only, each Ⓖ

* **L2999** Lower extremity orthoses, not otherwise specified Ⓑ

Foot (Orthopedic Shoes) (L3000-L3649)

Inserts

✪ **L3000** Foot, insert, removable, molded to patient model, 'UCB' type, Berkeley shell, each Ⓖ

If both feet casted and supplied with an orthosis, bill L3000-LT and L3000-RT

IOM: 100-02, 15, 290

✪ **L3001** Foot, insert, removable, molded to patient model, Spenco, each Ⓖ

IOM: 100-02, 15, 290

✪ **L3002** Foot, insert, removable, molded to patient model, Plastazote or equal, each Ⓖ

IOM: 100-02, 15, 290

✪ **L3003** Foot, insert, removable, molded to patient model, silicone gel, each Ⓑ

IOM: 100-02, 15, 290

✪ **L3010** Foot, insert, removable, molded to patient model, longitudinal arch support, each Ⓖ

IOM: 100-02, 15, 290

▶ New	↻ Revised	✔ Reinstated	deleted Deleted	⊘ Not covered or valid by Medicare
✪ Special coverage instructions		* Carrier discretion	Ⓑ Bill Part B MAC	Ⓖ Bill DME MAC

⊗ **L3020** Foot, insert, removable, molded to patient model, longitudinal/metatarsal support, each ⑧

IOM: 100-02, 15, 290

⊗ **L3030** Foot, insert, removable, formed to patient foot, each ⑧

IOM: 100-02, 15, 290

✳ **L3031** Foot, insert/plate, removable, addition to lower extremity orthosis, high strength, lightweight material, all hybrid lamination/prepreg composite, each ⑧

Arch Support, Removable, Premolded

⊗ **L3040** Foot, arch support, removable, premolded, longitudinal, each ⑧

IOM: 100-02, 15, 290

⊗ **L3050** Foot, arch support, removable, premolded, metatarsal, each ⑧

IOM: 100-02, 15, 290

⊗ **L3060** Foot, arch support, removable, premolded, longitudinal/metatarsal, each ⑥

IOM: 100-02, 15, 290

Arch Support, Non-removable, Attached to Shoe

⊗ **L3070** Foot, arch support, non-removable attached to shoe, longitudinal, each ⑧

IOM: 100-02, 15, 290

⊗ **L3080** Foot, arch support, non-removable attached to shoe, metatarsal, each ⑧

IOM: 100-02, 15, 290

⊗ **L3090** Foot, arch support, non-removable attached to shoe, longitudinal/metatarsal, each ⑥

IOM: 100-02, 15, 290

⊗ **L3100** Hallus-valgus night dynamic splint, prefabricated, off-the-shelf ⑧

IOM: 100-02, 15, 290

Abduction and Rotation Bars

⊗ **L3140** Foot, abduction rotation bar, including shoes ⑧

IOM: 100-02, 15, 290

⊗ **L3150** Foot, abduction rotation bar, without shoes ⑧

IOM: 100-02, 15, 290

✳ **L3160** Foot, adjustable shoe-styled positioning device ⑧

⊗ **L3170** Foot, plastic, silicone or equal, heel stabilizer, prefabricated, off-the-shelf, each ⑧

IOM: 100-02, 15, 290

Orthopedic Footwear

⊗ **L3201** Orthopedic shoe, oxford with supinator or pronator, infant ⑧

IOM: 100-02, 15, 290

⊗ **L3202** Orthopedic shoe, oxford with supinator or pronator, child ⑧

IOM: 100-02, 15, 290

⊗ **L3203** Orthopedic shoe, oxford with supinator or pronator, junior ⑧

IOM: 100-02, 15, 290

⊗ **L3204** Orthopedic shoe, hightop with supinator or pronator, infant ⑧

IOM: 100-02, 15, 290

⊗ **L3206** Orthopedic shoe, hightop with supinator or pronator, child ⑧

IOM: 100-02, 15, 290

⊗ **L3207** Orthopedic shoe, hightop with supinator or pronator, junior ⑧

IOM: 100-02, 15, 290

⊗ **L3208** Surgical boot, infant, each ⑧

IOM: 100-02, 15, 100

⊗ **L3209** Surgical boot, each, child ⑧

IOM: 100-02, 15, 100

⊗ **L3211** Surgical boot, each, junior ⑧

IOM: 100-02, 15, 100

⊗ **L3212** Benesch boot, pair, infant ⑧

IOM: 100-02, 15, 100

⊗ **L3213** Benesch boot, pair, child ⑧

IOM: 100-02, 15, 100

⊗ **L3214** Benesch boot, pair, junior ⑧

IOM: 100-02, 15, 100

⊘ **L3215** Orthopedic footwear, ladies shoe, oxford, each ⑧

⊘ **L3216** Orthopedic footwear, ladies shoe, depth inlay, each ⑥

⊘ **L3217** Orthopedic footwear, ladies shoe, hightop, depth inlay, each ⑧

⊘ **L3219** Orthopedic footwear, mens shoe, oxford, each ⑥

⊘ **L3221** Orthopedic footwear, mens shoe, depth inlay, each ⑧

▶ New   ⟳ Revised   ✔ Reinstated   ~~deleted~~ Deleted   ⊘ Not covered or valid by Medicare

⊗ Special coverage instructions   ✳ Carrier discretion   ⑧ Bill Part B MAC   ⑥ Bill DME MAC

⊘ **L3222** Orthopedic footwear, mens shoe, hightop, depth inlay, each ⑬

✿ **L3224** Orthopedic footwear, ladies shoe, oxford, used as an integral part of a brace (orthosis) ⑬

IOM: 100-02, 15, 290

✿ **L3225** Orthopedic footwear, mens shoe, oxford, used as an integral part of a brace (orthosis) ⑬

IOM: 100-02, 15, 290

✿ **L3230** Orthopedic footwear, custom shoe, depth inlay, each ⑬

IOM: 100-02, 15, 290

✿ **L3250** Orthopedic footwear, custom molded shoe, removable inner mold, prosthetic shoe, each ⑬

IOM: 100-02, 15, 290

✿ **L3251** Foot, shoe molded to patient model, silicone shoe, each ⑬

IOM: 100-02, 15, 290

✿ **L3252** Foot, shoe molded to patient model, Plastazote (or similar), custom fabricated, each ⑬

IOM: 100-02, 15, 290

✿ **L3253** Foot, molded shoe Plastazote (or similar), custom fitted, each ⑬

IOM: 100-02, 15, 290

✿ **L3254** Non-standard size or width ⑬

IOM: 100-02, 15, 290

✿ **L3255** Non-standard size or length ⑬

IOM: 100-02, 15, 290

✿ **L3257** Orthopedic footwear, additional charge for split size ⑬

IOM: 100-02, 15, 290

✿ **L3260** Surgical boot/shoe, each ⑬

IOM: 100-02, 15, 100

✽ **L3265** Plastazote sandal, each ⑬

Shoe Lifts

✿ **L3300** Lift, elevation, heel, tapered to metatarsals, per inch ⑬

IOM: 100-02, 15, 290

✿ **L3310** Lift, elevation, heel and sole, Neoprene, per inch ⑬

IOM: 100-02, 15, 290

✿ **L3320** Lift, elevation, heel and sole, cork, per inch ⑬

IOM: 100-02, 15, 290

✿ **L3330** Lift, elevation, metal extension (skate) ⑬

IOM: 100-02, 15, 290

✿ **L3332** Lift, elevation, inside shoe, tapered, up to one-half inch ⑬

IOM: 100-02, 15, 290

✿ **L3334** Lift, elevation, heel, per inch ⑬

IOM: 100-02, 15, 290

Shoe Wedges

✿ **L3340** Heel wedge, SACH ⑬

IOM: 100-02, 15, 290

✿ **L3350** Heel wedge ⑬

IOM: 100-02, 15, 290

✿ **L3360** Sole wedge, outside sole ⑬

IOM: 100-02, 15, 290

✿ **L3370** Sole wedge, between sole ⑬

IOM: 100-02, 15, 290

✿ **L3380** Clubfoot wedge ⑬

IOM: 100-02, 15, 290

✿ **L3390** Outflare wedge ⑬

IOM: 100-02, 15, 290

✿ **L3400** Metatarsal bar wedge, rocker ⑬

IOM: 100-02, 15, 290

✿ **L3410** Metatarsal bar wedge, between sole ⑬

IOM: 100-02, 15, 290

✿ **L3420** Full sole and heel wedge, between sole ⑬

IOM: 100-02, 15, 290

Shoe Heels

✿ **L3430** Heel, counter, plastic reinforced ⑬

IOM: 100-02, 15, 290

✿ **L3440** Heel, counter, leather reinforced ⑬

IOM: 100-02, 15, 290

✿ **L3450** Heel, SACH cushion type ⑬

IOM: 100-02, 15, 290

✿ **L3455** Heel, new leather, standard ⑬

IOM: 100-02, 15, 290

✿ **L3460** Heel, new rubber, standard ⑬

IOM: 100-02, 15, 290

✿ **L3465** Heel, Thomas with wedge ⑬

IOM: 100-02, 15, 290

✿ **L3470** Heel, Thomas extended to ball ⑬

IOM: 100-02, 15, 290

▶ New   ↻ Revised   ✔ Reinstated   ~~deleted~~ Deleted   ⊘ Not covered or valid by Medicare
✿ Special coverage instructions   ✽ Carrier discretion   ⑨ Bill Part B MAC   ⑬ Bill DME MAC

✪ **L3480** Heel, pad and depression for spur Ⓑ

IOM: 100-02, 15, 290

✪ **L3485** Heel, pad, removable for spur Ⓑ

IOM: 100-02, 15, 290

Orthopedic Shoe Additions: Other

✪ **L3500** Orthopedic shoe addition, insole, leather Ⓑ

IOM: 100-02, 15, 290

✪ **L3510** Orthopedic shoe addition, insole, rubber Ⓑ

IOM: 100-02, 15, 290

✪ **L3520** Orthopedic shoe addition, insole, felt covered with leather Ⓑ

IOM: 100-02, 15, 290

✪ **L3530** Orthopedic shoe addition, sole, half Ⓑ

IOM: 100-02, 15, 290

✪ **L3540** Orthopedic shoe addition, sole, full Ⓑ

IOM: 100-02, 15, 290

✪ **L3550** Orthopedic shoe addition, toe tap standard Ⓑ

IOM: 100-02, 15, 290

✪ **L3560** Orthopedic shoe addition, toe tap, horseshoe Ⓑ

IOM: 100-02, 15, 290

✪ **L3570** Orthopedic shoe addition, special extension to instep (leather with eyelets) Ⓑ

IOM: 100-02, 15, 290

✪ **L3580** Orthopedic shoe addition, convert instep to Velcro closure Ⓑ

IOM: 100-02, 15, 290

✪ **L3590** Orthopedic shoe addition, convert firm shoe counter to soft counter Ⓑ

IOM: 100-02, 15, 290

✪ **L3595** Orthopedic shoe addition, March bar Ⓑ

IOM: 100-02, 15, 290

Transfer or Replacement

✪ **L3600** Transfer of an orthosis from one shoe to another, caliper plate, existing Ⓑ

IOM: 100-02, 15, 290

✪ **L3610** Transfer of an orthosis from one shoe to another, caliper plate, new Ⓑ

IOM: 100-02, 15, 290

✪ **L3620** Transfer of an orthosis from one shoe to another, solid stirrup, existing Ⓑ

IOM: 100-02, 15, 290

✪ **L3630** Transfer of an orthosis from one shoe to another, solid stirrup, new Ⓑ

IOM: 100-02, 15, 290

✪ **L3640** Transfer of an orthosis from one shoe to another, Dennis Browne splint (Riveton), both shoes Ⓑ

IOM: 100-02, 15, 290

✪ **L3649** Orthopedic shoe, modification, addition or transfer, not otherwise specified Ⓑ

IOM: 100-02, 15, 290

Orthotic Devices: Upper Limb

NOTE: The procedures in this section are considered as base or basic procedures and may be modified by listing procedures from the Additions section and adding them to the base procedure.

Shoulder

✳ **L3650** Shoulder orthosis, figure of eight design abduction restrainer, prefabricated, off-the-shelf Ⓑ

✳ **L3660** Shoulder orthosis, figure of eight design abduction restrainer, canvas and webbing, prefabricated, off-the-shelf Ⓑ

✳ **L3670** Shoulder orthosis, acromio/clavicular (canvas and webbing type), prefabricated, off-the-shelf Ⓑ

✳ **L3671** Shoulder orthosis, shoulder joint design, without joints, may include soft interface, straps, custom fabricated, includes fitting and adjustment Ⓑ

✳ **L3674** Shoulder orthosis, abduction positioning (airplane design), thoracic component and support bar, with or without nontorsion joint/turnbuckle, may include soft interface, straps, custom fabricated, includes fitting and adjustment Ⓑ

✳ **L3675** Shoulder orthosis, vest type abduction restrainer, canvas webbing type or equal, prefabricated, off-the-shelf Ⓑ

✪ **L3677** Shoulder orthosis, shoulder joint design, without joints, may include soft interface, straps, prefabricated item that has been trimmed, bent, molded, assembled, or otherwise customized to fit a specific patient by an individual with expertise Ⓑ

✳ **L3678** Shoulder orthosis, shoulder joint design, without joints, may include soft interface, straps, prefabricated, off-the-shelf Ⓑ

▶ New   ⟲ Revised   ✔ Reinstated   ~~deleted~~ Deleted   ⊘ Not covered or valid by Medicare

✪ Special coverage instructions   ✳ Carrier discretion   Ⓟ Bill Part B MAC   Ⓑ Bill DME MAC

Elbow

✻ **L3702** Elbow orthosis, without joints, may include soft interface, straps, custom fabricated, includes fitting and adjustment ⓑ

✻ **L3710** Elbow orthosis, elastic with metal joints, prefabricated, off-the-shelf ⓑ

✻ **L3720** Elbow orthosis, double upright with forearm/arm cuffs, free motion, custom fabricated ⓑ

✻ **L3730** Elbow orthosis, double upright with forearm/arm cuffs, extension/flexion assist, custom fabricated ⓖ

✻ **L3740** Elbow orthosis, double upright with forearm/arm cuffs, adjustable position lock with active control, custom fabricated ⓑ

↩ ✻ **L3760** Elbow orthosis (EO), with adjustable position locking joint(s), prefabricated, item that has been trimmed, bent, molded, assembled, or otherwise customized to fit a specific patient by an individual with expertise ⓑ

▶ ✻ **L3761** Elbow orthosis (EO), with adjustable position locking joint(s), prefabricated, off-the-shelf

✻ **L3762** Elbow orthosis, rigid, without joints, includes soft interface material, prefabricated, off-the-shelf ⓑ

✻ **L3763** Elbow wrist hand orthosis, rigid, without joints, may include soft interface, straps, custom fabricated, includes fitting and adjustment ⓑ

✻ **L3764** Elbow wrist hand orthosis, includes one or more nontorsion joints, elastic bands, turnbuckles, may include soft interface, straps, custom fabricated, includes fitting and adjustment ⓑ

✻ **L3765** Elbow wrist hand finger orthosis, rigid, without joints, may include soft interface, straps, custom fabricated, includes fitting and adjustment ⓑ

✻ **L3766** Elbow wrist hand finger orthosis, includes one or more nontorsion joints, elastic bands, turnbuckles, may include soft interface, straps, custom fabricated, includes fitting and adjustment ⓑ

Wrist-Hand-Finger Orthosis (WHFO)

✻ **L3806** Wrist hand finger orthosis, includes one or more nontorsion joint(s), turnbuckles, elastic bands/springs, may include soft interface material, straps, custom fabricated, includes fitting and adjustment ⓑ

✻ **L3807** Wrist hand finger orthosis, without joint(s), prefabricated item that has been trimmed, bent, molded, assembled, or otherwise customized to fit a specific patient by an individual with expertise ⓑ

✻ **L3808** Wrist hand finger orthosis, rigid without joints, may include soft interface material; straps, custom fabricated, includes fitting and adjustment ⓑ

✻ **L3809** Wrist hand finger orthosis, without joint(s), prefabricated, off-the-shelf, any type ⓑ

⊘ **L3891** Addition to upper extremity joint, wrist or elbow, concentric adjustable torsion style mechanism for custom fabricated orthotics only, each ⓑ

✻ **L3900** Wrist hand finger orthosis, dynamic flexor hinge, reciprocal wrist extension/ flexion, finger flexion/extension, wrist or finger driven, custom fabricated ⓑ

✻ **L3901** Wrist hand finger orthosis, dynamic flexor hinge, reciprocal wrist extension/ flexion, finger flexion/extension, cable driven, custom fabricated ⓑ

✻ **L3904** Wrist hand finger orthosis, external powered, electric, custom fabricated ⓑ

Other Upper Extremity Orthotics

✻ **L3905** Wrist hand orthosis, includes one or more nontorsion joints, elastic bands, turnbuckles, may include soft interface, straps, custom fabricated, includes fitting and adjustment ⓑ

✻ **L3906** Wrist hand orthosis, without joints, may include soft interface, straps, custom fabricated, includes fitting and adjustment ⓑ

✻ **L3908** Wrist hand orthosis, wrist extension control cock-up, non-molded, prefabricated, off-the-shelf ⓑ

✻ **L3912** Hand finger orthosis (HFO), flexion glove with elastic finger control, prefabricated, off-the-shelf ⓑ

✻ **L3913** Hand finger orthosis, without joints, may include soft interface, straps, custom fabricated, includes fitting and adjustment ⓑ

✻ **L3915** Wrist hand orthosis, includes one or more nontorsion joint(s), elastic bands, turnbuckles, may include soft interface, straps, prefabricated item that has been trimmed, bent, molded, assembled, or otherwise customized to fit a specific patient by an individual with expertise ⓑ

▶ **New** ↩ **Revised** ✔ **Reinstated** deleted **Deleted** ⊘ **Not covered or valid by Medicare**
✿ **Special coverage instructions** ✻ **Carrier discretion** ⓟ **Bill Part B MAC** ⓑ **Bill DME MAC**

* **L3916** Wrist hand orthosis, includes one or more nontorsion joint(s), elastic bands, turnbuckles, may include soft interface, straps, prefabricated, off-the-shelf Ⓑ

* **L3917** Hand orthosis, metacarpal fracture orthosis, prefabricated item that has been trimmed, bent, molded, assembled, or otherwise customized to fit a specific patient by an individual with expertise Ⓑ

* **L3918** Hand orthosis, metacarpal fracture orthosis, prefabricated, off-the-shelf Ⓑ

* **L3919** Hand orthosis, without joints, may include soft interface, straps, custom fabricated, includes fitting and adjustment Ⓑ

* **L3921** Hand finger orthosis, includes one or more nontorsion joints, elastic bands, turnbuckles, may include soft interface, straps, custom fabricated, includes fitting and adjustment Ⓑ

* **L3923** Hand finger orthosis, without joints, may include soft interface, straps, prefabricated item that has been trimmed, bent, molded, assembled, or otherwise customized to fit a specific patient by an individual with expertise Ⓑ

* **L3924** Hand finger orthosis, without joints, may include soft interface, straps, prefabricated, off-the-shelf Ⓑ

* **L3925** Finger orthosis, proximal interphalangeal (PIP)/distal interphalangeal (DIP), non torsion joint/spring, extension/flexion, may include soft interface material, prefabricated, off-the-shelf Ⓑ

* **L3927** Finger orthosis, proximal interphalangeal (PIP)/distal interphalangeal (DIP), without joint/spring, extension/flexion (e.g., static or ring type), may include soft interface material, prefabricated, off-the-shelf Ⓑ

* **L3929** Hand finger orthosis, includes one or more nontorsion joint(s), turnbuckles, elastic bands/springs, may include soft interface material, straps, prefabricated item that has been trimmed, bent, molded, assembled, or otherwise customized to fit a specific patient by an individual with expertise Ⓑ

* **L3930** Hand finger orthosis, includes one or more nontorsion joint(s), turnbuckles, elastic bands/springs, may include soft interface material, straps, prefabricated, off-the-shelf Ⓑ

* **L3931** Wrist hand finger orthosis, includes one or more nontorsion joint(s), turnbuckles, elastic bands/springs, may include soft interface material, straps, prefabricated, includes fitting and adjustment Ⓑ

* **L3933** Finger orthosis, without joints, may include soft interface, custom fabricated, includes fitting and adjustment Ⓑ

* **L3935** Finger orthosis, nontorsion joint, may include soft interface, custom fabricated, includes fitting and adjustment Ⓑ

* **L3956** Addition of joint to upper extremity orthosis, any material, per joint Ⓑ

Shoulder-Elbow-Wrist-Hand Orthotics (SEWHO) (L3960-L3973)

* **L3960** Shoulder elbow wrist hand orthosis, abduction positioning, airplane design, prefabricated, includes fitting and adjustment Ⓑ

* **L3961** Shoulder elbow wrist hand orthosis, shoulder cap design, without joints, may include soft interface, straps, custom fabricated, includes fitting and adjustment Ⓑ

* **L3962** Shoulder elbow wrist hand orthosis, abduction positioning, Erb's palsy design, prefabricated, includes fitting and adjustment Ⓑ

* **L3967** Shoulder elbow wrist hand orthosis, abduction positioning (airplane design), thoracic component and support bar, without joints, may include soft interface, straps, custom fabricated, includes fitting and adjustment Ⓑ

* **L3971** Shoulder elbow wrist hand orthosis, shoulder cap design, includes one or more nontorsion joints, elastic bands, turnbuckles, may include soft interface, straps, custom fabricated, includes fitting and adjustment Ⓑ

* **L3973** Shoulder elbow wrist hand orthosis, abduction positioning (airplane design), thoracic component and support bar, includes one or more nontorsion joints, elastic bands, turnbuckles, may include soft interface, straps, custom fabricated, includes fitting and adjustment Ⓑ

▶ New   ↻ Revised   ✔ Reinstated   ~~deleted~~ Deleted   ⊘ Not covered or valid by Medicare
✪ Special coverage instructions   ✳ Carrier discretion   Ⓟ Bill Part B MAC   Ⓑ Bill DME MAC

Shoulder-Elbow-Wrist-Hand-Finger Orthotics

✳ **L3975** Shoulder elbow wrist hand finger orthosis, shoulder cap design, without joints, may include soft interface, straps, custom fabricated, includes fitting and adjustment Ⓑ

✳ **L3976** Shoulder elbow wrist hand finger orthosis, abduction positioning (airplane design), thoracic component and support bar, without joints, may include soft interface, straps, custom fabricated, includes fitting and adjustment Ⓑ

✳ **L3977** Shoulder elbow wrist hand finger orthosis, shoulder cap design, includes one or more nontorsion joints, elastic bands, turnbuckles, may include soft interface, straps, custom fabricated, includes fitting and adjustment Ⓑ

✳ **L3978** Shoulder elbow wrist hand finger orthosis, abduction positioning (airplane design), thoracic component and support bar, includes one or more nontorsion joints, elastic bands, turnbuckles, may include soft interface, straps, custom fabricated, includes fitting and adjustment Ⓑ

Fracture Orthorics

✳ **L3980** Upper extremity fracture orthosis, humeral, prefabricated, includes fitting and adjustment Ⓑ

✳ **L3981** Upper extremity fracture orthosis, humeral, prefabricated, includes shoulder cap design, with or without joints, forearm section, may include soft interface, straps, includes fitting and adjustments Ⓑ

✳ **L3982** Upper extremity fracture orthosis, radius/ulnar, prefabricated, includes fitting and adjustment Ⓑ

✳ **L3984** Upper extremity fracture orthosis, wrist, prefabricated, includes fitting and adjustment Ⓑ

✳ **L3995** Addition to upper extremity orthosis, sock, fracture or equal, each Ⓑ

✳ **L3999** Upper limb orthosis, not otherwise specified Ⓑ

Repairs

✳ **L4000** Replace girdle for spinal orthosis (CTLSO or SO) Ⓑ

✳ **L4002** Replacement strap, any orthosis, includes all components, any length, any type Ⓑ

✳ **L4010** Replace trilateral socket brim Ⓑ

✳ **L4020** Replace quadrilateral socket brim, molded to patient model Ⓑ

✳ **L4030** Replace quadrilateral socket brim, custom fitted Ⓑ

✳ **L4040** Replace molded thigh lacer, for custom fabricated orthosis only Ⓑ

✳ **L4045** Replace non-molded thigh lacer, for custom fabricated orthosis only Ⓑ

✳ **L4050** Replace molded calf lacer, for custom fabricated orthosis only Ⓑ

✳ **L4055** Replace non-molded calf lacer, for custom fabricated orthosis only Ⓑ

✳ **L4060** Replace high roll cuff Ⓑ

✳ **L4070** Replace proximal and distal upright for KAFO Ⓑ

✳ **L4080** Replace metal bands KAFO, proximal thigh Ⓑ

✳ **L4090** Replace metal bands KAFO-AFO, calf or distal thigh Ⓑ

✳ **L4100** Replace leather cuff KAFO, proximal thigh Ⓑ

✳ **L4110** Replace leather cuff KAFO-AFO, calf or distal thigh Ⓑ

✳ **L4130** Replace pretibial shell Ⓑ

✪ **L4205** Repair of orthotic device, labor component, per 15 minutes Ⓑ

IOM: 100-02, 15, 110.2

✪ **L4210** Repair of orthotic device, repair or replace minor parts Ⓑ

IOM: 100-02, 15, 110.2; 100-02, 15, 120

Ancillary Orthotic Services

✳ **L4350** Ankle control orthosis, stirrup style, rigid, includes any type interface (e.g., pneumatic, gel), prefabricated, off-the-shelf Ⓑ

▶ **New**   ↻ **Revised**   ✔ **Reinstated**   ~~deleted~~ **Deleted**   ⊘ **Not covered or valid by Medicare**

✪ **Special coverage instructions**   ✳ **Carrier discretion**   Ⓟ **Bill Part B MAC**   Ⓑ **Bill DME MAC**

✳ **L4360** Walking boot, pneumatic and/or vacuum, with or without joints, with or without interface material, prefabricated item that has been trimmed, bent, molded, assembled, or otherwise customized to fit a specific patient by an individual with expertise Ⓑ

Noncovered when walking boots used primarily to relieve pressure, especially on sole of foot, or are used for patients with foot ulcers

✳ **L4361** Walking boot, pneumatic and/or vacuum, with or without joints, with or without interface material, prefabricated, off-the-shelf Ⓑ

✳ **L4370** Pneumatic full leg splint, prefabricated, off-the-shelf Ⓑ

✳ **L4386** Walking boot, non-pneumatic, with or without joints, with or without interface material, prefabricated item that has been trimmed, bent, molded, assembled, or otherwise customized to fit a specific patient by an individual with expertise Ⓑ

✳ **L4387** Walking boot, non-pneumatic, with or without joints, with or without interface material, prefabricated, off-the-shelf Ⓑ

✳ **L4392** Replacement, soft interface material, static AFO Ⓑ

✳ **L4394** Replace soft interface material, foot drop splint Ⓑ

✳ **L4396** Static or dynamic ankle foot orthosis, including soft interface material, adjustable for fit, for positioning, may be used for minimal ambulation, prefabricated item that has been trimmed, bent, molded, assembled, or otherwise customized to fit a specific patient by an individual with expertise Ⓑ

✳ **L4397** Static or dynamic ankle foot orthosis, including soft interface material, adjustable for fit, for positioning, may be used for minimal ambulation, prefabricated, off-the-shelf Ⓑ

✳ **L4398** Foot drop splint, recumbent positioning device, prefabricated, off-the-shelf Ⓑ

✳ **L4631** Ankle foot orthosis, walking boot type, varus/valgus correction, rocker bottom, anterior tibial shell, soft interface, custom arch support, plastic or other material, includes straps and closures, custom fabricated Ⓑ

PROSTHETICS (L5000-L9999)

Lower Limb (L5000-L5999)

NOTE: The procedures in this section are considered as base or basic procedures and may be modified by listing items/procedures or special materials from the Additions section and adding them to the base procedure.

Partial Foot

✪ **L5000** Partial foot, shoe insert with longitudinal arch, toe filler Ⓑ

IOM: 100-02, 15, 290

✪ **L5010** Partial foot, molded socket, ankle height, with toe filler Ⓑ

IOM: 100-02, 15, 290

✪ **L5020** Partial foot, molded socket, tibial tubercle height, with toe filler Ⓑ

IOM: 100-02, 15, 290

Ankle

✳ **L5050** Ankle, Symes, molded socket, SACH foot Ⓑ

✳ **L5060** Ankle, Symes, metal frame, molded leather socket, articulated ankle/foot Ⓑ

Below Knee

✳ **L5100** Below knee, molded socket, shin, SACH foot Ⓑ

✳ **L5105** Below knee, plastic socket, joints and thigh lacer, SACH foot Ⓑ

Knee Disarticulation

✳ **L5150** Knee disarticulation (or through knee), molded socket, external knee joints, shin, SACH foot Ⓑ

✳ **L5160** Knee disarticulation (or through knee), molded socket, bent knee configuration, external knee joints, shin, SACH foot Ⓑ

Above Knee

✳ **L5200** Above knee, molded socket, single axis constant friction knee, shin, SACH foot Ⓑ

✳ **L5210** Above knee, short prosthesis, no knee joint ('stubbies'), with foot blocks, no ankle joints, each Ⓑ

▶ New   ↻ Revised   ✔ Reinstated   ~~deleted~~ Deleted   ⊘ Not covered or valid by Medicare
✪ Special coverage instructions   ✳ Carrier discretion   Ⓟ Bill Part B MAC   Ⓑ Bill DME MAC

✳ **L5220** Above knee, short prosthesis, no knee joint ('stubbies'), with articulated ankle/foot, dynamically aligned, each Ⓑ

✳ **L5230** Above knee, for proximal femoral focal deficiency, constant friction knee, shin, SACH foot Ⓑ

Hip Disarticulation

✳ **L5250** Hip disarticulation, Canadian type; molded socket, hip joint, single axis constant friction knee, shin, SACH foot Ⓑ

✳ **L5270** Hip disarticulation, tilt table type; molded socket, locking hip joint, single axis constant friction knee, shin, SACH foot Ⓑ

Hemipelvectomy

✳ **L5280** Hemipelvectomy, Canadian type; molded socket, hip joint, single axis constant friction knee, shin, SACH foot Ⓑ

Endoskeletal

✳ **L5301** Below knee, molded socket, shin, SACH foot, endoskeletal system Ⓑ

✳ **L5312** Knee disarticulation (or through knee), molded socket, single axis knee, pylon, sach foot, endoskeletal system Ⓑ

✳ **L5321** Above knee, molded socket, open end, SACH foot, endoskeletal system, single axis knee Ⓑ

✳ **L5331** Hip disarticulation, Canadian type, molded socket, endoskeletal system, hip joint, single axis knee, SACH foot Ⓑ

✳ **L5341** Hemipelvectomy, Canadian type, molded socket, endoskeletal system, hip joint, single axis knee, SACH foot Ⓑ

Immediate Postsurgical or Early Fitting Procedures

✳ **L5400** Immediate post surgical or early fitting, application of initial rigid dressing, including fitting, alignment, suspension, and one cast change, below knee Ⓑ

✳ **L5410** Immediate post surgical or early fitting, application of initial rigid dressing, including fitting, alignment and suspension, below knee, each additional cast change and realignment Ⓑ

✳ **L5420** Immediate post surgical or early fitting, application of initial rigid dressing, including fitting, alignment and suspension and one cast change 'AK' or knee disarticulation Ⓑ

✳ **L5430** Immediate postsurgical or early fitting, application of initial rigid dressing, including fitting, alignment, and suspension, 'AK' or knee disarticulation, each additional cast change and realignment Ⓑ

✳ **L5450** Immediate post surgical or early fitting, application of non-weight bearing rigid dressing, below knee Ⓑ

✳ **L5460** Immediate post surgical or early fitting, application of non-weight bearing rigid dressing, above knee Ⓑ

Initial Prosthesis

✳ **L5500** Initial, below knee 'PTB' type socket, non-alignable system, pylon, no cover, SACH foot, plaster socket, direct formed Ⓑ

✳ **L5505** Initial, above knee-knee disarticulation, ischial level socket, non-alignable system, pylon, no cover, SACH foot, plaster socket, direct formed Ⓑ

Preparatory Prosthesis

✳ **L5510** Preparatory, below knee 'PTB' type socket, non-alignable system, pylon, no cover, SACH foot, plaster socket, molded to model Ⓑ

✳ **L5520** Preparatory, below knee 'PTB' type socket, non-alignable system, pylon, no cover, SACH foot, thermoplastic or equal, direct formed Ⓑ

✳ **L5530** Preparatory, below knee 'PTB' type socket, non-alignable system, pylon, no cover, SACH foot, thermoplastic or equal, molded to model Ⓑ

✳ **L5535** Preparatory, below knee 'PTB' type socket, non-alignable system, no cover, SACH foot, prefabricated, adjustable open end socket Ⓑ

✳ **L5540** Preparatory, below knee 'PTB' type socket, non-alignable system, pylon, no cover, SACH foot, laminated socket, molded to model Ⓑ

✳ **L5560** Preparatory, above knee - knee disarticulation, ischial level socket, non-alignable system, pylon, no cover, SACH foot, plaster socket, molded to model Ⓑ

✳ **L5570** Preparatory, above knee - knee disarticulation, ischial level socket, non-alignable system, pylon, no cover, SACH foot, thermoplastic or equal, direct formed Ⓑ

▶ New   ↻ Revised   ✔ Reinstated   ~~deleted~~ Deleted   ⊘ Not covered or valid by Medicare
✪ Special coverage instructions   ✳ Carrier discretion   Ⓑ Bill Part B MAC   Ⓑ Bill DME MAC

* **L5580** Preparatory, above knee - knee disarticulation, ischial level socket, non-alignable system, pylon, no cover, SACH foot, thermoplastic or equal, molded to model Ⓑ

* **L5585** Preparatory, above knee - knee disarticulation, ischial level socket, non-alignable system, pylon, no cover, SACH foot, prefabricated adjustable open end socket Ⓑ

* **L5590** Preparatory, above knee - knee disarticulation, ischial level socket, non-alignable system, pylon, no cover, SACH foot, laminated socket, molded to model Ⓑ

* **L5595** Preparatory, hip disarticulation-hemipelvectomy, pylon, no cover, SACH foot, thermoplastic or equal, molded to patient model Ⓑ

* **L5600** Preparatory, hip disarticulation-hemipelvectomy, pylon, no cover, SACH foot, laminated socket, molded to patient model Ⓑ

Additions to Lower Extremity

* **L5610** Addition to lower extremity, endoskeletal system, above knee, hydracadence system Ⓑ

* **L5611** Addition to lower extremity, endoskeletal system, above knee-knee disarticulation, 4 bar linkage, with friction swing phase control Ⓑ

* **L5613** Addition to lower extremity, endoskeletal system, above knee-knee disarticulation, 4 bar linkage, with hydraulic swing phase control Ⓑ

* **L5614** Addition to lower extremity, exoskeletal system, above knee-knee disarticulation, 4 bar linkage, with pneumatic swing phase control Ⓑ

* **L5616** Addition to lower extremity, endoskeletal system, above knee, universal multiplex system, friction swing phase control Ⓑ

* **L5617** Addition to lower extremity, quick change self-aligning unit, above knee or below knee, each Ⓑ

Additions to Test Sockets

* **L5618** Addition to lower extremity, test socket, Symes Ⓑ

* **L5620** Addition to lower extremity, test socket, below knee Ⓑ

* **L5622** Addition to lower extremity, test socket, knee disarticulation Ⓑ

* **L5624** Addition to lower extremity, test socket, above knee Ⓑ

* **L5626** Addition to lower extremity, test socket, hip disarticulation Ⓑ

* **L5628** Addition to lower extremity, test socket, hemipelvectomy Ⓑ

Additions to Socket Variations

* **L5629** Addition to lower extremity, below knee, acrylic socket Ⓑ

* **L5630** Addition to lower extremity, Symes type, expandable wall socket Ⓑ

* **L5631** Addition to lower extremity, above knee or knee disarticulation, acrylic socket Ⓑ

* **L5632** Addition to lower extremity, Symes type, 'PTB' brim design socket Ⓑ

* **L5634** Addition to lower extremity, Symes type, posterior opening (Canadian) socket Ⓑ

* **L5636** Addition to lower extremity, Symes type, medial opening socket Ⓑ

* **L5637** Addition to lower extremity, below knee, total contact Ⓑ

* **L5638** Addition to lower extremity, below knee, leather socket Ⓑ

* **L5639** Addition to lower extremity, below knee, wood socket Ⓑ

* **L5640** Addition to lower extremity, knee disarticulation, leather socket Ⓑ

* **L5642** Addition to lower extremity, above knee, leather socket Ⓑ

* **L5643** Addition to lower extremity, hip disarticulation, flexible inner socket, external frame Ⓑ

* **L5644** Addition to lower extremity, above knee, wood socket Ⓑ

* **L5645** Addition to lower extremity, below knee, flexible inner socket, external frame Ⓑ

* **L5646** Addition to lower extremity, below knee, air, fluid, gel or equal, cushion socket Ⓑ

* **L5647** Addition to lower extremity, below knee, suction socket Ⓑ

* **L5648** Addition to lower extremity, above knee, air, fluid, gel or equal, cushion socket Ⓑ

* **L5649** Addition to lower extremity, ischial containment/narrow M-L socket Ⓑ

* **L5650** Additions to lower extremity, total contact, above knee or knee disarticulation socket Ⓑ

▶ New   ↻ Revised   ✔ Reinstated   ~~deleted~~ Deleted   ⊘ Not covered or valid by Medicare

✺ Special coverage instructions   ✱ Carrier discretion   Ⓟ Bill Part B MAC   Ⓑ Bill DME MAC

✳ **L5651** Addition to lower extremity, above knee, flexible inner socket, external frame Ⓑ

✳ **L5652** Addition to lower extremity, suction suspension, above knee or knee disarticulation socket Ⓑ

✳ **L5653** Addition to lower extremity, knee disarticulation, expandable wall socket Ⓑ

Additions to Socket Insert and Suspension

✳ **L5654** Addition to lower extremity, socket insert, Symes, (Kemblo, Pelite, Aliplast, Plastazote or equal) Ⓑ

✳ **L5655** Addition to lower extremity, socket insert, below knee (Kemblo, Pelite, Aliplast, Plastazote or equal) Ⓑ

✳ **L5656** Addition to lower extremity, socket insert, knee disarticulation (Kemblo, Pelite, Aliplast, Plastazote or equal) Ⓑ

✳ **L5658** Addition to lower extremity, socket insert, above knee (Kemblo, Pelite, Aliplast, Plastazote or equal) Ⓑ

✳ **L5661** Addition to lower extremity, socket insert, multi-durometer Symes Ⓑ

✳ **L5665** Addition to lower extremity, socket insert, multi-durometer, below knee Ⓑ

✳ **L5666** Addition to lower extremity, below knee, cuff suspension Ⓑ

✳ **L5668** Addition to lower extremity, below knee, molded distal cushion Ⓑ

✳ **L5670** Addition to lower extremity, below knee, molded supracondylar suspension ('PTS' or similar) Ⓑ

✳ **L5671** Addition to lower extremity, below knee/above knee suspension locking mechanism (shuttle, lanyard or equal), excludes socket insert Ⓑ

✳ **L5672** Addition to lower extremity, below knee, removable medial brim suspension Ⓑ

✳ **L5673** Addition to lower extremity, below knee/above knee, custom fabricated from existing mold or prefabricated, socket insert, silicone gel, elastomeric or equal, for use with locking mechanism Ⓑ

✳ **L5676** Additions to lower extremity, below knee, knee joints, single axis, pair Ⓑ

✳ **L5677** Additions to lower extremity, below knee, knee joints, polycentric, pair Ⓑ

✳ **L5678** Additions to lower extremity, below knee, joint covers, pair Ⓑ

✳ **L5679** Addition to lower extremity, below knee/above knee, custom fabricated from existing mold or prefabricated, socket insert, silicone gel, elastomeric or equal, not for use with locking mechanism Ⓑ

✳ **L5680** Addition to lower extremity, below knee, thigh lacer, non-molded Ⓑ

✳ **L5681** Addition to lower extremity, below knee/above knee, custom fabricated socket insert for congenital or atypical traumatic amputee, silicone gel, elastomeric or equal, for use with or without locking mechanism, initial only (for other than initial, use code L5673 or L5679) Ⓑ

✳ **L5682** Addition to lower extremity, below knee, thigh lacer, gluteal/ischial, molded Ⓑ

✳ **L5683** Addition to lower extremity, below knee/above knee, custom fabricated socket insert for other than congenital or atypical traumatic amputee, silicone gel, elastomeric, or equal, for use with or without locking mechanism, initial only (for other than initial, use code L5673 or L5679) Ⓑ

✳ **L5684** Addition to lower extremity, below knee, fork strap Ⓑ

✳ **L5685** Addition to lower extremity prosthesis, below knee, suspension/sealing sleeve, with or without valve, any material, each Ⓑ

✳ **L5686** Addition to lower extremity, below knee, back check (extension control) Ⓑ

✳ **L5688** Addition to lower extremity, below knee, waist belt, webbing Ⓑ

✳ **L5690** Addition to lower extremity, below knee, waist belt, padded and lined Ⓑ

✳ **L5692** Addition to lower extremity, above knee, pelvic control belt, light Ⓑ

✳ **L5694** Addition to lower extremity, above knee, pelvic control belt, padded and lined Ⓑ

✳ **L5695** Addition to lower extremity, above knee, pelvic control, sleeve suspension, neoprene or equal, each Ⓑ

✳ **L5696** Addition to lower extremity, above knee or knee disarticulation, pelvic joint Ⓑ

✳ **L5697** Addition to lower extremity, above knee or knee disarticulation, pelvic band Ⓑ

✳ **L5698** Addition to lower extremity, above knee or knee disarticulation, Silesian bandage Ⓑ

✳ **L5699** All lower extremity prostheses, shoulder harness Ⓑ

▶ New   ↻ Revised   ✔ Reinstated   ~~deleted~~ Deleted   ⊘ Not covered or valid by Medicare
✪ Special coverage instructions   ✳ Carrier discretion   Ⓟ Bill Part B MAC   Ⓑ Bill DME MAC

Replacement Sockets

* **L5700** Replacement, socket, below knee, molded to patient model Ⓑ

* **L5701** Replacement, socket, above knee/knee disarticulation, including attachment plate, molded to patient model Ⓑ

* **L5702** Replacement, socket, hip disarticulation, including hip joint, molded to patient model Ⓑ

* **L5703** Ankle, Symes, molded to patient model, socket without solid ankle cushion heel (SACH) foot, replacement only Ⓑ

Protective Covers

* **L5704** Custom shaped protective cover, below knee Ⓑ

* **L5705** Custom shaped protective cover, above knee Ⓑ

* **L5706** Custom shaped protective cover, knee disarticulation Ⓑ

* **L5707** Custom shaped protective cover, hip disarticulation Ⓑ

Additions to Exoskeletal-Knee-Shin System

* **L5710** Addition, exoskeletal knee-shin system, single axis, manual lock Ⓑ

* **L5711** Additions exoskeletal knee-shin system, single axis, manual lock, ultra-light material Ⓑ

* **L5712** Addition, exoskeletal knee-shin system, single axis, friction swing and stance phase control (safety knee) Ⓑ

* **L5714** Addition, exoskeletal knee-shin system, single axis, variable friction swing phase control Ⓑ

* **L5716** Addition, exoskeletal knee-shin system, polycentric, mechanical stance phase lock Ⓑ

* **L5718** Addition, exoskeletal knee-shin system, polycentric, friction swing and stance phase control Ⓑ

* **L5722** Addition, exoskeletal knee-shin system, single axis, pneumatic swing, friction stance phase control Ⓑ

* **L5724** Addition, exoskeletal knee-shin system, single axis, fluid swing phase control Ⓑ

* **L5726** Addition, exoskeletal knee-shin system, single axis, external joints, fluid swing phase control Ⓑ

* **L5728** Addition, exoskeletal knee-shin system, single axis, fluid swing and stance phase control Ⓑ

* **L5780** Addition, exoskeletal knee-shin system, single axis, pneumatic/hydra pneumatic swing phase control Ⓑ

Vacuum Pumps

* **L5781** Addition to lower limb prosthesis, vacuum pump, residual limb volume management and moisture evacuation system Ⓑ

* **L5782** Addition to lower limb prosthesis, vacuum pump, residual limb volume management and moisture evacuation system, heavy duty Ⓑ

Component Modification

* **L5785** Addition, exoskeletal system, below knee, ultra-light material (titanium, carbon fiber, or equal) Ⓑ

* **L5790** Addition, exoskeletal system, above knee, ultra-light material (titanium, carbon fiber, or equal) Ⓑ

* **L5795** Addition, exoskeletal system, hip disarticulation, ultra-light material (titanium, carbon fiber, or equal) Ⓑ

Endoskeletal

* **L5810** Addition, endoskeletal knee-shin system, single axis, manual lock Ⓑ

* **L5811** Addition, endoskeletal knee-shin system, single axis, manual lock, ultralight material Ⓑ

* **L5812** Addition, endoskeletal knee-shin system, single axis, friction swing and stance phase control (safety knee) Ⓑ

* **L5814** Addition, endoskeletal knee-shin system, polycentric, hydraulic swing phase control, mechanical stance phase lock Ⓑ

* **L5816** Addition, endoskeletal knee-shin system, polycentric, mechanical stance phase lock Ⓑ

* **L5818** Addition, endoskeletal knee-shin system, polycentric, friction swing, and stance phase control Ⓑ

* **L5822** Addition, endoskeletal knee-shin system, single axis, pneumatic swing, friction stance phase control Ⓑ

* **L5824** Addition, endoskeletal knee-shin system, single axis, fluid swing phase control Ⓑ

* **L5826** Addition, endoskeletal knee-shin system, single axis, hydraulic swing phase control, with miniature high activity frame Ⓑ

▶ **New**   ↻ **Revised**   ✔ **Reinstated**   ~~deleted~~ **Deleted**   ⊘ **Not covered or valid by Medicare**

✪ **Special coverage instructions**   * **Carrier discretion**   Ⓑ **Bill Part B MAC**   Ⓑ **Bill DME MAC**

* **L5828** Addition, endoskeletal knee-shin system, single axis, fluid swing and stance phase control ⑧

* **L5830** Addition, endoskeletal knee-shin system, single axis, pneumatic/swing phase control ⑧

* **L5840** Addition, endoskeletal knee/shin system, 4-bar linkage or multiaxial, pneumatic swing phase control ⑧

* **L5845** Addition, endoskeletal, knee-shin system, stance flexion feature, adjustable ⑧

* **L5848** Addition to endoskeletal, knee-shin system, fluid stance extension, dampening feature, with or without adjustability ⑧

* **L5850** Addition, endoskeletal system, above knee or hip disarticulation, knee extension assist ⑧

* **L5855** Addition, endoskeletal system, hip disarticulation, mechanical hip extension assist ⑧

* **L5856** Addition to lower extremity prosthesis, endoskeletal knee-shin system, microprocessor control feature, swing and stance phase; includes electronic sensor(s), any type ⑧

* **L5857** Addition to lower extremity prosthesis, endoskeletal knee-shin system, microprocessor control feature, swing phase only; includes electronic sensor(s), any type ⑧

* **L5858** Addition to lower extremity prosthesis, endoskeletal knee shin system, microprocessor control feature, stance phase only, includes electronic sensor(s), any type ⑧

* **L5859** Addition to lower extremity prosthesis, endoskeletal knee-shin system, powered and programmable flexion/extension assist control, includes any type motor(s) ⑧

* **L5910** Addition, endoskeletal system, below knee, alignable system ⑧

* **L5920** Addition, endoskeletal system, above knee or hip disarticulation, alignable system ⑧

* **L5925** Addition, endoskeletal system, above knee, knee disarticulation or hip disarticulation, manual lock ⑧

* **L5930** Addition, endoskeletal system, high activity knee control frame ⑧

* **L5940** Addition, endoskeletal system, below knee, ultra-light material (titanium, carbon fiber or equal) ⑧

* **L5950** Addition, endoskeletal system, above knee, ultra-light material (titanium, carbon fiber or equal) ⑧

* **L5960** Addition, endoskeletal system, hip disarticulation, ultra-light material (titanium, carbon fiber, or equal) ⑧

* **L5961** Addition, endoskeletal system, polycentric hip joint, pneumatic or hydraulic control, rotation control, with or without flexion, and/or extension control ⑧

* **L5962** Addition, endoskeletal system, below knee, flexible protective outer surface covering system ⑧

* **L5964** Addition, endoskeletal system, above knee, flexible protective outer surface covering system ⑧

* **L5966** Addition, endoskeletal system, hip disarticulation, flexible protective outer surface covering system ⑧

Additions to Ankle and/or Foot

* **L5968** Addition to lower limb prosthesis, multiaxial ankle with swing phase active dorsiflexion feature ⑧

* **L5969** Addition, endoskeletal ankle-foot or ankle system, power assist, includes any type motor(s) ⑧

* **L5970** All lower extremity prostheses, foot, external keel, SACH foot ⑧

* **L5971** All lower extremity prosthesis, solid ankle cushion keel (SACH) foot, replacement only ⑧

* **L5972** All lower extremity prostheses (foot, flexible keel) ⑧

* **L5973** Endoskeletal ankle foot system, microprocessor controlled feature, dorsiflexion and/or plantar flexion control, includes power source ⑧

* **L5974** All lower extremity prostheses, foot, single axis ankle/foot ⑧

* **L5975** All lower extremity prostheses, combination single axis ankle and flexible keel foot ⑧

* **L5976** All lower extremity prostheses, energy storing foot (Seattle Carbon Copy II or equal) ⑧

* **L5978** All lower extremity prostheses, foot, multiaxial ankle/foot ⑧

* **L5979** All lower extremity prostheses, multiaxial ankle, dynamic response foot, one piece system ⑧

▶ **New**   ↻ **Revised**   ✔ **Reinstated**   ~~deleted~~ **Deleted**   ⊘ **Not covered or valid by Medicare**

✪ **Special coverage instructions**   ✱ **Carrier discretion**   ⑨ **Bill Part B MAC**   ⑧ **Bill DME MAC**

* **L5980** All lower extremity prostheses, flex foot system ⑥

* **L5981** All lower extremity prostheses, flexwalk system or equal ⑥

* **L5982** All exoskeletal lower extremity prostheses, axial rotation unit ⑥

* **L5984** All endoskeletal lower extremity prostheses, axial rotation unit, with or without adjustability ⑥

* **L5985** All endoskeletal lower extremity prostheses, dynamic prosthetic pylon ⑥

* **L5986** All lower extremity prostheses, multiaxial rotation unit ('MCP' or equal) ⑥

* **L5987** All lower extremity prostheses, shank foot system with vertical loading pylon ⑥

* **L5988** Addition to lower limb prosthesis, vertical shock reducing pylon feature ⑥

* **L5990** Addition to lower extremity prosthesis, user adjustable heel height ⑥

* **L5999** Lower extremity prosthesis, not otherwise specified ⑥

Upper Limb (L6000-L7600)

NOTE: The procedures in L6000-L6599 are considered as base or basic procedures and may be modified by listing procedures from the additions sections. The base procedures include only standard friction wrist and control cable system unless otherwise specified.

Partial Hand

* **L6000** Partial hand, thumb remaining ⑥

* **L6010** Partial hand, little and/or ring finger remaining ⑥

* **L6020** Partial hand, no finger remaining ⑥

* **L6026** Transcarpal/metacarpal or partial hand disarticulation prosthesis, external power, self-suspended, inner socket with removable forearm section, electrodes and cables, two batteries, charger, myoelectric control of terminal device, excludes terminal device(s) ⑥

Wrist Disarticulation

* **L6050** Wrist disarticulation, molded socket, flexible elbow hinges, triceps pad ⑥

* **L6055** Wrist disarticulation, molded socket with expandable interface, flexible elbow hinges, triceps pad ⑥

Below Elbow

* **L6100** Below elbow, molded socket, flexible elbow hinge, triceps pad ⑥

* **L6110** Below elbow, molded socket, (Muenster or Northwestern suspension types) ⑥

* **L6120** Below elbow, molded double wall split socket, step-up hinges, half cuff ⑥

* **L6130** Below elbow, molded double wall split socket, stump activated locking hinge, half cuff ⑥

Elbow Disarticulation

* **L6200** Elbow disarticulation, molded socket, outside locking hinge, forearm ⑥

* **L6205** Elbow disarticulation, molded socket with expandable interface, outside locking hinges, forearm ⑥

Above Elbow

* **L6250** Above elbow, molded double wall socket, internal locking elbow, forearm ⑥

Shoulder Disarticulation

* **L6300** Shoulder disarticulation, molded socket, shoulder bulkhead, humeral section, internal locking elbow, forearm ⑥

* **L6310** Shoulder disarticulation, passive restoration (complete prosthesis) ⑥

* **L6320** Shoulder disarticulation, passive restoration (shoulder cap only) ⑥

Interscapular Thoracic

* **L6350** Interscapular thoracic, molded socket, shoulder bulkhead, humeral section, internal locking elbow, forearm ⑥

* **L6360** Interscapular thoracic, passive restoration (complete prosthesis) ⑥

* **L6370** Interscapular thoracic, passive restoration (shoulder cap only) ⑥

Immediate and Early Postsurgical Procedures

* **L6380** Immediate post surgical or early fitting, application of initial rigid dressing, including fitting alignment and suspension of components, and one cast change, wrist disarticulation or below elbow ⑥

▶ New   ↻ Revised   ✔ Reinstated   ~~deleted~~ Deleted   ⊘ Not covered or valid by Medicare
✪ Special coverage instructions   * Carrier discretion   Ⓑ Bill Part B MAC   ⑥ Bill DME MAC

* **L6382** Immediate post surgical or early fitting, application of initial rigid dressing including fitting alignment and suspension of components, and one cast change, elbow disarticulation or above elbow ⑧

* **L6384** Immediate post surgical or early fitting, application of initial rigid dressing including fitting alignment and suspension of components, and one cast change, shoulder disarticulation or interscapular thoracic ⑧

* **L6386** Immediate post surgical or early fitting, each additional cast change and realignment ⑧

* **L6388** Immediate post surgical or early fitting, application of rigid dressing only ⑧

Molded Socket

* **L6400** Below elbow, molded socket, endoskeletal system, including soft prosthetic tissue shaping ⑧

* **L6450** Elbow disarticulation, molded socket, endoskeletal system, including soft prosthetic tissue shaping ⑧

* **L6500** Above elbow, molded socket, endoskeletal system, including soft prosthetic tissue shaping ⑧

* **L6550** Shoulder disarticulation, molded socket, endoskeletal system, including soft prosthetic tissue shaping ⑧

* **L6570** Interscapular thoracic, molded socket, endoskeletal system, including soft prosthetic tissue shaping ⑧

Preparatory Prosthetic

* **L6580** Preparatory, wrist disarticulation or below elbow, single wall plastic socket, friction wrist, flexible elbow hinges, figure of eight harness, humeral cuff, Bowden cable control, USMC or equal pylon, no cover, molded to patient model ⑧

* **L6582** Preparatory, wrist disarticulation or below elbow, single wall socket, friction wrist, flexible elbow hinges, figure of eight harness, humeral cuff, Bowden cable control, USMC or equal pylon, no cover, direct formed ⑧

* **L6584** Preparatory, elbow disarticulation or above elbow, single wall plastic socket, friction wrist, locking elbow, figure of eight harness, fair lead cable control, USMC or equal pylon, no cover, molded to patient model ⑧

* **L6586** Preparatory, elbow disarticulation or above elbow, single wall socket, friction wrist, locking elbow, figure of eight harness, fair lead cable control, USMC or equal pylon, no cover, direct formed ⑧

* **L6588** Preparatory, shoulder disarticulation or interscapular thoracic, single wall plastic socket, shoulder joint, locking elbow, friction wrist, chest strap, fair lead cable control, USMC or equal pylon, no cover, molded to patient model ⑧

* **L6590** Preparatory, shoulder disarticulation or interscapular thoracic, single wall socket, shoulder joint, locking elbow, friction wrist, chest strap, fair lead cable control, USMC or equal pylon, no cover, direct formed ⑧

Additions to Upper Limb

NOTE: The following procedures/modifications/components may be added to other base procedures. The items in this section should reflect the additional complexity of each modification procedure, in addition to base procedure, at the time of the original order.

* **L6600** Upper extremity additions, polycentric hinge, pair ⑧

* **L6605** Upper extremity additions, single pivot hinge, pair ⑧

* **L6610** Upper extremity additions, flexible metal hinge, pair ⑧

* **L6611** Addition to upper extremity prosthesis, external powered, additional switch, any type ⑧

* **L6615** Upper extremity addition, disconnect locking wrist unit ⑧

* **L6616** Upper extremity addition, additional disconnect insert for locking wrist unit, each ⑧

* **L6620** Upper extremity addition, flexion/extension wrist unit, with or without friction ⑧

* **L6621** Upper extremity prosthesis addition, flexion/extension wrist with or without friction, for use with external powered terminal device ⑧

* **L6623** Upper extremity addition, spring assisted rotational wrist unit with latch release ⑧

PROSTHETICS

* **L6624** Upper extremity addition, flexion/extension and rotation wrist unit ⑥

* **L6625** Upper extremity addition, rotation wrist unit with cable lock ⑥

* **L6628** Upper extremity addition, quick disconnect hook adapter, Otto Bock or equal ⑥

* **L6629** Upper extremity addition, quick disconnect lamination collar with coupling piece, Otto Bock or equal ⑥

* **L6630** Upper extremity addition, stainless steel, any wrist ⑥

* **L6632** Upper extremity addition, latex suspension sleeve, each ⑥

* **L6635** Upper extremity addition, lift assist for elbow ⑥

* **L6637** Upper extremity addition, nudge control elbow lock ⑥

* **L6638** Upper extremity addition to prosthesis, electric locking feature, only for use with manually powered elbow ⑥

* **L6640** Upper extremity additions, shoulder abduction joint, pair ⑥

* **L6641** Upper extremity addition, excursion amplifier, pulley type ⑥

* **L6642** Upper extremity addition, excursion amplifier, lever type ⑥

* **L6645** Upper extremity addition, shoulder flexion-abduction joint, each ⑥

* **L6646** Upper extremity addition, shoulder joint, multipositional locking, flexion, adjustable abduction friction control, for use with body powered or external powered system ⑥

* **L6647** Upper extremity addition, shoulder lock mechanism, body powered actuator ⑥

* **L6648** Upper extremity addition, shoulder lock mechanism, external powered actuator ⑥

* **L6650** Upper extremity addition, shoulder universal joint, each ⑥

* **L6655** Upper extremity addition, standard control cable, extra ⑥

* **L6660** Upper extremity addition, heavy duty control cable ⑥

* **L6665** Upper extremity addition, Teflon, or equal, cable lining ⑥

* **L6670** Upper extremity addition, hook to hand, cable adapter ⑥

* **L6672** Upper extremity addition, harness, chest or shoulder, saddle type ⑥

* **L6675** Upper extremity addition, harness, (e.g., figure of eight type), single cable design ⑥

* **L6676** Upper extremity addition, harness, (e.g., figure of eight type), dual cable design ⑥

* **L6677** Upper extremity addition, harness, triple control, simultaneous operation of terminal device and elbow ⑥

* **L6680** Upper extremity addition, test socket, wrist disarticulation or below elbow ⑥

* **L6682** Upper extremity addition, test socket, elbow disarticulation or above elbow ⑥

* **L6684** Upper extremity addition, test socket, shoulder disarticulation or interscapular thoracic ⑥

* **L6686** Upper extremity addition, suction socket ⑥

* **L6687** Upper extremity addition, frame type socket, below elbow or wrist disarticulation ⑥

* **L6688** Upper extremity addition, frame type socket, above elbow or elbow disarticulation ⑥

* **L6689** Upper extremity addition, frame type socket, shoulder disarticulation ⑥

* **L6690** Upper extremity addition, frame type socket, interscapular-thoracic ⑥

* **L6691** Upper extremity addition, removable insert, each ⑥

* **L6692** Upper extremity addition, silicone gel insert or equal, each ⑥

* **L6693** Upper extremity addition, locking elbow, forearm counterbalance ⑥

* **L6694** Addition to upper extremity prosthesis, below elbow/above elbow, custom fabricated from existing mold or prefabricated, socket insert, silicone gel, elastomeric or equal, for use with locking mechanism ⑥

* **L6695** Addition to upper extremity prosthesis, below elbow/above elbow, custom fabricated from existing mold or prefabricated, socket insert, silicone gel, elastomeric or equal, not for use with locking mechanism ⑥

* **L6696** Addition to upper extremity prosthesis, below elbow/above elbow, custom fabricated socket insert for congenital or atypical traumatic amputee, silicone gel, elastomeric or equal, for use with or without locking mechanism, initial only (for other than initial, use code L6694 or L6695) ⑥

▶ New   ↻ Revised   ✔ Reinstated   deleted Deleted   ⃠ Not covered or valid by Medicare
☼ Special coverage instructions   ✳ Carrier discretion   Ⓟ Bill Part B MAC   Ⓓ Bill DME MAC

279

PROSTHETICS   L6624 — L6696

✳ **L6697**   Addition to upper extremity prosthesis, below elbow/above elbow, custom fabricated socket insert for other than congenital or atypical traumatic amputee, silicone gel, elastomeric or equal, for use with or without locking mechanism, initial only (for other than initial, use code L6694 or L6695) Ⓑ

✳ **L6698**   Addition to upper extremity prosthesis, below elbow/above elbow, lock mechanism, excludes socket insert Ⓓ

Terminal Devices (L6703-L6882)

✳ **L6703**   Terminal device, passive hand/mitt, any material, any size Ⓓ

✳ **L6704**   Terminal device, sport/recreational/work attachment, any material, any size Ⓑ

✳ **L6706**   Terminal device, hook, mechanical, voluntary opening, any material, any size, lined or unlined Ⓓ

✳ **L6707**   Terminal device, hook, mechanical, voluntary closing, any material, any size, lined or unlined Ⓓ

✳ **L6708**   Terminal device, hand, mechanical, voluntary opening, any material, any size Ⓑ

✳ **L6709**   Terminal device, hand, mechanical, voluntary closing, any material, any size Ⓓ

✳ **L6711**   Terminal device, hook, mechanical, voluntary opening, any material, any size, lined or unlined, pediatric Ⓓ

✳ **L6712**   Terminal device, hook, mechanical, voluntary closing, any material, any size, lined or unlined, pediatric Ⓓ

✳ **L6713**   Terminal device, hand, mechanical, voluntary opening, any material, any size, pediatric Ⓑ

✳ **L6714**   Terminal device, hand, mechanical, voluntary closing, any material, any size, pediatric Ⓓ

✳ **L6715**   Terminal device, multiple articulating digit, includes motor(s), initial issue or replacement Ⓓ

✳ **L6721**   Terminal device, hook or hand, heavy duty, mechanical, voluntary opening, any material, any size, lined or unlined Ⓑ

✳ **L6722**   Terminal device, hook or hand, heavy duty, mechanical, voluntary closing, any material, any size, lined or unlined Ⓑ

✿ **L6805**   Addition to terminal device, modifier wrist unit Ⓑ

IOM: 100-02, 15, 120; 100-04, 3, 10.4

✿ **L6810**   Addition to terminal device, precision pinch device Ⓑ

IOM: 100-02, 15, 120; 100-04, 3, 10.4

✳ **L6880**   Electric hand, switch or myoelectric controlled, independently articulating digits, any grasp pattern or combination of grasp patterns, includes motor(s) Ⓑ

✳ **L6881**   Automatic grasp feature, addition to upper limb electric prosthetic terminal device Ⓑ

✿ **L6882**   Microprocessor control feature, addition to upper limb prosthetic terminal device Ⓑ

IOM: 100-02, 15, 120; 100-04, 3, 10.4

Replacement Sockets

✳ **L6883**   Replacement socket, below elbow/wrist disarticulation, molded to patient model, for use with or without external power Ⓑ

✳ **L6884**   Replacement socket, above elbow/elbow disarticulation, molded to patient model, for use with or without external power Ⓑ

✳ **L6885**   Replacement socket, shoulder disarticulation/interscapular thoracic, molded to patient model, for use with or without external power Ⓑ

Hand Restoration

✳ **L6890**   Addition to upper extremity prosthesis, glove for terminal device, any material, prefabricated, includes fitting and adjustment Ⓑ

✳ **L6895**   Addition to upper extremity prosthesis, glove for terminal device, any material, custom fabricated Ⓑ

✳ **L6900**   Hand restoration (casts, shading and measurements included), partial hand, with glove, thumb or one finger remaining Ⓑ

✳ **L6905**   Hand restoration (casts, shading and measurements included), partial hand, with glove, multiple fingers remaining Ⓑ

✳ **L6910**   Hand restoration (casts, shading and measurements included), partial hand, with glove, no fingers remaining Ⓑ

✳ **L6915**   Hand restoration (shading, and measurements included), replacement glove for above Ⓑ

▶ **New**   ↻ **Revised**   ✔ **Reinstated**   ~~deleted~~ **Deleted**   ⊘ **Not covered or valid by Medicare**

✿ **Special coverage instructions**   ✳ **Carrier discretion**   Ⓑ **Bill Part B MAC**   Ⓓ **Bill DME MAC**

External Power

* **L6920** Wrist disarticulation, external power, self-suspended inner socket, removable forearm shell, Otto Bock or equal switch, cables, two batteries and one charger, switch control of terminal device Ⓑ

* **L6925** Wrist disarticulation, external power, self-suspended inner socket, removable forearm shell, Otto Bock or equal electrodes, cables, two batteries and one charger, myoelectronic control of terminal device Ⓑ

* **L6930** Below elbow, external power, self-suspended inner socket, removable forearm shell, Otto Bock or equal switch, cables, two batteries and one charger, switch control of terminal device Ⓑ

* **L6935** Below elbow, external power, self-suspended inner socket, removable forearm shell, Otto Bock or equal electrodes, cables, two batteries and one charger, myoelectronic control of terminal device Ⓑ

* **L6940** Elbow disarticulation, external power, molded inner socket, removable humeral shell, outside locking hinges, forearm, Otto Bock or equal switch, cables, two batteries and one charger, switch control of terminal device Ⓑ

* **L6945** Elbow disarticulation, external power, molded inner socket, removable humeral shell, outside locking hinges, forearm, Otto Bock or equal electrodes, cables, two batteries and one charger, myoelectronic control of terminal device Ⓑ

* **L6950** Above elbow, external power, molded inner socket, removable humeral shell, internal locking elbow, forearm, Otto Bock or equal switch, cables, two batteries and one charger, switch control of terminal device Ⓑ

* **L6955** Above elbow, external power, molded inner socket, removable humeral shell, internal locking elbow, forearm, Otto Bock or equal electrodes, cables, two batteries and one charger, myoelectronic control of terminal device Ⓑ

* **L6960** Shoulder disarticulation, external power, molded inner socket, removable shoulder shell, shoulder bulkhead, humeral section, mechanical elbow, forearm, Otto Bock or equal switch, cables, two batteries and one charger, switch control of terminal device Ⓑ

* **L6965** Shoulder disarticulation, external power, molded inner socket, removable shoulder shell, shoulder bulkhead, humeral section, mechanical elbow, forearm, Otto Bock or equal electrodes, cables, two batteries and one charger, myoelectronic control of terminal device Ⓑ

* **L6970** Interscapular-thoracic, external power, molded inner socket, removable shoulder shell, shoulder bulkhead, humeral section, mechanical elbow, forearm, Otto Bock or equal switch, cables, two batteries and one charger, switch control of terminal device Ⓑ

* **L6975** Interscapular-thoracic, external power, molded inner socket, removable shoulder shell, shoulder bulkhead, humeral section, mechanical elbow, forearm, Otto Bock or equal electrodes, cables, two batteries and one charger, myoelectronic control of terminal device Ⓑ

Additions to Electronic Hand or Hook

* **L7007** Electric hand, switch or myoelectric controlled, adult Ⓖ

* **L7008** Electric hand, switch or myoelectric controlled, pediatric Ⓑ

* **L7009** Electric hook, switch or myoelectric controlled, adult Ⓖ

* **L7040** Prehensile actuator, switch controlled Ⓖ

* **L7045** Electric hook, switch or myoelectric controlled, pediatric Ⓑ

Additions to Electronic Elbow

* **L7170** Electronic elbow, Hosmer or equal, switch controlled Ⓑ

* **L7180** Electronic elbow, microprocessor sequential control of elbow and terminal device Ⓖ

* **L7181** Electronic elbow, microprocessor simultaneous control of elbow and terminal device Ⓖ

* **L7185** Electronic elbow, adolescent, Variety Village or equal, switch controlled Ⓑ

* **L7186** Electronic elbow, child, Variety Village or equal, switch controlled Ⓑ

* **L7190** Electronic elbow, adolescent, Variety Village or equal, myoelectronically controlled Ⓑ

* **L7191** Electronic elbow, child, Variety Village or equal, myoelectronically controlled Ⓑ

▶ **New**   ↻ **Revised**   ✔ **Reinstated**   ~~deleted~~ **Deleted**   ⊘ **Not covered or valid by Medicare**
✪ **Special coverage instructions**   ✳ **Carrier discretion**   Ⓑ **Bill Part B MAC**   Ⓖ **Bill DME MAC**

Wrist

* L7259   Electronic wrist rotator, any type Ⓑ

Battery Components

* L7360   Six volt battery, each Ⓑ
* L7362   Battery charger, six volt, each Ⓑ
* L7364   Twelve volt battery, each Ⓑ
* L7366   Battery charger, twelve volt, each Ⓑ
* L7367   Lithium ion battery, rechargeable, replacement Ⓑ
* L7368   Lithium ion battery charger, replacement only Ⓑ

Additions

* L7400   Addition to upper extremity prosthesis, below elbow/wrist disarticulation, ultralight material (titanium, carbon fiber or equal) Ⓑ
* L7401   Addition to upper extremity prosthesis, above elbow disarticulation, ultralight material (titanium, carbon fiber or equal) Ⓑ
* L7402   Addition to upper extremity prosthesis, shoulder disarticulation/interscapular thoracic, ultralight material (titanium, carbon fiber or equal) Ⓑ
* L7403   Addition to upper extremity prosthesis, below elbow/wrist disarticulation, acrylic material Ⓑ
* L7404   Addition to upper extremity prosthesis, above elbow disarticulation, acrylic material Ⓑ
* L7405   Addition to upper extremity prosthesis, shoulder disarticulation/interscapular thoracic, acrylic material Ⓑ

Other/Repair

* L7499   Upper extremity prosthesis, not otherwise specified Ⓑ
⊘ L7510   Repair of prosthetic device, repair or replace minor parts Ⓥ Ⓑ

     IOM: 100-02, 15, 110.2; 100-02, 15, 120; 100-04, 32, 100

* L7520   Repair prosthetic device, labor component, per 15 minutes Ⓥ Ⓑ
⊘ L7600   Prosthetic donning sleeve, any material, each Ⓑ

General

Prosthetic Socket Insert

▶ * L7700   Gasket or seal, for use with prosthetic socket insert, any type, each

Penile Prosthetics

⊘ L7900   Male vacuum erection system Ⓑ
⊘ L7902   Tension ring, for vacuum erection device, any type, replacement only, each Ⓑ

Breast Prosthetics

⊘ L8000   Breast prosthesis, mastectomy bra, without integrated breast prosthesis form, any size, any type Ⓑ

     IOM: 100-02, 15, 120

⊘ L8001   Breast prosthesis, mastectomy bra, with integrated breast prosthesis form, unilateral, any size, any type Ⓑ

     IOM: 100-02, 15, 120

⊘ L8002   Breast prosthesis, mastectomy bra, with integrated breast prosthesis form, bilateral, any size, any type Ⓑ

     IOM: 100-02, 15, 120

⊘ L8010   Breast prosthesis, mastectomy sleeve Ⓑ

     IOM: 100-02, 15, 120

⊘ L8015   External breast prosthesis garment, with mastectomy form, post mastectomy Ⓑ

     IOM: 100-02, 15, 120

⊘ L8020   Breast prosthesis, mastectomy form Ⓑ

     IOM: 100-02, 15, 120

⊘ L8030   Breast prosthesis, silicone or equal, without integral adhesive Ⓑ

     IOM: 100-02, 15, 120

⊘ L8031   Breast prosthesis, silicone or equal, with integral adhesive Ⓑ

     IOM: 100-02, 15, 120

* L8032   Nipple prosthesis, reusable, any type, each Ⓑ
⊘ L8035   Custom breast prosthesis, post mastectomy, molded to patient model Ⓑ

     IOM: 100-02, 15, 120

* L8039   Breast prosthesis, not otherwise specified Ⓑ

▶ **New**   ⟲ **Revised**   ✔ **Reinstated**   ~~deleted~~ **Deleted**   ⊘ **Not covered or valid by Medicare**

⊘ **Special coverage instructions**   * **Carrier discretion**   Ⓑ **Bill Part B MAC**   Ⓑ **Bill DME MAC**

Nasal, Orbital, Auricular Prostherics

✳ **L8040** Nasal prosthesis, provided by a non-physician ⑧

✳ **L8041** Midfacial prosthesis, provided by a non-physician ⑧

✳ **L8042** Orbital prosthesis, provided by a non-physician ⑧

✳ **L8043** Upper facial prosthesis, provided by a non-physician ⑧

✳ **L8044** Hemi-facial prosthesis, provided by a non-physician ⑧

✳ **L8045** Auricular prosthesis, provided by a non-physician ⑧

✳ **L8046** Partial facial prosthesis, provided by a non-physician ⑧

✳ **L8047** Nasal septal prosthesis, provided by a non-physician ⑧

✳ **L8048** Unspecified maxillofacial prosthesis, by report, provided by a non-physician ⑧

✳ **L8049** Repair or modification of maxillofacial prosthesis, labor component, 15 minute increments, provided by a non-physician ⑧

Trusses

✿ **L8300** Truss, single with standard pad ⑧

IOM: 100-02, 15, 120; 100-03, 4, 280.11; 100-03, 4, 280.12; 100-04, 4, 240

✿ **L8310** Truss, double with standard pads ⑧

IOM: 100-02, 15, 120; 100-03, 4, 280.11; 100-03, 4, 280.12; 100-04, 4, 240

✿ **L8320** Truss, addition to standard pad, water pad ⑧

IOM: 100-02, 15, 120; 100-03, 4, 280.11; 100-03, 4, 280.12; 100-04, 4, 240

✿ **L8330** Truss, addition to standard pad, scrotal pad ⑧

IOM: 100-02, 15, 120; 100-03, 4, 280.11; 100-03, 4, 280.12; 100-04, 4, 240

Prosthetic Socks

✿ **L8400** Prosthetic sheath, below knee, each ⑧

IOM: 100-02, 15, 200

✿ **L8410** Prosthetic sheath, above knee, each ⑧

IOM: 100-02, 15, 200

✿ **L8415** Prosthetic sheath, upper limb, each ⑧

IOM: 100-02, 15, 200

✳ **L8417** Prosthetic sheath/sock, including a gel cushion layer, below knee or above knee, each ⑧

✿ **L8420** Prosthetic sock, multiple ply, below knee, each ⑧

IOM: 100-02, 15, 200

✿ **L8430** Prosthetic sock, multiple ply, above knee, each ⑧

IOM: 100-02, 15, 200

✿ **L8435** Prosthetic sock, multiple ply, upper limb, each ⑧

IOM: 100-02, 15, 200

✿ **L8440** Prosthetic shrinker, below knee, each ⑧

IOM: 100-02, 15, 200

✿ **L8460** Prosthetic shrinker, above knee, each ⑧

IOM: 100-02, 15, 200

✿ **L8465** Prosthetic shrinker, upper limb, each ⑧

IOM: 100-02, 15, 200

✿ **L8470** Prosthetic sock, single ply, fitting, below knee, each ⑧

IOM: 100-02, 15, 200

✿ **L8480** Prosthetic sock, single ply, fitting, above knee, each ⑧

IOM: 100-02, 15, 200

✿ **L8485** Prosthetic sock, single ply, fitting, upper limb, each ⑧

IOM: 100-02, 15, 200

Unlisted

✳ **L8499** Unlisted procedure for miscellaneous prosthetic services ⑨ ⑧

Prosthetic Implants (L8500-L9900)

Larynx, Tracheoesophageal

✿ **L8500** Artificial larynx, any type ⑧

IOM: 100-02, 15, 120; 100-03, 1, 50.2; 100-04, 4, 240

✿ **L8501** Tracheostomy speaking valve ⑧

IOM: 100-03, 1, 50.4

✳ **L8505** Artificial larynx replacement battery/accessory, any type ⑧

✳ **L8507** Tracheo-esophageal voice prosthesis, patient inserted, any type, each ⑧

✳ **L8509** Tracheo-esophageal voice prosthesis, inserted by a licensed health care provider, any type ⑨ ⑧

✿ **L8510** Voice amplifier ⑧

IOM: 100-03, 1, 50.2

✳ **L8511** Insert for indwelling tracheoesophageal prosthesis, with or without valve, replacement only, each ⑨ ⑧

▶ New	↻ Revised	✔ Reinstated	~~deleted~~ Deleted	⊘ Not covered or valid by Medicare
✿ Special coverage instructions		✳ Carrier discretion	⑨ Bill Part B MAC	⑧ Bill DME MAC

⁕ **L8512** Gelatin capsules or equivalent, for use with tracheoesophageal voice prosthesis, replacement only, per 10 ⑨ ⑬

⁕ **L8513** Cleaning device used with tracheoesophageal voice prosthesis, pipet, brush, or equal, replacement only, each ⑨ ⑬

⁕ **L8514** Tracheoesophageal puncture dilator, replacement only, each ⑨ ⑬

⁕ **L8515** Gelatin capsule, application device for use with tracheoesophageal voice prosthesis, each ⑨ ⑬

Breast

✪ **L8600** Implantable breast prosthesis, silicone or equal ⑬

IOM: 100-02, 15, 120; 100-3, 2, 140.2

Bulking Agents

✪ **L8603** Injectable bulking agent, collagen implant, urinary tract, 2.5 ml syringe, includes shipping and necessary supplies ⑬

Bill on paper, acquisition cost invoice required

IOM: 100-03, 4, 280.1

⁕ **L8604** Injectable bulking agent, dextranomer/hyaluronic acid copolymer implant, urinary tract, 1 ml, includes shipping and necessary supplies ⑬

⁕ **L8605** Injectable bulking agent, dextranomer/hyaluronic acid copolymer implant, anal canal, 1 ml, includes shipping and necessary supplies ⑬

✪ **L8606** Injectable bulking agent, synthetic implant, urinary tract, 1 ml syringe, includes shipping and necessary supplies ⑬

Bill on paper, acquisition cost invoice required

IOM: 100-03, 4, 280.1

✪ **L8607** Injectable bulking agent for vocal cord medialization, 0.1 ml, includes shipping and necessary supplies ⑬

IOM: 100-03, 4, 280.1

Eye and Ear

⁕ **L8609** Artificial cornea ⑬

✪ **L8610** Ocular implant ⑬

IOM: 100-02, 15, 120

✪ **L8612** Aqueous shunt ⑬

IOM: 100-02, 15, 120

Cross Reference Q0074

✪ **L8613** Ossicula implant ⑨

IOM: 100-02, 15, 120

✪ **L8614** Cochlear device, includes all internal and external components ⑬

IOM: 100-02, 15, 120; 100-03, 1, 50.3

✪ **L8615** Headset/headpiece for use with cochlear implant device, replacement ⑨

IOM: 100-03, 1, 50.3

✪ **L8616** Microphone for use with cochlear implant device, replacement ⑨

IOM: 100-03, 1, 50.3

✪ **L8617** Transmitting coil for use with cochlear implant device, replacement ⑬

IOM: 100-03, 1, 50.3

↻ ✪ **L8618** Transmitter cable for use with cochlear implant device or auditory osseointegrated device, replacement ⑨

IOM: 100-03, 1, 50.3

✪ **L8619** Cochlear implant, external speech processor and controller, integrated system, replacement ⑬

IOM: 100-03, 1, 50.3

⁕ **L8621** Zinc air battery for use with cochlear implant device and auditory osseointegrated sound processors, replacement, each ⑨

⁕ **L8622** Alkaline battery for use with cochlear implant device, any size, replacement, each ⑬

⁕ **L8623** Lithium ion battery for use with cochlear implant device speech processor, other than ear level, replacement, each ⑬

↻ ⁕ **L8624** Lithium ion battery for use with cochlear implant or auditory osseointegrated device speech processor, ear level, replacement, each ⑬

▶ ✪ **L8625** External recharging system for battery for use with cochlear implant or auditory osseointegrated device, replacement only, each

IOM: 103-03, PART 1, 50.3

✪ **L8627** Cochlear implant, external speech processor, component, replacement ⑬

IOM: 103-03, PART 1, 50.3

✪ **L8628** Cochlear implant, external controller component, replacement ⑨

IOM: 103-03, PART 1, 50.3

▶ New	↻ Revised	✔ Reinstated	~~deleted~~ Deleted	⊘ Not covered or valid by Medicare
✪ Special coverage instructions		⁕ Carrier discretion	⑬ Bill Part B MAC	⑬ Bill DME MAC

✪ **L8629** Transmitting coil and cable, integrated, for use with cochlear implant device, replacement Ⓑ

IOM: 103-03, PART 1, 50.3

Hand and Foot

✪ **L8630** Metacarpophalangeal joint implant Ⓑ

IOM: 100-02, 15, 120

✪ **L8631** Metacarpal phalangeal joint replacement, two or more pieces, metal (e.g., stainless steel or cobalt chrome), ceramic-like material (e.g., pyrocarbon), for surgical implantation (all sizes, includes entire system) Ⓑ

IOM: 100-02, 15, 120

✪ **L8641** Metatarsal joint implant Ⓑ

IOM: 100-02, 15, 120

✪ **L8642** Hallux implant Ⓑ

May be billed by ambulatory surgical center or surgeon

IOM: 100-02, 15, 120

Cross Reference Q0073

✪ **L8658** Interphalangeal joint spacer, silicone or equal, each Ⓑ

IOM: 100-02, 15, 120

✪ **L8659** Interphalangeal finger joint replacement, 2 or more pieces, metal (e.g., stainless steel or cobalt chrome), ceramic-like material (e.g., pyrocarbon) for surgical implantation, any size Ⓑ

IOM: 100-02, 15, 120

Vascular

✪ **L8670** Vascular graft material, synthetic, implant Ⓑ

IOM: 100-02, 15, 120

Neurostimulator

✪ **L8679** Implantable neurostimulator, pulse generator, any type Ⓑ

IOM: 100-03, 4, 280.4

⊘ **L8680** Implantable neurostimulator electrode, each Ⓑ

Related CPT codes: 43647, 63650, 63655, 64553, 64555, 64560, 64561, 64565, 64573, 64575, 64577, 64580, 64581.

✪ **L8681** Patient programmer (external) for use with implantable programmable neurostimulator pulse generator, replacement only Ⓑ

IOM: 100-03, 4, 280.4

✪ **L8682** Implantable neurostimulator radiofrequency receiver Ⓑ

IOM: 100-03, 4, 280.4

✪ **L8683** Radiofrequency transmitter (external) for use with implantable neurostimulator radiofrequency receiver Ⓑ

IOM: 100-03, 4, 280.4

✪ **L8684** Radiofrequency transmitter (external) for use with implantable sacral root neurostimulator receiver for bowel and bladder management, replacement Ⓑ

IOM: 100-03, 4, 280.4

⊘ **L8685** Implantable neurostimulator pulse generator, single array, rechargeable, includes extension Ⓑ

Related CPT codes: 61885, 64590, 63685.

⊘ **L8686** Implantable neurostimulator pulse generator, single array, non-rechargeable, includes extension Ⓑ

Related CPT codes: 61885, 64590, 63685.

⊘ **L8687** Implantable neurostimulator pulse generator, dual array, rechargeable, includes extension Ⓑ

Related CPT codes: 64590, 63685, 61886.

⊘ **L8688** Implantable neurostimulator pulse generator, dual array, non-rechargeable, includes extension Ⓑ

Related CPT codes: 61885, 64590, 63685.

✪ **L8689** External recharging system for battery (internal) for use with implantable neurostimulator, replacement only Ⓑ

IOM: 100-03, 4, 280.4

Miscellaneous Orthotic and Prosthetic Components, Services, and Supplies

✳ **L8690** Auditory osseointegrated device, includes all internal and external components Ⓑ

Related CPT codes: 69714, 69715, 69717, 69718.

↻ ✳ **L8691** Auditory osseointegrated device, external sound processor, excludes transducer/actuator, replacement only, each Ⓑ

⊘ **L8692** Auditory osseointegrated device, external sound processor, used without osseointegration, body worn, includes headband or other means of external attachment Ⓑ

▶ **New**   ↻ **Revised**   ✔ **Reinstated**   ~~deleted~~ **Deleted**   ⊘ **Not covered or valid by Medicare**
✪ **Special coverage instructions**   ✳ **Carrier discretion**   Ⓑ **Bill Part B MAC**   Ⓓ **Bill DME MAC**

✳ **L8693** Auditory osseointegrated device abutment, any length, replacement only Ⓑ

▶ ✳ **L8694** Auditory osseointegrated device, transducer/actuator, replacement only, each

✿ **L8695** External recharging system for battery (external) for use with implantable neurostimulator, replacement only Ⓑ

IOM: 100-03, 4, 280.4

✿ **L8696** Antenna (external) for use with implantable diaphragmatic/phrenic nerve stimulation device, replacement, each Ⓑ

✳ **L8699** Prosthetic implant, not otherwise specified Ⓑ

✳ **L9900** Orthotic and prosthetic supply, accessory, and/or service component of another HCPCS "L" code

---

▶ **New**   ↻ **Revised**   ✔ **Reinstated**   deleted **Deleted**   ⊘ **Not covered or valid by Medicare**
✿ **Special coverage instructions**   ✳ **Carrier discretion**   Ⓑ **Bill Part B MAC**   Ⓑ **Bill DME MAC**

OTHER MEDICAL SERVICES (M0000-M0301)

○ **M0075** Cellular therapy ⑬

○ **M0076** Prolotherapy ⑬

Prolotherapy stimulates production of new ligament tissue. Not covered by Medicare.

○ **M0100** Intragastric hypothermia using gastric freezing ⑬

○ **M0300** IV chelation therapy (chemical endarterectomy) ⑬

○ **M0301** Fabric wrapping of abdominal aneurysm ⑬

Treatment for abdominal aneurysms that involves wrapping aneurysms with cellophane or fascia lata. Fabric wrapping of abdominal aneurysms is not a covered Medicare procedure.

▶ **New**   ↻ **Revised**   ✔ **Reinstated**   deleted **Deleted**   ○ **Not covered or valid by Medicare**

✿ **Special coverage instructions**   ✳ **Carrier discretion**   ⑬ **Bill Part B MAC**   ⑬ **Bill DME MAC**

LABORATORY SERVICES (P0000-P9999)

Chemistry and toxicology Tests

⊛ **P2028**   Cephalin floculation, blood Ⓑ

This code appears on a CMS list of codes that represent obsolete and unreliable tests and procedures. Verify before reporting.

IOM: 100-03, 4, 300.1,

⊛ **P2029**   Congo red, blood Ⓑ

This code appears on a CMS list of codes that represent obsolete and unreliable tests and procedures. Verify before reporting.

IOM: 100-03, 4, 300.1,

⊘ **P2031**   Hair analysis (excluding arsenic) Ⓑ

IOM: 100-03, 4, 300.1,

⊛ **P2033**   Thymol turbidity, blood Ⓑ

This code appears on a CMS list of codes that represent obsolete and unreliable tests and procedures. Verify before reporting.

IOM: 100-03, 4, 300.1,

⊛ **P2038**   Mucoprotein, blood (seromucoid) (medical necessity procedure) Ⓑ

This code appears on a CMS list of codes that represent obsolete and unreliable tests and procedures. Verify before reporting.

IOM: 100-03, 4, 300.1,

Pathology Screening Tests

⊛ **P3000**   Screening Papanicolaou smear, cervical or vaginal, up to three smears, by technician under physician supervision Ⓑ

Co-insurance and deductible waived

Assign for Pap smear ordered for screening purposes only, conventional method, performed by technician

IOM: 100-03, 3, 190.2

⊛ **P3001**   Screening Papanicolaou smear, cervical or vaginal, up to three smears, requiring interpretation by physician Ⓑ

Co-insurance and deductible waived

Report professional component for Pap smears requiring physician interpretation. There are CPT codes assigned for diagnostic Paps, such as, 88141; HCPCS are for screening Paps.

IOM: 100-03, 3, 190.2

Microbiology Tests

⊘ **P7001**   Culture, bacterial, urine; quantitative, sensitivity study Ⓑ

Cross Reference CPT

Miscellaneous Pathology

⊛ **P9010**   Blood (whole), for transfusion, per unit Ⓑ

Blood furnished on an outpatient basis, subject to Medicare Part B blood deductible; applicable to first 3 pints of whole blood or equivalent units of packed red cells in calendar year

IOM: 100-01, 3, 20.5; 100-02, 1, 10

⊛ **P9011**   Blood, split unit Ⓑ

Reports all splitting activities of any blood component

IOM: 100-01, 3, 20.5; 100-02, 1, 10

⊛ **P9012**   Cryoprecipitate, each unit Ⓑ

IOM: 100-01, 3, 20.5; 100-02, 1, 10

⊛ **P9016**   Red blood cells, leukocytes reduced, each unit Ⓑ

IOM: 100-01, 3, 20.5; 100-02, 1, 10

⊛ **P9017**   Fresh frozen plasma (single donor), frozen within 8 hours of collection, each unit Ⓑ

IOM: 100-01, 3, 20.5; 100-02, 1, 10

⊛ **P9019**   Platelets, each unit Ⓑ

IOM: 100-01, 3, 20.5; 100-02, 1, 10

⊛ **P9020**   Platelet rich plasma, each unit Ⓑ

IOM: 100-01, 3, 20.5; 100-02, 1, 10

⊛ **P9021**   Red blood cells, each unit Ⓑ

IOM: 100-01, 3, 20.5; 100-02, 1, 10

⊛ **P9022**   Red blood cells, washed, each unit Ⓑ

IOM: 100-01, 3, 20.5; 100-02, 1, 10

⊛ **P9023**   Plasma, pooled multiple donor, solvent/detergent treated, frozen, each unit Ⓑ

IOM: 100-01, 3, 20.5; 100-02, 1, 10

⊛ **P9031**   Platelets, leukocytes reduced, each unit Ⓑ

IOM: 100-01, 3, 20.5; 100-02, 1, 10

⊛ **P9032**   Platelets, irradiated, each unit Ⓑ

IOM: 100-01, 3, 20.5; 100-02, 1, 10

⊛ **P9033**   Platelets, leukocytes reduced, irradiated, each unit Ⓑ

IOM: 100-01, 3, 20.5; 100-02, 1, 10

▶ New	⟳ Revised	✔ Reinstated	deleted Deleted	⊘ Not covered or valid by Medicare
⊛ Special coverage instructions		✳ Carrier discretion	Ⓑ Bill Part B MAC	Ⓓ Bill DME MAC

⊛ **P9034** Platelets, pheresis, each unit Ⓑ

IOM: 100-01, 3, 20.5; 100-02, 1, 10

⊛ **P9035** Platelets, pheresis, leukocytes reduced, each unit Ⓑ

IOM: 100-01, 3, 20.5; 100-02, 1, 10

⊛ **P9036** Platelets, pheresis, irradiated, each unit Ⓑ

IOM: 100-01, 3, 20.5; 100-02, 1, 10

⊛ **P9037** Platelets, pheresis, leukocytes reduced, irradiated, each unit Ⓑ

IOM: 100-01, 3, 20.5; 100-02, 1, 10

⊛ **P9038** Red blood cells, irradiated, each unit Ⓑ

IOM: 100-01, 3, 20.5; 100-02, 1, 10

⊛ **P9039** Red blood cells, deglycerolized, each unit Ⓑ

IOM: 100-01, 3, 20.5; 100-02, 1, 10

⊛ **P9040** Red blood cells, leukocytes reduced, irradiated, each unit Ⓑ

IOM: 100-01, 3, 20.5; 100-02, 1, 10

✳ **P9041** Infusion, albumin (human), 5%, 50 ml Ⓑ

⊛ **P9043** Infusion, plasma protein fraction (human), 5%, 50 ml Ⓑ

IOM: 100-01, 3, 20.5; 100-02, 1, 10

⊛ **P9044** Plasma, cryoprecipitate reduced, each unit Ⓑ

IOM: 100-01, 3, 20.5; 100-02, 1, 10

✳ **P9045** Infusion, albumin (human), 5%, 250 ml Ⓑ

✳ **P9046** Infusion, albumin (human), 25%, 20 ml Ⓑ

✳ **P9047** Infusion, albumin (human), 25%, 50 ml Ⓑ

✳ **P9048** Infusion, plasma protein fraction (human), 5%, 250 ml Ⓑ

✳ **P9050** Granulocytes, pheresis, each unit Ⓑ

⊛ **P9051** Whole blood or red blood cells, leukocytes reduced, CMV-negative, each unit Ⓑ

⊛ **P9052** Platelets, HLA-matched leukocytes reduced, apheresis/pheresis, each unit Ⓑ

⊛ **P9053** Platelets, pheresis, leukocytes reduced, CMV-negative, irradiated, each unit Ⓑ

Freezing and thawing are reported separately, see Transmittal 1487 (Hospital outpatient)

⊛ **P9054** Whole blood or red blood cells, leukocytes reduced, frozen, deglycerol, washed, each unit Ⓑ

⊛ **P9055** Platelets, leukocytes reduced, CMV-negative, apheresis/pheresis, each unit Ⓑ

⊛ **P9056** Whole blood, leukocytes reduced, irradiated, each unit Ⓑ

⊛ **P9057** Red blood cells, frozen/deglycerolized/washed, leukocytes reduced, irradiated, each unit Ⓑ

⊛ **P9058** Red blood cells, leukocytes reduced, CMV-negative, irradiated, each unit Ⓑ

⊛ **P9059** Fresh frozen plasma between 8-24 hours of collection, each unit Ⓑ

⊛ **P9060** Fresh frozen plasma, donor retested, each unit Ⓑ

⊛ **P9070** Plasma, pooled multiple donor, pathogen reduced, frozen, each unit Ⓑ

⊛ **P9071** Plasma (single donor), pathogen reduced, frozen, each unit Ⓑ

IOM: 100-01, 3, 20.5; 100-02, 1, 10

~~P9072~~ ~~Platelets, pheresis, pathogen reduced or rapid bacterial tested, each unit~~ ✖

▶ ⊛ **P9073** Platelets, pheresis, pathogen-reduced, each unit

IOM: 100-01, 3, 20.5; 100-02, 1, 10

▶ ⊛ **P9100** Pathogen(s) test for platelets

IOM: 100-03, 4, 300.1

Travel Allowance for Specimen Collection

⊛ **P9603** Travel allowance one way in connection with medically necessary laboratory specimen collection drawn from home bound or nursing home bound patient; prorated miles actually traveled Ⓑ

Fee for clinical laboratory travel (P9603) is $1.025 per mile for CY2015.

IOM: 100-04, 16, 60

⊛ **P9604** Travel allowance one way in connection with medically necessary laboratory specimen collection drawn from home bound or nursing home bound patient; prorated trip charge Ⓑ

For CY2010, the fee for clinical laboratory travel is $10.30 per flat rate trip for CY2015.

IOM: 100-04, 16, 60

▶ New   ↻ Revised   ✔ Reinstated   ~~deleted~~ Deleted   ⊘ Not covered or valid by Medicare

⊛ Special coverage instructions   ✳ Carrier discretion   Ⓑ Bill Part B MAC   Ⓑ Bill DME MAC

Catheterization for Specimen Collection

⊕ **P9612** Catheterization for collection of specimen, single patient, all places of service ⑧

NCCI edits indicate that when 51701 is comprehensive or is a Column 1 code, P9612 cannot be reported. When the catheter insertion is a component of another procedure, do not report straight catheterization separately.

IOM: 100-04, 16, 60

⊕ **P9615** Catheterization for collection of specimen(s) (multiple patients) ⑧

IOM: 100-04, 16, 60

TEMPORARY CODES ASSIGNED BY CMS
(Q0000-Q9999)

Cardiokymography

⊗ **Q0035** Cardiokymography Ⓑ

Report modifier 26 if professional component only

IOM: 100-03, 1, 20.24

Infusion Therapy

⊗ **Q0081** Infusion therapy, using other than chemotherapeutic drugs, per visit Ⓑ

IV piggyback only assigned one time per patient encounter per day. Report for hydration or the intravenous administration of antibiotics, anti-emetics, or analgesics. Bill on paper. Requires a report.

IOM: 100-03, 4, 280.14

Chemotherapy Administration

✳ **Q0083** Chemotherapy administration by other than infusion technique only (e.g., subcutaneous, intramuscular, push), per visit Ⓑ

⊗ **Q0084** Chemotherapy administration by infusion technique only, per visit Ⓑ

IOM: 100-03, 4, 280.14

✳ **Q0085** Chemotherapy administration by both infusion technique and other technique(s) (e.g., subcutaneous, intramuscular, push), per visit Ⓑ

Smear Preparation

⊗ **Q0091** Screening Papanicolaou smear; obtaining, preparing and conveyance of cervical or vaginal smear to laboratory Ⓑ

Medicare does not cover comprehensive preventive medicine services; however, services described by G0101 and Q0091 (only for Medicare patients) are covered. Includes the services necessary to procure and transport the specimen to the laboratory.

IOM: 100-03, 3, 190.2

Portable X-ray Setup

⊗ **Q0092** Set-up portable x-ray equipment Ⓑ

IOM: 100-04, 13, 90

Miscellaneous Lab Services

✳ **Q0111** Wet mounts, including preparations of vaginal, cervical or skin specimens Ⓑ

✳ **Q0112** All potassium hydroxide (KOH) preparations Ⓑ

✳ **Q0113** Pinworm examinations Ⓑ

✳ **Q0114** Fern test Ⓑ

✳ **Q0115** Post-coital direct, qualitative examinations of vaginal or cervical mucous Ⓑ

Drugs

✳ **Q0138** Injection, ferumoxytol, for treatment of iron deficiency anemia, 1 mg (non-ESRD use) Ⓑ

Feraheme is FDA approved for chronic kidney disease.

✳ **Q0139** Injection, ferumoxytol, for treatment of iron deficiency anemia, 1 mg (for ESRD on dialysis) Ⓑ

⊘ **Q0144** Azithromycin dihydrate, oral, capsules/powder, 1 gm Ⓑ Ⓓ

✳ **Q0161** Chlorpromazine hydrochloride, 5 mg, oral, FDA approved prescription anti-emetic, for use as a complete therapeutic substitute for an IV anti-emetic at the time of chemotherapy treatment, not to exceed a 48 hour dosage regimen Ⓓ

⊗ **Q0162** Ondansetron 1 mg, oral, FDA-approved prescription anti-emetic, for use as a complete therapeutic substitute for an iv anti-emetic at the time of chemotherapy treatment, not to exceed a 48 hour dosage regimen Ⓓ

⊗ **Q0163** Diphenhydramine hydrochloride, 50 mg, oral, FDA approved prescription anti-emetic, for use as a complete therapeutic substitute for an IV anti-emetic at time of chemotherapy treatment not to exceed a 48 hour dosage regimen Ⓓ

▶ New   ↻ Revised   ✔ Reinstated   ~~deleted~~ Deleted   ⊘ Not covered or valid by Medicare

⊗ Special coverage instructions   ✳ Carrier discretion   Ⓑ Bill Part B MAC   Ⓓ Bill DME MAC

⊘ **Q0164** Prochlorperazine maleate, 5 mg, oral, FDA approved prescription anti-emetic, for use as a complete therapeutic substitute for an IV anti-emetic at the time of chemotherapy treatment, not to exceed a 48 hour dosage regimen Ⓑ

⊘ **Q0166** Granisetron hydrochloride, 1 mg, oral, FDA approved prescription anti-emetic, for use as a complete therapeutic substitute for an IV anti-emetic at the time of chemotherapy treatment, not to exceed a 24 hour dosage regimen Ⓑ

⊘ **Q0167** Dronabinol, 2.5 mg, oral, FDA approved prescription anti-emetic, for use as a complete therapeutic substitute for an IV anti-emetic at the time of chemotherapy treatment, not to exceed a 48 hour dosage regimen Ⓑ

⊘ **Q0169** Promethazine hydrochloride, 12.5 mg, oral, FDA approved prescription anti-emetic, for use as a complete therapeutic substitute for an IV anti-emetic at the time of chemotherapy treatment, not to exceed a 48 hour dosage regimen Ⓑ

⊘ **Q0173** Trimethobenzamide hydrochloride, 250 mg, oral, FDA approved prescription anti-emetic, for use as a complete therapeutic substitute for an IV anti-emetic at the time of chemotherapy treatment, not to exceed a 48 hour dosage regimen Ⓑ

⊘ **Q0174** Thiethylperazine maleate, 10 mg, oral, FDA approved prescription anti-emetic, for use as a complete therapeutic substitute for an IV anti-emetic at the time of chemotherapy treatment, not to exceed a 48 hour dosage regimen Ⓑ

⊘ **Q0175** Perphenazine, 4 mg, oral, FDA approved prescription anti-emetic, for use as a complete therapeutic substitute for an IV anti-emetic at the time of chemotherapy treatment, not to exceed a 48 hour dosage regimen Ⓑ

⊘ **Q0177** Hydroxyzine pamoate, 25 mg, oral, FDA approved prescription anti-emetic, for use as a complete therapeutic substitute for an IV anti-emetic at the time of chemotherapy treatment, not to exceed a 48 hour dosage regimen Ⓑ

⊘ **Q0180** Dolasetron mesylate, 100 mg, oral, FDA approved prescription anti-emetic, for use as a complete therapeutic substitute for an IV anti-emetic at the time of chemotherapy treatment, not to exceed a 24 hour dosage regimen Ⓑ

⊘ **Q0181** Unspecified oral dosage form, FDA approved prescription anti-emetic, for use as a complete therapeutic substitute for a IV anti-emetic at the time of chemotherapy treatment, not to exceed a 48 hour dosage regimen Ⓑ

Ventricular Assist Devices

▶ ⊘ **Q0477** Power module patient cable for use with electric or electric/pneumatic ventricular assist device, replacement only

⊘ **Q0478** Power adapter for use with electric or electric/pneumatic ventricular assist device, vehicle type Ⓑ

CMS has determined the reasonable useful lifetime is one year. Add modifier RA to claims to report when battery is replaced because it was lost, stolen, or irreparably damaged.

⊘ **Q0479** Power module for use with electric or electric/pneumatic ventricular assist device, replacemment only Ⓑ

CMS has determined the reasonable useful lifetime is one year. Add modifier RA in cases where the battery is being replaced because it was lost, stolen, or irreparably damaged.

⊘ **Q0480** Driver for use with pneumatic ventricular assist device, replacement only Ⓑ

⊘ **Q0481** Microprocessor control unit for use with electric ventricular assist device, replacement only Ⓑ

⊘ **Q0482** Microprocessor control unit for use with electric/pneumatic combination ventricular assist device, replacement only Ⓑ

⊘ **Q0483** Monitor/display module for use with electric ventricular assist device, replacement only Ⓑ

⊘ **Q0484** Monitor/display module for use with electric or electric/pneumatic ventricular assist device, replacement only Ⓑ

⊘ **Q0485** Monitor control cable for use with electric ventricular assist device, replacement only Ⓑ

⊘ **Q0486** Monitor control cable for use with electric/pneumatic ventricular assist device, replacement only Ⓑ

⊘ **Q0487** Leads (pneumatic/electrical) for use with any type electric/pneumatic ventricular assist device, replacement only Ⓑ

✪ **Q0488** Power pack base for use with electric ventricular assist device, replacement only ⑧

✪ **Q0489** Power pack base for use with electric/pneumatic ventricular assist device, replacement only ⑧

✪ **Q0490** Emergency power source for use with electric ventricular assist device, replacement only ⑧

✪ **Q0491** Emergency power source for use with electric/pneumatic ventricular assist device, replacement only ⑧

✪ **Q0492** Emergency power supply cable for use with electric ventricular assist device, replacement only ⑧

✪ **Q0493** Emergency power supply cable for use with electric/pneumatic ventricular assist device, replacement only ⑧

✪ **Q0494** Emergency hand pump for use with electric or electric/pneumatic ventricular assist device, replacement only ⑧

✪ **Q0495** Battery/power pack charger for use with electric or electric/pneumatic ventricular assist device, replacement only ⑧

✪ **Q0496** Battery, other than lithium-ion, for use with electric or electric/pneumatic ventricular assist device, replacement only ⑧

Reasonable useful lifetime is 6 months (CR3931).

✪ **Q0497** Battery clips for use with electric or electric/pneumatic ventricular assist device, replacement only ⑧

✪ **Q0498** Holster for use with electric or electric/pneumatic ventricular assist device, replacement only ⑧

✪ **Q0499** Belt/vest/bag for use to carry external peripheral components of any type ventricular assist device, replacement only ⑧

✪ **Q0500** Filters for use with electric or electric/pneumatic ventricular assist device, replacement only ⑧

✪ **Q0501** Shower cover for use with electric or electric/pneumatic ventricular assist device, replacement only ⑧

✪ **Q0502** Mobility cart for pneumatic ventricular assist device, replacement only ⑧

✪ **Q0503** Battery for pneumatic ventricular assist device, replacement only, each ⑧

Reasonable useful lifetime is 6 months (CR3931).

✪ **Q0504** Power adapter for pneumatic ventricular assist device, replacement only, vehicle type ⑧

✪ **Q0506** Battery, lithium-ion, for use with electric or electric/pneumatic, ventricular assist device, replacement only ⑧

Reasonable useful lifetime is 12 months. Add -RA for replacement if lost, stolen, or irreparable damage.

✪ **Q0507** Miscellaneous supply or accessory for use with an external ventricular assist device ⑧

✪ **Q0508** Miscellaneous supply or accessory for use with an implanted ventricular assist device ⑧

✪ **Q0509** Miscellaneous supply or accessory for use with any implanted ventricular assist device for which payment was not made under Medicare Part A ⑧

Pharmacy: Supply and Dispensing Fee

✪ **Q0510** Pharmacy supply fee for initial immunosuppressive drug(s), first month following transplant ⑧

✪ **Q0511** Pharmacy supply fee for oral anti-cancer, oral anti-emetic or immunosuppressive drug(s); for the first prescription in a 30-day period ⑧

✪ **Q0512** Pharmacy supply fee for oral anti-cancer, oral anti-emetic or immunosuppressive drug(s); for a subsequent prescription in a 30-day period ⑧

✪ **Q0513** Pharmacy dispensing fee for inhalation drug(s); per 30 days ⑧

✪ **Q0514** Pharmacy dispensing fee for inhalation drug(s); per 90 days ⑧

Sermorelin Acetate

✪ **Q0515** Injection, sermorelin acetate, 1 microgram ⑧

IOM: 100-02, 15, 50

New Technology: Intraocular Lens

✪ **Q1004** New technology intraocular lens category 4 as defined in Federal Register notice ⑧

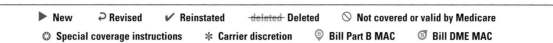

▶ New   ↩ Revised   ✔ Reinstated   ~~deleted~~ Deleted   ⊘ Not covered or valid by Medicare
✪ Special coverage instructions   ✳ Carrier discretion   ⑧ Bill Part B MAC   ⑨ Bill DME MAC

⊘ **Q1005** New technology intraocular lens category 5 as defined in Federal Register notice ⑨

Solutions and Drugs

⊘ **Q2004** Irrigation solution for treatment of bladder calculi, for example renacidin, per 500 ml ⑧

IOM: 100-02, 15, 50

↻⊘ **Q2009** Injection, fosphenytoin, 50 mg phenytoin equivalent ⑧

IOM: 100-02, 15, 50

⊘ **Q2017** Injection, teniposide, 50 mg ⑧

IOM: 100-02, 15, 50

⊘ **Q2026** Injection, radiesse, 0.1 ml ⑧

⊘ **Q2028** Injection, sculptra, 0.5 mg ⑧

⊘ **Q2034** Influenza virus vaccine, split virus, for intramuscular use (Agriflu) Sipuleucel-t, minimum of 50 million autologous CD54+ cells activated with PAP-GM-CSF, including leukapheresis and all other preparatory procedures, per infusion ⑧

IOM: 100-02, 15, 50

⊘ **Q2035** Influenza virus vaccine, split virus, when administered to individuals 3 years of age and older, for intramuscular use (Afluria) ⑧

Preventive service; no deductible

IOM: 100-02, 15, 50

⊘ **Q2036** Influenza virus vaccine, split virus, when administered to individuals 3 years of age and older, for intramuscular use (Flulaval) ⑨

Preventive service; no deductible

IOM: 100-02, 15, 50

⊘ **Q2037** Influenza virus vaccine, split virus, when administered to individuals 3 years of age and older, for intramuscular use (Fluvirin) ⑧

Preventive service; no deductible

IOM: 100-02, 15, 50

⊘ **Q2038** Influenza virus vaccine, split virus, when administered to individuals 3 years of age or older, for intramuscular use (Fluzone) ⑧

Preventive service; no deductible

IOM: 100-02, 15, 50

⊘ **Q2039** Influenza virus vaccine, not otherwise specified ⑧

Preventive service; no deductible

IOM: 100-02, 15, 50

▶ ✳ **Q2040** Tisagenlecleucel, up to 250 million car-positive viable T cells, including leukapheresis and dose preparation procedures, per infusion

⊘ **Q2043** Sipuleucel-T, minimum of 50 million autologous CD54+ cells activated with PAP-GM-CSF, including leukapheresis and all other preparatory procedures, per infusion ⑧

✳ **Q2049** Injection, doxorubicin hydrochloride, liposomal, imported lipodox, 10 mg ⑨ ⑧

⊘ **Q2050** Injection, doxorubicin hydrochloride, liposomal, not otherwise specified, 10 mg ⑨ ⑧

IOM: 100-02, 15, 50

⊘ **Q2052** Services, supplies and accessories used in the home under the Medicare intravenous immune globulin (IVIG) demonstration ⑧

Brachytherapy Radioelements

⊘ **Q3001** Radioelements for brachytherapy, any type, each ⑧

IOM: 100-04, 12, 70; 100-04, 13, 20

Telehealth

✳ **Q3014** Telehealth originating site facility fee ⑨

Effective January of each year, the fee for telehealth services is increased by the Medicare Economic Index (MEI). The telehealth originating facility site fee (HCPCS code Q3014) for 2011 was 80 percent of the lesser of the actual charge or $24.10.

Drugs

⊘ **Q3027** Injection, interferon beta-1a, 1 mcg for intramuscular use ⑧

IOM: 100-02, 15, 50

⊘ **Q3028** Injection, interferon beta-1a, 1 mcg for subcutaneous use ⑧

▶ New	↻ Revised	✔ Reinstated	~~deleted~~ Deleted	⊘ Not covered or valid by Medicare
⊘ Special coverage instructions		✳ Carrier discretion	⑨ Bill Part B MAC	⑧ Bill DME MAC

Skin Test

⊕ **Q3031**   Collagen skin test ⑧
IOM: 100-03, 4, 280.1

Supplies: Cast

Q4001-Q4051: Payment on a reasonable charge basis is required for splints, casts by regulations contained in 42 CFR 405.501.

✳ **Q4001**   Casting supplies, body cast adult, with or without head, plaster ⑧

✳ **Q4002**   Cast supplies, body cast adult, with or without head, fiberglass ⑧

✳ **Q4003**   Cast supplies, shoulder cast, adult (11 years +), plaster ⑧

✳ **Q4004**   Cast supplies, shoulder cast, adult (11 years +), fiberglass ⑧

✳ **Q4005**   Cast supplies, long arm cast, adult (11 years +), plaster ⑧

✳ **Q4006**   Cast supplies, long arm cast, adult (11 years +), fiberglass ⑧

✳ **Q4007**   Cast supplies, long arm cast, pediatric (0-10 years), plaster ⑧

✳ **Q4008**   Cast supplies, long arm cast, pediatric (0-10 years), fiberglass ⑧

✳ **Q4009**   Cast supplies, short arm cast, adult (11 years +), plaster ⑧

✳ **Q4010**   Cast supplies, short arm cast, adult (11 years +), fiberglass ⑧

✳ **Q4011**   Cast supplies, short arm cast, pediatric (0-10 years), plaster ⑧

✳ **Q4012**   Cast supplies, short arm cast, pediatric (0-10 years), fiberglass ⑧

✳ **Q4013**   Cast supplies, gauntlet cast (includes lower forearm and hand), adult (11 years +), plaster ⑧

✳ **Q4014**   Cast supplies, gauntlet cast (includes lower forearm and hand), adult (11 years +), fiberglass ⑧

✳ **Q4015**   Cast supplies, gauntlet cast (includes lower forearm and hand), pediatric (0-10 years), plaster ⑧

✳ **Q4016**   Cast supplies, gauntlet cast (includes lower forearm and hand), pediatric (0-10 years), fiberglass ⑧

✳ **Q4017**   Cast supplies, long arm splint, adult (11 years +), plaster ⑧

✳ **Q4018**   Cast supplies, long arm splint, adult (11 years +), fiberglass ⑧

✳ **Q4019**   Cast supplies, long arm splint, pediatric (0-10 years), plaster ⑧

✳ **Q4020**   Cast supplies, long arm splint, pediatric (0-10 years), fiberglass ⑧

✳ **Q4021**   Cast supplies, short arm splint, adult (11 years +), plaster ⑧

✳ **Q4022**   Cast supplies, short arm splint, adult (11 years +), fiberglass ⑧

✳ **Q4023**   Cast supplies, short arm splint, pediatric (0-10 years), plaster ⑧

✳ **Q4024**   Cast supplies, short arm splint, pediatric (0-10 years), fiberglass ⑧

✳ **Q4025**   Cast supplies, hip spica (one or both legs), adult (11 years +), plaster ⑧

✳ **Q4026**   Cast supplies, hip spica (one or both legs), adult (11 years +), fiberglass ⑧

✳ **Q4027**   Cast supplies, hip spica (one or both legs), pediatric (0-10 years), plaster ⑧

✳ **Q4028**   Cast supplies, hip spica (one or both legs), pediatric (0-10 years), fiberglass ⑧

✳ **Q4029**   Cast supplies, long leg cast, adult (11 years +), plaster ⑧

✳ **Q4030**   Cast supplies, long leg cast, adult (11 years +), fiberglass ⑧

✳ **Q4031**   Cast supplies, long leg cast, pediatric (0-10 years), plaster ⑧

✳ **Q4032**   Cast supplies, long leg cast, pediatric (0-10 years), fiberglass ⑧

✳ **Q4033**   Cast supplies, long leg cylinder cast, adult (11 years +), plaster ⑧

✳ **Q4034**   Cast supplies, long leg cylinder cast, adult (11 years +), fiberglass ⑧

✳ **Q4035**   Cast supplies, long leg cylinder cast, pediatric (0-10 years), plaster ⑧

✳ **Q4036**   Cast supplies, long leg cylinder cast, pediatric (0-10 years), fiberglass ⑧

✳ **Q4037**   Cast supplies, short leg cast, adult (11 years +), plaster ⑧

✳ **Q4038**   Cast supplies, short leg cast, adult (11 years +), fiberglass ⑧

✳ **Q4039**   Cast supplies, short leg cast, pediatric (0-10 years), plaster ⑧

✳ **Q4040**   Cast supplies, short leg cast, pediatric (0-10 years), fiberglass ⑧

✳ **Q4041**   Cast supplies, long leg splint, adult (11 years +), plaster ⑧

✳ **Q4042**   Cast supplies, long leg splint, adult (11 years +), fiberglass ⑧

✳ **Q4043**   Cast supplies, long leg splint, pediatric (0-10 years), plaster ⑧

✳ **Q4044**   Cast supplies, long leg splint, pediatric (0-10 years), fiberglass ⑧

▶ New   ↻ Revised   ✔ Reinstated   ~~deleted~~ Deleted   ⊘ Not covered or valid by Medicare

⊕ Special coverage instructions   ✳ Carrier discretion   ⑧ Bill Part B MAC   ⑨ Bill DME MAC

✳ **Q4045** Cast supplies, short leg splint, adult (11 years +), plaster ⑧

✳ **Q4046** Cast supplies, short leg splint, adult (11 years +), fiberglass ⑧

✳ **Q4047** Cast supplies, short leg splint, pediatric (0-10 years), plaster ⑧

✳ **Q4048** Cast supplies, short leg splint, pediatric (0-10 years), fiberglass ⑧

✳ **Q4049** Finger splint, static ⑧

✳ **Q4050** Cast supplies, for unlisted types and materials of casts ⑧

✳ **Q4051** Splint supplies, miscellaneous (includes thermoplastics, strapping, fasteners, padding and other supplies) ⑧

Drugs

✳ **Q4074** Iloprost, inhalation solution, FDA-approved final product, non-compounded, administered through DME, unit dose form, up to 20 micrograms ⑨ ⑧

⊗ **Q4081** Injection, epoetin alfa, 100 units (for ESRD on dialysis) ⑧

✳ **Q4082** Drug or biological, not otherwise classified, Part B drug competitive acquisition program (CAP) ⑧

Skin Substitutes

✳ **Q4100** Skin substitute, not otherwise specified ⑧

✳ **Q4101** Apligraf, per square centimeter ⑧

✳ **Q4102** Oasis Wound Matrix, per square centimeter ⑧

✳ **Q4103** Oasis Burn Matrix, per square centimeter ⑧

✳ **Q4104** Integra Bilayer Matrix Wound Dressing (BMWD), per square centimeter ⑧

✳ **Q4105** Integra Dermal Regeneration Template (DRT,) or integra omnigraft dermal regeneration matrix, per square centimeter ⑧

✳ **Q4106** Dermagraft, per square centimeter ⑧

✳ **Q4107** Graftjacket, per square centimeter ⑧

✳ **Q4108** Integra Matrix, per square centimeter ⑧

✳ **Q4110** Primatrix, per square centimeter ⑧

✳ **Q4111** GammaGraft, per square centimeter ⑧

✳ **Q4112** Cymetra, injectable, 1 cc ⑧

✳ **Q4113** GraftJacket Xpress, injectable, 1 cc ⑧

✳ **Q4114** Integra Flowable Wound Matrix, injectable, 1 cc ⑧

✳ **Q4115** Alloskin, per square centimeter ⑧

✳ **Q4116** Alloderm, per square centimeter ⑧

✳ **Q4117** Hyalomatrix, per square centimeter ⑧

IOM: 100-02, 15, 50

✳ **Q4118** Matristem micromatrix, 1 mg ⑧

↩ ✳ **Q4121** Theraskin, per square centimeter ⑧

✳ **Q4122** Dermacell, per square centimeter ⑧

✳ **Q4123** AlloSkin RT, per square centimeter ⑧

✳ **Q4124** Oasis Ultra Tri-layer Wound Matrix, per square centimeter ⑧

✳ **Q4125** Arthroflex, per square centimeter ⑧

✳ **Q4126** Memoderm, dermaspan, tranzgraft or integuply, per square centimeter ⑧

✳ **Q4127** Talymed, per square centimeter ⑧

✳ **Q4128** FlexHD, Allopatch HD, or Matrix HD, per square centimeter ⑧

✳ **Q4130** Strattice TM, per square centimeter ⑧

✳ **Q4131** Epifix, per square centimeter ⑧

↩ ✳ **Q4132** Grafix core and GrafixPL core, per square centimeter ⑧

↩ ✳ **Q4133** Grafix prime and GrafixPL prime, per square centimeter ⑧

✳ **Q4134** Hmatrix, per square centimeter ⑧

✳ **Q4135** Mediskin, per square centimeter ⑧

✳ **Q4136** Ez-derm, per square centimeter ⑧

✳ **Q4137** Amnioexcel or biodexcel, per square centimeter ⑧

✳ **Q4138** Biodfence dryflex, per square centimeter ⑧

✳ **Q4139** Amniomatrix or biodmatrix, injectable, 1 cc ⑧

✳ **Q4140** Biodfence, per square centimeter ⑧

✳ **Q4141** Alloskin ac, per square centimeter ⑧

✳ **Q4142** XCM biologic tissue matrix, per square centimeter ⑧

✳ **Q4143** Repriza, per square centimeter ⑧

✳ **Q4145** Epifix, injectable, 1 mg ⑧

✳ **Q4146** Tensix, per square centimeter ⑧

✳ **Q4147** Architect, architect PX, or architect FX, extracellular matrix, per square centimeter ⑧

↩ ✳ **Q4148** Neox cord 1K, Neox cord RT, or Clarix cord 1K, per square centimeter ⑧

✳ **Q4149** Excellagen, 0.1 cc ⑧

✳ **Q4150** AlloWrap DS or dry, per square centimeter ⑧

✳ **Q4151** Amnioband or guardian, per square centimeter ⑨

✳ **Q4152** DermaPure, per square centimeter ⑧

✳ **Q4153** Dermavest and Plurivest, per square centimeter ⑨

✳ **Q4154** Biovance, per square centimeter ⑧

✳ **Q4155** Neoxflo or clarixflo, 1 mg ⑨

↻ ✳ **Q4156** NEOX 100 or Clarix 100, per square centimeter ⑨

✳ **Q4157** Revitalon, per square centimeter ⑧

↻ ✳ **Q4158** Kerecis Omega3, per square centimeter ⑨

✳ **Q4159** Affinity, per square centimeter ⑧

✳ **Q4160** Nushield, per square centimeter ⑧

✳ **Q4161** Bio-ConneKt Wound Matrix, per square centimeter ⑧

↻ ✳ **Q4162** Woundex flow, BioSkin flow 0.5 cc ⑨

↻ ✳ **Q4163** Woundex, BioSkin per square centimeter ⑧

✳ **Q4164** Helicoll, per square centimeter ⑧

✳ **Q4165** Keramatrix, per square centimeter ⑧

✳ **Q4166** Cytal, per square centimeter

✳ **Q4167** TruSkin, per square centimeter

✳ **Q4168** AmnioBand, 1 mg

✳ **Q4169** Artacent wound, per square centimeter

✳ **Q4170** Cygnus, per square centimeter

✳ **Q4171** Interfyl, 1 mg

↻ ✳ **Q4172** Puraply or puraply am, per square centimeter

✳ **Q4173** PalinGen or PalinGen XPlus, per square centimeter

✳ **Q4174** PalinGen or ProMatrX, 0.36 mg per 0.25 cc

✳ **Q4175** Miroderm, per square centimeter

▶ ✳ **Q4176** Neopatch, per square centimeter

▶ ✳ **Q4177** Floweramnioflo, 0.1 cc

▶ ✳ **Q4178** Floweramniopatch, per square centimeter

▶ ✳ **Q4179** Flowerderm, per square centimeter

▶ ✳ **Q4180** Revita, per square centimeter

▶ ✳ **Q4181** Amnio wound, per square centimeter

▶ ✳ **Q4182** Transcyte, per square centimeter

Hospice Care

⊛ **Q5001** Hospice or home health care provided in patient's home/residence ⑧

⊛ **Q5002** Hospice or home health care provided in assisted living facility ⑧

⊛ **Q5003** Hospice care provided in nursing long term care facility (LTC) or non-skilled nursing facility (NF) ⑨

⊛ **Q5004** Hospice care provided in skilled nursing facility (SNF) ⑧

⊛ **Q5005** Hospice care provided in inpatient hospital ⑧

⊛ **Q5006** Hospice care provided in inpatient hospice facility ⑧

Hospice care provided in an inpatient hospice facility. These are residential facilities, which are places for patients to live while receiving routine home care or continuous home care. These hospice residential facilities are not certified by Medicare or Medicaid for provision of General Inpatient (GIP) or respite care, and regulations at 42 CFR 418.202(e) do not allow provision of GIP or respite care at hospice residential facilities.

⊛ **Q5007** Hospice care provided in long term care facility ⑧

⊛ **Q5008** Hospice care provided in inpatient psychiatric facility ⑧

⊛ **Q5009** Hospice or home health care provided in place not otherwise specified (NOS) ⑧

⊛ **Q5010** Hospice home care provided in a hospice facility ⑧

Biosimilar Drugs

⊛ **Q5101** Injection, filgrastim (G-CSF), biosimilar, 1 microgram ⑧ ⑧

↻ ⊛ **Q5102** Injection, infliximab, biosimilar, 10 mg ⑧ ⑧

IOM: 100-02, 15, 50

Contrast Agents

↻ ✳ **Q9950** Injection, sulfur hexafluoride lipid microspheres, per ml ⑧

⊛ **Q9951** Low osmolar contrast material, 400 or greater mg/ml iodine concentration, per ml ⑧

IOM: 100-04, 12, 70; 100-04, 13, 20; 100-04, 13, 90

⊛ **Q9953** Injection, iron-based magnetic resonance contrast agent, per ml ⑧

IOM: 100-04, 12, 70; 100-04, 13, 20; 100-04, 13, 90

| ▶ New | ↻ Revised | ✔ Reinstated | deleted Deleted | ⊘ Not covered or valid by Medicare |
| ⊛ Special coverage instructions | ✳ Carrier discretion | ⑧ Bill Part B MAC | ⑧ Bill DME MAC |

⊙ **Q9954**   Oral magnetic resonance contrast agent, per 100 ml ⑬

IOM: 100-04, 12, 70; 100-04, 13, 20; 100-04, 13, 90

✳ **Q9955**   Injection, perflexane lipid microspheres, per ml ⑱

✳ **Q9956**   Injection, octafluoropropane microspheres, per ml ⑱

✳ **Q9957**   Injection, perflutren lipid microspheres, per ml ⑱

⊙ **Q9958**   High osmolar contrast material, up to 149 mg/ml iodine concentration, per ml ⑬

IOM: 100-04, 12, 70; 100-04, 13, 20; 100-04, 13, 90

⊙ **Q9959**   High osmolar contrast material, 150-199 mg/ml iodine concentration, per ml ⑬

IOM: 100-04, 12, 70; 100-04, 13, 20; 100-04, 13, 90

⊙ **Q9960**   High osmolar contrast material, 200-249 mg/ml iodine concentration, per ml ⑱

IOM: 100-04, 12, 70; 100-04, 13, 20; 100-04, 13, 90

⊙ **Q9961**   High osmolar contrast material, 250-299 mg/ml iodine concentration, per ml ⑱

IOM: 100-04, 12, 70; 100-04, 13, 20; 100-04, 13, 90

⊙ **Q9962**   High osmolar contrast material, 300-349 mg/ml iodine concentration, per ml ⑱

IOM: 100-04, 12, 70; 100-04, 13, 20; 100-04, 13, 90

⊙ **Q9963**   High osmolar contrast material, 350-399 mg/ml iodine concentration, per ml ⑱

IOM: 100-04, 12, 70; 100-04, 13, 20; 100-04, 13, 90

⊙ **Q9964**   High osmolar contrast material, 400 or greater mg/ml iodine concentration, per ml ⑬

IOM: 100-04, 12, 70; 100-04, 13, 20; 100-04, 13, 90

⊙ **Q9965**   Low osmolar contrast material, 100-199 mg/ml iodine concentration, per ml ⑬

IOM: 100-04, 12, 70; 100-04, 13, 20; 100-04, 13, 90

⊙ **Q9966**   Low osmolar contrast material, 200-299 mg/ml iodine concentration, per ml ⑬

IOM: 100-04, 12, 70; 100-04, 13, 20; 100-04, 13, 90

⊙ **Q9967**   Low osmolar contrast material, 300-399 mg/ml iodine concentration, per ml ⑬

IOM: 100-04, 12, 70; 100-04, 13, 20; 100-04, 13, 90

✳ **Q9968**   Injection, non-radioactive, non-contrast, visualization adjunct (e.g., Methylene Blue, Isosulfan Blue), 1 mg ⑬

⊙ **Q9969**   Tc-99m from non-highly enriched uranium source, full cost recovery add-on, per study dose ⑱

Radiopharmaceuticals

⊙ **Q9982**   Flutemetamol F18, diagnostic, per study dose, up to 5 millicuries ⑱

⊙ **Q9983**   Florbetaben F18, diagnostic, per study dose, up to 8.1 millicuries ⑱

Miscellaneous

~~Q9984~~   ~~Levonorgestrel-releasing intrauterine contraceptive system (kyleena), 19.5 mg~~   ✖

Cross Reference J7296

~~Q9985~~   ~~Injection, hydroxyprogesterone caproate, not otherwise specified, 10 mg~~   ✖

Cross Reference J1729

~~Q9986~~   ~~Injection, hydroxyprogesterone caproate, (makena), 10 mg~~   ✖

Cross Reference J1726

~~Q9987~~   ~~Pathogen(s) test for platelets~~   ✖

Cross Reference P9100

~~Q9988~~   ~~Platelets, pheresis, pathogen-reduced, each unit~~   ✖

Cross Reference P9073

~~Q9989~~   ~~Ustekinumab, for intravenous injection, 1 mg~~   ✖

Cross Reference J3358

▶ **New**   ↻ **Revised**   ✔ **Reinstated**   ~~deleted~~ **Deleted**   ⦸ **Not covered or valid by Medicare**
⊙ **Special coverage instructions**   ✳ **Carrier discretion**   ⑱ **Bill Part B MAC**   ⑬ **Bill DME MAC**

DIAGNOSTIC RADIOLOGY SERVICES
(R0000-R9999)

Transportation/Setup of Portable Equipment

⊛ **R0070** Transportation of portable x-ray equipment and personnel to home or nursing home, per trip to facility or location, one patient seen ⑥

CMS Transmittal B03-049; specific instructions to contractors on pricing

IOM: 100-04, 13, 90; 100-04, 13, 90.3

⊛ **R0075** Transportation of portable x-ray equipment and personnel to home or nursing home, per trip to facility or location, more than one patient seen ⑧

This code would not apply to the x-ray equipment if stored at the location where the x-ray was performed (e.g., a nursing home).

IOM: 100-04, 13, 90; 100-04, 13, 90.3

⊛ **R0076** Transportation of portable ECG to facility or location, per patient ⑥

EKG procedure code 93000 or 93005 must be submitted on same claim as transportation code. Bundled status on physician fee schedule

IOM: 100-01, 5, 90.2; 100-02, 15, 80; 100-03, 1, 20.15; 100-04, 13, 90; 100-04, 16, 10; 100-04, 16, 110.4

▶ New   ↻ Revised   ✔ Reinstated   ~~deleted~~ Deleted   ⊘ Not covered or valid by Medicare
⊛ Special coverage instructions   ✳ Carrier discretion   ⑥ Bill Part B MAC   ⑧ Bill DME MAC

TEMPORARY NATIONAL CODES ESTABLISHED BY PRIVATE PAYERS (S0000-S9999)

NOTE: Medicare and other federal payers do not recognize "S" codes; however, S codes may be useful for claims to some private insurers.

Non-Medicare Drugs

⊘ **S0012** Butorphanol tartrate, nasal spray, 25 mg

⊘ **S0014** Tacrine hydrochloride, 10 mg

⊘ **S0017** Injection, aminocaproic acid, 5 grams

⊘ **S0020** Injection, bupivacaine hydrochloride, 30 ml

⊘ **S0021** Injection, cefoperazone sodium, 1 gram

⊘ **S0023** Injection, cimetidine hydrochloride, 300 mg

⊘ **S0028** Injection, famotidine, 20 mg

⊘ **S0030** Injection, metronidazole, 500 mg

⊘ **S0032** Injection, nafcillin sodium, 2 grams

⊘ **S0034** Injection, ofloxacin, 400 mg

⊘ **S0039** Injection, sulfamethoxazole and trimethoprim, 10 ml

⊘ **S0040** Injection, ticarcillin disodium and clavulanate potassium, 3.1 grams

⊘ **S0073** Injection, aztreonam, 500 mg

⊘ **S0074** Injection, cefotetan disodium, 500 mg

⊘ **S0077** Injection, clindamycin phosphate, 300 mg

⊘ **S0078** Injection, fosphenytoin sodium, 750 mg

⊘ **S0080** Injection, pentamidine isethionate, 300 mg

⊘ **S0081** Injection, piperacillin sodium, 500 mg

⊘ **S0088** Imatinib, 100 mg

⊘ **S0090** Sildenafil citrate, 25 mg

⊘ **S0091** Granisetron hydrochloride, 1 mg (for circumstances falling under the Medicare Statute, use Q0166)

⊘ **S0092** Injection, hydromorphone hydrochloride, 250 mg (loading dose for infusion pump)

⊘ **S0093** Injection, morphine sulfate, 500 mg (loading dose for infusion pump)

⊘ **S0104** Zidovudine, oral, 100 mg

⊘ **S0106** Bupropion HCl sustained release tablet, 150 mg, per bottle of 60 tablets

⊘ **S0108** Mercaptopurine, oral, 50 mg

⊘ **S0109** Methadone, oral, 5 mg

⊘ **S0117** Tretinoin, topical, 5 grams

⊘ **S0119** Ondansetron, oral, 4 mg (for circumstances falling under the Medicare statute, use HCPCS Q code)

⊘ **S0122** Injection, menotropins, 75 IU

⊘ **S0126** Injection, follitropin alfa, 75 IU

⊘ **S0128** Injection, follitropin beta, 75 IU

⊘ **S0132** Injection, ganirelix acetate, 250 mcg

⊘ **S0136** Clozapine, 25 mg

⊘ **S0137** Didanosine (DDI), 25 mg

⊘ **S0138** Finasteride, 5 mg

⊘ **S0139** Minoxidil, 10 mg

⊘ **S0140** Saquinavir, 200 mg

⊘ **S0142** Colistimethate sodium, inhalation solution administered through DME, concentrated form, per mg

⊘ **S0145** Injection, pegylated interferon alfa-2a, 180 mcg per ml

⊘ **S0148** Injection, pegylated interferon ALFA-2b, 10 mcg

⊘ **S0155** Sterile dilutant for epoprostenol, 50 ml

⊘ **S0156** Exemestane, 25 mg

⊘ **S0157** Becaplermin gel 0.01%, 0.5 gm

⊘ **S0160** Dextroamphetamine sulfate, 5 mg

⊘ **S0164** Injection, pantoprazole sodium, 40 mg

⊘ **S0166** Injection, olanzapine, 2.5 mg

⊘ **S0169** Calcitrol, 0.25 microgram

⊘ **S0170** Anastrozole, oral, 1 mg

⊘ **S0171** Injection, bumetanide, 0.5 mg

⊘ **S0172** Chlorambucil, oral, 2 mg

⊘ **S0174** Dolasetron mesylate, oral 50 mg (for circumstances falling under the Medicare Statute, use Q0180)

⊘ **S0175** Flutamide, oral, 125 mg

⊘ **S0176** Hydroxyurea, oral, 500 mg

⊘ **S0177** Levamisole hydrochloride, oral, 50 mg

⊘ **S0178** Lomustine, oral, 10 mg

⊘ **S0179** Megestrol acetate, oral, 20 mg

⊘ **S0182** Procarbazine hydrochloride, oral, 50 mg

⊘ **S0183** Prochlorperazine maleate, oral, 5 mg (for circumstances falling under the Medicare Statute, use Q0164)

⊘ **S0187** Tamoxifen citrate, oral, 10 mg

⊘ **S0189** Testosterone pellet, 75 mg

⊘ **S0190** Mifepristone, oral, 200 mg

⊘ **S0191** Misoprostol, oral 200 mcg

▶ New   ⟲ Revised   ✔ Reinstated   ~~deleted~~ Deleted   ⊘ Not covered or valid by Medicare
⊕ Special coverage instructions   ✳ Carrier discretion   Ⓑ Bill Part B MAC   Ⓖ Bill DME MAC

⊘ **S0194** Dialysis/stress vitamin supplement, oral, 100 capsules

⊘ **S0197** Prenatal vitamins, 30-day supply

Provider Services

⊘ **S0199** Medically induced abortion by oral ingestion of medication including all associated services and supplies (e.g., patient counseling, office visits, confirmation of pregnancy by HCG, ultrasound to confirm duration of pregnancy, ultrasound to confirm completion of abortion) except drugs

⊘ **S0201** Partial hospitalization services, less than 24 hours, per diem

⊘ **S0207** Paramedic intercept, non-hospital-based ALS service (non-voluntary), non-transport

⊘ **S0208** Paramedic intercept, hospital-based ALS service (non-voluntary), non-transport

⊘ **S0209** Wheelchair van, mileage, per mile

⊘ **S0215** Non-emergency transportation; mileage per mile

⊘ **S0220** Medical conference by a physician with interdisciplinary team of health professionals or representatives of community agencies to coordinate activities of patient care (patient is present); approximately 30 minutes

⊘ **S0221** Medical conference by a physician with interdisciplinary team of health professionals or representatives of community agencies to coordinate activities of patient care (patient is present); approximately 60 minutes

⊘ **S0250** Comprehensive geriatric assessment and treatment planning performed by assessment team

⊘ **S0255** Hospice referral visit (advising patient and family of care options) performed by nurse, social worker, or other designated staff

⊘ **S0257** Counseling and discussion regarding advance directives or end of life care planning and decisions, with patient and/or surrogate (list separately in addition to code for appropriate evaluation and management service)

⊘ **S0260** History and physical (outpatient or office) related to surgical procedure (list separately in addition to code for appropriate evaluation and management service)

⊘ **S0265** Genetic counseling, under physician supervision, each 15 minutes

⊘ **S0270** Physician management of patient home care, standard monthly case rate (per 30 days)

⊘ **S0271** Physician management of patient home care, hospice monthly case rate (per 30 days)

⊘ **S0272** Physician management of patient home care, episodic care monthly case rate (per 30 days)

⊘ **S0273** Physician visit at member's home, outside of a capitation arrangement

⊘ **S0274** Nurse practitioner visit at member's home, outside of a capitation arrangement

⊘ **S0280** Medical home program, comprehensive care coordination and planning, initial plan

⊘ **S0281** Medical home program, comprehensive care coordination and planning, maintenance of plan

⊘ **S0285** Colonoscopy consultation performed prior to a screening colonoscopy procedure

⊘ **S0302** Completed Early Periodic Screening Diagnosis and Treatment (EPSDT) service (list in addition to code for appropriate evaluation and management service)

⊘ **S0310** Hospitalist services (list separately in addition to code for appropriate evaluation and management service)

⊘ **S0311** Comprehensive management and care coordination for advanced illness, per calendar month

⊘ **S0315** Disease management program; initial assessment and initiation of the program

⊘ **S0316** Disease management program; follow-up/reassessment

⊘ **S0317** Disease management program; per diem

⊘ **S0320** Telephone calls by a registered nurse to a disease management program member for monitoring purposes; per month

⊘ **S0340** Lifestyle modification program for management of coronary artery disease, including all supportive services; first quarter/stage

⊘ **S0341** Lifestyle modification program for management of coronary artery disease, including all supportive services; second or third quarter/stage

---

▶ New   ↻ Revised   ✔ Reinstated   ~~deleted~~ Deleted   ⊘ Not covered or valid by Medicare

✪ Special coverage instructions   ✳ Carrier discretion   Ⓑ Bill Part B MAC   Ⓑ Bill DME MAC

⊘ **S0342** Lifestyle modification program for management of coronary artery disease, including all supportive services; fourth quarter/stage

⊘ **S0353** Treatment planning and care coordination management for cancer, initial treatment

⊘ **S0354** Treatment planning and care coordination management for cancer, established patient with a change of regimen

⊘ **S0390** Routine foot care; removal and/or trimming of corns, calluses and/or nails and preventive maintenance in specific medical conditions (e.g., diabetes), per visit

⊘ **S0395** Impression casting of a foot performed by a practitioner other than the manufacturer of the orthotic

⊘ **S0400** Global fee for extracorporeal shock wave lithotripsy treatment of kidney stone(s)

Vision Supplies

⊘ **S0500** Disposable contact lens, per lens

⊘ **S0504** Single vision prescription lens (safety, athletic, or sunglass), per lens

⊘ **S0506** Bifocal vision prescription lens (safety, athletic, or sunglass), per lens

⊘ **S0508** Trifocal vision prescription lens (safety, athletic, or sunglass), per lens

⊘ **S0510** Non-prescription lens (safety, athletic, or sunglass), per lens

⊘ **S0512** Daily wear specialty contact lens, per lens

⊘ **S0514** Color contact lens, per lens

⊘ **S0515** Scleral lens, liquid bandage device, per lens

⊘ **S0516** Safety eyeglass frames

⊘ **S0518** Sunglasses frames

⊘ **S0580** Polycarbonate lens (list this code in addition to the basic code for the lens)

⊘ **S0581** Nonstandard lens (list this code in addition to the basic code for the lens)

⊘ **S0590** Integral lens service, miscellaneous services reported separately

⊘ **S0592** Comprehensive contact lens evaluation

⊘ **S0595** Dispensing new spectacle lenses for patient supplied frame

⊘ **S0596** Phakic intraocular lens for correction of refractive error

Screening and Examinations

⊘ **S0601** Screening proctoscopy

⊘ **S0610** Annual gynecological examination, new patient

⊘ **S0612** Annual gynecological examination, established patient

⊘ **S0613** Annual gynecological examination; clinical breast examination without pelvic evaluation

⊘ **S0618** Audiometry for hearing aid evaluation to determine the level and degree of hearing loss

⊘ **S0620** Routine ophthalmological examination including refraction; new patient

Many non-Medicare vision plans may require code for routine encounter, no complaints

⊘ **S0621** Routine ophthalmological examination including refraction; established patient

Many non-Medicare vision plans may require code for routine encounter, no complaints

⊘ **S0622** Physical exam for college, new or established patient (list separately) in addition to appropriate evaluation and management code

Provider Services and Supplies

⊘ **S0630** Removal of sutures; by a physician other than the physician who originally closed the wound

⊘ **S0800** Laser in situ keratomileusis (LASIK)

⊘ **S0810** Photorefractive keratectomy (PRK)

⊘ **S0812** Phototherapeutic keratectomy (PTK)

⊘ **S1001** Deluxe item, patient aware (list in addition to code for basic item)

⊘ **S1002** Customized item (list in addition to code for basic item)

⊘ **S1015** IV tubing extension set

⊘ **S1016** Non-PVC (polyvinyl chloride) intravenous administration set, for use with drugs that are not stable in PVC (e.g., paclitaxel)

⊘ **S1030** Continuous noninvasive glucose monitoring device, purchase (for physician interpretation of data, use CPT code)

| ▶ **New** | ↻ **Revised** | ✔ **Reinstated** | ~~deleted~~ **Deleted** | ⊘ **Not covered or valid by Medicare** |
| ✿ **Special coverage instructions** | | ✳ **Carrier discretion** | Ⓑ **Bill Part B MAC** | Ⓖ **Bill DME MAC** |

⊘ **S1031** Continuous noninvasive glucose monitoring device, rental, including sensor, sensor replacement, and download to monitor (for physician interpretation of data, use CPT code)

⊘ **S1034** Artificial pancreas device system (e.g., low glucose suspend (LGS) feature) including continuous glucose monitor, blood glucose device, insulin pump and computer algorithm that communicates with all of the devices

⊘ **S1035** Sensor; invasive (e.g., subcutaneous), disposable, for use with artificial pancreas device system

⊘ **S1036** Transmitter; external, for use with artificial pancreas device system

⊘ **S1037** Receiver (monitor); external, for use with artificial pancreas device system

⊘ **S1040** Cranial remolding orthosis, pediatric, rigid, with soft interface material, custom fabricated, includes fitting and adjustment(s)

⊘ **S1090** Mometasone furoate sinus implant, 370 micrograms

⊘ **S2053** Transplantation of small intestine and liver allografts

⊘ **S2054** Transplantation of multivisceral organs

⊘ **S2055** Harvesting of donor multivisceral organs, with preparation and maintenance of allografts; from cadaver donor

⊘ **S2060** Lobar lung transplantation

⊘ **S2061** Donor lobectomy (lung) for transplantation, living donor

⊘ **S2065** Simultaneous pancreas kidney transplantation

⊘ **S2066** Breast reconstruction with gluteal artery perforator (GAP) flap, including harvesting of the flap, microvascular transfer, closure of donor site and shaping the flap into a breast, unilateral

⊘ **S2067** Breast reconstruction of a single breast with "stacked" deep inferior epigastric perforator (DIEP) flap(s) and/or gluteal artery perforator (GAP) flap(s), including harvesting of the flap(s), microvascular transfer, closure of donor site(s) and shaping the flap into a breast, unilateral

⊘ **S2068** Breast reconstruction with deep inferior epigastric perforator (DIEP) flap, or superficial inferior epigastric artery (SIEA) flap, including harvesting of the flap, microvascular transfer, closure of donor site and shaping the flap into a breast, unilateral

⊘ **S2070** Cystourethroscopy, with ureteroscopy and/or pyeloscopy; with endoscopic laser treatment of ureteral calculi (includes ureteral catheterization)

⊘ **S2079** Laparoscopic esophagomyotomy (Heller type)

⊘ **S2080** Laser-assisted uvulopalatoplasty (LAUP)

⊘ **S2083** Adjustment of gastric band diameter via subcutaneous port by injection or aspiration of saline

⊘ **S2095** Transcatheter occlusion or embolization for tumor destruction, percutaneous, any method, using yttrium-90 microspheres

⊘ **S2102** Islet cell tissue transplant from pancreas; allogeneic

⊘ **S2103** Adrenal tissue transplant to brain

⊘ **S2107** Adoptive immunotherapy i.e. development of specific anti-tumor reactivity (e.g., tumor-infiltrating lymphocyte therapy) per course of treatment

⊘ **S2112** Arthroscopy, knee, surgical for harvesting of cartilage (chondrocyte cells)

⊘ **S2115** Osteotomy, periacetabular, with internal fixation

⊘ **S2117** Arthroereisis, subtalar

⊘ **S2118** Metal-on-metal total hip resurfacing, including acetabular and femoral components

⊘ **S2120** Low density lipoprotein (LDL) apheresis using heparin-induced extracorporeal LDL precipitation

⊘ **S2140** Cord blood harvesting for transplantation, allogeneic

⊘ **S2142** Cord blood-derived stem cell transplantation, allogeneic

⊘ **S2150** Bone marrow or blood-derived stem cells (peripheral or umbilical), allogeneic or autologous, harvesting, transplantation, and related complications; including: pheresis and cell preparation/storage; marrow ablative therapy; drugs, supplies, hospitalization with outpatient follow-up; medical/surgical, diagnostic, emergency, and rehabilitative services; and the number of days of pre- and post-transplant care in the global definition

---

▶ **New**   ↵ **Revised**   ✔ **Reinstated**   ~~deleted~~ **Deleted**   ⊘ **Not covered or valid by Medicare**

✪ **Special coverage instructions**   ✳ **Carrier discretion**   Ⓟ **Bill Part B MAC**   Ⓑ **Bill DME MAC**

⊘ **S2152** Solid organ(s), complete or segmental, single organ or combination of organs; deceased or living donor(s), procurement, transplantation, and related complications; including: drugs; supplies; hospitalization with outpatient follow-up; medical/surgical, diagnostic, emergency, and rehabilitative services, and the number of days of pre- and post-transplant care in the global definition

⊘ **S2202** Echosclerotherapy

⊘ **S2205** Minimally invasive direct coronary artery bypass surgery involving mini-thoracotomy or mini-sternotomy surgery, performed under direct vision; using arterial graft(s), single coronary arterial graft

⊘ **S2206** Minimally invasive direct coronary artery bypass surgery involving mini-thoracotomy or mini-sternotomy surgery, performed under direct vision; using arterial graft(s), two coronary arterial grafts

⊘ **S2207** Minimally invasive direct coronary artery bypass surgery involving mini-thoracotomy or mini-sternotomy surgery, performed under direct vision; using venous graft only, single coronary venous graft

⊘ **S2208** Minimally invasive direct coronary artery bypass surgery involving mini-thoracotomy or mini-sternotomy surgery, performed under direct vision; using single arterial and venous graft(s), single venous graft

⊘ **S2209** Minimally invasive direct coronary artery bypass surgery involving mini-thoracotomy or mini-sternotomy surgery, performed under direct vision; using two arterial grafts and single venous graft

⊘ **S2225** Myringotomy, laser-assisted

⊘ **S2230** Implantation of magnetic component of semi-implantable hearing device on ossicles in middle ear

⊘ **S2235** Implantation of auditory brain stem implant

⊘ **S2260** Induced abortion, 17 to 24 weeks

⊘ **S2265** Induced abortion, 25 to 28 weeks

⊘ **S2266** Induced abortion, 29 to 31 weeks

⊘ **S2267** Induced abortion, 32 weeks or greater

⊘ **S2300** Arthroscopy, shoulder, surgical; with thermally-induced capsulorrhaphy

⊘ **S2325** Hip core decompression

⊘ **S2340** Chemodenervation of abductor muscle(s) of vocal cord

⊘ **S2341** Chemodenervation of adductor muscle(s) of vocal cord

⊘ **S2342** Nasal endoscopy for post-operative debridement following functional endoscopic sinus surgery, nasal and/or sinus cavity(s), unilateral or bilateral

⊘ **S2348** Decompression procedure, percutaneous, of nucleus pulpous of intervertebral disc, using radiofrequency energy, single or multiple levels, lumbar

⊘ **S2350** Diskectomy, anterior, with decompression of spinal cord and/or nerve root(s), including osteophytectomy; lumbar, single interspace

⊘ **S2351** Diskectomy, anterior, with decompression of spinal cord and/or nerve root(s) including osteophytectomy; lumbar, each additional interspace (list separately in addition to code for primary procedure)

⊘ **S2400** Repair, congenital diaphragmatic hernia in the fetus using temporary tracheal occlusion, procedure performed in utero

⊘ **S2401** Repair, urinary tract obstruction in the fetus, procedure performed in utero

⊘ **S2402** Repair, congenital cystic adenomatoid malformation in the fetus, procedure performed in utero

⊘ **S2403** Repair, extralobar pulmonary sequestration in the fetus, procedure performed in utero

⊘ **S2404** Repair, myelomeningocele in the fetus, procedure performed in utero

⊘ **S2405** Repair of sacrococcygeal teratoma in the fetus, procedure performed in utero

⊘ **S2409** Repair, congenital malformation of fetus, procedure performed in utero, not otherwise classified

⊘ **S2411** Fetoscopic laser therapy for treatment of twin-to-twin transfusion syndrome

⊘ **S2900** Surgical techniques requiring use of robotic surgical system (list separately in addition to code for primary procedure)

⊘ **S3000** Diabetic indicator; retinal eye exam, dilated, bilateral

⊘ **S3005** Performance measurement, evaluation of patient self assessment, depression

⊘ **S3600** STAT laboratory request (situations other than S3601)

⊘ **S3601** Emergency STAT laboratory charge for patient who is homebound or residing in a nursing facility

✪ **S3620** Newborn metabolic screening panel, includes test kit, postage and the laboratory tests specified by the state for inclusion in this panel (e.g., galactose; hemoglobin, electrophoresis; hydroxyprogesterone, 17-D; phenylalanine (PKU); and thyroxine, total)

⊘ **S3630** Eosinophil count, blood, direct

⊘ **S3645** HIV-1 antibody testing of oral mucosal transudate

⊘ **S3650** Saliva test, hormone level; during menopause

⊘ **S3652** Saliva test, hormone level; to assess preterm labor risk

⊘ **S3655** Antisperm antibodies test (immunobead)

⊘ **S3708** Gastrointestinal fat absorption study

⊘ **S3722** Dose optimization by area under the curve (AUC) analysis, for infusional 5-fluorouracil

Genetic Testing

⊘ **S3800** Genetic testing for amyotrophic lateral sclerosis (ALS)

⊘ **S3840** DNA analysis for germline mutations of the RET proto-oncogene for susceptibility to multiple endocrine neoplasia type 2

⊘ **S3841** Genetic testing for retinoblastoma

⊘ **S3842** Genetic testing for von Hippel-Lindau disease

⊘ **S3844** DNA analysis of the connexin 26 gene (GJB2) for susceptibility to congenital, profound deafness

⊘ **S3845** Genetic testing for alpha-thalassemia

⊘ **S3846** Genetic testing for hemoglobin E beta-thalassemia

⊘ **S3849** Genetic testing for Niemann-Pick disease

⊘ **S3850** Genetic testing for sickle cell anemia

⊘ **S3852** DNA analysis for APOE epilson 4 allele for susceptibility to Alzheimer's disease

⊘ **S3853** Genetic testing for myotonic muscular dystrophy

⊘ **S3854** Gene expression profiling panel for use in the management of breast cancer treatment

⊘ **S3861** Genetic testing, sodium channel, voltage-gated, type V, alpha subunit (SCN5A) and variants for suspected Brugada syndrome

⊘ **S3865** Comprehensive gene sequence analysis for hypertrophic cardiomyopathy

⊘ **S3866** Genetic analysis for a specific gene mutation for hypertrophic cardiomyopathy (HCM) in an individual with a known HCM mutation in the family

⊘ **S3870** Comparative genomic hybridization (CGH) microarray testing for developmental delay, autism spectrum disorder and/or intellectual disability

Other Tests

⊘ **S3900** Surface electromyography (EMG)

⊘ **S3902** Ballistrocardiogram

⊘ **S3904** Masters two step

Bill on paper. Requires a report.

Obstetric and Fertility Services

⊘ **S4005** Interim labor facility global (labor occurring but not resulting in delivery)

⊘ **S4011** In vitro fertilization; including but not limited to identification and incubation of mature oocytes, fertilization with sperm, incubation of embryo(s), and subsequent visualization for determination of development

⊘ **S4013** Complete cycle, gamete intrafallopian transfer (GIFT), case rate

⊘ **S4014** Complete cycle, zygote intrafallopian transfer (ZIFT), case rate

⊘ **S4015** Complete in vitro fertilization cycle, not otherwise specified, case rate

⊘ **S4016** Frozen in vitro fertilization cycle, case rate

⊘ **S4017** Incomplete cycle, treatment cancelled prior to stimulation, case rate

⊘ **S4018** Frozen embryo transfer procedure cancelled before transfer, case rate

⊘ **S4020** In vitro fertilization procedure cancelled before aspiration, case rate

⊘ **S4021** In vitro fertilization procedure cancelled after aspiration, case rate

⊘ **S4022** Assisted oocyte fertilization, case rate

⊘ **S4023** Donor egg cycle, incomplete, case rate

▶ New	↻ Revised	✔ Reinstated	~~deleted~~ Deleted	⊘ Not covered or valid by Medicare
✪ Special coverage instructions	✳ Carrier discretion	Ⓥ Bill Part B MAC	Ⓓ Bill DME MAC	

⊘ **S4025** Donor services for in vitro fertilization (sperm or embryo), case rate

⊘ **S4026** Procurement of donor sperm from sperm bank

⊘ **S4027** Storage of previously frozen embryos

⊘ **S4028** Microsurgical epididymal sperm aspiration (MESA)

⊘ **S4030** Sperm procurement and cryopreservation services; initial visit

⊘ **S4031** Sperm procurement and cryopreservation services; subsequent visit

⊘ **S4035** Stimulated intrauterine insemination (IUI), case rate

⊘ **S4037** Cryopreserved embryo transfer, case rate

⊘ **S4040** Monitoring and storage of cryopreserved embryos, per 30 days

⊘ **S4042** Management of ovulation induction (interpretation of diagnostic tests and studies, non-face-to-face medical management of the patient), per cycle

⊘ **S4981** Insertion of levonorgestrel-releasing intrauterine system

⊘ **S4989** Contraceptive intrauterine device (e.g., Progestasert IUD), including implants and supplies

Therapeutic Substances and Medications

⊘ **S4990** Nicotine patches, legend

⊘ **S4991** Nicotine patches, non-legend

⊘ **S4993** Contraceptive pills for birth control

Only billed by Family Planning Clinics

⊘ **S4995** Smoking cessation gum

⊘ **S5000** Prescription drug, generic

⊘ **S5001** Prescription drug, brand name

⊘ **S5010** 5% dextrose and 0.45% normal saline, 1000 ml

⊘ **S5012** 5% dextrose with potassium chloride, 1000 ml

⊘ **S5013** 5% dextrose/0.45% normal saline with potassium chloride and magnesium sulfate, 1000 ml

⊘ **S5014** 5% dextrose/0.45% normal saline with potassium chloride and magnesium sulfate, 1500 ml

Home Care Services

⊘ **S5035** Home infusion therapy, routine service of infusion device (e.g., pump maintenance)

⊘ **S5036** Home infusion therapy, repair of infusion device (e.g., pump repair)

⊘ **S5100** Day care services, adult; per 15 minutes

⊘ **S5101** Day care services, adult; per half day

⊘ **S5102** Day care services, adult; per diem

⊘ **S5105** Day care services, center-based; services not included in program fee, per diem

⊘ **S5108** Home care training to home care client, per 15 minutes

⊘ **S5109** Home care training to home care client, per session

⊘ **S5110** Home care training, family; per 15 minutes

⊘ **S5111** Home care training, family; per session

⊘ **S5115** Home care training, non-family; per 15 minutes

⊘ **S5116** Home care training, non-family; per session

⊘ **S5120** Chore services; per 15 minutes

⊘ **S5121** Chore services; per diem

⊘ **S5125** Attendant care services; per 15 minutes

⊘ **S5126** Attendant care services; per diem

⊘ **S5130** Homemaker service, NOS; per 15 minutes

⊘ **S5131** Homemaker service, NOS; per diem

⊘ **S5135** Companion care, adult (e.g., IADL/ADL); per 15 minutes

⊘ **S5136** Companion care, adult (e.g., IADL/ADL); per diem

⊘ **S5140** Foster care, adult; per diem

⊘ **S5141** Foster care, adult; per month

⊘ **S5145** Foster care, therapeutic, child; per diem

⊘ **S5146** Foster care, therapeutic, child; per month

⊘ **S5150** Unskilled respite care, not hospice; per 15 minutes

⊘ **S5151** Unskilled respite care, not hospice; per diem

⊘ **S5160** Emergency response system; installation and testing

⊘ **S5161** Emergency response system; service fee, per month (excludes installation and testing)

⊘ **S5162** Emergency response system; purchase only

▶ New	↻ Revised	✔ Reinstated	~~deleted~~ Deleted	⊘ Not covered or valid by Medicare
✪ Special coverage instructions		✳ Carrier discretion	Ⓑ Bill Part B MAC	Ⓓ Bill DME MAC

⊘ **S5165** Home modifications; per service

⊘ **S5170** Home delivered meals, including preparation; per meal

⊘ **S5175** Laundry service, external, professional; per order

⊘ **S5180** Home health respiratory therapy, initial evaluation

⊘ **S5181** Home health respiratory therapy, NOS, per diem

⊘ **S5185** Medication reminder service, non-face-to-face; per month

⊘ **S5190** Wellness assessment, performed by non-physician

⊘ **S5199** Personal care item, NOS, each

Home Infusion Therapy

⊘ **S5497** Home infusion therapy, catheter care/maintenance, not otherwise classified; includes administrative services, professional pharmacy services, care coordination, and all necessary supplies and equipment (drugs and nursing visits coded separately), per diem

⊘ **S5498** Home infusion therapy, catheter care/maintenance, simple (single lumen), includes administrative services, professional pharmacy services, care coordination and all necessary supplies and equipment, (drugs and nursing visits coded separately), per diem

⊘ **S5501** Home infusion therapy, catheter care/maintenance, complex (more than one lumen), includes administrative services, professional pharmacy services, care coordination, and all necessary supplies and equipment (drugs and nursing visits coded separately), per diem

⊘ **S5502** Home infusion therapy, catheter care/maintenance, implanted access device, includes administrative services, professional pharmacy services, care coordination, and all necessary supplies and equipment, (drugs and nursing visits coded separately), per diem (use this code for interim maintenance of vascular access not currently in use)

⊘ **S5517** Home infusion therapy, all supplies necessary for restoration of catheter patency or declotting

⊘ **S5518** Home infusion therapy, all supplies necessary for catheter repair

⊘ **S5520** Home infusion therapy, all supplies (including catheter) necessary for a peripherally inserted central venous catheter (PICC) line insertion

Bill on paper. Requires a report.

⊘ **S5521** Home infusion therapy, all supplies (including catheter) necessary for a midline catheter insertion

⊘ **S5522** Home infusion therapy, insertion of peripherally inserted central venous catheter (PICC), nursing services only (no supplies or catheter included)

⊘ **S5523** Home infusion therapy, insertion of midline central venous catheter, nursing services only (no supplies or catheter included)

Insulin Services

⊘ **S5550** Insulin, rapid onset, 5 units

⊘ **S5551** Insulin, most rapid onset (Lispro or Aspart); 5 units

⊘ **S5552** Insulin, intermediate acting (NPH or Lente); 5 units

⊘ **S5553** Insulin, long acting; 5 units

⊘ **S5560** Insulin delivery device, reusable pen; 1.5 ml size

⊘ **S5561** Insulin delivery device, reusable pen; 3 ml size

⊘ **S5565** Insulin cartridge for use in insulin delivery device other than pump; 150 units

⊘ **S5566** Insulin cartridge for use in insulin delivery device other than pump; 300 units

⊘ **S5570** Insulin delivery device, disposable pen (including insulin); 1.5 ml size

⊘ **S5571** Insulin delivery device, disposable pen (including insulin); 3 ml size

Imaging

⊘ **S8030** Scleral application of tantalum ring(s) for localization of lesions for proton beam therapy

⊘ **S8035** Magnetic source imaging

⊘ **S8037** Magnetic resonance cholangiopancreatography (MRCP)

⊘ **S8040** Topographic brain mapping

⊘ **S8042** Magnetic resonance imaging (MRI), low-field

▶ New	⟲ Revised	✔ Reinstated	~~deleted~~ Deleted	⊘ Not covered or valid by Medicare
✪ Special coverage instructions	✳ Carrier discretion	⑧ Bill Part B MAC	⑨ Bill DME MAC	

⊘ **S8055** Ultrasound guidance for multifetal pregnancy reduction(s), technical component (only to be used when the physician doing the reduction procedure does not perform the ultrasound, guidance is included in the CPT code for multifetal pregnancy reduction - 59866)

⊘ **S8080** Scintimammography (radioimmunoscintigraphy of the breast), unilateral, including supply of radiopharmaceutical

⊘ **S8085** Fluorine-18 fluorodeoxyglucose (F-18 FDG) imaging using dual-head coincidence detection system (non-dedicated PET scan)

⊘ **S8092** Electron beam computed tomography (also known as ultrafast CT, cine CT)

Assistive Breathing Supplies

⊘ **S8096** Portable peak flow meter

⊘ **S8097** Asthma kit (including but not limited to portable peak expiratory flow meter, instructional video, brochure, and/or spacer)

⊘ **S8100** Holding chamber or spacer for use with an inhaler or nebulizer; without mask

⊘ **S8101** Holding chamber or spacer for use with an inhaler or nebulizer; with mask

⊘ **S8110** Peak expiratory flow rate (physician services)

⊘ **S8120** Oxygen contents, gaseous, 1 unit equals 1 cubic foot

⊘ **S8121** Oxygen contents, liquid, 1 unit equals 1 pound

⊘ **S8130** Interferential current stimulator, 2 channel

⊘ **S8131** Interferential current stimulator, 4 channel

⊘ **S8185** Flutter device

⊘ **S8186** Swivel adapter

⊘ **S8189** Tracheostomy supply, not otherwise classified

⊘ **S8210** Mucus trap

Miscellaneous Supplies and Services

⊘ **S8265** Haberman feeder for cleft lip/palate

⊘ **S8270** Enuresis alarm, using auditory buzzer and/or vibration device

⊘ **S8301** Infection control supplies, not otherwise specified

⊘ **S8415** Supplies for home delivery of infant

⊘ **S8420** Gradient pressure aid (sleeve and glove combination), custom made

⊘ **S8421** Gradient pressure aid (sleeve and glove combination), ready made

⊘ **S8422** Gradient pressure aid (sleeve), custom made, medium weight

⊘ **S8423** Gradient pressure aid (sleeve), custom made, heavy weight

⊘ **S8424** Gradient pressure aid (sleeve), ready made

⊘ **S8425** Gradient pressure aid (glove), custom made, medium weight

⊘ **S8426** Gradient pressure aid (glove), custom made, heavy weight

⊘ **S8427** Gradient pressure aid (glove), ready made

⊘ **S8428** Gradient pressure aid (gauntlet), ready made

⊘ **S8429** Gradient pressure exterior wrap

⊘ **S8430** Padding for compression bandage, roll

⊘ **S8431** Compression bandage, roll

⊘ **S8450** Splint, prefabricated, digit (specify digit by use of modifier)

⊘ **S8451** Splint, prefabricated, wrist or ankle

⊘ **S8452** Splint, prefabricated, elbow

⊘ **S8460** Camisole, post-mastectomy

⊘ **S8490** Insulin syringes (100 syringes, any size)

⊘ **S8930** Electrical stimulation of auricular acupuncture points; each 15 minutes of personal one-on-one contact with the patient

⊘ **S8940** Equestrian/Hippotherapy, per session

⊘ **S8948** Application of a modality (requiring constant provider attendance) to one or more areas; low-level laser; each 15 minutes

⊘ **S8950** Complex lymphedema therapy, each 15 minutes

⊘ **S8990** Physical or manipulative therapy performed for maintenance rather than restoration

⊘ **S8999** Resuscitation bag (for use by patient on artificial respiration during power failure or other catastrophic event)

⊘ **S9001** Home uterine monitor with or without associated nursing services

⊘ **S9007** Ultrafiltration monitor

⊘ **S9024** Paranasal sinus ultrasound

▶ New   ↻ Revised   ✔ Reinstated   ~~deleted~~ Deleted   ⊘ Not covered or valid by Medicare

✪ Special coverage instructions   ✷ Carrier discretion   ⑧ Bill Part B MAC   ⑧ Bill DME MAC

⊘ **S9025** Omnicardiogram/cardiointegram

⊘ **S9034** Extracorporeal shockwave lithotripsy for gall stones (if performed with ERCP, use 43265)

⊘ **S9055** Procuren or other growth factor preparation to promote wound healing

⊘ **S9056** Coma stimulation per diem

⊘ **S9061** Home administration of aerosolized drug therapy (e.g., pentamidine); administrative services, professional pharmacy services, care coordination, all necessary supplies and equipment (drugs and nursing visits coded separately), per diem

⊘ **S9083** Global fee urgent care centers

⊘ **S9088** Services provided in an urgent care center (list in addition to code for service)

⊘ **S9090** Vertebral axial decompression, per session

⊘ **S9097** Home visit for wound care

⊘ **S9098** Home visit, phototherapy services (e.g., Bili-Lite), including equipment rental, nursing services, blood draw, supplies, and other services, per diem

⊘ **S9110** Telemonitoring of patient in their home, including all necessary equipment; computer system, connections, and software; maintenance; patient education and support; per month

⊘ **S9117** Back school, per visit

⊘ **S9122** Home health aide or certified nurse assistant, providing care in the home; per hour

⊘ **S9123** Nursing care, in the home; by registered nurse, per hour (use for general nursing care only, not to be used when CPT codes 99500-99602 can be used)

⊘ **S9124** Nursing care, in the home; by licensed practical nurse, per hour

⊘ **S9125** Respite care, in the home, per diem

⊘ **S9126** Hospice care, in the home, per diem

⊘ **S9127** Social work visit, in the home, per diem

⊘ **S9128** Speech therapy, in the home, per diem

⊘ **S9129** Occupational therapy, in the home, per diem

⊘ **S9131** Physical therapy; in the home, per diem

⊘ **S9140** Diabetic management program, follow-up visit to non-MD provider

⊘ **S9141** Diabetic management program, follow-up visit to MD provider

⊘ **S9145** Insulin pump initiation, instruction in initial use of pump (pump not included)

⊘ **S9150** Evaluation by ocularist

⊘ **S9152** Speech therapy, re-evaluation

Home Management of Pregnancy

⊘ **S9208** Home management of preterm labor, including administrative services, professional pharmacy services, care coordination, and all necessary supplies or equipment (drugs and nursing visits coded separately), per diem (do not use this code with any home infusion per diem code)

⊘ **S9209** Home management of preterm premature rupture of membranes (PPROM), including administrative services, professional pharmacy services, care coordination, and all necessary supplies or equipment (drugs and nursing visits coded separately), per diem (do not use this code with any home infusion per diem code)

⊘ **S9211** Home management of gestational hypertension, includes administrative services, professional pharmacy services, care coordination, and all necessary supplies and equipment (drugs and nursing visits coded separately); per diem (do not use this code with any home infusion per diem code)

⊘ **S9212** Home management of postpartum hypertension, includes administrative services, professional pharmacy services, care coordination, and all necessary supplies and equipment (drugs and nursing visits coded separately), per diem (do not use this code with any home infusion per diem code)

⊘ **S9213** Home management of preeclampsia, includes administrative services, professional pharmacy services, care coordination, and all necessary supplies and equipment (drugs and nursing services coded separately); per diem (do not use this code with any home infusion per diem code)

▶ **New** ↻ **Revised** ✔ **Reinstated** ~~deleted~~ **Deleted** ⊘ **Not covered or valid by Medicare**

✪ **Special coverage instructions** ✳ **Carrier discretion** Ⓟ **Bill Part B MAC** Ⓓ **Bill DME MAC**

⊘ **S9214** Home management of gestational diabetes, includes administrative services, professional pharmacy services, care coordination, and all necessary supplies and equipment (drugs and nursing visits coded separately); per diem (do not use this code with any home infusion per diem code)

Home Infusion Therapy

⊘ **S9325** Home infusion therapy, pain management infusion; administrative services, professional pharmacy services, care coordination, and all necessary supplies and equipment, (drugs and nursing visits coded separately), per diem (do not use this code with S9326, S9327 or S9328)

⊘ **S9326** Home infusion therapy, continuous (twenty-four hours or more) pain management infusion; administrative services, professional pharmacy services, care coordination, and all necessary supplies and equipment (drugs and nursing visits coded separately), per diem

⊘ **S9327** Home infusion therapy, intermittent (less than twenty-four hours) pain management infusion; administrative services, professional pharmacy services, care coordination, and all necessary supplies and equipment (drugs and nursing visits coded separately), per diem

⊘ **S9328** Home infusion therapy, implanted pump pain management infusion; administrative services, professional pharmacy services, care coordination, and all necessary supplies and equipment (drugs and nursing visits coded separately), per diem

⊘ **S9329** Home infusion therapy, chemotherapy infusion; administrative services, professional pharmacy services, care coordination, and all necessary supplies and equipment (drugs and nursing visits coded separately), per diem (do not use this code with S9330 or S9331)

⊘ **S9330** Home infusion therapy, continuous (twenty-four hours or more) chemotherapy infusion; administrative services, professional pharmacy services, care coordination, and all necessary supplies and equipment (drugs and nursing visits coded separately), per diem

⊘ **S9331** Home infusion therapy, intermittent (less than twenty-four hours) chemotherapy infusion; administrative services, professional pharmacy services, care coordination, and all necessary supplies and equipment (drugs and nursing visits coded separately), per diem

⊘ **S9335** Home therapy, hemodialysis; administrative services, professional pharmacy services, care coordination, and all necessary supplies and equipment (drugs and nursing services coded separately), per diem

⊘ **S9336** Home infusion therapy, continuous anticoagulant infusion therapy (e.g., heparin), administrative services, professional pharmacy services, care coordination, and all necessary supplies and equipment (drugs and nursing visits coded separately), per diem

⊘ **S9338** Home infusion therapy, immunotherapy, administrative services, professional pharmacy services, care coordination, and all necessary supplies and equipment (drug and nursing visits coded separately), per diem

⊘ **S9339** Home therapy; peritoneal dialysis, administrative services, professional pharmacy services, care coordination and all necessary supplies and equipment (drugs and nursing visits coded separately), per diem

⊘ **S9340** Home therapy; enteral nutrition; administrative services, professional pharmacy services, care coordination, and all necessary supplies and equipment (enteral formula and nursing visits coded separately), per diem

⊘ **S9341** Home therapy; enteral nutrition via gravity; administrative services, professional pharmacy services, care coordination, and all necessary supplies and equipment (enteral formula and nursing visits coded separately), per diem

⊘ **S9342** Home therapy; enteral nutrition via pump; administrative services, professional pharmacy services, care coordination, and all necessary supplies and equipment (enteral formula and nursing visits coded separately), per diem

---

▶ **New**　　↩ **Revised**　　✔ **Reinstated**　　~~deleted~~ **Deleted**　　⊘ **Not covered or valid by Medicare**

⊗ **Special coverage instructions**　　✳ **Carrier discretion**　　Ⓑ **Bill Part B MAC**　　Ⓑ **Bill DME MAC**

⊘ **S9343** Home therapy; enteral nutrition via bolus; administrative services, professional pharmacy services, care coordination, and all necessary supplies and equipment (enteral formula and nursing visits coded separately), per diem

⊘ **S9345** Home infusion therapy, anti-hemophilic agent infusion therapy (e.g., Factor VIII); administrative services, professional pharmacy services, care coordination, and all necessary supplies and equipment (drugs and nursing visits coded separately), per diem

⊘ **S9346** Home infusion therapy, alpha-1-proteinase inhibitor (e.g., Prolastin); administrative services, professional pharmacy services, care coordination, and all necessary supplies and equipment (drugs and nursing visits coded separately), per diem

⊘ **S9347** Home infusion therapy, uninterrupted, long-term, controlled rate intravenous or subcutaneous infusion therapy (e.g., Epoprostenol); administrative services, professional pharmacy services, care coordination, and all necessary supplies and equipment (drugs and nursing visits coded separately), per diem

⊘ **S9348** Home infusion therapy, sympathomimetic/inotropic agent infusion therapy (e.g., Dobutamine); administrative services, professional pharmacy services, care coordination, all necessary supplies and equipment (drugs and nursing visits coded separately), per diem

⊘ **S9349** Home infusion therapy, tocolytic infusion therapy; administrative services, professional pharmacy services, care coordination, and all necessary supplies and equipment (drugs and nursing visits coded separately), per diem

⊘ **S9351** Home infusion therapy, continuous or intermittent anti-emetic infusion therapy; administrative services, professional pharmacy services, care coordination, and all necessary supplies and equipment (drugs and visits coded separately), per diem

⊘ **S9353** Home infusion therapy, continuous insulin infusion therapy; administrative services, professional pharmacy services, care coordination, and all necessary supplies and equipment (drugs and nursing visits coded separately), per diem

⊘ **S9355** Home infusion therapy, chelation therapy; administrative services, professional pharmacy services, care coordination, and all necessary supplies and equipment (drugs and nursing visits coded separately), per diem

⊘ **S9357** Home infusion therapy, enzyme replacement intravenous therapy; (e.g., Imiglucerase); administrative services, professional pharmacy services, care coordination, and all necessary supplies and equipment (drugs and nursing visits coded separately), per diem

⊘ **S9359** Home infusion therapy, anti-tumor necrosis factor intravenous therapy; (e.g., Infliximab); administrative services, professional pharmacy services, care coordination, and all necessary supplies and equipment (drugs and nursing visits coded separately), per diem

⊘ **S9361** Home infusion therapy, diuretic intravenous therapy; administrative services, professional pharmacy services, care coordination, and all necessary supplies and equipment (drugs and nursing visits coded separately), per diem

⊘ **S9363** Home infusion therapy, anti-spasmotic therapy; administrative services, professional pharmacy services, care coordination, and all necessary supplies and equipment (drugs and nursing visits coded separately), per diem

⊘ **S9364** Home infusion therapy, total parenteral nutrition (TPN); administrative services, professional pharmacy services, care coordination, and all necessary supplies and equipment including standard TPN formula (lipids, specialty amino acid formulas, drugs other than in standard formula, and nursing visits coded separately) per diem (do not use with home infusion codes S9365-S9368 using daily volume scales)

⊘ **S9365** Home infusion therapy, total parenteral nutrition (TPN); one liter per day, administrative services, professional pharmacy services, care coordination, and all necessary supplies and equipment including standard TPN formula (lipids, specialty amino acid formulas, drugs other than in standard formula and nursing visits coded separately), per diem

---

▶ New   ↻ Revised   ✔ Reinstated   ~~deleted~~ Deleted   ⊘ Not covered or valid by Medicare

✪ Special coverage instructions   ✳ Carrier discretion   Ⓑ Bill Part B MAC   Ⓓ Bill DME MAC

⊘ **S9366** Home infusion therapy, total parenteral nutrition (TPN); more than one liter but no more than two liters per day, administrative services, professional pharmacy services, care coordination, and all necessary supplies and equipment including standard TPN formula; (lipids, specialty amino acid formulas, drugs other than in standard formula and nursing visits coded separately), per diem

⊘ **S9367** Home infusion therapy, total parenteral nutrition (TPN); more than two liters but no more than three liters per day, administrative services, professional pharmacy services, care coordination, and all necessary supplies and equipment including standard TPN formula (lipids, specialty amino acid formulas, drugs other than in standard formula and nursing visits coded separately), per diem

⊘ **S9368** Home infusion therapy, total parenteral nutrition (TPN); more than three liters per day, administrative services, professional pharmacy services, care coordination, and all necessary supplies and equipment (including standard TPN formula; lipids, specialty amino acid formulas, drugs other than in standard formula and nursing visits coded separately), per diem

⊘ **S9370** Home therapy, intermittent anti-emetic injection therapy; administrative services, professional pharmacy services, care coordination, and all necessary supplies and equipment (drugs and nursing visits coded separately), per diem

⊘ **S9372** Home therapy; intermittent anticoagulant injection therapy (e.g., heparin); administrative services, professional pharmacy services, care coordination, and all necessary supplies and equipment (drugs and nursing visits coded separately), per diem (do not use this code for flushing of infusion devices with heparin to maintain patency)

⊘ **S9373** Home infusion therapy, hydration therapy; administrative services, professional pharmacy services, care coordination, and all necessary supplies and equipment (drugs and nursing visits coded separately), per diem (do not use with hydration therapy codes S9374-S9377 using daily volume scales)

⊘ **S9374** Home infusion therapy, hydration therapy; one liter per day, administrative services, professional pharmacy services, care coordination, and all necessary supplies and equipment (drugs and nursing visits coded separately), per diem

⊘ **S9375** Home infusion therapy, hydration therapy; more than one liter but no more than two liters per day, administrative services, professional pharmacy services, care coordination, and all necessary supplies and equipment (drugs and nursing visits coded separately), per diem

⊘ **S9376** Home infusion therapy, hydration therapy; more than two liters but no more than three liters per day, administrative services, professional pharmacy services, care coordination, and all necessary supplies and equipment (drugs and nursing visits coded separately), per diem

⊘ **S9377** Home infusion therapy, hydration therapy; more than three liters per day, administrative services, professional pharmacy services, care coordination, and all necessary supplies (drugs and nursing visits coded separately), per diem

⊘ **S9379** Home infusion therapy, infusion therapy, not otherwise classified; administrative services, professional pharmacy services, care coordination, and all necessary supplies and equipment (drugs and nursing visits coded separately), per diem

Miscellaneous Supplies and Services

⊘ **S9381** Delivery or service to high risk areas requiring escort or extra protection, per visit

⊘ **S9401** Anticoagulation clinic, inclusive of all services except laboratory tests, per session

⊘ **S9430** Pharmacy compounding and dispensing services

⊘ **S9433** Medical food nutritionally complete, administered orally, providing 100% of nutritional intake

⊘ **S9434** Modified solid food supplements for inborn errors of metabolism

⊘ **S9435** Medical foods for inborn errors of metabolism

⊘ **S9436** Childbirth preparation/Lamaze classes, non-physician provider, per session

| ▶ New | ↻ Revised | ✔ Reinstated | ~~deleted~~ Deleted | ⊘ Not covered or valid by Medicare |
| ✿ Special coverage instructions | ✳ Carrier discretion | ⑧ Bill Part B MAC | ⑨ Bill DME MAC | |

⊘ **S9437** Childbirth refresher classes, non-physician provider, per session

⊘ **S9438** Cesarean birth classes, non-physician provider, per session

⊘ **S9439** VBAC (vaginal birth after cesarean) classes, non-physician provider, per session

⊘ **S9441** Asthma education, non-physician provider, per session

⊘ **S9442** Birthing classes, non-physician provider, per session

⊘ **S9443** Lactation classes, non-physician provider, per session

⊘ **S9444** Parenting classes, non-physician provider, per session

⊘ **S9445** Patient education, not otherwise classified, non-physician provider, individual, per session

⊘ **S9446** Patient education, not otherwise classified, non-physician provider, group, per session

⊘ **S9447** Infant safety (including CPR) classes, non-physician provider, per session

⊘ **S9449** Weight management classes, non-physician provider, per session

⊘ **S9451** Exercise classes, non-physician provider, per session

⊘ **S9452** Nutrition classes, non-physician provider, per session

⊘ **S9453** Smoking cessation classes, non-physician provider, per session

⊘ **S9454** Stress management classes, non-physician provider, per session

⊘ **S9455** Diabetic management program, group session

⊘ **S9460** Diabetic management program, nurse visit

⊘ **S9465** Diabetic management program, dietitian visit

⊘ **S9470** Nutritional counseling, dietitian visit

⊘ **S9472** Cardiac rehabilitation program, non-physician provider, per diem

⊘ **S9473** Pulmonary rehabilitation program, non-physician provider, per diem

⊘ **S9474** Enterostomal therapy by a registered nurse certified in enterostomal therapy, per diem

⊘ **S9475** Ambulatory setting substance abuse treatment or detoxification services, per diem

⊘ **S9476** Vestibular rehabilitation program, non-physician provider, per diem

⊘ **S9480** Intensive outpatient psychiatric services, per diem

⊘ **S9482** Family stabilization services, per 15 minutes

⊘ **S9484** Crisis intervention mental health services, per hour

⊘ **S9485** Crisis intervention mental health services, per diem

Home Therapy Services

⊘ **S9490** Home infusion therapy, corticosteroid infusion; administrative services, professional pharmacy services, care coordination, and all necessary supplies and equipment (drugs and nursing visits coded separately), per diem

⊘ **S9494** Home infusion therapy, antibiotic, antiviral, or antifungal therapy; administrative services, professional pharmacy services, care coordination, and all necessary supplies and equipment (drugs and nursing visits coded separately) per diem (do not use this code with home infusion codes for hourly dosing schedules S9497-S9504)

⊘ **S9497** Home infusion therapy, antibiotic, antiviral, or antifungal therapy; once every 3 hours; administrative services, professional pharmacy services, care coordination, and all necessary supplies and equipment (drugs and nursing visits coded separately), per diem

⊘ **S9500** Home infusion therapy, antibiotic, antiviral, or antifungal therapy; once every 24 hours; administrative services, professional pharmacy services, care coordination, and all necessary supplies and equipment (drugs and nursing visits coded separately), per diem

⊘ **S9501** Home infusion therapy, antibiotic, antiviral, or antifungal therapy; once every 12 hours; administrative services, professional pharmacy services, care coordination, and all necessary supplies and equipment (drugs and nursing visits coded separately), per diem

⊘ **S9502** Home infusion therapy, antibiotic, antiviral, or antifungal therapy; once every 8 hours, administrative services, professional pharmacy services, care coordination, and all necessary supplies and equipment (drugs and nursing visits coded separately), per diem

▶ New   ↩ Revised   ✔ Reinstated   ~~deleted~~ Deleted   ⊘ Not covered or valid by Medicare
✪ Special coverage instructions   ✳ Carrier discretion   Ⓟ Bill Part B MAC   Ⓑ Bill DME MAC

⊘ **S9503**   Home infusion therapy, antibiotic, antiviral, or antifungal; once every 6 hours; administrative services, professional pharmacy services, care coordination, and all necessary supplies and equipment (drugs and nursing visits coded separately), per diem

⊘ **S9504**   Home infusion therapy, antibiotic, antiviral, or antifungal; once every 4 hours; administrative services, professional pharmacy services, care coordination, and all necessary supplies and equipment (drugs and nursing visits coded separately), per diem

⊘ **S9529**   Routine venipuncture for collection of specimen(s), single home bound, nursing home, or skilled nursing facility patient

⊘ **S9537**   Home therapy; hematopoietic hormone injection therapy (e.g., erythropoietin, G-CSF, GM-CSF); administrative services, professional pharmacy services, care coordination, and all necessary supplies and equipment (drugs and nursing visits coded separately), per diem

⊘ **S9538**   Home transfusion of blood product(s); administrative services, professional pharmacy services, care coordination, and all necessary supplies and equipment (blood products, drugs, and nursing visits coded separately), per diem

⊘ **S9542**   Home injectable therapy; not otherwise classified, including administrative services, professional pharmacy services, care coordination, and all necessary supplies and equipment (drugs and nursing visits coded separately), per diem

⊘ **S9558**   Home injectable therapy; growth hormone, including administrative services, professional pharmacy services, care coordination, and all necessary supplies and equipment (drugs and nursing visits coded separately), per diem

⊘ **S9559**   Home injectable therapy; interferon, including administrative services, professional pharmacy services, care coordination, and all necessary supplies and equipment (drugs and nursing visits coded separately), per diem

⊘ **S9560**   Home injectable therapy; hormonal therapy (e.g., Leuprolide, Goserelin), including administrative services, professional pharmacy services, care coordination, and all necessary supplies and equipment (drugs and nursing visits coded separately), per diem

⊘ **S9562**   Home injectable therapy, palivizumab, including administrative services, professional pharmacy services, care coordination, and all necessary supplies and equipment (drugs and nursing visits coded separately), per diem

⊘ **S9590**   Home therapy, irrigation therapy (e.g., sterile irrigation of an organ or anatomical cavity); including administrative services, professional pharmacy services, care coordination, and all necessary supplies and equipment (drugs and nursing visits coded separately), per diem

⊘ **S9810**   Home therapy; professional pharmacy services for provision of infusion, specialty drug administration, and/or disease state management, not otherwise classified, per hour (do not use this code with any per diem code)

Other Services and Fees

⊘ **S9900**   Services by journal-listed Christian Science Practitioner for the purpose of healing, per diem

⊘ **S9901**   Services by a journal-listed Christian Science nurse, per hour

⊘ **S9960**   Ambulance service, conventional air service, nonemergency transport, one way (fixed wing)

⊘ **S9961**   Ambulance service, conventional air service, nonemergency transport, one way (rotary wing)

⊘ **S9970**   Health club membership, annual

⊘ **S9975**   Transplant related lodging, meals and transportation, per diem

⊘ **S9976**   Lodging, per diem, not otherwise classified

⊘ **S9977**   Meals, per diem, not otherwise specified

⊘ **S9981**   Medical records copying fee, administrative

⊘ **S9982**   Medical records copying fee, per page

⊘ **S9986**   Not medically necessary service (patient is aware that service not medically necessary)

▶ **New**   ↻ **Revised**   ✔ **Reinstated**   ~~deleted~~ **Deleted**   ⊘ **Not covered or valid by Medicare**
✪ **Special coverage instructions**   ✳ **Carrier discretion**   Ⓟ **Bill Part B MAC**   Ⓑ **Bill DME MAC**

⊘ **S9988**   Services provided as part of a Phase I clinical trial

⊘ **S9989**   Services provided outside of the United States of America (list in addition to code(s) for services(s))

⊘ **S9990**   Services provided as part of a Phase II clinical trial

⊘ **S9991**   Services provided as part of a Phase III clinical trial

⊘ **S9992**   Transportation costs to and from trial location and local transportation costs (e.g., fares for taxicab or bus) for clinical trial participant and one caregiver/companion

⊘ **S9994**   Lodging costs (e.g., hotel charges) for clinical trial participant and one caregiver/companion

⊘ **S9996**   Meals for clinical trial participant and one caregiver/companion

⊘ **S9999**   Sales tax

▶ New   ⤾ Revised   ✔ Reinstated   ~~deleted~~ Deleted   ⊘ Not covered or valid by Medicare
✪ Special coverage instructions   ✻ Carrier discretion   Ⓑ Bill Part B MAC   Ⓑ Bill DME MAC

DIAGNOSTIC RADIOLOGY SERVICES   S9988 — S9999

315

TEMPORARY NATIONAL CODES ESTABLISHED BY MEDICAID (T1000-T9999)

Not Valid For Medicare

⊘ **T1000** Private duty/independent nursing service(s) - licensed, up to 15 minutes

⊘ **T1001** Nursing assessment/evaluation

⊘ **T1002** RN services, up to 15 minutes

⊘ **T1003** LPN/LVN services, up to 15 minutes

⊘ **T1004** Services of a qualified nursing aide, up to 15 minutes

⊘ **T1005** Respite care services, up to 15 minutes

⊘ **T1006** Alcohol and/or substance abuse services, family/couple counseling

⊘ **T1007** Alcohol and/or substance abuse services, treatment plan development and/or modification

⊘ **T1009** Child sitting services for children of the individual receiving alcohol and/or substance abuse services

⊘ **T1010** Meals for individuals receiving alcohol and/or substance abuse services (when meals not included in the program)

⊘ **T1012** Alcohol and/or substance abuse services, skills development

⊘ **T1013** Sign language or oral interpretive services, per 15 minutes

⊘ **T1014** Telehealth transmission, per minute, professional services bill separately

⊘ **T1015** Clinic visit/encounter, all-inclusive

⊘ **T1016** Case Management, each 15 minutes

⊘ **T1017** Targeted Case Management, each 15 minutes

⊘ **T1018** School-based individualized education program (IEP) services, bundled

⊘ **T1019** Personal care services, per 15 minutes, not for an inpatient or resident of a hospital, nursing facility, ICF/MR or IMD, part of the individualized plan of treatment (code may not be used to identify services provided by home health aide or certified nurse assistant)

⊘ **T1020** Personal care services, per diem, not for an inpatient or resident of a hospital, nursing facility, ICF/MR or IMD, part of the individualized plan of treatment (code may not be used to identify services provided by home health aide or certified nurse assistant)

⊘ **T1021** Home health aide or certified nurse assistant, per visit

⊘ **T1022** Contracted home health agency services, all services provided under contract, per day

⊘ **T1023** Screening to determine the appropriateness of consideration of an individual for participation in a specified program, project or treatment protocol, per encounter

⊘ **T1024** Evaluation and treatment by an integrated, specialty team contracted to provide coordinated care to multiple or severely handicapped children, per encounter

⊘ **T1025** Intensive, extended multidisciplinary services provided in a clinic setting to children with complex medical, physical, mental and psychosocial impairments, per diem

⊘ **T1026** Intensive, extended multidisciplinary services provided in a clinic setting to children with complex medical, physical, medical and psychosocial impairments, per hour

⊘ **T1027** Family training and counseling for child development, per 15 minutes

⊘ **T1028** Assessment of home, physical and family environment, to determine suitability to meet patient's medical needs

⊘ **T1029** Comprehensive environmental lead investigation, not including laboratory analysis, per dwelling

⊘ **T1030** Nursing care, in the home, by registered nurse, per diem

⊘ **T1031** Nursing care, in the home, by licensed practical nurse, per diem

⊘ **T1040** Medicaid certified community behavioral health clinic services, per diem

⊘ **T1041** Medicaid certified community behavioral health clinic services, per month

⊘ **T1502** Administration of oral, intramuscular and/or subcutaneous medication by health care agency/professional, per visit

⊘ **T1503** Administration of medication, other than oral and/or injectable, by a health care agency/professional, per visit

⊘ **T1505** Electronic medication compliance management device, includes all components and accessories, not otherwise classified

---

▶ New   ↻ Revised   ✔ Reinstated   ~~deleted~~ Deleted   ⊘ Not covered or valid by Medicare
❂ Special coverage instructions   ✳ Carrier discretion   Ⓑ Bill Part B MAC   Ⓓ Bill DME MAC

⊘ **T1999** Miscellaneous therapeutic items and supplies, retail purchases, not otherwise classified; identify product in "remarks"

⊘ **T2001** Non-emergency transportation; patient attendant/escort

⊘ **T2002** Non-emergency transportation; per diem

⊘ **T2003** Non-emergency transportation; encounter/trip

⊘ **T2004** Non-emergency transport; commercial carrier, multi-pass

⊘ **T2005** Non-emergency transportation: stretcher van

⊘ **T2007** Transportation waiting time, air ambulance and non-emergency vehicle, one-half (1/2) hour increments

⊘ **T2010** Preadmission screening and resident review (PASRR) level I identification screening, per screen

⊘ **T2011** Preadmission screening and resident review (PASRR) level II evaluation, per evaluation

⊘ **T2012** Habilitation, educational, waiver; per diem

⊘ **T2013** Habilitation, educational, waiver; per hour

⊘ **T2014** Habilitation, prevocational, waiver; per diem

⊘ **T2015** Habilitation, prevocational, waiver; per hour

⊘ **T2016** Habilitation, residential, waiver; per diem

⊘ **T2017** Habilitation, residential, waiver; 15 minutes

⊘ **T2018** Habilitation, supported employment, waiver; per diem

⊘ **T2019** Habilitation, supported employment, waiver; per 15 minutes

⊘ **T2020** Day habilitation, waiver; per diem

⊘ **T2021** Day habilitation, waiver; per 15 minutes

⊘ **T2022** Case management, per month

⊘ **T2023** Targeted case management; per month

⊘ **T2024** Service assessment/plan of care development, waiver

⊘ **T2025** Waiver services; not otherwise specified (NOS)

⊘ **T2026** Specialized childcare, waiver; per diem

⊘ **T2027** Specialized childcare, waiver; per 15 minutes

⊘ **T2028** Specialized supply, not otherwise specified, waiver

⊘ **T2029** Specialized medical equipment, not otherwise specified, waiver

⊘ **T2030** Assisted living, waiver; per month

⊘ **T2031** Assisted living; waiver, per diem

⊘ **T2032** Residential care, not otherwise specified (NOS), waiver; per month

⊘ **T2033** Residential care, not otherwise specified (NOS), waiver; per diem

⊘ **T2034** Crisis intervention, waiver; per diem

⊘ **T2035** Utility services to support medical equipment and assistive technology/devices, waiver

⊘ **T2036** Therapeutic camping, overnight, waiver; each session

⊘ **T2037** Therapeutic camping, day, waiver; each session

⊘ **T2038** Community transition, waiver; per service

⊘ **T2039** Vehicle modifications, waiver; per service

⊘ **T2040** Financial management, self-directed, waiver; per 15 minutes

⊘ **T2041** Supports brokerage, self-directed, waiver; per 15 minutes

⊘ **T2042** Hospice routine home care; per diem

⊘ **T2043** Hospice continuous home care; per hour

⊘ **T2044** Hospice inpatient respite care; per diem

⊘ **T2045** Hospice general inpatient care; per diem

⊘ **T2046** Hospice long term care, room and board only; per diem

⊘ **T2048** Behavioral health; long-term care residential (non-acute care in a residential treatment program where stay is typically longer than 30 days), with room and board, per diem

⊘ **T2049** Non-emergency transportation; stretcher van, mileage; per mile

⊘ **T2101** Human breast milk processing, storage and distribution only

⊘ **T4521** Adult sized disposable incontinence product, brief/diaper, small, each

IOM: 100-03, 4, 280.1

⊘ **T4522** Adult sized disposable incontinence product, brief/diaper, medium, each

IOM: 100-03, 4, 280.1

▶ New   ⟲ Revised   ✔ Reinstated   ~~deleted~~ Deleted   ⊘ Not covered or valid by Medicare

✪ Special coverage instructions   ✳ Carrier discretion   Ⓟ Bill Part B MAC   Ⓑ Bill DME MAC

⊘ **T4523** Adult sized disposable incontinence product, brief/diaper, large, each

IOM: 100-03, 4, 280.1

⊘ **T4524** Adult sized disposable incontinence product, brief/diaper, extra large, each

IOM: 100-03, 4, 280.1

⊘ **T4525** Adult sized disposable incontinence product, protective underwear/pull-on, small size, each

IOM: 100-03, 4, 280.1

⊘ **T4526** Adult sized disposable incontinence product, protective underwear/pull-on, medium size, each

IOM: 100-03, 4, 280.1

⊘ **T4527** Adult sized disposable incontinence product, protective underwear/pull-on, large size, each

IOM: 100-03, 4, 280.1

⊘ **T4528** Adult sized disposable incontinence product, protective underwear/pull-on, extra large size, each

IOM: 100-03, 4, 280.1

⊘ **T4529** Pediatric sized disposable incontinence product, brief/diaper, small/medium size, each

IOM: 100-03, 4, 280.1

⊘ **T4530** Pediatric sized disposable incontinence product, brief/diaper, large size, each

IOM: 100-03, 4, 280.1

⊘ **T4531** Pediatric sized disposable incontinence product, protective underwear/pull-on, small/medium size, each

IOM: 100-03, 4, 280.1

⊘ **T4532** Pediatric sized disposable incontinence product, protective underwear/pull-on, large size, each

IOM: 100-03, 4, 280.1

⊘ **T4533** Youth sized disposable incontinence product, brief/diaper, each

IOM: 100-03, 4, 280.1

⊘ **T4534** Youth sized disposable incontinence product, protective underwear/pull-on, each

IOM: 100-03, 4, 280.1

⊘ **T4535** Disposable liner/shield/guard/pad/undergarment, for incontinence, each

IOM: 100-03, 4, 280.1

⊘ **T4536** Incontinence product, protective underwear/pull-on, reusable, any size, each

IOM: 100-03, 4, 280.1

⊘ **T4537** Incontinence product, protective underpad, reusable, bed size, each

IOM: 100-03, 4, 280.1

⊘ **T4538** Diaper service, reusable diaper, each diaper

IOM: 100-03, 4, 280.1

⊘ **T4539** Incontinence product, diaper/brief, reusable, any size, each

IOM: 100-03, 4, 280.1

⊘ **T4540** Incontinence product, protective underpad, reusable, chair size, each

IOM: 100-03, 4, 280.1

⊘ **T4541** Incontinence product, disposable underpad, large, each

⊘ **T4542** Incontinence product, disposable underpad, small size, each

⊘ **T4543** Adult sized disposable incontinence product, protective brief/diaper, above extra large, each

IOM: 100-03, 4, 280.1

⊘ **T4544** Adult sized disposable incontinence product, protective underwear/pull-on, above extra large, each

IOM: 100-03, 4, 280.1

⊘ **T5001** Positioning seat for persons with special orthopedic needs, supply, not otherwise specified

⊘ **T5999** Supply, not otherwise specified

▶ **New** ⟳ **Revised** ✔ **Reinstated** ~~deleted~~ **Deleted** ⊘ **Not covered or valid by Medicare**
✿ **Special coverage instructions** ✳ **Carrier discretion** Ⓑ **Bill Part B MAC** Ⓑ **Bill DME MAC**

VISION SERVICES (V0000-V2999)

Frames

✪ **V2020** Frames, purchases ⑧

Includes cost of frame/replacement and dispensing fee. One unit of service represents one pair of eyeglass frames.

IOM: 100-02, 15, 120

⊘ **V2025** Deluxe frame ⑧

Not a benefit. Billing deluxe frames-submit V2020 on one line; V2025 on second line

IOM: 100-04, 1, 30.3.5

If a CPT procedure code for supply of spectacles or a permanent prosthesis is reported, recode with the specific lens type listed below.

Single Vision Lenses

❋ **V2100** Sphere, single vision, plano to plus or minus 4.00, per lens ⑧

❋ **V2101** Sphere, single vision, plus or minus 4.12 to plus or minus 7.00d, per lens ⑧

❋ **V2102** Sphere, single vision, plus or minus 7.12 to plus or minus 20.00d, per lens ⑧

❋ **V2103** Spherocylinder, single vision, plano to plus or minus 4.00d sphere, .12 to 2.00d cylinder, per lens ⑧

❋ **V2104** Spherocylinder, single vision, plano to plus or minus 4.00d sphere, 2.12 to 4.00d cylinder, per lens ⑧

❋ **V2105** Spherocylinder, single vision, plano to plus or minus 4.00d sphere, 4.25 to 6.00d cylinder, per lens ⑧

❋ **V2106** Spherocylinder, single vision, plano to plus or minus 4.00d sphere, over 6.00d cylinder, per lens ⑧

❋ **V2107** Spherocylinder, single vision, plus or minus 4.25 to plus or minus 7.00 sphere, .12 to 2.00d cylinder, per lens ⑧

❋ **V2108** Spherocylinder, single vision, plus or minus 4.25d to plus or minus 7.00d sphere, 2.12 to 4.00d cylinder, per lens ⑧

❋ **V2109** Spherocylinder, single vision, plus or minus 4.25 to plus or minus 7.00d sphere, 4.25 to 6.00d cylinder, per lens ⑧

❋ **V2110** Sperocylinder, single vision, plus or minus 4.25 to 7.00d sphere, over 6.00d cylinder, per lens ⑧

❋ **V2111** Spherocylinder, single vision, plus or minus 7.25 to plus or minus 12.00d sphere, .25 to 2.25d cylinder, per lens ⑧

❋ **V2112** Spherocylinder, single vision, plus or minus 7.25 to plus or minus 12.00d sphere, 2.25d to 4.00d cylinder, per lens ⑧

❋ **V2113** Spherocylinder, single vision, plus or minus 7.25 to plus or minus 12.00d sphere, 4.25 to 6.00d cylinder, per lens ⑧

❋ **V2114** Spherocylinder, single vision, sphere over plus or minus 12.00d, per lens ⑧

❋ **V2115** Lenticular, (myodisc), per lens, single vision ⑧

❋ **V2118** Aniseikonic lens, single vision ⑧

✪ **V2121** Lenticular lens, per lens, single ⑧

IOM: 100-02, 15, 120; 100-04, 3, 10.4

❋ **V2199** Not otherwise classified, single vision lens ⑧

Bill on paper. Requires report of type of single vision lens and optical lab invoice.

Bifocal Lenses

❋ **V2200** Sphere, bifocal, plano to plus or minus 4.00d, per lens ⑧

❋ **V2201** Sphere, bifocal, plus or minus 4.12 to plus or minus 7.00d, per lens ⑧

❋ **V2202** Sphere, bifocal, plus or minus 7.12 to plus or minus 20.00d, per lens ⑧

❋ **V2203** Spherocylinder, bifocal, plano to plus or minus 4.00d sphere, .12 to 2.00d cylinder, per lens ⑧

❋ **V2204** Spherocylinder, bifocal, plano to plus or minus 4.00d sphere, 2.12 to 4.00d cylinder, per lens ⑧

❋ **V2205** Spherocylinder, bifocal, plano to plus or minus 4.00d sphere, 4.25 to 6.00d cylinder, per lens ⑧

❋ **V2206** Spherocylinder, bifocal, plano to plus or minus 4.00d sphere, over 6.00d cylinder, per lens ⑧

❋ **V2207** Spherocylinder, bifocal, plus or minus 4.25 to plus or minus 7.00d sphere, .12 to 2.00d cylinder, per lens ⑧

❋ **V2208** Spherocylinder, bifocal, plus or minus 4.25 to plus or minus 7.00d sphere, 2.12 to 4.00d cylinder, per lens ⑧

▶ New ↩ Revised ✔ Reinstated ~~deleted~~ Deleted ⊘ Not covered or valid by Medicare ✪ Special coverage instructions ❋ Carrier discretion ⑨ Bill Part B MAC ⑧ Bill DME MAC

✳ **V2209** Spherocylinder, bifocal, plus or minus 4.25 to plus or minus 7.00d sphere, 4.25 to 6.00d cylinder, per lens Ⓑ

✳ **V2210** Spherocylinder, bifocal, plus or minus 4.25 to plus or minus 7.00d sphere, over 6.00d cylinder, per lens Ⓑ

✳ **V2211** Spherocylinder, bifocal, plus or minus 7.25 to plus or minus 12.00d sphere, .25 to 2.25d cylinder, per lens Ⓑ

✳ **V2212** Spherocylinder, bifocal, plus or minus 7.25 to plus or minus 12.00d sphere, 2.25 to 4.00d cylinder, per lens Ⓑ

✳ **V2213** Spherocylinder, bifocal, plus or minus 7.25 to plus or minus 12.00d sphere, 4.25 to 6.00d cylinder, per lens Ⓑ

✳ **V2214** Spherocylinder, bifocal, sphere over plus or minus 12.00d, per lens Ⓑ

✳ **V2215** Lenticular (myodisc), per lens, bifocal Ⓑ

✳ **V2218** Aniseikonic, per lens, bifocal Ⓑ

✳ **V2219** Bifocal seg width over 28 mm Ⓑ

✳ **V2220** Bifocal add over 3.25d Ⓑ

⊘ **V2221** Lenticular lens, per lens, bifocal Ⓑ

IOM: 100-02, 15, 120; 100-04, 3, 10.4

✳ **V2299** Specialty bifocal (by report) Ⓑ

Bill on paper. Requires report of type of specialty bifocal lens and optical lab invoice.

Trifocal Lenses

✳ **V2300** Sphere, trifocal, plano to plus or minus 4.00d, per lens Ⓑ

✳ **V2301** Sphere, trifocal, plus or minus 4.12 to plus or minus 7.00d per lens Ⓑ

✳ **V2302** Sphere, trifocal, plus or minus 7.12 to plus or minus 20.00, per lens Ⓑ

✳ **V2303** Spherocylinder, trifocal, plano to plus or minus 4.00d sphere, .12 to 2.00d cylinder, per lens Ⓑ

✳ **V2304** Spherocylinder, trifocal, plano to plus or minus 4.00d sphere, 2.25-4.00d cylinder, per lens Ⓑ

✳ **V2305** Spherocylinder, trifocal, plano to plus or minus 4.00d sphere, 4.25 to 6.00 cylinder, per lens Ⓑ

✳ **V2306** Spherocylinder, trifocal, plano to plus or minus 4.00d sphere, over 6.00d cylinder, per lens Ⓑ

✳ **V2307** Spherocylinder, trifocal, plus or minus 4.25 to plus or minus 7.00d sphere, .12 to 2.00d cylinder, per lens Ⓑ

✳ **V2308** Spherocylinder, trifocal, plus or minus 4.25 to plus or minus 7.00d sphere, 2.12 to 4.00d cylinder, per lens Ⓑ

✳ **V2309** Spherocylinder, trifocal, plus or minus 4.25 to plus or minus 7.00d sphere, 4.25 to 6.00d cylinder, per lens Ⓑ

✳ **V2310** Spherocylinder, trifocal, plus or minus 4.25 to plus or minus 7.00d sphere, over 6.00d cylinder, per lens Ⓑ

✳ **V2311** Spherocylinder, trifocal, plus or minus 7.25 to plus or minus 12.00d sphere, .25 to 2.25d cylinder, per lens Ⓑ

✳ **V2312** Spherocylinder, trifocal, plus or minus 7.25 to plus or minus 12.00d sphere, 2.25 to 4.00d cylinder, per lens Ⓑ

✳ **V2313** Spherocylinder, trifocal, plus or minus 7.25 to plus or minus 12.00d sphere, 4.25 to 6.00d cylinder, per lens Ⓑ

✳ **V2314** Spherocylinder, trifocal, sphere over plus or minus 12.00d, per lens Ⓑ

✳ **V2315** Lenticular, (myodisc), per lens, trifocal Ⓑ

✳ **V2318** Aniseikonic lens, trifocal Ⓑ

✳ **V2319** Trifocal seg width over 28 mm Ⓑ

✳ **V2320** Trifocal add over 3.25d Ⓑ

⊘ **V2321** Lenticular lens, per lens, trifocal Ⓑ

IOM: 100-02, 15, 120; 100-04, 3, 10.4

✳ **V2399** Specialty trifocal (by report) Ⓑ

Bill on paper. Requires report of type of trifocal lens and optical lab invoice.

Variable Asphericity/Sphericity Lenses

✳ **V2410** Variable asphericity lens, single vision, full field, glass or plastic, per lens Ⓑ

✳ **V2430** Variable asphericity lens, bifocal, full field, glass or plastic, per lens Ⓑ

✳ **V2499** Variable sphericity lens, other type Ⓑ

Bill on paper. Requires report of other ptical lab invoice.

Contact Lenses

If a CPT procedure code for supply of contact lens is reported, recode with specific lens type listed below (per lens).

✳ **V2500** Contact lens, PMMA, spherical, per lens Ⓑ

Requires prior authorization for patients under age 21.

✳ **V2501** Contact lens, PMMA, toric or prism ballast, per lens ⑧

Requires prior authorization for clients under age 21.

✳ **V2502** Contact lens, PMMA, bifocal, per lens ⑧

Requires prior authorization for clients under age 21. Bill on paper. Requires optical lab invoice.

✳ **V2503** Contact lens PMMA, color vision deficiency, per lens ⑧

Requires prior authorization for clients under age 21. Bill on paper. Requires optical lab invoice.

✳ **V2510** Contact lens, gas permeable, spherical, per lens ⑧

Requires prior authorization for clients under age 21.

✳ **V2511** Contact lens, gas permeable, toric, prism ballast, per lens ⑧

Requires prior authorization for clients under age 21.

✳ **V2512** Contact lens, gas permeable, bifocal, per lens ⑧

Requires prior authorization for clients under age 21.

✳ **V2513** Contact lens, gas permeable, extended wear, per lens ⑧

Requires prior authorization for clients under age 21.

❂ **V2520** Contact lens, hydrophilic, spherical, per lens ⑨ ⑧

Requires prior authorization for clients under age 21.

IOM: 100-03, 1, 80.1; 100-03, 1, 80.4

❂ **V2521** Contact lens, hydrophilic, toric, or prism ballast, per lens ⑨ ⑧

Requires prior authorization for clients under age 21.

IOM: 100-03, 1, 80.1; 100-03, 1, 80.4

❂ **V2522** Contact lens, hydrophilic, bifocal, per lens ⑨ ⑧

Requires prior authorization for clients under age 21.

IOM: 100-03, 1, 80.1; 100-03, 1, 80.4

❂ **V2523** Contact lens, hydrophilic, extended wear, per lens ⑧ ⑧

Requires prior authorization for clients under age 21.

IOM: 100-03, 1, 80.1; 100-03, 1, 80.4

✳ **V2530** Contact lens, scleral, gas impermeable, per lens (for contact lens modification, see 92325) ⑧

Requires prior authorization for clients under age 21.

❂ **V2531** Contact lens, scleral, gas permeable, per lens (for contact lens modification, see 92325) ⑧

Requires prior authorization for clients under age 21. Bill on paper. Requires optical lab invoice.

IOM: 100-03, 1, 80.5

✳ **V2599** Contact lens, other type ⑨ ⑧

Requires prior authorization for clients under age 21. Bill on paper. Requires report of other type of contact lens and optical invoice.

Low Vision Aids

If a CPT procedure code for supply of low vision aid is reported, recode with specific systems listed below.

✳ **V2600** Hand held low vision aids and other nonspectacle mounted aids ⑧

Requires prior authorization.

✳ **V2610** Single lens spectacle mounted low vision aids ⑧

Requires prior authorization.

✳ **V2615** Telescopic and other compound lens system, including distance vision telescopic, near vision telescopes and compound microscopic lens system ⑧

Requires prior authorization. Bill on paper. Requires optical lab invoice.

Prosthetic Eye

❂ **V2623** Prosthetic eye, plastic, custom ⑧

DME regional carrier. Requires prior authorization. Bill on paper. Requires optical lab invoice.

✳ **V2624** Polishing/resurfacing of ocular prosthesis ⑧

Requires prior authorization. Bill on paper. Requires optical lab invoice.

✳ **V2625** Enlargement of ocular prosthesis ⑧

Requires prior authorization. Bill on paper. Requires optical lab invoice.

▶ New ⮌ Revised ✔ Reinstated ~~deleted~~ Deleted ⊘ Not covered or valid by Medicare
❂ Special coverage instructions ✳ Carrier discretion ⑨ Bill Part B MAC ⑧ Bill DME MAC

✳ **V2626** Reduction of ocular prosthesis Ⓑ

Requires prior authorization. Bill on paper. Requires optical lab invoice.

⊘ **V2627** Scleral cover shell Ⓑ

DME regional carrier

Requires prior authorization. Bill on paper. Requires optical lab invoice.

IOM: 100-03, 4, 280.2

✳ **V2628** Fabrication and fitting of ocular conformer Ⓑ

Requires prior authorization. Bill on paper. Requires optical lab invoice.

✳ **V2629** Prosthetic eye, other type Ⓑ

Requires prior authorization. Bill on paper. Requires optical lab invoice.

Intraocular Lenses

⊘ **V2630** Anterior chamber intraocular lens Ⓑ

IOM: 100-02, 15, 120

⊘ **V2631** Iris supported intraocular lens Ⓑ

IOM: 100-02, 15, 120

⊘ **V2632** Posterior chamber intraocular lens Ⓑ

IOM: 100-02, 15, 120

Miscellaneous Vision Services

✳ **V2700** Balance lens, per lens Ⓑ

⊘ **V2702** Deluxe lens feature Ⓑ

IOM: 100-02, 15, 120; 100-04, 3, 10.4

✳ **V2710** Slab off prism, glass or plastic, per lens Ⓑ

✳ **V2715** Prism, per lens Ⓑ

✳ **V2718** Press-on lens, Fresnel prism, per lens Ⓑ

✳ **V2730** Special base curve, glass or plastic, per lens Ⓑ

⊘ **V2744** Tint, photochromatic, per lens Ⓑ

Requires prior authorization.

IOM: 100-02, 15, 120; 100-04, 3, 10.4

⊘ **V2745** Addition to lens, tint, any color, solid, gradient or equal, excludes photochroatic, any lens material, per lens Ⓑ

Includes photochromatic lenses (V2744) used as sunglasses, which are prescribed in addition to regular prosthetic lenses for aphakic patient will be denied as not medically necessary.

IOM: 100-02, 15, 120; 100-04, 3, 10.4

⊘ **V2750** Anti-reflective coating, per lens Ⓑ

Requires prior authorization.

IOM: 100-02, 15, 120; 100-04, 3, 10.4

⊘ **V2755** U-V lens, per lens Ⓑ

IOM: 100-02, 15, 120; 100-04, 3, 10.4

✳ **V2756** Eye glass case Ⓑ

✳ **V2760** Scratch resistant coating, per lens Ⓑ

⊘ **V2761** Mirror coating, any type, solid, gradient or equal, any lens material, per lens Ⓑ

IOM: 100-02, 15, 120; 100-04, 3, 10.4

⊘ **V2762** Polarization, any lens material, per lens Ⓑ

IOM: 100-02, 15, 120; 100-04, 3, 10.4

✳ **V2770** Occluder lens, per lens Ⓑ

Requires prior authorization.

✳ **V2780** Oversize lens, per lens Ⓑ

Requires prior authorization.

✳ **V2781** Progressive lens, per lens Ⓑ

Requires prior authorization.

⊘ **V2782** Lens, index 1.54 to 1.65 plastic or 1.60 to 1.79 glass, excludes polycarbonate, per lens Ⓑ

Do not bill in addition to V2784

IOM: 100-02, 15, 120; 100-04, 3, 10.4

⊘ **V2783** Lens, index greater than or equal to 1.66 plastic or greater than or equal to 1.80 glass, excludes polycarbonate, per lens Ⓑ

Do not bill in addition to V2784

IOM: 100-02, 15, 120; 100-04, 3, 10.4

⊘ **V2784** Lens, polycarbonate or equal, any index, per lens Ⓑ

Covered only for patients with functional vision in one eye-in this situation, an impact-resistant material is covered for both lenses if eyeglasses are covered. Claims with V2784 that do not meet this coverage criterion will be denied as not medically necessary.

IOM: 100-02, 15, 120; 100-04, 3, 10.4

▶ **New** ↻ **Revised** ✔ **Reinstated** ~~deleted~~ **Deleted** ⊘ **Not covered or valid by Medicare**
⊘ **Special coverage instructions** ✳ **Carrier discretion** Ⓑ **Bill Part B MAC** Ⓓ **Bill DME MAC**

✳ **V2785** Processing, preserving and transporting corneal tissue ⑬

For ASC, bill on paper. Must attach eye bank invoice to claim.

For Hospitals, bill charges for corneal tissue to receive cost based reimbursement.

IOM: 100-4, 4, 200.1

✺ **V2786** Specialty occupational multifocal lens, per lens ⑬

IOM: 100-02, 15, 120; 100-04, 3, 10.4

⊘ **V2787** Astigmatism correcting function of intraocular lens ⑬

⊘ **V2788** Presbyopia correcting function of intraocular lens ⑬

✳ **V2790** Amniotic membrane for surgical reconstruction, per procedure ⑬

✳ **V2797** Vision supply, accessory and/or service component of another HCPCS vision code ⑬

✳ **V2799** Vision item or service, miscellaneous ⑬

Bill on paper. Requires report of miscellaneous service and optical lab invoice.

HEARING SERVICES (V5000-V5999)

NOTE: These codes are for non-physician services.

Assessments and Evaluations

⊘ **V5008** Hearing screening ⑬

IOM: 100-02, 16, 90

⊘ **V5010** Assessment for hearing aid ⑬

⊘ **V5011** Fitting/orientation/checking of hearing aid ⑬

⊘ **V5014** Repair/modification of a hearing aid ⑬

⊘ **V5020** Conformity evaluation ⑬

Monaural Hearing Aid

⊘ **V5030** Hearing aid, monaural, body worn, air conduction ⑬

⊘ **V5040** Hearing aid, monaural, body worn, bone conduction ⑬

⊘ **V5050** Hearing aid, monaural, in the ear ⑬

⊘ **V5060** Hearing aid, monaural, behind the ear ⑬

Miscellaneous Services and Supplies

⊘ **V5070** Glasses, air conduction ⑬

⊘ **V5080** Glasses, bone conduction ⑬

⊘ **V5090** Dispensing fee, unspecified hearing aid ⑬

⊘ **V5095** Semi-implantable middle ear hearing prosthesis ⑬

⊘ **V5100** Hearing aid, bilateral, body worn ⑬

⊘ **V5110** Dispensing fee, bilateral ⑬

Hearing Aids

⊘ **V5120** Binaural, body ⑬

⊘ **V5130** Binaural, in the ear ⑬

⊘ **V5140** Binaural, behind the ear ⑬

⊘ **V5150** Binaural, glasses ⑬

⊘ **V5160** Dispensing fee, binaural ⑬

⊘ **V5170** Hearing aid, CROS, in the ear ⑬

⊘ **V5180** Hearing aid, CROS, behind the ear ⑬

⊘ **V5190** Hearing aid, CROS, glasses ⑬

⊘ **V5200** Dispensing fee, CROS ⑬

⊘ **V5210** Hearing aid, BICROS, in the ear ⑬

⊘ **V5220** Hearing aid, BICROS, behind the ear ⑬

⊘ **V5230** Hearing aid, BICROS, glasses ⑬

⊘ **V5240** Dispensing fee, BICROS ⑬

⊘ **V5241** Dispensing fee, monaural hearing aid, any type ⑬

⊘ **V5242** Hearing aid, analog, monaural, CIC (completely in the ear canal) ⑬

⊘ **V5243** Hearing aid, analog, monaural, ITC (in the canal) ⑬

⊘ **V5244** Hearing aid, digitally programmable analog, monaural, CIC ⑬

⊘ **V5245** Hearing aid, digitally programmable, analog, monaural, ITC ⑬

⊘ **V5246** Hearing aid, digitally programmable analog, monaural, ITE (in the ear) ⑬

⊘ **V5247** Hearing aid, digitally programmable analog, monaural, BTE (behind the ear) ⑬

⊘ **V5248** Hearing aid, analog, binaural, CIC ⑬

⊘ **V5249** Hearing aid, analog, binaural, ITC ⑬

⊘ **V5250** Hearing aid, digitally programmable analog, binaural, CIC ⑬

⊘ **V5251** Hearing aid, digitally programmable analog, binaural, ITC ⑬

⊘ **V5252** Hearing aid, digitally programmable, binaural, ITE ⑬

▶ New   ↻ Revised   ✔ Reinstated   ~~deleted~~ Deleted   ⊘ Not covered or valid by Medicare
✺ Special coverage instructions   ✳ Carrier discretion   ⑬ Bill Part B MAC   ⑬ Bill DME MAC

⊘ **V5253** Hearing aid, digitally programmable, binaural, BTE ⑧

⊘ **V5254** Hearing aid, digital, monaural, CIC ⑧

⊘ **V5255** Hearing aid, digital, monaural, ITC ⑧

⊘ **V5256** Hearing aid, digital, monaural, ITE ⑧

⊘ **V5257** Hearing aid, digital, monaural, BTE ⑧

⊘ **V5258** Hearing aid, digital, binaural, CIC ⑧

⊘ **V5259** Hearing aid, digital, binaural, ITC ⑧

⊘ **V5260** Hearing aid, digital, binaural, ITE ⑧

⊘ **V5261** Hearing aid, digital, binaural, BTE ⑧

⊘ **V5262** Hearing aid, disposable, any type, monaural ⑧

⊘ **V5263** Hearing aid, disposable, any type, binaural ⑧

⊘ **V5264** Ear mold/insert, not disposable, any type ⑧

⊘ **V5265** Ear mold/insert, disposable, any type ⑧

⊘ **V5266** Battery for use in hearing device ⑧

⊘ **V5267** Hearing aid or assistive listening device/supplies/accessories, not otherwise specified ⑧

Assistive Listening Devices

⊘ **V5268** Assistive listening device, telephone amplifier, any type ⑧

⊘ **V5269** Assistive listening device, alerting, any type ⑧

⊘ **V5270** Assistive listening device, television amplifier, any type ⑧

⊘ **V5271** Assistive listening device, television caption decoder ⑧

⊘ **V5272** Assistive listening device, TDD ⑧

⊘ **V5273** Assistive listening device, for use with cochlear implant ⑧

⊘ **V5274** Assistive listening device, not otherwise specified ⑧

⊘ **V5275** Ear impression, each ⑧

⊘ **V5281** Assistive listening device, personal FM/DM system, monaural, (1 receiver, transmitter, microphone), any type ⑧

⊘ **V5282** Assistive listening device, personal FM/DM system, binaural, (2 receivers, transmitter, microphone), any type ⑧

⊘ **V5283** Assistive listening device, personal FM/DM neck, loop induction receiver ⑧

⊘ **V5284** Assistive listening device, personal FM/DM, ear level receiver ⑧

⊘ **V5285** Assistive listening device, personal FM/DM, direct audio input receiver ⑧

⊘ **V5286** Assistive listening device, personal blue tooth FM/DM receiver ⑧

⊘ **V5287** Assistive listening device, personal FM/DM receiver, not otherwise specified ⑧

⊘ **V5288** Assistive listening device, personal FM/DM transmitter assistive listening device ⑧

⊘ **V5289** Assistive listening device, personal FM/DM adapter/boot coupling device for receiver, any type ⑧

⊘ **V5290** Assistive listening device, transmitter microphone, any type ⑧

Other Supllies and Miscellaneous Services

⊘ **V5298** Hearing aid, not otherwise classified ⑧

✺ **V5299** Hearing service, miscellaneous ⑧

IOM: 100-02, 16, 90

Repair/Modification

⊘ **V5336** Repair/modification of augmentative communicative system or device (excludes adaptive hearing aid) ⑧

Speech, Language, and Pathology Screening

These codes are for non-physician services.

⊘ **V5362** Speech screening ⑧

⊘ **V5363** Language screening ⑧

⊘ **V5364** Dysphagia screening ⑧

▶ New   ↻ Revised   ✔ Reinstated   ~~deleted~~ Deleted   ⊘ Not covered or valid by Medicare
✺ Special coverage instructions   ✳ Carrier discretion   ⑧ Bill Part B MAC   ⑧ Bill DME MAC

APPENDIX A

Jurisdiction List for DMEPOS HCPCS Codes

Deleted codes are valid for dates of service on or before the date of deletion. The jurisdiction list includes codes that are not payable by Medicare. Please consult the Medicare contractor in whose jurisdiction a claim would be filed in order to determine coverage under Medicare.

NOTE: All Local Carrier language has been changed to Part B MAC

HCPCS	DESCRIPTION	JURISDICTION
A0021 - A0999	Ambulance Services	Part B MAC
A4206 - A4209	Medical, Surgical, and Self- Administered Injection Supplies	Part B MAC if incident to a physician's service (not separately payable). If other, DME MAC.
A4210	Needle Free Injection Device	DME MAC
A4211	Medical, Surgical, and Self-Administered Injection Supplies	Part B MAC if incident to a physician's service (not separately payable). If other, DME MAC.
A4212	Non Coring Needle or Stylet with or without Catheter	Part B MAC
A4213 - A4215	Medical, Surgical, and Self-Administered Injection Supplies	Part B MAC if incident to a physician's service (not separately payable). If other, DME MAC.
A4216 - A4218	Saline	Part B MAC if incident to a physician's service (not separately payable). If other, DME MAC.
A4220	Refill Kit for Implantable Pump	Part B MAC
A4221 - A4236	Self-Administered Injection and Diabetic Supplies	DME MAC
A4244 - A4250	Medical, Surgical, and Self-Administered Injection Supplies	Part B MAC if incident to a physician's service (not separately payable). If other, DME MAC.
A4252 - A4259	Diabetic Supplies	DME MAC
A4261	Cervical Cap for Contraceptive Use	Part B MAC
A4262 - A4263	Lacrimal Duct Implants	Part B MAC
A4264	Contraceptive Implant	Part B MAC
A4265	Paraffin	Part B MAC if incident to a physician's service (not separately payable). If other, DME MAC.
A4266 - A4269	Contraceptives	Part B MAC
A4270	Endoscope Sheath	Part B MAC
A4280	Accessory for Breast Prosthesis	DME MAC
A4281 - A4286	Accessory for Breast Pump	DME MAC
A4290	Sacral Nerve Stimulation Test Lead	Part B MAC
A4300 - A4301	Implantable Catheter	Part B MAC
A4305 - A4306	Disposable Drug Delivery System	Part B MAC if incident to a physician's service (not separately payable). If other, DME MAC.

HCPCS	DESCRIPTION	JURISDICTION
A4310 - A4358	Incontinence Supplies/ Urinary Supplies	If provided in the physician's office for a temporary condition, the item is incident to the physician's service & billed to the Part B MAC. If provided in the physician's office or other place of service for a permanent condition, the item is a prosthetic device & billed to the DME MAC.
A4360 - A4435	Urinary Supplies	If provided in the physician's office for a temporary condition, the item is incident to the physician's service & billed to the Part B MAC. If provided in the physician's office or other place of service for a permanent condition, the item is a prosthetic device & billed to the DME MAC.
A4450 - A4456	Tape; Adhesive Remover	Part B MAC if incident to a physician's service (not separately payable), or if supply for implanted prosthetic device. If other, DME MAC.
A4458-A4459	Enema Bag/System	DME MAC
A4461-A4463	Surgical Dressing Holders	Part B MAC if incident to a physician's service (not separately payable). If other, DME MAC.
A4465 - A4467	Non-elastic Binder and Garment, Strap, Covering	DME MAC
A4470	Gravlee Jet Washer	Part B MAC
A4480	Vabra Aspirator	Part B MAC
A4481	Tracheostomy Supply	Part B MAC if incident to a physician's service (not separately payable). If other, DME MAC.
A4483	Moisture Exchanger	DME MAC
A4490 - A4510	Surgical Stockings	DME MAC
A4520	Diapers	DME MAC
A4550	Surgical Trays	Part B MAC
A4553 - A4554	Underpads	DME MAC
A4555 - A4558	Electrodes; Lead Wires; Conductive Paste	Part B MAC if incident to a physician's service (not separately payable). If other, DME MAC.
A4559	Coupling Gel	Part B MAC if incident to a physician's service (not separately payable). If other, DME MAC.
A4561 - A4562	Pessary	Part B MAC

HCPCS	DESCRIPTION	JURISDICTION
A4565-A4566	Sling	Part B MAC
A4570	Splint	Part B MAC
A4575	Topical Hyperbaric Oxygen Chamber, Disposable	DME MAC
A4580 - A4590	Casting Supplies & Material	Part B MAC
A4595	TENS Supplies	Part B MAC if incident to a physician's service (not separately payable). If other, DME MAC.
A4600	Sleeve for Intermittent Limb Compression Device	DME MAC
A4601-A4602	Lithium Replacement Batteries	DME MAC
A4604	Tubing for Positive Airway Pressure Device	DME MAC
A4605	Tracheal Suction Catheter	DME MAC
A4606	Oxygen Probe for Oximeter	DME MAC
A4608	Transtracheal Oxygen Catheter	DME MAC
A4611 - A4613	Oxygen Equipment Batteries and Supplies	DME MAC
A4614	Peak Flow Rate Meter	Part B MAC if incident to a physician's service (not separately payable). If other, DME MAC.
A4615 - A4629	Oxygen & Tracheostomy Supplies	Part B MAC if incident to a physician's service (not separately payable). If other, DME MAC.
A4630 - A4640	DME Supplies	DME MAC
A4641 - A4642	Imaging Agent; Contrast Material	Part B MAC
A4648	Tissue Marker, Implanted	Part B MAC
A4649	Miscellaneous Surgical Supplies	Part B MAC if incident to a physician's service (not separately payable), or if supply for implanted prosthetic device or implanted DME. If other, DME MAC.
A4650	Implantable Radiation Dosimeter	Part B MAC
A4651 - A4932	Supplies for ESRD	DME MAC (not separately payable)
A5051 - A5093	Additional Ostomy Supplies	If provided in the physician's office for a temporary condition, the item is incident to the physician's service & billed to the Part B MAC. If provided in the physician's office or other place of service for a permanent condition, the item is a prosthetic device & billed to the DME MAC.

HCPCS	DESCRIPTION	JURISDICTION
A5102 - A5200	Additional Incontinence and Ostomy Supplies	If provided in the physician's office for a temporary condition, the item is incident to the physician's service & billed to the Part B MAC. If provided in the physician's office or other place of service for a permanent condition, the item is a prosthetic device & billed to the DME MAC.
A5500 - A5513	Therapeutic Shoes	DME MAC
A6000	Non-Contact Wound Warming Cover	DME MAC
A6010-A6024	Surgical Dressing	Part B MAC if incident to a physician's service (not separately payable) or if supply for implanted prosthetic device or implanted DME. If other, DME MAC.
A6025	Silicone Gel Sheet	Part B MAC if incident to a physician's service (not separately payable) or if supply for implanted prosthetic device or implanted DME. If other, DME MAC.
A6154 - A6411	Surgical Dressing	Part B MAC if incident to a physician's service (not separately payable) or if supply for implanted prosthetic device or implanted DME. If other, DME MAC.
A6412	Eye Patch	Part B MAC if incident to a physician's service (not separately payable) or if supply for implanted prosthetic device or implanted DME. If other, DME MAC.
A6413	Adhesive Bandage	Part B MAC if incident to a physician's service (not separately payable) or if supply for implanted prosthetic device or implanted DME. If other, DME MAC.
A6441 - A6512	Surgical Dressings	Part B MAC if incident to a physician's service (not separately payable) or if supply for implanted prosthetic device or implanted DME. If other, DME MAC.
A6513	Compression Burn Mask	DME MAC
A6530 - A6549	Compression Gradient Stockings	DME MAC
A6550	Supplies for Negative Pressure Wound Therapy Electrical Pump	DME MAC
A7000 - A7002	Accessories for Suction Pumps	DME MAC
A7003 - A7039	Accessories for Nebulizers, Aspirators and Ventilators	DME MAC
A7040 - A7041	Chest Drainage Supplies	Part B MAC
A7044 - A7047	Respiratory Accessories	DME MAC
A7048	Vacuum Drainage Supply	Part B MAC

HCPCS	DESCRIPTION	JURISDICTION
A7501-A7527	Tracheostomy Supplies	DME MAC
A8000-A8004	Protective Helmets	DME MAC
A9150	Non-Prescription Drugs	Part B MAC
A9152 - A9153	Vitamins	Part B MAC
A9155	Artificial Saliva	Part B MAC
A9180	Lice Infestation Treatment	Part B MAC
A9270	Noncovered Items or Services	DME MAC
A9272	Disposable Wound Suction Pump	DME MAC
A9273	Hot Water Bottles, Ice Caps or Collars, and Heat and/or Cold Wraps	DME MAC
A9274 - A9278	Glucose Monitoring	DME MAC
A9279	Monitoring Feature/ Device	DME MAC
A9280	Alarm Device	DME MAC
A9281	Reaching/Grabbing Device	DME MAC
A9282	Wig	DME MAC
A9283	Foot Off Loading Device	DME MAC
A9284- A9286	Non-electric Spirometer, Inversion Devices and Hygienic Items	DME MAC
A9300	Exercise Equipment	DME MAC
A9500 - A9700	Supplies for Radiology Procedures	Part B MAC
A9900	Miscellaneous DME Supply or Accessory	Part B MAC if used with implanted DME. If other, DME MAC.
A9901	Delivery	DME MAC
A9999	Miscellaneous DME Supply or Accessory	Part B MAC if used with implanted DME. If other, DME MAC.
B4034 - B9999	Enteral and Parenteral Therapy	DME MAC
D0120 - D9999	Dental Procedures	Part B MAC
E0100 - E0105	Canes	DME MAC
E0110 - E0118	Crutches	DME MAC
E0130 - E0159	Walkers	DME MAC
E0160 - E0175	Commodes	DME MAC
E0181 - E0199	Decubitus Care Equipment	DME MAC
E0200 - E0239	Heat/Cold Applications	DME MAC
E0240 - E0248	Bath and Toilet Aids	DME MAC
E0249	Pad for Heating Unit	DME MAC
E0250 - E0304	Hospital Beds	DME MAC
E0305 - E0326	Hospital Bed Accessories	DME MAC
E0328 - E0329	Pediatric Hospital Beds	DME MAC

HCPCS	DESCRIPTION	JURISDICTION
E0350 - E0352	Electronic Bowel Irrigation System	DME MAC
E0370	Heel Pad	DME MAC
E0371 - E0373	Decubitus Care Equipment	DME MAC
E0424 - E0484	Oxygen and Related Respiratory Equipment	DME MAC
E0485 - E0486	Oral Device to Reduce Airway Collapsibility	DME MAC
E0487	Electric Spirometer	DME MAC
E0500	IPPB Machine	DME MAC
E0550 - E0585	Compressors/Nebulizers	DME MAC
E0600	Suction Pump	DME MAC
E0601	CPAP Device	DME MAC
E0602 - E0604	Breast Pump	DME MAC
E0605	Vaporizer	DME MAC
E0606	Drainage Board	DME MAC
E0607	Home Blood Glucose Monitor	DME MAC
E0610 - E0615	Pacemaker Monitor	DME MAC
E0616	Implantable Cardiac Event Recorder	Part B MAC
E0617	External Defibrillator	DME MAC
E0618 - E0619	Apnea Monitor	DME MAC
E0620	Skin Piercing Device	DME MAC
E0621 - E0636	Patient Lifts	DME MAC
E0637 - E0642	Standing Devices/Lifts	DME MAC
E0650 - E0676	Pneumatic Compressor and Appliances	DME MAC
E0691 - E0694	Ultraviolet Light Therapy Systems	DME MAC
E0700	Safety Equipment	DME MAC
E0705	Transfer Board	DME MAC
E0710	Restraints	DME MAC
E0720 - E0745	Electrical Nerve Stimulators	DME MAC
E0746	EMG Device	Part B MAC
E0747 - E0748	Osteogenic Stimulators	DME MAC
E0749	Implantable Osteogenic Stimulators	Part B MAC
E0755- E0770	Stimulation Devices	DME MAC
E0776	IV Pole	DME MAC
E0779 - E0780	External Infusion Pumps	DME MAC
E0781	Ambulatory Infusion Pump	DME MAC
E0782 - E0783	Infusion Pumps, Implantable	Part B MAC
E0784	Infusion Pumps, Insulin	DME MAC

HCPCS	DESCRIPTION	JURISDICTION
E0785 - E0786	Implantable Infusion Pump Catheter	Part B MAC
E0791	Parenteral Infusion Pump	DME MAC
E0830	Ambulatory Traction Device	DME MAC
E0840 - E0900	Traction Equipment	DME MAC
E0910 - E0930	Trapeze/Fracture Frame	DME MAC
E0935 - E0936	Passive Motion Exercise Device	DME MAC
E0940	Trapeze Equipment	DME MAC
E0941	Traction Equipment	DME MAC
E0942 - E0945	Orthopedic Devices	DME MAC
E0946 - E0948	Fracture Frame	DME MAC
E0950 - E1298	Wheelchairs	DME MAC
E1300 - E1310	Whirlpool Equipment	DME MAC
E1352 - E1392	Additional Oxygen Related Equipment	DME MAC
E1399	Miscellaneous DME	Part B MAC if implanted DME. If other, DME MAC.
E1405 - E1406	Additional Oxygen Equipment	DME MAC
E1500 - E1699	Artificial Kidney Machines and Accessories	DME MAC (not separately payable)
E1700 - E1702	TMJ Device and Supplies	DME MAC
E1800 - E1841	Dynamic Flexion Devices	DME MAC
E1902	Communication Board	DME MAC
E2000	Gastric Suction Pump	DME MAC
E2100 - E2101	Blood Glucose Monitors with Special Features	DME MAC
E2120	Pulse Generator for Tympanic Treatment of Inner Ear	DME MAC
E2201 - E2397	Wheelchair Accessories	DME MAC
E2402	Negative Pressure Wound Therapy Pump	DME MAC
E2500 - E2599	Speech Generating Device	DME MAC
E2601 - E2633	Wheelchair Cushions and Accessories	DME MAC
E8000 - E8002	Gait Trainers	DME MAC
G0008 - G0329	Misc. Professional Services	Part B MAC
G0333	Dispensing Fee	DME MAC
G0337 - G0365	Misc. Professional Services	Part B MAC
G0372	Misc. Professional Services	Part B MAC
G0378 - G0490 G0493-G9862	Misc. Professional Services	Part B MAC

HCPCS	DESCRIPTION	JURISDICTION
J0120 - J3570	Injection	Part B MAC if incident to a physician's service or used in an implanted infusion pump. If other, DME MAC.
J3590	Unclassified Biologicals	Part B MAC
J7030 - J7131	Miscellaneous Drugs and Solutions	Part B MAC if incident to a physician's service or used in an implanted infusion pump. If other, DME MAC.
J7175-J7179	Clotting Factors	Part B MAC
J7180 - J7195	Antihemophilic Factor	Part B MAC
J7196 - J7197	Antithrombin III	Part B MAC
J7198	Anti-inhibitor; per I.U.	Part B MAC
J7199 - J7209	Other Hemophilia Clotting Factors	Part B MAC
J7297 - J7307	Contraceptives	Part B MAC
J7308 - J7309	Aminolevulinic Acid HCL	Part B MAC
J7310	Ganciclovir, Long-Acting Implant	Part B MAC
J7311 - J7316	Ophthalmic Drugs	Part B MAC
J7320 - J7328	Hyaluronan	Part B MAC
J7330	Autologous Cultured Chondrocytes, Implant	Part B MAC
J7336	Capsaicin	Part B MAC
J7340	Carbidopa/Levodopa	Part B MAC if incident to a physician's service or used in an implanted infusion pump. If other, DME MAC.
J7342	Ciprofloxacin otic	Part B MAC
J7500 - J7599	Immunosuppressive Drugs	Part B MAC if incident to a physician's service or used in an implanted infusion pump. If other, DME MAC.
J7604 - J7699	Inhalation Solutions	Part B MAC if incident to a physician's service. If other, DME MAC.
J7799 -J7999	NOC Drugs, Other than Inhalation Drugs	Part B MAC if incident to a physician's service or used in an implanted infusion pump. If other, DME MAC.
J8498	Anti-emetic Drug	DME MAC
J8499	Prescription Drug, Oral, Non Chemotherapeutic	Part B MAC if incident to a physician's service. If other, DME MAC.
J8501 - J8999	Oral Anti-Cancer Drugs	DME MAC
J9000 - J9999	Chemotherapy Drugs	Part B MAC if incident to a physician's service or used in an implanted infusion pump. If other, DME MAC.
K0001 - K0108	Wheelchairs	DME MAC
K0195	Elevating Leg Rests	DME MAC
K0455	Infusion Pump used for Uninterrupted Administration of Epoprostenal	DME MAC

HCPCS	DESCRIPTION	JURISDICTION
K0462	Loaner Equipment	DME MAC
K0552	External Infusion Pump Supplies	DME MAC
K0601 - K0605	External Infusion Pump Batteries	DME MAC
K0606 - K0609	Defibrillator Accessories	DME MAC
K0669	Wheelchair Cushion	DME MAC
K0672	Soft Interface for Orthosis	DME MAC
K0730	Inhalation Drug Delivery System	DME MAC
K0733	Power Wheelchair Accessory	DME MAC
K0738	Oxygen Equipment	DME MAC
K0739	Repair or Nonroutine Service for DME	Part B MAC if implanted DME. If other, DME MAC
K0740	Repair or Nonroutine Service for Oxygen Equipment	DME MAC
K0743 - K0746	Suction Pump and Dressings	DME MAC
K0800 - K0899	Power Mobility Devices	DME MAC
K0900	Custom DME, other than Wheelchair	DME MAC
L0112 - L4631	Orthotics	DME MAC
L5000 - L5999	Lower Limb Prosthetics	DME MAC
L6000 - L7499	Upper Limb Prosthetics	DME MAC
L7510 - L7520	Repair of Prosthetic Device	Part B MAC if repair of implanted prosthetic device. If other, DME MAC.
L7600	Prosthetic Donning Sleeve	DME MAC
L7900-L7902	Vacuum Erection System	DME MAC
L8000 - L8485	Prosthetics	DME MAC
L8499	Unlisted Procedure for Miscellaneous Prosthetic Services	Part B MAC if implanted prosthetic device. If other, DME MAC.
L8500 - L8501	Artificial Larynx; Tracheostomy Speaking Valve	DME MAC
L8505	Artificial Larynx Accessory	DME MAC
L8507	Voice Prosthesis, Patient Inserted	DME MAC
L8509	Voice Prosthesis, Inserted by a Licensed Health Care Provider	Part B MAC for dates of service on or after 10/01/2010. DME MAC for dates of service prior to 10/01/2010
L8510	Voice Prosthesis	DME MAC
L8511 - L8515	Voice Prosthesis	Part B MAC if used with tracheoesophageal voice prostheses inserted by a licensed health care provider. If other, DME MAC

HCPCS	DESCRIPTION	JURISDICTION
L8600 - L8699	Prosthetic Implants	Part B MAC
L9900	Miscellaneous Orthotic or Prosthetic Component or Accessory	Part B MAC if used with implanted prosthetic device. If other, DME MAC.
M0075 - M0301	Medical Services	Part B MAC
P2028 - P9615	Laboratory Tests	Part B MAC
Q0035	Influenza Vaccine; Cardiokymography	Part B MAC
Q0081	Infusion Therapy	Part B MAC
Q0083 - Q0085	Chemotherapy Administration	Part B MAC
Q0091	Smear Preparation	Part B MAC
Q0092	Portable X-ray Setup	Part B MAC
Q0111 - Q0115	Miscellaneous Lab Services	Part B MAC
Q0138-Q0139	Ferumoxytol Injection	Part B MAC
Q0144	Azithromycin Dihydrate	Part B MAC if incident to a physician's service. If other, DME MAC.
Q0161 - Q0181	Anti-emetic	DME MAC
Q0478 - Q0509	Ventricular Assist Devices	Part B MAC
Q0510 - Q0514	Drug Dispensing Fees	DME MAC
Q0515	Sermorelin Acetate	Part B MAC
Q1004 - Q1005	New Technology IOL	Part B MAC
Q2004	Irrigation Solution	Part B MAC
Q2009	Fosphenytoin	Part B MAC
Q2017	Teniposide	Part B MAC
Q2026-Q2028	Injectable Dermal Fillers	Part B MAC
Q2034 - Q2039	Influenza Vaccine	Part B MAC
Q2043	Sipuleucel-T	Part B MAC
Q2049-Q2050	Doxorubicin	Part B MAC if incident to a physician's service or used in an implanted infusion pump. If other, DME MAC.
Q2052	IVIG Demonstration	DME MAC
Q3001	Supplies for Radiology Procedures	Part B MAC
Q3014	Telehealth Originating Site Facility Fee	Part B MAC
Q3027 - Q3028	Vaccines	Part B MAC
Q3031	Collagen Skin Test	Part B MAC
Q4001 - Q4051	Splints and Casts	Part B MAC
Q4074	Inhalation Drug	Part B MAC if incident to a physician's service. If other, DME MAC.
Q4081	Epoetin	Part B MAC
Q4082	Drug Subject to Competitive Acquisition Program	Part B MAC
Q4100 - Q4175	Skin Substitutes	Part B MAC

HCPCS	DESCRIPTION	JURISDICTION
Q5001 - Q5010	Hospice Services	Part B MAC
Q5101-Q5102	Injection	Part B MAC if incident to a physician's service or used in an implanted infusion pump. If other, DME MAC.
Q9950 - Q9954	Imaging Agents	Part B MAC
Q9955 - Q9957	Microspheres	Part B MAC
Q9958 - Q9969	Imaging Agents	Part B MAC
Q9982-Q9983	Supplies for Radiology Procedures	Part B MAC
R0070 - R0076	Diagnostic Radiology Services	Part B MAC
V2020 - V2025	Frames	DME MAC
V2100 - V2513	Lenses	DME MAC
V2520 - V2523	Hydrophilic Contact Lenses	Part B MAC if incident to a physician's service. If other, DME MAC.
V2530 - V2531	Contact Lenses, Scleral	DME MAC
V2599	Contact Lens, Other Type	Part B MAC if incident to a physician's service. If other, DME MAC.
V2600 - V2615	Low Vision Aids	DME MAC

HCPCS	DESCRIPTION	JURISDICTION
V2623 - V2629	Prosthetic Eyes	DME MAC
V2630 - V2632	Intraocular Lenses	Part B MAC
V2700 - V2780	Miscellaneous Vision Service	DME MAC
V2781	Progressive Lens	DME MAC
V2782 - V2784	Lenses	DME MAC
V2785	Processing—Corneal Tissue	Part B MAC
V2786	Lens	DME MAC
V2787 - V2788	Intraocular Lenses	Part B MAC
V2790	Amniotic Membrane	Part B MAC
V2797	Vision Supply	DME MAC
V2799	Miscellaneous Vision Service	DME MAC
V5008 - V5299	Hearing Services	Part B MAC
V5336	Repair/Modification of Augmentative Communicative System or Device	DME MAC
V5362 - V5364	Speech Screening	Part B MAC